Pain

BEST PRACTICE &
RESEARCH COMPENDIUM

For Elsevier:

Commissioning Editor: Alison Taylor
Development Editor: Kim Benson
Development: Louisa Welch
Production Manager: Susan Stuart
Project Manager: Helius
Cover Design: Marie Prime

Pain

BEST PRACTICE & RESEARCH COMPENDIUM

Edited by

Harald Breivik MD DMSc FRCA

Professor of Anaesthesiology, Rikshospitalet Medical Centre,
Oslo, Norway

Michael Shipley MA MD FRCP

Consultant Rheumatologist, Centre for Rheumatology, University College Hospital,
London, UK

ELSEVIER

EDINBURGH LONDON NEW YORK OXFORD
PHILADELPHIA ST LOUIS SYDNEY TORONTO 2007

ELSEVIER

ISBN: 978-0-08-044684-4

British Library Cataloguing in Publication Data
A catalogue record for this book is available from the British Library.

Library of Congress Cataloging in Publication Data
A catalog record for this book is available from the Library of Congress.

Note

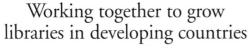

Working together to grow
libraries in developing countries

www.elsevier.com | www.bookaid.org | www.sabre.org

ELSEVIER   BOOK AID International   Sabre Foundation

your source for books,
journals and multimedia
in the health sciences
www.elsevierhealth.com

The
publisher's
policy is to use
paper manufactured
from sustainable forests

Printed in Spain

Contents

Contributors

Laurie Allan MD
Northwick Park Hospital and St Marks
NHS Trust
Harrow, UK

Anne-Françoise Allaz MD
Professor of Internal Medicine
Internal Medicine of Rehabilitation, and
Multidisciplinary Pain Centre
Geneva University Hospital
Geneva, Switzerland

Andrew Baranowski BscHons, MBBS,
FRCA, MD
Consultant in Pain Medicine
National Hospital for Neurology and
Neurosurgery
London, UK

Les Barnsley BMed(Hons), GradDipEpi,
PhD, FRACP, FAFRM(RACP)
Associate Professor
Department of Medicine
University of Sydney
Head, Department of Rheumatology
Concord Hospital
Sydney, Australia

Robert M. Bennett MD, FRCP
Professor of Medicine
Department of Medicine
Oregon Health and Science University
Portland, OR, USA

Nikolai Bogduk BSc(Med), MB, BS,
PhD, MD, DSc, DipPainMed,
FFPM(ANZCA)
Director, Department of Clinical
Research
Royal Newcastle Hospital
Newcastle, Australia

Claire Bombardier MD, PhD
Professor
Institute for Work and Health
Toronto, Canada

Harald Breivik MD, DMedSci, FRCA
Professor of Anaesthesiology
University of Oslo, Faculty of Medicine
Rikshospitalet Medical Centre
Department of Anaesthesiology
Oslo, Norway

Matthew D. Caldwell MD
Clinical Assistant Professor
Department of Anesthesiology
University of Michigan
Ann Arbor, MI, USA

Marco A. Campello PT, PhD
Acting Director
Occupational and Industrial
Orthopaedic Center
NYU Hospital for Joint Diseases
New York, USA

Christine Cedraschi PhD
Research and Clinical Psychologist
Clinical Pharmacology and Toxicology,
Multidisciplinary Pain Centre, and
Internal Medicine of Rehabilitation
Geneva University Hospital
Geneva, Switzerland

Daniel J. Clauw MD
Professor of Internal Medicine
Rheumatology
University of Michigan
Ann Arbor, MI, USA

Lesley A. Colvin MBChB, FRCA, PhD
Senior Lecturer/Consultant in
Anaesthesia and Pain Medicine
Department of Anaesthesia, Critical
Care and Pain Medicine
Western General Hospital
Edinburgh, UK

Peter Croft MSc, MD, MRCGP
Professor of Primary Care Epidemiology
Primary Care Musculoskeletal Research
Centre
Keele University
Keele, UK

Geert Crombez PhD
Professor of Health Psychology
Department of Experimental, Clinical
and Health Psychology
Ghent University
Ghent, Belgium

Michele Curatolo MD, PhD
Professor
Head, Division of Pain Therapy
Department of Anaesthesiology
University Hospital of Bern
Bern, Switzerland

Pierre Dayer MD
Professor of Internal Medicine, and
Clinical Pharmacology and Toxicology
Clinical Pharmacology and Toxicology,
and Multidisciplinary Pain Centre
Geneva University Hospital
Geneva, Switzerland

Paul L. I. Dellemijn MD
Máxima Medical Centre
Veldhoven, The Netherlands

Jules A. Desmeules MD
Associate Professor
Internal Medicine and Clinical
Pharmacologist and Toxicologist
Clinical Pharmacology and Toxicology,
and Multidisciplinary Pain Centre
Geneva University Hospital
Geneva, Switzerland

Krysia Dziedzic PhD, MCSP
arc Senior Lecturer in Physiotherapy
Primary Care Musculoskeletal Research
Centre
Keele University
Keele, UK

Clara C. Faura MD
Instituto de Neurosciencias
Universidad Miguel Hernández-CSIC
Alicante, Spain

Robert Ferrari MD, FRCPC, FACP
Clinical Professor
Department of Medicine
University of Alberta Hospital
Edmonton
Alberta, Canada

Karin Ø. Forseth MD, DMedSci
Consultant Rheumatologist
Section for Treatment Abroad
Department of Rheumatology
Rikshospitalet Medical Centre
Oslo, Norway

Bernard Fouquet MD
Fédération Universitaire
Interhospitalière de Médecine Physique
et de Réadaptation
Hôpital Trousseau
Tours, France

Liesbet Goubert PhD
Postdoctoral Fellow
Department of Experimental, Clinical
and Health Psychology
Ghent University
Ghent, Belgium

Jan T. Gran MD, DMedSci
Professor of Rheumatology
University of Oslo, Medical Faculty
Department of Rheumatology
Rikshospitalet Medical Centre
Oslo, Norway

Edwin Y. Hanada MD, FRCPC
Assistant Professor
Division of Physical Medicine and
Rehabilitation
Dalhousie University/Nova Scotia
Rehabilitation Centre
Halifax, Canada

Richard E. Harris PhD
Research Investigator
Chronic Pain and Fatigue Research
Center
University of Michigan
Ann Arbor, MI, USA

Håkon Haugtomt MD
Rikshospitalet University Clinic
Department of Anaesthesiology
Oslo, Norway

Elaine M. Hay MD, FRCP
Professor of Community Rheumatology
Primary Care Musculoskeletal Research
Centre
Keele University
Keele, UK

Wilfried K. Ilias MD
Hospital of the Hospitaller Order of St
John Of God
Vienna, Austria

Aage Indahl MD, PhD
Hospital for Rehabilitering – Stavern
Rikshospitalet-Radiumhospitalet
Medical Center
Oslo, Norway

Troels S. Jensen MD
Aarhus University Hospital
Aarhus, Denmark

Joanne L. Jordan BSc, MSc, MA
Research Assistant: Systematic Reviews
Primary Care Musculoskeletal Research
Centre
Keele University
Keele, UK

Ellen Jørum MD, PhD
Head of Laboratory for Clinical
Neurophysiology
Rikshospitalet Medical Centre
Oslo, Norway

Eija Kalso MD, DMedSci
Department of Anaesthesia and
Intensive Care Medicine
Pain Clinic
Helsinki University Central Hospital
Helsinki, Finland

Peter J. Keel MD
Director of Outpatient Clinic for
Psychiatry and Psychosomatics
Associate Professor of Psychiatry
Bethesda-Spital
Basel, Switzerland

Nicholas A. S. Kendall PhD,
DipClinPsych, MNZCCP
Senior Lecturer
Orthopaedic Surgery and
Musculoskeletal Medicine
Christchurch School of Medicine
Christchurch, New Zealand

Bruce L Kidd DM, FRCP
Professor of Rheumatology
Barts & The London, Queen Mary
School of Medicine
London, UK

Bart Koes PhD
Professor
Department of General Practice
Erasmus University
Rotterdam, The Netherlands

Gunnvald Kvarstein MD, DMedSci
Rikshospitalet Medical Centre
Department of Anaesthesiology
Oslo, Norway

Susan M. Lord BMedSci, BMed, PhD,
FANZCA, FFPM(ANZCA)
Staff Specialist
Division of Anaesthesia, Intensive Care
and Pain Management
John Hunter Hospital
Newcastle, Australia

Mary McLoone MBBS, FRCA
Advanced Pain Trainee
National Hospital for Neurology and
Neurosurgery
London, UK

Geir Niemi MD, DMedSci
Rikshospitalet University Clinic
Department of Anaesthesiology
Oslo, Norway

Margareta Nordin PT, DrSci
Research Professor
Departments of Orthopaedics and
Environmental Medicine
School of Medicine
New York University
New York, USA

Serge Perrot MD
Hospital Tarnier
Paris, France

Markus Pietrek MD
Consultant Orthopaedic and Spine
Surgeon
Orthopaedic Department
Marienhospital
Wickede, Germany

Valérie Piguet MD
Consultant
Clinical Pharmacology and Toxicology,
and Multidisciplinary Pain Centre
Geneva University Hospital
Geneva, Switzerland

Leon H. Plaghki MD
Cliniques Universitaires St Luc
Université Catholique de Louvain
Brussels, Belgium

Ian Power BSc(Hons), MBChB, FRCA,
MD, FFPMANZCA, FANZCA, FRCSEd,
FRCP(Edin)
Professor of Anaesthesia
Critical Care and Pain Medicine
College of Medicine and Veterinary
Medicine
University of Edinburgh
Edinburgh, UK

Srinivas G. Rao MD, PhD
Chief Scientific Officer
Cypress Bioscience, Inc.
San Diego, CA, USA

Victoria Rollason PharmD, PhD
Clinical Pharmacologist and Toxicologist
Clinical Pharmacology and Toxicology,
and Multidisciplinary Pain Centre
Geneva University Hospital
Geneva, Switzerland

Luis Romundstad MD
Rikshospitalet University Clinic
Department of Anaesthesiology
Oslo, Norway

Anthony S. Russell BChir, MB, FRCPC,
FACP
Professor Emeritus
Department of Rheumatic Diseases
University of Alberta
Edmonton
Alberta, Canada

Hans-Georg Schaible DrMed
Department of Physiology
University of Jena
Jena, Germany

Michael Shipley MA, MD, FRCP
Consultant Rheumatologist
Centre for Rheumatology
University College Hospital
London, UK

Julius Sim BA, MSc, PhD
Professor of Health Care Research
Primary Care Musculoskeletal Research
Centre
Keele University
Keele, UK

Tuulikki Sokka MD, PhD
Research Assistant Professor
Jyväskylä Central Hospital
Jyväskylä, Finland

Cathy Speed BMedSci, BMBS,
Dip Sports Med, MA, PhD, FRCP,
FFSEM(I)(UK)
Honorary Consultant in Rheumatology
Sports and Exercise Medicine
Addenbrooke's Hospital
Cambridge, UK

Audun Stubhaug MD, DMedSci
University of Oslo, Faculty of Medicine
Rikshospitalet Medical Centre
Department of Anaesthesiology
Oslo, Norway

Gorazd Svetičič MD
Resident, Division of Pain Therapy
Department of Anaesthesiology
University Hospital of Bern
Bern, Switzerland

Horacio Vanegas MD, PhD
Professor of Physiology and Biophysics
Instituto Venezolano de Investigaciones
Cientificas (IVIC)
Caracas, Venezuela

Maurits van Tulder PhD
Senior Investigator
EMGO Institute and Department of
Clinical Epidemiology and Biostatistics
VU University Medical Centre
Amsterdam, The Netherlands,
and Institute for Work and Health
Toronto, Canada

Johan W. S. Vlaeyen PhD
Professor of Behavioural Medicine
Department of Clinical, Medical and
Experimental Psychology
Maastricht University
Maastricht, The Netherlands

Sherri Weiser PhD
Research Assistant Professor
Department of Orthopaedics and
Environmental Health Sciences
Program of Ergonomics and
Biomechanics
New York University
New York, USA

Amanda C. de C. Williams MSc, PhD,
CPsychol
Reader in Clinical Health Psychology
Sub-Department of Clinical Health
Psychology
University College London
London, UK

Christopher L. Wu MD
Associate Professor of Anesthesiology
The John Hopkins Hospital
Baltimore, MD, USA

Michael Zenz MD
BG-University Hospital Bergmannsheil
Bochum, Germany

Preface

This book, which is unique in the literature, represents the first attempt to build a bridge between specialists in acute pain, the anaesthesiologists, and specialists in chronic pain, the rheumatologists. Rheumatologists mainly specialize in the management of chronic pain conditions but often see their patients in acute pain. Conversely, more and more anaesthetists are involved in the management of patients with chronic pain conditions. This compendium comprises updated reviews on pain topics from *Best Practice and Research Clinical Rheumatology* and *Best Practice and Research Clinical Anaesthesiology* as well as chapters written de novo. We are confident that this book will be helpful for these two groups of clinicians who see patients with acute and chronic pain from two different practice standpoints. The book discusses basic principles of pain, diagnosis, the recognition of 'red' flags indicating a greater risk of serious causes and 'yellow' flags indicating a greater risk of developing more chronic pain, and the evidence-based management of a variety of conditions.

We believe that many other healthcare professionals, specialists, general practitioners, physical therapists, nurses and psychologists will benefit from this unique and valuable collection of reviews of topics on acute and chronic pain.

An important lesson is that there are many conflicting opinions and views on pathophysiology and management of pain, whether based on 'evidence base' or 'experts' opinion'. We confess that we do not agree with every opinion expressed in this book, nor have we tried to influence the authors of the chapters to agree with us, although, when required, mild editorial advice has been offered.

We hope that you will enjoy the book and that you will find its content – prepared by some of the world's leading experts on pain management – to be of help to you.

Harald Breivik
Michael Shipley

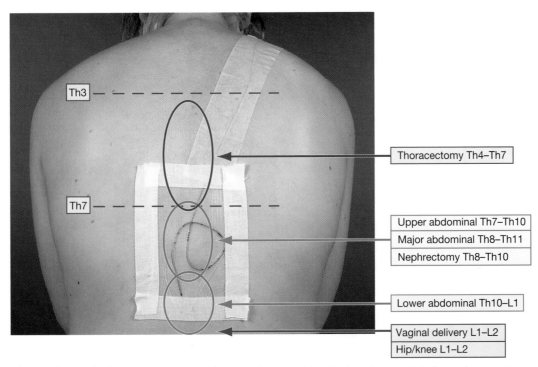

Plate I. The standard triple component epidural solution containing bupivacaine 1 mg/mL, fentanyl 2 μg/mL and adrenalin 2 μg/mL causes segmental epidural analgesia when the drugs reach the spinal cord dorsal horn at the appropriate segmental level. Placement of the epidural catheter at an optimal segmental site, appropriate for the type and site of surgery, is therefore decisive for the quality of the analgesia produced.

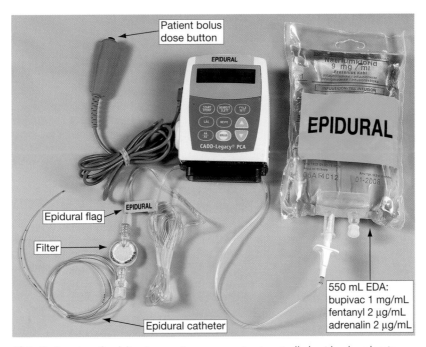

Plate II. A system for delivering continuous or patient-controlled epidural analgesia. The closed system reduces the risk of bacterial contamination.

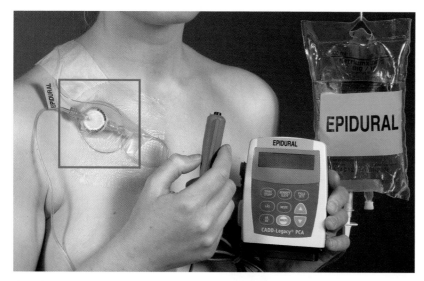

Plate III Strict hygienic precautions are necessary. Fix the epidural catheter with transparent adhesive covers. Do not change the tubing or filter unless they are contaminated. Inspect for signs of local inflammation (redness) and examine for local tenderness at the insertion site at least once daily. If there are signs of catheter site or catheter track infection, remove the catheter, culture the tip of the catheter and start antibiotics early.

Fix epi-catheter with Tegaderm/Opsite, and tape edges carefully

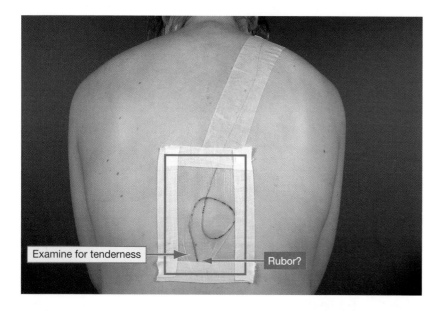

Plate IV. Analysis of components of chronic pain after mastectomy.

An area of *hypoaesthesia* is a result of section of the peripheral sensory nerves. This is a sign of nerve injury.

A *trigger area* where *hyperexcitable peripheral nerves* cause *ectopic discharges*, and pain occurring *spontaneously* or after *stimulation by pressure or movement*. This type of pain may be relieved by a sodium-channel blocker; lidocaine topically or intravenously.

An area of *allodynia* (i.e. pain provoked by light touch) indicates central nervous system sensitization. Lidocaine, NMDA blockers or opioids may reduce this pain component. An area of *spontaneous, burning pain*, is most likely due to central maladaptation and dysfunction of pain-modulating neurons. Amitriptyline, gabapentin, pregabalin and opioids may reduce this pain component.

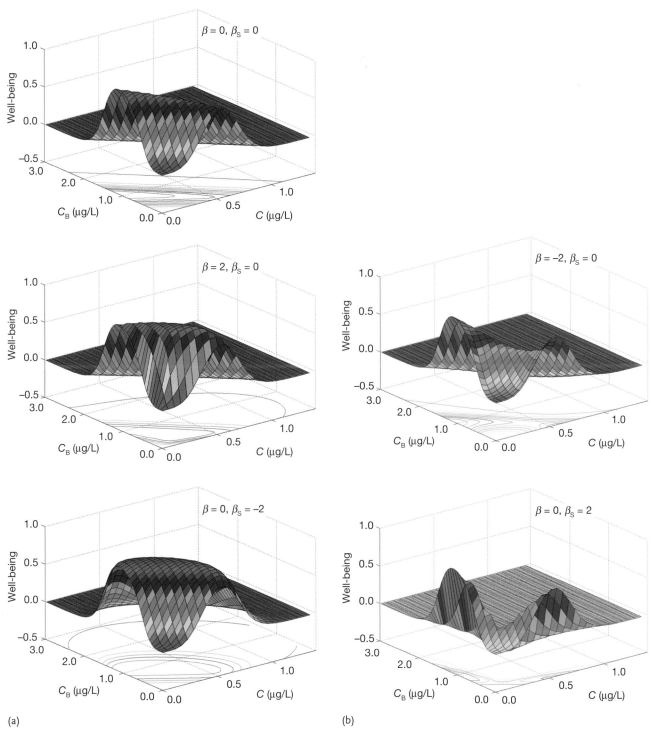

(a)   (b)

Plate V. (a) Well-being surface for various values of the interaction parameter for positive effect (β) and negative (β_S) effect. The effect of the parameters on the shape of the well-being surface assessed by the sensitivity analysis is consistent with the interpretation in terms of synergy and antagonism and with common clinical knowledge. Considering the interaction parameter, a synergism in the positive effect ($\beta > 0$) or antagonism in negative effect ($\beta_S < 0$) results in the surface that reaches a higher well-being value than a zero interaction constellation, and forms a plateau. This means that the same effect can be reached by more than just one drug concentration combination of drugs A and B. (b) In the same way, the interactions between the negative effects can be interpreted in terms of synergy and antagonism: a positive value of β_S indicates synergy between the negative effects, while a negative value indicates antagonism. In the latter case, the surface reaches lower well-being values for a given combination of drugs, and forms a depression. This means that a single drug results in a better effect than a combination. C is the concentration of drug A and C_B is the concentration of drug B in the effect compartment.

SECTION 1

Introduction

Chapter 1

Bridging the gap between pain management as a specialty and rheumatology

Harald Breivik and Michael Shipley

Pain management has always been a primary objective of anaesthesiology, pain-free surgery by general or regional anaesthesia being a prerequisite for advances in surgery during the last 150 years. Effective and low-risk relief of dynamic pain after surgery allows an accelerated rehabilitation of bodily functions after the insult of surgical trauma.

From their practice of acute pain relief, anaesthetists developed expertise in relieving severe cancer pain, based on their pharmacological knowledge and skills in regional nerve blocks with local anaesthetics and neurololytic agents. Gradually anaesthetists also became involved in the relief of chronic non-cancer pain. Eventually, a subspecialty of pain management developed in the specialty of anaesthesiology.[1] This has involved the acquisition of specific diagnostic and psychosocial skills, although many anaesthetically trained pain specialists work closely with other specialists as part of a multidisciplinary team. Now pain management is an officially recognized subspecialty in several countries. This subspecialty can be obtained by anaesthesiologists, neurologists, neurosurgeons, psychiatrists, rheumatologists and those in other mainstream specialities. Requirements by the health authorities for practical training and documentation of adequate knowledge have been established in, for instance, Finland, Sweden, Turkey and several other countries. In several countries, such as the UK and Ireland, and the five Nordic countries (Denmark, Finland, Iceland, Norway and Sweden), subspecialty training in advanced pain management is being offered – by the Royal Colleges in the UK and Ireland, and by the Scandinavian Society of Anaesthesiology and Intensive Care Medicine in the Nordic countries.[2] Although rheumatologists are pain-management specialists by means of training in their specialty, only a small minority of those who have obtained subspecialty recognition as pain-management specialists in Finland and Sweden are rheumatologists. The

International Association for the Study of Pain (IASP) has about 7000 individual members, half of whom are anaesthetists, but only 70 of whom were rheumatologists in 2005.[3] Almost 10% of 4839 patients with chronic pain interviewed in 16 European countries in 2003 stated that they were treated by a rheumatologist, 23% had been seen by a 'pain-management specialist', but only 2% were currently being treated by a 'pain specialist'.[4]

Management of pain is a major part of clinical rheumatology, and musculoskeletal pain has a high prevalence worldwide and increases with increasing age.[5] There is good evidence that it is more common than it was 40 years ago.[6] Rheumatologists have long been experienced in working with a team of clinicians – physiotherapists, occupational therapists, podiatrists and psychologists – all of whom have an important role in managing pain. Rheumatologists are trained in the skills of clinical diagnosis and in the use of medications for pain control. They were amongst the earliest specialty to study drugs methodically and to use the double-blind trial protocol. Intra-articular and soft-tissue injection techniques are central to their management of many of the commoner conditions that present to a rheumatologist. Some see themselves as physicians who should focus their skills on treating the more severe inflammatory and autoimmune conditions and thereby reduce damage and chronic pain. However, the British Society for Rheumatology (and other national societies to a greater or lesser extent) recognized a decade or so ago that, in order to increase the distribution of rheumatologists more evenly across the UK and to improve the quality of patient care, they would need to take on a much wider remit, including the management of local soft-tissue problems and of chronic pain. This is happening and is an appropriate use of their listening and diagnostic skills. As a specialty rheumatologists have been slow to take up the use of imaging as a means of more accurately guiding injections. The next generation of rheumatologists will be trained in ultrasound diagnosis and in the use of ultrasound-guided injections.[7] Those who use injections for spinal pain will acquire radiology licences to enable the more accurate positioning of the therapeutic agent. These developments are long overdue and should be welcomed.

All patients with acute and chronic pain require the input of a wide variety of practitioners. Rheumatologists are particularly likely to see people with chronic musculoskeletal pain. Pain is a complex process influenced by genetic, environmental and cultural factors, as well as socio-economic status and psychological factors.[5] In acute pain, what might be called 'guided self-management' by the patient is appropriate to avoid 'medicalizing' what is often a short-lived and reversible problem. As pain becomes more chronic it changes and a wider variety of skills is needed from a variety of specialists, physical therapists and behavioural psychologists. Early intervention, targeted at 'at-risk' individuals, has been effective in, for example, acute low back pain, and a variety of evidence-based guidelines are available worldwide.[8] Chronic pain does not fit well into the traditional medical model of disease, and recognizing this and putting into practice a wider psychosocial approach that recognizes the complex interplay of physical, psychological and social factors is a challenge to pain specialists, generalists and patients.[9] Helping primary care physicians to use this approach in the often time-constrained circumstances of their practice and to reduce the use of medical resources by this often frequently attending group of challenging patients will be an important step for pain specialists to engage in.

The role of the patient in his or her own care is central. Pain is personal and is best recorded in a self-reporting approach using questionnaires. These can be simple and used in daily practice. Many patients in rheumatological practice see pain as their greatest problem and feel that it is often only poorly managed. The balance between adequate pain control and the avoidance or minimizing of side-effects is essential. The choice which a patient faces from orthodox medical and complementary practitioners is enormous and often confusing. The way that these approaches are used often reflects the desperation of the patient. There are many factors that influence an individual patient's ability to cope with pain and that need to be addressed.[10] Illness behaviour and psychological distress strongly influence the onset and persistence of chronic widespread pain.[11, 12] The mechanisms underlying chronic pain are discussed in this book. Our knowledge is increasing, but there are many aspects of chronic pain and associated problems, such as chronic fatigue, that are what are often called 'medically unexplained symptoms'. This requires specialist management and great care in communicating with the patient. Cognitive–behavioural therapy may be an essential part of helping patients with such complex phenomena to come to terms with and manage their pain, despite their symptoms.[13]

The evidence base for many of the techniques used in managing pain is poor. It is undoubtedly improving, but much more needs to be done, and we have asked each author who has contributed to this book to specify what information is evidence based and to suggest what research needs to be undertaken.

This compendium on the management of pain comprises selected and updated papers about pain management from *Best Practice and Research in Rheumatology* and *Best Practice and Research in Anaesthesiology* published during the last decade. The papers illustrate that there is a growing understanding and mutual interaction between these two clinical specialities, one dealing primarily with acute pain, the other primarily with chronic non-cancer pain. Thus, these papers cover pain problems from two different pain 'worlds'. The management strategies for acute pain cannot necessarily be used for chronic non-cancer pain of patients with rheumatological disorders. Disease-modifying treatments occupy a major part of the treatment armamentarium of the rheumatologist, and the reduction of pain and an improvement in function are sensitive variables indicating the success of such treatment. However, it appears from a recent large-scale, computer-assisted telephone survey of the prevalence, treatment and impact of chronic pain in Europe that many patients were concerned that their doctor was mainly occupied with specific treatment of the underlying cause of the pain, and too little concerned with relieving the pain.[4]

On the other hand, anaesthesiology-based pain specialists are less well trained in rehabilitation in chronic painful diseases such as rheumatoid arthritis and osteoarthrosis. Thus more interaction between pain-interested rheumatologists and anaesthesiologists is needed, and this must be beneficial for both specialities and their patients. We hope that the present compendium on various aspects of the management of acute and chronic pain will be of value and have some impact on both anaesthesiologists and rheumatologists, and on the wider group of practitioners who play such a vital role in helping people to manage and live with chronic pain.

REFERENCES

1. Breivik H. The future role of the anaesthesiologist in pain management. *Acta Anaesthesiol Scand* 2005; **49**: 922–926.
2. Breivik H, Lindahl SG. Training programme in advanced pain medicine for Nordic anaesthesiologists. *Acta Anaesthesiol Scand* 2001; **45**: 1191–1192.
3. Available at: http://www.iasp-pain.org (accessed 28 August 2006).
4. Breivik H, Collette B, Ventafridda V et al. Survey of chronic pain in Europe: Prevalence, impact on daily life, and treatment. *Eur J Pain* 2006; **10**: 287–333.
5. Brooks P. Issues with chronic musculoskeletal pain [Editorial] *Rheumatology* 2005; **44**: 831–833.
6. Harkness EF, Macfarlane GJ, Silman AJ et al. Is musculoskeletal pain more common now than 40 years ago? Two population-based cross-sectional studies. *Rheumatology* 2005; **44**: 890–895.
7. Cunnington J, Hide G, Kane D. Training in musculoskeletal ultrasound by UK rheumatologists: when is now, but how? [Editorial]. *Rheumatology* 2005; **44**: 1470–1472.
8. Koes BW, Van Tulder M, Osteso R et al. Clinical guidelines for the management of low back pain in primary care – an international comparison. *Spine* 2001; **26**: 2504–2513.
9. Foster NE, Pincus T, Underwood MR et al. Understanding the process of care for musculoskeletal conditions – why a biomedical approach is inadequate [Editorial]. *Rheumatology* 2003; **42**: 401–403.
10. Rahman A, Ambler G, Underwood M et al. Important determinants of self-efficacy in patients with chronic musculoskeletal pain. *J Rheumatol* 2004; **31**: 1187–1192.
11. McBeth J, MacFarlane GJ, Benjamin S et al. Features of somatisation predict the onset of chronic widespread pain. *Arthritis Rheum* 2001; **44**: 940–946.
12. McBeth J, MacFarlane GJ, Hunt IM et al. Risk factors for persistent chronic widespread pain: a community based study. *Rheumatology* 2001; **40**: 95–101.
13. Rosendal MR, Oelsen F, Fink P. Management of medically unexplained symptoms [Editorial]. *BMJ* 2005; **330**: 4–5.

SECTION 2

Science and psychology of pain

Chapter 2
Science and psychology of pain

Johan W. S. Vlaeyen, Geert Crombez and Liesbet Goubert

INTRODUCTION

Pain, including headache, stomach ache and musculoskeletal pain, is among the most common somatic complaints. Fortunately, pain is long-lasting, severe and interferes with activities of daily life in only a minority of patients. Persons with chronic invalidating pain frequently present to healthcare providers. Often they experience anxiety and depression, irritation, frustration and helplessness, and suffer from insomnia and excessive medication use. It is well known that this group of chronic sufferers is difficult to treat – there is no immediate and definitive solution available for the pain problem. Therefore, the objectives of treatment consist of learning to control the somatic complaints and to improve quality of life.

In this chapter the importance of cognitive and behavioural processes in the experience of chronic pain, and the resulting problems encountered in performing daily activities are discussed. First, pain is discussed from within a traditional perspective that assumes a direct and immediate relationship between tissue damage, pain experience and disability. Pain problems are then considered within a biopsychosocial perspective. Implications for the treatment of patients with chronic pain problems are outlined. We summarize theoretically grounded and effective treatment strategies in patients with pain, and conclude with emergent themes for future research and for the improvement of clinical practice.

THE BIOMEDICAL MODEL

A traditional biomedical perspective considers pain as a direct consequence of an underlying pathology. The French philosopher René Descartes was one of the first to describe pain by means of a mechanical model. In this model there are direct and unique pain pathways from the peripheral nervous system to the brain, in the same way the bell in a church tower rings when the rope attached to it is pulled. For Descartes, pain was a reflex of the mind upon nociceptive stimulation of the body.

Pain was treated as a symptom, isomorphically related to the severity of the underlying pathology of the organism. According to this perspective, pain treatment mainly consists of two acts: localization of the underlying pathology, and removal of the pathology with an appropriate remedy or cure. In the absence of bodily damage, the mind was assumed to be at fault, and a psychological pathology was inferred.

This model has been extremely influential. The same assumptions are made in, for example, the specificity theory of pain. This theory assumes that specific receptors or bundles of nerve fibres exist that transmit information about tissue damage (nociception) in an unambiguous way to the brain. It is not surprising that, due to these characteristics, one speaks of 'pain receptors', 'pain nerves' and 'pain centres'. This biomedical perspective has undoubtedly generated medical successes. However, many experiences cannot be explained by the specificity theory. First, no receptors or specific nerves exist that are uniquely sensitive for (information about) tissue damage. At most, there is specialization: some receptors or peripheral nerves are more sensitive than others in transmitting information about tissue damage. Second, research has not been successful in locating specific pain centres in the cortex, as is the case for other perceptual systems. In the historical experiments done by Penfield, electrical stimulation of the visual or auditory cortex in patients with epilepsy evoked visual and auditory sensations, respectively. Pain sensations provoked by electrical stimulation were so unusual that it was concluded that 'pain [probably] has little, if any, true cortical representation'.[1] In addition, ablation studies showed that pain is not exclusively located in the cortex. Specific lesions in the brain seldom led to a selective deficit in pain sensation. Today it is assumed that the processing and integration of nociceptive information occurs in different specialized areas of the brain.

Patients often make sense of their pain within the traditional biomedical model, and these beliefs often are referred to as 'pain myths'[2] (Box 2.1). These myths clearly illustrate that patients are inclined to medicalize their pain problems, and to

> **Box 2.1.** Myths about chronic pain
>
> - Pain always means that there is a physical injury
> - When physicians do not detect the cause of the pain, pain is imaginary
> - Pain always means that one has to rest, take medication or go to the physician
> - When psychological remedies are able to relieve the pain, then pain is imaginary
> - If I could live without pain, then I would be completely happy

reject psychological understandings of their pain. The rejection of psychological explanations is understandable. In Western cultures dominant psychological accounts of pain are strongly associated with understandings of simulation, secondary gain and personal weakness.[3]

A rejection of the belief that psychological and social variables influence pain is understandable, but erroneous. The answers formulated within the biomedical perspective are incomplete. The effects of complex physiological processes and psychological and social variables on pain are disregarded for the sake of convenience and parsimony. In most natural situations, the relationships between tissue damage and pain are, however, far from perfect. Patients with the same injury may experience pain differently, and some individuals with similar kinds of injury may report no complaints at all. Often psychological and social variables may (partially) account for these discrepancies.

A Kuhnian shift of paradigm occurred with the gate control theory proposed by Ronald Melzack and Patrick Wall.[4] They pioneered the idea that the dorsal horn of the spinal cord functioned as a gate, by which the transmission of information about tissue damage may be facilitated (the gate opens) or inhibited (the gate closes). At the peripheral level, the opening of the gate was proposed to be dependent on the relative activity of two groups of nerve fibres. The first group comprises thick nerve fibres that are specialized in transmitting information about

tissue damage (nociception) and tend to open the gate. The second group consists of fibres specialized in transmitting tactile information, and these tend to close the gate. The idea that descending pathways also modulated the gate was revolutionary. Melzack and Wall proposed that psychological variables such as attention, fear and expectations affected the gate mechanism through descending pathways. The gate control theory gave rise to intriguing and innovative findings in pain research. The descending, pain-inhibiting circuits were identified, and their physiological and pharmacological features were unravelled. Often the pain inhibition by these circuits was based on endogenous opioids. In addition, the environmental triggers for activation of these circuits were identified. First, extremely stressful (life-threatening) situations were found to activate the endogenous circuitry and made animals less sensitive to pain (stress-induced analgesia). Second, it was found that directing attention towards or away from pain influenced the gate mechanism in the spinal cord, and as a consequence directly affected the transmission of nociception to the brain. The gate control theory metaphorically 'opened' the gate for psychology. The perception of pain was no longer assumed to be a passive registration process, but was conceptualized as the end product of a series of active and constructive sensory, cognitive and affective–motivational processes.

Clinical practice promptly followed this scientific revolution. Pain was no longer equated with tissue damage. In 1986 the International Association for the Study of Pain defined pain as 'an unpleasant sensory and emotional experience associated with actual or potential tissue damage, or described in terms of such damage'. This definition meant a radical break with the traditional biomedical model. A direct relationship between tissue damage and pain was no longer assumed. It is sufficient if the experience is worded *as if* it concerns tissue damage. Furthermore, the gate control theory has proven a useful metaphor for patients with chronic pain to transcend dualistic thinking about organic and psychogenic pain, and to challenge the pain myths (Table 2.1). The finding that psychological factors influence pain positively or negatively is labelled as normal instead of pathological. In addition, the patient is no

Table 2.1. Factors that open and close the gate

Type of variable	Variables that open the gate	Variables that close the gate
Physical	Extent of injury	Medication
	Sensitivity of the central nervous system	Counterstimulation
	Too high/low activity level	Adjusted activity level
Affective	Depression	Relaxation
	Fear	Positive emotions
	Aggression	Calm
Cognitive	Attention to pain	Distraction
	Boredom	Engagement
	Negative attitude towards pain	Positive attitude towards pain

longer seen as a passive victim of his body. The patient himself can take control and can have an active role in the modulation of nociceptive information.

BIOPSYCHOSOCIAL MODEL

The American internist and psychiatrist George Engel argued strongly in favour of a broad biopsychosocial perspective on illness.[5] This perspective acknowledges that the origin of illness is *complex* and *multifactorial.* It was a plea to take into consideration not only biomedical variables, but also psychological (behaviour, emotions, beliefs and coping strategies, experience of social support) and social variables (social network, socio-economic status) in illness. Generally, a distinction is made between different types of causal factors. Some are *predisposing factors* (e.g. hereditary capacities, poor living conditions). Others are *initiating factors* (e.g. an accident, a virus). Finally, there are reinforcing or *maintaining factors* (e.g. insomnia as a consequence of pain). A combination of these factors determines:

- whether the body deviates from the normal, healthy body, and whether someone develops a *disease*
- how severe symptoms are experienced and how a person experiences his or her *illness*
- how a person behaves when he or she is ill, and whether the patient experiences interference in performing daily social activities (*sick-role*, dysfunction).

In the context of pain, a sharp distinction has to be made between biomedical factors (disease), the pain complaints (illness) and the disability in daily life (dysfunction). Although these constructs are interrelated, in most natural situations and most medical disorders they overlap only partially. In patients with chronic low back pain, low correlations are found between biomedical signs of pathology, reported pain severity and reported functional disability.[6, 7] The biopsychosocial perspective goes beyond the gate control theory of Melzack and Wall. It not only emphasizes that the relationship between tissue damage and pain is far from absolute, but it also firmly argues that the relationship between the experience of pain and functional disability is far from perfect. Disability can be different in patients with equal pain intensity, whereas people without disability may report intense pain. Finally, moderate levels of pain may be accompanied by severe disability in daily life. In summary, disability is one of the most substantial consequences of pain without being completely reducible to pain. Inevitably, this means that other processes are yet to be identified to explain the severity of pain and the extent of disability.

Considering the loose relationship between pain intensity and disability, a paramount question is then what exactly are the characteristics of patients with chronic pain? The presence of a pain symptom is necessary but not sufficient. Just as important are a high level of emotional suffering and a high level of functional disability due to pain. In addition to pain, patients with a pain disorder report complaints in the social, affective and cognitive arenas. High prevalences of social phobia, agoraphobia, blood phobia and thanatophobia are found.[8] Other affective problems, such as depression,[9] anger[10] and frustration,[11] are often present. Pain, fear and depression may each have a negative impact on daily cognitive functioning. Patients complain of problems of attention and concentration[12] and memory problems.[13] Several answers have been formulated to the question of how patients become trapped in this vicious circle of physical, emotional, cognitive and behavioural problems. Some of these answers are discussed below.

Operant conditioning perspective

In the 1960s the American psychologist Wilbert Fordyce pointed to the importance of the behavioural dysfunction of the patient in analysing the pain problem and treatment.[14] According to him, the pain behaviour of the patient, rather than the pain complaint, needs to be the central issue. In proposing this approach he acknowledged that the relationship between the pain experience and the dysfunction is often far from perfect. Pain behaviour was defined as behaviour from which outsiders may infer that a person suffers from pain. This behaviour may vary considerably: painful grimace, moaning, taking pain medication, a disordered posture, bed rest, avoidance behaviour, isolation, work leave, etc. It is highly likely that some behaviours have a communicative function. The origin of other behaviours is self-protective and recuperative. The patient tries to minimize the pain by his behaviour. Therefore, not all pain behaviour can be considered to have a communicative function.[15]

In addition, according to Fordyce,[16, 17] pain behaviours are likely to come under the control of short-term consequences through *operant conditioning* principles. Acute pain elicits evolutionarily determined self-protective behaviours. When these behaviours are able to diminish pain, they are likely to increase in frequency. A patient who experiences that escaping having to undertake certain activities reduces pain, will stop doing these activities and will avoid them on future occasions. Performing tasks during intense pain is a frustrating and difficult experience. Others may criticize the patient because tasks are not performed as expected. By no longer performing those activities the patient may escape his or her own feelings of frustration and avoids criticism from others. The patient may also avoid some annoying tasks or responsibilities because of pain. In all the above-mentioned situations the pain behaviour is maintained through avoidance of negative consequences; this is called *negative reinforcement.*

Pain behaviour may also be maintained through *positive reinforcement.* Partners and family members may reinforce pain behaviour by the way they give attention to the patient.[18] Support for and comprehension of partners and family members for the pain complaint should, however, not be banned. Pain behaviour occurs less in patients with sufficient support of family members. A possible explanation is that in these families support and attention is given not only in difficult situations, but also in situations where no pain behaviour is exhibited, or in situations in which the patient successfully copes with the pain. Indirect evidence for the role of positive reinforcement is provided by a study in which patients with chronic pain were asked to perform physical tasks in the absence or presence of his or her spouse. In the presence of solicitous spouses, patients' pain behaviours increased, whereas the presence of punishing spouses tended to decrease pain behaviours compared with situations in which no spouses were present.[19] Furthermore, a number of experimental studies have shown that verbal reports of pain intensity experienced from a repeated noxious stimulus of equal intensity can be modified through operant conditioning. Subjects who received verbal positive reinforcement from the experimenter after each trial if their report of pain intensity exceeded that of the previous trial reported significantly greater pain than did non-reinforced subjects.[20] Interestingly, the effects of upward conditioning of pain reports appear to extinguish much more slowly in patients with chronic pain than in healthy controls.[21]

Operant treatment may be applied if excessive pain behaviour is identified.[16] The objective of operant treatment is to promote 'healthy' behaviour, leaving less opportunity for pain behaviour to occur. Therefore, environmental influences must be controlled. This means that all practitioners, including the referring general practitioner and specialist, must pay more attention to healthy behaviours (e.g. resuming daily activities) than to pain behaviours. Initially, operant treatments were performed on inpatients, but in less marked pain behaviour treatment is also possible in an outpatient department. Operant treatments are usually highly structured, and consist of a number of essential parts: presentation of a rationale, determining treatment goals, establishing a baseline, and choosing the starting level of treatment and the intermediate stages in the direction of the final goal. This information results in a (preferably written) treatment agreement, after which the actual treatment begins, with the application of reinforcement schemes. For an extensive description the reader is referred to the chapter by Sanders.[22] In extreme cases of pain behaviour, the behaviour repertoire of the patient may contain too little healthy behaviour. In this case healthy behaviours must be reconstructed step by step (shaping). Vlaeyen et al[23] have described a programme for a patient who was unable to stand or sit still due to chronic back pain. In 17 steps, the difference between the baseline behaviour and the target behaviour (sit still on a chair) was narrowed, starting with running in place without arm movements, via standing with and without movements, and ending with sitting on a normal chair. Each approach to the target behaviour was systematically reinforced (successive approximation). Apart from some technical aspects of the performance, operant treatment may also be considered as an attitude of the practitioner who pays attention to healthy behaviour, and, in this way, helps to redirect attention from pain to daily functioning.

Because the partners of patients may influence pain behaviour to a considerable extent, they should be involved as much as possible. They may be involved in a relatively intensive training programme, in which they learn to identify pain behaviour and healthy behaviour and to pay more attention to the capabilities of their partners than to pain behaviour.[24] Partners may also be involved in communication skills training of the patient through which direct communication may be stimulated at the expense of the indirect communicative function of pain behaviour.[25]

Psychophysiological reactivity

Emotional events, stress and pain have an influence on our physiological systems such as heartbeat, respiration and muscle tension. In many circumstances these psychophysiological reactions are adaptive and functional. In anxiety and fear these reactions are part of an energetic and motor preparation for fight or flight. When in pain, muscles may become tightened to avoid further pain increases. Sustained muscle contraction is, however, accompanied by a reduction of oxygen in the muscles and a hypersensitivity of the receptors, which may paradoxically increase pain. Evidence exists that a prolonged elevated muscle tension may cause pain, even long after the tension in the muscles is released. However, it is still unclear how important this mechanism is in the maintenance of pain problems.

Although the nature of the psychophysiological responses strongly depends on situational characteristics, strong and consistent individual differences in physiological reactions to stress exist. This phenomenon has been labelled *response stereotypy*. Response stereotypy has been investigated extensively in chronic pain. Indeed, a clinical hypothesis is that pain patients react to stressful situations with an automatic tensing of the muscles in the painful area. Although for a long time reliable data in favour of this hypothesis were lacking,[26] several methodologically sound studies have now been reported. Flor et al[27] investigated the relationship between physiological parameters and both personally relevant and general stressors in several groups of patients with chronic pain. Compared with non-pain patients, only patients with pain in the maxillary joint showed a stronger increase in the electromyographic (EMG) values for the maxillary joint muscles in the personal stress situation (talking about important life events). Patients with chronic low back pain particularly responded by tensing the back muscles in the same stress situation. This type of response stereotypy has also been shown to be associated with increased pain.[28]

The aim of relaxation exercises is to reduce muscle tension and psychophysiological reactivity. A commonly used technique is *applied relaxation*,[29] by which the patient learns to relax in an increasingly shorter span of time and, subsequently, to apply the relaxation response in the diverse situations in which stress usually increases. Training can take place both individually and in groups, and consists of three phases: reconceptualization, skills training and generalization. Skills training starts with *progressive* relaxation, in which the patient learns to feel the difference between tensed and relaxed muscle groups, and subsequently to relax the muscle groups. Thereafter, so-called 'cues' are introduced. The goal of this phase is to bring about a conditioning between a cue (e.g. the word 'relax', a visual stimulus) and the relaxed state. By means of these cues, the patient learns to execute the relaxation response during the performance of daily activities, which facilitates generalization. Sometimes training is supported by EMG biofeedback.[30] To date, there is relatively little empirical support for the effectiveness of relaxation exercises with or without biofeedback, except for headache patients.[31] One of the reasons for the limited effectiveness of this approach relates to the fact that most treatments pay little attention to the implementation of the learnt relaxation response in personally relevant stressful situations.

Cognitive perspective

Psychophysiological reactions and behaviours cannot be separated from the context in which the individual is situated and its meaning to them. The cognitive processes involved in this process of making sense of pain have been elaborated on extensively by Turk and co-workers.[32, 33] Cognitive processes have a substantial impact on pain. Attention is an important factor, but so are the individual's attributions and expectations regarding the possibility of controlling the pain experience.

Attention

It makes sense that pain interrupts ongoing activities and demands attention, even in situations where the current concern of the individual is not related to pain. Pain is an evolutionary signal of bodily threat that urges escape. Despite the fact that in many situations of chronic pain, pain may be considered a 'false alarm', pain continues to interrupt attention. Research has revealed that the interrupting quality of pain is amplified by its intensity, its novelty and unpredictability, and its threat value.[34] Pain may also become the focus of attention because of its immediate relevance to the current goals of the individual. There are many examples in which the processing of pain-related information has priority over and is of immediate relevance to the goal of the individual. Patients may attempt to avoid the worsening of pain during physical activity. Patients may worry about the ineffectiveness of previous medical interventions, and continue to search for other ways to manage their pain.[35] These examples have in common that the current goal of the individual is related to pain. In such situations a hypervigilance to pain or pain-related information emerges.[36] Attention is automatically shifted to pain or cues for pain[37] and, once detected, attention dwells on the pain and it is difficult to disengage from.[38] Hypervigilance to pain is largely automatic and emerges when pain has a high threat value. It is an unintentional and efficient process that occurs when the individual's current concern is to escape and avoid pain. Evidence shows that hypervigilance can be controlled, but that control is far from optimal and not without costs. Studies have revealed that attempts to suppress pain or fear may prove futile, and may lead to a paradoxical increase in pain or anxious thoughts once the attempts to suppress them are stopped.[39] Both the interrupting quality of pain and hypervigilance to pain are related to attributions about pain and expectations about the possibilities of having control of the situation.

Attributions and catastrophizing about pain

Attributions refer to the interpretation of events and the search for possible explanations for the complaints. For patients with chronic pain it is often difficult to make sense of the pain. Pain is of little diagnostic value for either the patient or the physician. Pain is experienced as useless. Patients struggle with the 'mysterious' origin of their pain.[40] Frequently, patients catastrophize about their pain. Although the criteria for catastrophizing about pain have never been stated explicitly, it has been broadly conceived of as an exaggerated negative orientation towards actual or anticipated pain experiences ('Pain is the worst that can happen to me').[41] Experimental studies have shown that a catastrophic style of thinking is related to higher pain intensity, worrying about pain, feelings of helplessness and difficulty in directing attention away from pain.[42] Catastrophizing about pain is also related to the personality characteristic of negative affectivity, a general negative orientation towards oneself and the world. However, research has indicated that catastrophizing about pain may not be equated with the degree of this personality characteristic.[43] Furthermore, particular situations may facilitate catastrophizing about pain. Poor communication between the patient and caregiver may, for example, give rise to catastrophizing about pain ('After many investigations the specialist still has not made a diagnosis; my condition will be so serious that he still has not dared to say something.').[44]

Expectations and perceived control

Patients have expectations about which situations exacerbate pain and about the long-term consequences of pain. These expectations instigate avoidance behaviour.[45] A particular expectation in patients with chronic back pain is the fear of movement, which is (erroneously) assumed to be a possible cause of (re)injury.[46] This is called *kinesiophobia*.[47] The research findings can be summarized as follows (for a review see Vlaeyen and Linton[48]):

- in patients suffering from chronic musculoskeletal pain, pain-related fear is associated with impaired physical performance[46, 49–52] and increased self-reported disability[53, 54]
- in the open population pain-related fear predicts future disability and health status[55–57]
- in acute patients with acute lower back pain, pain-related fear predicts future occupational disability[58]
- educational interventions aimed at reducing negative attitudes and beliefs that mediate avoidance behaviour reduce absence from work due to lower back pain.[59, 60]

Self-efficacy is the confidence someone has in his or her own abilities to perform specific tasks successfully.[61, 62] This implies that the extent of self-efficacy may vary according to the type of task. In this way, experienced self-efficacy for the performance of relaxation exercises may vary considerably from the self-efficacy for the performance of physical activities. Self-efficacy has been shown to be related to the extent to which patients suffer from their pain.[63]

Coping

Coping is defined as the way in which an individual reacts to situations that need adaptation in order to eliminate or reduce a stressor. Often a distinction is made between problem-focused strategies and emotion-focused strategies, or between active and passive coping strategies. In the context of pain, problem-focused coping strategies aim at solving or fixing the pain problem. Emotion-focused coping strategies aim at reducing pain intensity or pain-associated distress. Few studies have systematically investigated the effectiveness of different pain coping strategies. Furthermore, results do not support the hypothesis that one particular way of coping is superior. A flexible use of different coping strategies may be preferable.

Although coping is a clinically, intuitively appealing construct, theoretical research related to coping in general, or coping with pain, has been less convincing.[64] One of the main reasons for this is that research is often limited to a structural approach in which coping attempts are categorized and unduly related to outcome variables. What is needed is a dynamic and functional framework that makes sense of the different ways in which individuals respond to specific challenges in their environment.[65] A comprehensive understanding of the goal that patients want to accomplish is then necessary. Taking these considerations into account, one may often conclude that patients with chronic pain are stuck in their coping with pain. They repeatedly and actively search for a solution that will remove the underlying cause of the pain. They consult several physicians, hoping that these experts will solve their problem. Taking medication may be considered as a form of emotion-focused coping in order to control the symptoms. All these strategies to cope with pain are, however, doomed to fail in patients with chronic pain: there is no ready-made solution for the pain. Many patients may then be characterized by a perseverant use of coping strategies, despite repeated experiences of failure and frustration. It may be more advisable to accept the pain problem as insoluble and to direct coping attempts at the pain-related disability.[66] There is some merit in the idea that patients should shift their focus from coping with pain towards coping with disability. Obviously, such a shift is not readily accomplished. It may imply another view of oneself and the future. It may imply a change in the identity of the person;[35] ambitions and life goals will have to be adjusted, and a new meaning of life will have to be found.

Cognitive treatments focus primarily on pain or stress, and aim at changing attributions and expectations concerning the patient's pain control. Most of the time these treatments are offered as part of a comprehensive treatment plan. The most commonly applied are pain-oriented hypnotherapeutic skills training,[67] stress-oriented cognitive therapy according to Beck[68] and problem-solving skills training.[69, 70] Hypnotherapeutic skills training teaches patients how they can intensively make use of self-suggestions and imagination to influence pain. Patients are told that the approach involves techniques everyone knows from daily life, and often uses spontaneously and unconsciously, but which they will now learn to use consciously. Symptom transformation relates to changing pain intensity, changing the modality of the pain experience in another sensation, and changing the locus of pain. In incompatible sensory imagination, attention is directed towards a pleasant bodily sensation, such as relaxation or a pleasant phantasm or memory.[71]

Beck's cognitive therapy assumes that mood disorders are primarily the result of a dysfunctional style of thinking. If people think about themselves and their experiences in a very negative way, their chances of experiencing a negative mood are greater. If pain patients consider the pain experience as a catastrophe, pain is experienced as more negative in comparison with a situation where they accept pain. The goal of treatment is to defy and modify dysfunctional cognitive styles. The patient is asked to record in a diary typical thoughts that arise during difficult situations and activities. Next, thoughts are subjected to a so-called rational self-analysis.[72]

A third cognitive treatment that has been recently applied to chronic pain is aimed at teaching the patient to cope with stress and everyday problems: problem-solving skills training. This training is based on the treatment proposed by D'Zurilla and Goldfried.[73] The training consists of the following steps:

1. problem orientation
2. problem definition and problem formulation
3. considering many solutions
4. making decisions
5. carrying out and evaluating the solution.

Up to now the application of problem-solving skills in pain patients has been scant. Linton and co-workers[74] added problem-solving skills to a multimodal programme for employees with an increased risk of chronic back pain, and found positive effects in the short and the long term. Adding a problem-solving skills training to an operant treatment results in prompter resumption of work and less functional disability.[70]

Exposure in vivo

A relatively large subgroup of back pain patients reports cognitions related to fear of movement and (re)injury. For example: 'It is really not safe for a person with a condition like mine to be physically active'. In this case the patient may be asked how convinced he or she is of this thought, and to what extent he or she has experience of this outcome with a gradual resumption of activities. For most patients the latter is not the case, and the thought is a consequence of the experience that pain complaints increase with vigorous activity. 'It hurts' and 'Activity is dangerous for my body' become synonyms. Just as in phobias these cognitions lead to persistent avoidance behaviour. Thus such patients no longer have the opportunity to correct the faulty expectations about the occurrence of (re)injury. By means of exposure in vivo, a successful and frequently used technique in phobias, patients are exposed to situations they fear, and their expectations are corrected.

For patients with kinesiophobia this implies that an inventory is made of activities that are considered 'dangerous' for the back. For example, photographs of daily activities can be arranged on a 'fear thermometer'.[75] Subsequently, clear and unambiguous information is provided about the importance of being physically active and the absence of vulnerability, in accordance with the prevailing guidelines. Finally, patients are encouraged to perform the feared activities in gradually more difficult situations. This kind of exposure strongly resembles so-called behaviour experiments. Basically, it is a cognitive therapy in which the patient, together with the therapist, searches for rational and functional alternatives to catastrophic thoughts and beliefs. The patient is encouraged to test new hypotheses concerning the relationship between doing movements and the occurrence of pain and injury in practice.

As mentioned before, negative consequences of movements are often overestimated and abilities to perform a number of activities underestimated.[76] During a behaviour experiment the expectations of the patient before the experiment are compared with the experience afterwards. In this way, new conclusions are made about relationships between events. The effectiveness has so far been established using single-case experimental designs, during which exposure in vivo is followed or preceded by operant graded activity or a no-treatment waiting period. Analyses showed that improvements in the dependent variables only occurred during the graded exposure in vivo treatment and not during operant graded activity, irrespective of the order of interventions.[77, 78] A study using an ambulant activity monitor showed that the results are generalized to the home situation.[79] Another finding was that in fearful back pain patients, exposure was superior in reducing functional disability compared with graded activity and education.[80] Similar results were also obtained for patients suffering long-standing complex regional pain syndrome.[81]

Effectiveness of cognitive–behaviour therapy

A number of systematic reviews on the effectiveness of behaviour therapy for patients with a pain disorder show that cognitive–behaviour therapy is effective. A meta-analysis of 25 controlled studies of behaviour therapy in adult patients with a pain disorder, excluding headache, included studies that were published during the period 1974–1996, and compared cognitive–behavioural treatments with a waiting-list condition or an alternative treatment.[82] This meta-analysis included 1672 patients with back pain, rheumatoid arthritis, shoulder pain and fibromyalgia, with an average pain duration of 12.3 years. In more than half of the studies, treatment was provided in groups. The treatments were spread across a mean period of 7 weeks, and the mean duration of treatment was 16 hours. When the cognitive–behavioural method was compared with a waiting-list condition, the largest effects were on the following variables: pain experience, mood and affect, cognitive coping and appraisal, pain behaviour and level of physical activities, and fulfilling social roles. Compared with alternative treatments, cognitive–behaviour therapy was superior on the domains pain experience, coping and fulfilling of a social role. Another meta-analysis of studies in which behavioural treatments were conducted in patients with back pain only, showed similar results.[83] The results of this meta-analysis were summarized in five categories, ranging from strong evidence for effectiveness (category 1) to strong evidence for ineffectiveness (category 5). Behavioural therapies were classified in categories 1 and 2, implying moderate to strong evidence for effectiveness.

No less than 78 studies with a total of 175 conditions (a total of 2866 patients) were selected in a meta-analysis of cognitive–behavioural treatments for headache. This analysis showed that cognitive therapy, relaxation exercises and EMG biofeedback (whether or not accompanied by relaxation therapy) were superior to no treatment or to attentional control.[31] Pharmacological and other treatments were better than no treatment at all. When analyses were limited to studies in which a headache diary was used, pharmacotherapy was no better than attentional control. From an evidence-based-medicine approach, cognitive–behaviour therapy is an effective treatment in patients with a pain disorder. In addition, research has indicated that these treatments are also cost-effective, emphasizing their importance for both the individual and society.[84]

SUMMARY

In the last decade the psychology of pain has evolved rapidly, and a gradual shift has occurred from a traditional approach, in which chronic pain problems were viewed as a mechanical problem to be fixed, or as an expression of an underlying psychogenic problem, to a more dynamic scientific approach. Within this biopsychosocial perspective chronic pain and its associated behaviour are considered to be the result of normal psychological processes: normal processes that are adaptive in acute pain, but dysfunctional in the abnormal situation of chronic pain. Patients may then become trapped into a vicious circle of physical, emotional, cognitive and behavioural problems.

Cognitive–behavioural treatment interventions for chronic pain have expanded considerably. It is now well established that these interventions are effective in reducing the enormous suffering that patients with chronic pain have to bear. In addition, these interventions have potential economic benefits in that they appear to be cost-effective as well. Despite these achievements, there is still room for improvement. First, there is a substantial proportion of patients who do not appear to benefit from the treatment interventions available. One way to progress is to better match the treatment to the relevant characteristics of the patients, rather than providing all patients

---

PRACTICE POINTS

- There are no one-to-one relationships between tissue damage, pain and disability.

- Catastrophic misinterpretations of pain may cause more distress than pain itself.

- Pain-related fear may be more disabling than pain itself.

- Paradoxically, chronic pain problems may be the result of a persistent, but unsuccessful, search for a solution to the pain.

- Attention-diversion techniques are effective only in low-fear patients.

- Cognitive–behavioural treatments are successful when modifying pain-related beliefs and in increasing functional and goal-directed activities.

with the same treatment 'package'.[85] Second, although the sizes of the effects of most cognitive–behavioural treatments for chronic pain are comparable with those in psychopathology, they are modest. Maybe we should invest in the development of effective secondary prevention strategies, which can include patients in whom the pain problem has not yet become too complex. This approach will need reliable identification of those at risk of developing a chronic condition and effective treatments. Third, still relatively little is known about the specific biobehavioural mechanisms that lead to chronic pain and pain disability. Novel imaging techniques, integrated with behavioural experimental research, may enhance our understanding and management of individuals with chronic pain.

RESEARCH AGENDA

- The identification of psychological risk factors to prevent the development of chronic pain disability.
- A better match between patient characteristics and treatment options.
- The pain-reducing effects of exposure to fear-eliciting situations.
- The application of cognitive–behavioural interventions in pain patients with medical diagnoses (cancer pain, neuropathic pain, etc.).
- The effectiveness of acceptance-based interventions for chronic pain.

REFERENCES

1. Penfield W, Boldrey E. Somatic motor and sensory representation in the cerebral cortex as studied by electrical stimulation. *Brain* 1937; **60**: 441.
2. Malec J, Glasgow RE, Ely R et al. Coping with pain: a self-management approach. *JSAS Catalog Selected Documents Psychol* 1977; **7**(113): Ms. No. 1601.
3. Eccleston C, Williams AC, Rogers WS. Patients' and professionals' understandings of the causes of chronic pain: blame, responsibility and identity protection. *Soc Sci Med* 1997; **45**: 699–709.
4. Melzack R, Wall PD. Pain mechanisms: a new theory. *Science* 1965; **150**: 971–979.
5. Engel GL. The clinical application of the biopsychosocial model. *Am J Psychiatry* 1980; **137**: 535–544.
6. Peters ML, Vlaeyen JW, Weber WE. The joint contribution of physical pathology, pain-related fear and catastrophizing to chronic back pain disability. *Pain* 2005; **113**: 45–50.
7. Waddell G. Volvo award in clinical sciences. A new clinical model for the treatment of low-back pain. *Spine* 1987; **12**: 632–644.
8. Asmundson GJ, Norton GR, Jacobson SJ. Social, blood/injury, and agoraphobic fears in patients with physically unexplained chronic pain: are they clinically significant? *Anxiety* 1996; **2**: 28–33.
9. Turk DC, Okifuji A, Scharff L. Chronic pain and depression: role of perceived impact and perceived control in different age cohorts. *Pain* 1995; **61**: 93–101.
10. Fernandez E, Turk DC. The scope and significance of anger in the experience of chronic pain. *Pain* 1995; **61**: 165–175.
11. Riley JL, Robinson ME, Wade JB. Sex differences in negative emotional responses to chronic pain. *J Pain* 2001; **2**: 354–359.
12. Kewman DG, Vaishampayan N, Zald D et al. Cognitive impairment in musculoskeletal pain patients. *Int J Psychiatry Med* 1991; **21**: 253–262.
13. Jamison RN, Sbrocco T, Parris WC. The influence of physical and psychosocial factors on accuracy of memory for pain in chronic pain patients. *Pain* 1989; **37**: 289–294.
14. Fordyce WE, Fowler RS, DeLateur B. An application of behavior modification technique to a problem of chronic pain. *Behav Res Ther* 1968; **6**: 105–107.
15. Williams AC. Facial expression of pain: an evolutionary account. *Behav Brain Sci* 2002; **25**: 439–455; 455–488 [discussion].
16. Fordyce WE. *Behavioral Methods for Chronic Pain and Illness.* Mosby, St. Louis, 1976.
17. Fordyce WE, Fowler RS Jr, Lehmann JF et al. Operant conditioning in the treatment of chronic pain. *Arch Phys Med Rehabil* 1973; **54**: 399–408.
18. Block AR. Investigation of the response of the spouse to chronic pain behavior. *Psychosom Med* 1981; **43**: 415–422.
19. Romano JM, Turner JA, Friedman LS et al. Sequential analysis of chronic pain behaviors and spouse responses. *J Consult Clin Psychol* 1992; **60**: 777–782.
20. Jolliffe CD, Nicholas MK. Verbally reinforcing pain reports: an experimental test of the operant model of chronic pain. *Pain* 2004; **107**: 167–175.
21. Flor H, Knost B, Birbaumer N. The role of operant conditioning in chronic pain: an experimental investigation. *Pain* 2002; **95**: 111–118.
22. Sanders S. Operant treatment. Back to basics. In: DC Turk, RJ Gatchel (eds), *Psychological Approaches to Pain Management. A Practitioner's Handbook.* Guilford Press, New York, 2002.
23. Vlaeyen JW, Groenman NH, Thomassen J et al. A behavioral treatment for sitting and standing intolerance in a patient with chronic low back pain [see Comments]. *Clin J Pain* 1989; **5**: 233–237.
24. Kole-Snijders AM, Vlaeyen JW, Goossens ME et al. Chronic low-back pain: what does cognitive coping skills training add to operant behavioral treatment? Results of a randomized clinical trial. *J Consult Clin Psychol* 1999; **67**: 931–944.
25. Keefe FJ, Caldwell DS, Baucom D et al. Spouse-assisted coping skills training in the management of knee pain in osteoarthritis: long-term followup results. *Arthritis Care Res* 1999; **12**: 101–111.
26. Flor H, Turk DC. Psychophysiology of chronic pain: do chronic pain patients exhibit symptom-specific psychophysiological responses? *Psychol Bull* 1989; **105**: 215–259.
27. Flor H, Birbaumer N, Schugens MM et al. Symptom-specific psychophysiological responses in chronic pain patients. *Psychophysiology* 1992; **29**: 452–460.
28. Burns JW, Wiegner S, Derleth M et al. Linking symptom-specific physiological reactivity to pain severity in chronic low back pain patients: a test of mediation and moderation models. *Health Psychol* 1997; **16**: 319–326.
29. Öst LG. Applied relaxation: description of an effective coping technique. *Scand J Behav Ther* 1988; **17**: 83–96.
30. Donaldson S, Romney D, Donaldson M et al. Randomized study of the application of single motor unit biofeedback training to chronic low back pain. *J Occupat Rehabil* 1994; **4**: 23–37.
31. Bogaards MC, ter Kuile MM. Treatment of recurrent tension headache: a meta-analytic review. *Clin J Pain* 1994; **10**: 174–190.
32. Turk DC, Meichenbaum D, Genest M. *Pain and Behavioral Medicine. A Cognitive–Behavioral Perspective.* Guilford Press, New York, 1983.
33. Turk DC, Rudy TE. Cognitive factors and persistent pain: a glimpse into Pandora's box. *Cog Ther Res* 1992; **16**: 99–122.
34. Eccleston C, Crombez G. Pain demands attention: a cognitive–affective model of the interruptive function of pain. *Psychol Bull* 1999; **125**: 356–366.
35. Aldrich S, Eccleston C, Crombez G. Worrying about chronic pain: vigilance to threat and misdirected problem solving. *Behav Res Ther* 2000; **38**: 457–470.
36. Crombez G, Van Damme S, Eccleston C. Hypervigilance to pain: an experimental and clinical analysis. *Pain* 2005; **116**: 4–7.
37. Peters ML, Vlaeyen JW, Kunnen AM. Is pain-related fear a predictor of somatosensory hypervigilance in chronic low back pain patients? *Behav Res Ther* 2002; **40**: 85–103.
38. Van Damme S, Crombez G, Eccleston C. Disengagement from pain: the role of catastrophic thinking about pain. *Pain* 2004; **107**: 70–76.
39. Koster EH, Rassin E, Crombez G et al. The paradoxical effects of suppressing anxious thoughts during imminent threat. *Behav Res Ther* 2003; **41**: 1113–1120.
40. Williams DA, Keefe FJ. Pain beliefs and the use of cognitive–behavioral coping strategies. *Pain* 1991; **46**: 185–190.
41. Sullivan MJL, Bishop SR, Pivik J. The pain catastrophizing scale: development and validation. *Psychol. Assess* 1995; **7**: 524–532.
42. Sullivan MJ, Thorn B, Haythornthwaite JA et al. Theoretical perspectives on the relation between catastrophizing and pain. *Clin J Pain* 201; **17**: 52–64.
43. Goubert L, Crombez G, Van Damme S. The role of neuroticism, pain catastrophizing and pain-related fear in vigilance to pain: a structural equations approach. *Pain* 2004; **107**: 234–241.

44. Houben RM, Gijsen A, Peterson J et al. Do health care providers' attitudes towards back pain predict their treatment recommendations? Differential predictive validity of implicit and explicit attitude measures. *Pain* 2005; **114**: 491–498.

45. Crombez G, Vervaet L, Lysens R et al Avoidance and confrontation of painful, back-straining movements in chronic back pain patients. *Behav Modif* 1998; **22**: 62–77.

46. Vlaeyen JW, Kole-Snijders AM, Boeren RG et al. Fear of movement/(re)injury in chronic low back pain and its relation to behavioral performance. Pain 1995; **62**: 363–372.

47. Kori SH, Miller RP, Todd DD. Kinesiophobia: a new view of chronic pain behavior. *Pain Management* 1990; **Jan/Feb**: 35–43.

48. Vlaeyen JWS, Linton SJ. Fear-avoidance and its consequences in chronic musculoskeletal pain: a state of the art. Pain 2000; **85**: 317–332.

49. Al-Obaidi SM, Nelson RM, Al-Awadhi S et al. The role of anticipation and fear of pain in the persistence of avoidance behavior in patients with chronic low back pain. Spine 2000; **25**: 1126–1131.

50. Crombez G, Vlaeyen JW, Heuts PH et al. Pain-related fear is more disabling than pain itself: evidence on the role of pain-related fear in chronic back pain disability. Pain 1999; **80**: 329–339.

51. Heuts PH, Vlaeyen JW, Roelofs J et al. Pain-related fear and daily functioning in patients with osteoarthritis. *Pain* 2004; **110**: 228–235.

52. Nederhand MJ, Ijzerman MJ, Hermens HJ et al. Predictive value of fear avoidance in developing chronic neck pain disability: consequences for clinical decision making. Arch Phys Med Rehabil 2004; **85**: 496–501.

53. Asmundson GJ, Norton GR, Allerdings MD. Fear and avoidance in dysfunctional chronic back pain patients. *Pain* 1997; **69**: 231–236.

54. Vlaeyen JWS, Kole Snijders AMJ, Rotteveel AM et al. The role of fear of movement/(re)injury in pain disability. *J Occup Rehabil* 1995; **5**: 235–252.

55. Buer N, Linton SJ. Fear-avoidance beliefs and catastrophizing: occurrence and risk factor in back pain and ADL in the general population. Pain 2002; **99**: 485–491.

56. Picavet HS, Vlaeyen JW, Schouten JS. Pain catastrophizing and kinesiophobia: predictors of chronic low back pain. *Am J Epidemiol* 2002; **156**: 1028–1034.

57. Severeijns R, van den Hout M, Vlaeyen J et al. Pain catastrophizing and general health status in a large Dutch community sample. *Pain* 2002; **99**: 367.

58. Fritz JM, George SZ, Delitto A. The role of fear-avoidance beliefs in acute low back pain: relationships with current and future disability and work status. *Pain* 2001; **94**: 7–15.

59. Buchbinder R, Jolley D, Wyatt M. Population based intervention to change back pain beliefs and disability: three part evaluation. *BMJ* 2001; **322**: 1516–1520.

60. Moore JE, Von Korff M, Cherkin D et al. A randomized trial of a cognitive–behavioral program for enhancing back pain self care in a primary care setting. *Pain* 2000; **88**: 145–153.

61. Bandura A. Self-efficacy: toward a unifying theory of behavioral change. *Psychol Rev* 1977; **84**: 191–215.

62. Dolce JJ, Doleys DM, Raczynski JM et al. The role of self-efficacy expectancies in the prediction of pain tolerance. *Pain* 1986; **27**: 261–272.

63. Turner JA, Ersek M, Kemp C. Self-efficacy for managing pain is associated with disability, depression, and pain coping among retirement community residents with chronic pain. *J Pain* 2005; **6**: 471–479.

64. Skinner EA, Edge K, Altman J et al. Searching for the structure of coping: a review and critique of category systems for classifying ways of coping. *Psychol Bull* 2003; **129**: 216–269.

65. Brandtstädter J, Rothermund K, Schmitz U. Maintaining self-integrity and efficacy through adulthood and later life: the adaptive functions of assimilative persistence and accommodative flexibility. In: Heckhausen J, Dweck CS (eds), *Motivation and Self-regulation Across the Life Span*. Cambridge University Press, Cambridge, 1998, pp. 365–388.

66. McCracken LM. Learning to live with the pain: acceptance of pain predicts adjustment in persons with chronic pain. *Pain* 1998; **74**: 21–27.

67. Gay MC, Philippot P, Luminet O. Differential effectiveness of psychological interventions for reducing osteoarthritis pain: a comparison of Erikson [correction of Erickson] hypnosis and Jacobson relaxation. *Eur J Pain* 2002; **6**: 1–16.

68. Turner JA, Clancy S, McQuade KJ et al Effectiveness of behavioral therapy for chronic low back pain: a component analysis. *J Consult Clin Psychol* 1990; **58**: 573–579.

69. Nezu AM, Perri MG. Social problem-solving therapy for unipolar depression: an initial dismantling investigation. *J Consult Clin Psychol* 1989; **57**: 408–413.

70. van den Hout JH, Vlaeyen JW, Heuts PH et al. Secondary prevention of work-related disability in nonspecific low back pain: does problem-solving therapy help? A randomized clinical trial. *Clin J Pain* 2003; **19**: 87–96.

71. Barber J. *Hypnosis and the Suggestive Management of Pain*. W. W. Norton, New York, 1996.

72. Turner JA, Jensen MP. Efficacy of cognitive therapy for chronic low back pain. *Pain* 1993; **52**: 169–177.

73. D'Zurilla TJ, Goldfried MR. Problem solving and behavior modification. *J Abnorm Psychol* 1971; **78**: 107–126.

74. Linton SJ, Bradley LA, Jensen I et al. The secondary prevention of low back pain: a controlled study with follow-up. Pain 1989; **36**: 197–207.

75. Kugler K, Wijn J, Geilen M et al. *The Photograph series of Daily Activities (PHODA)*. CD-ROM version 1.0. Institute for Rehabilitation Research and School for Physiotherapy, Heerlen, The Netherlands, 1999.

76. Goubert L, Francken G, Crombez G et al. Exposure to physical movement in chronic back pain patients: no evidence for generalization across different movements. *Behav Res Ther* 2002; **40**: 415–429.

77. Vlaeyen JW, de Jong J, Geilen M et al. Graded exposure in vivo in the treatment of pain-related fear: a replicated single-case experimental design in four patients with chronic low back pain. *Behav Res Ther* 2001; **39**: 151–166.

78. Vlaeyen JW, De Jong JR, Onghena P et al. Can pain-related fear be reduced? The application of cognitive–behavioural exposure in vivo. *Pain Res Manag* 202; **7**: 144–153.

79. Vlaeyen JW, De Jong J, Geilen M et al. The treatment of fear of movement/(re)injury in chronic low back pain: further evidence on the effectiveness of exposure in vivo. *Clin J Pain* 2002; **18**: 251–261.

80. de Jong JR, Vlaeyen JW, Onghena P et al. Fear of movement/(re)injury in chronic low back pain: education or exposure in vivo as mediator to fear reduction? *Clin J Pain* 2005; **21**: 9–17.

81. de Jong JR, Vlaeyen JW, Onghena P et al. Reduction of pain-related fear in complex regional pain syndrome type I: the application of graded exposure in vivo. *Pain* 2005; **116**: 264–275.

82. Morley S, Eccleston C, Williams A. Systematic review and meta-analysis of randomized controlled trials of cognitive behaviour therapy and behaviour therapy for chronic pain in adults, excluding headache. *Pain* 1999; **80**: 1–13.

83. van Tulder MW, Ostelo R, Vlaeyen JW et al. Behavioral treatment for chronic low back pain: a systematic review within the framework of the Cochrane Back Review Group. *Spine* 2001; **26**: 270–281.

84. Goossens ME, Rutten-Van Molken MP, Kole-Snijders AM et al. Health economic assessment of behavioural rehabilitation in chronic low back pain: a randomised clinical trial. *Health Econom* 1998; **7**: 39–51.

85. Vlaeyen JW, Morley S. Cognitive–behavioral treatments for chronic pain: what works for whom? *Clin J Pain* 2005; **21**: 1–8.

Chapter 3
The mechanisms of chronic pain

Bruce L. Kidd

INTRODUCTION

For the most part, pain and its underlying mechanisms have received curiously little attention from health professionals dealing with soft-tissue and other musculoskeletal disorders. A tacit acceptance that symptoms reflect underlying disease remains all too common despite abundant evidence to the contrary. Patients with atypical or extreme symptoms are regarded at best as being guilty of exaggeration and at worst are labelled as frankly hysterical or malingering. Clearly, this situation is not in the best interests of either the individual patient or, indeed, the wider health community.

This chapter is divided into three parts and summarizes pain concepts that have emerged over the last few years. The first section is clinically orientated and deals with general issues related to the classification and assessment of pain. The second section describes underlying cellular and molecular mechanisms, and the final section is primarily concerned with issues related to treatment. Overall, this chapter aims to show how an understanding of the mechanisms contributing to pain leads to both improved assessment and more effective therapy.

ASSESSING A PATIENT WITH CHRONIC MUSCULOSKELETAL PAIN

Classification

Pain states have traditionally been regarded as being either nociceptive or neuropathic, depending on the presence or absence of damage within neural pathways.[1] This somewhat restrictive classification is now being superseded by more broadly based schemes (Figure 3.1).

Nociceptive pain refers to transient symptoms arising in response to acute tissue injury and reflects activation of high-threshold sensory fibres (nociceptors) and corresponding activity in more central pathways. Under these conditions symptoms broadly reflect the initiating stimulus or injury.

Neuropathic pain occurs in the presence of nerve injury. Ectopic expression of ion channels, receptors and related

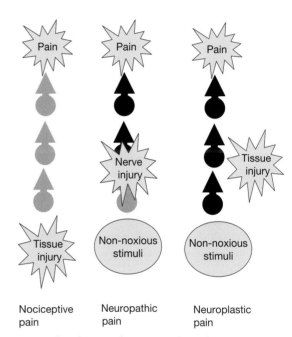

Figure 3.1. Classification of pain. Note that, whereas nociceptive pain is triggered by tissue injury, normally innocuous stimuli produce pain in neuropathic and neuroplastic conditions.

phenomena occurs in both injured and neighbouring non-injured neurons. The result is local sensory loss combined with more regional pain hypersensitivity.

Neuroplastic pain (also called inflammatory pain) is associated with altered excitability of nociceptive pathways and arises in response to mediators released from inflamed or damaged tissues. This has the effect of making everyday events such as standing or walking painful and is the most common pain state associated with persistent musculoskeletal disease.

There is currently debate as to whether to include a fourth category of pain, *functional pain*, to cover such medically unexplained disorders as fibromyalgia syndrome, irritable bowel syndrome and tension headache. In all these disorders evidence of peripheral pathology remains minimal and symptoms are considered to reflect disordered nociceptive processing at more central levels.

Neuroplastic pain

Individuals with musculoskeletal and other chronic diseases present with a wide constellation of symptoms and signs. For example, patients with arthritis complain of aching and throbbing, interspersed by sharp or stabbing pain.[2, 3] Other individuals simply complain that an area hurts or is sore. In sharp contrast to pain following an acute tissue injury, symptoms occur either spontaneously or following stimuli that are not normally painful, such as light touch or movement.

The term 'neuroplastic pain' is derived from the fact that symptoms arising from tissue injury are strongly influenced by changes to the sensitivity (plasticity) of underlying pain pathways. The magnitude of these changes will be contingent on additional somatic, environmental as well as genetic influences, all of which will serve to modify encoded information passing from the periphery through to higher centres in the brain (Figure 3.2). Consistent with this there is relatively poor correlation between objective markers of tissue injury, such as radiological score, and severity of pain, which is often more strongly associated with a range of psychosocial and other factors.[4]

In the presence of musculoskeletal injury or disease, multiple tissue factors serve to sensitize peripheral nociceptors.[5] This is most easily appreciated in the context of an inflammatory stimulus, when inflammatory mediators such as prostaglandins and other signalling molecules alter the threshold for activation of receptors. Clinically this leads to pain and tenderness (primary allodynia) at the site of injury, with symptoms and signs broadly reflecting the extent and severity of the underlying pathology.

The central terminals of primary nociceptive neurons synapse with small interneurons or longer projection neurons. Sensitization of neurons at this level results in enhanced pain perception at the site of injury, as well as the development of pain and tenderness in normal tissues both adjacent to (secondary allodynia) and removed from (referred pain) the primary site.[6]

The supraspinal compartment is less well defined and involves all higher centres from the level of the brainstem through to the cortex. Although supraspinal or cortical sensitization remains unproven, there is a good deal of empirical evidence from sensory testing and functional magnetic resonance imaging (MRI) to suggest the presence of such a phenomenon.[7] Environmental inputs are likely to play a regulatory role at this level and influence both overall pain perception as well as subsequent behavioural and emotional responses. The consequences are likely to be rather generalized discomfort, increased attention to symptoms and new pain-related behaviours.

Assessment of pain

When evaluating a patient with musculoskeletal pain it should be kept firmly in mind that symptoms will reflect not only the underlying pathology but also the sensitivity of underlying pain pathways. The purpose of the evaluation should therefore be to define: (a) the peripheral source of the pain, (b) additional factors likely to be influencing neural sensitivity and (c) the functional consequences and disability. Information from all these areas will then serve to inform therapeutic decisions.

The assessment should include an appraisal of the duration, intensity and character of the pain. The response to previous pharmacological and non-pharmacological interventions should be characterized, as should pain behaviours and disability. Psychosocial and environmental factors have been shown to have an important influence on pain perception and disability, but it has often been difficult for the non-specialist to assess these in any systematic way. The advent of 'yellow flags' has provided a useful tool for assessment, and individuals with these factors have been shown to have higher risk of prolonged pain and disability (Box 3.1).

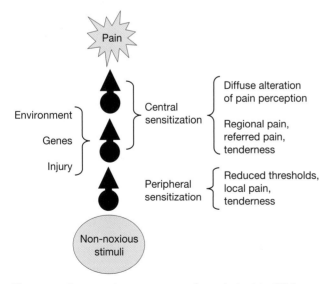

Figure 3.2. Causes and consequences of neural plasticity. Whilst tissue injury or inflammation can trigger nociceptor sensitization, other somatic, psychological and environmental influences are likely to determine the magnitude of any subsequent change.

Box 3.1. Yellow flags

- History of numerous episodes
- Duration of symptoms
- Intensity of symptoms
- Anxiety
- Depression
- Locus of control
- Catastrophizing
- Activity intolerance
- Dependence on passive therapies

Given the varied influences on pain perception it may also prove clinically useful to identify, where possible, underlying nociceptive mechanisms. Symptoms and signs limited to an area of inflammation or damage, for example, would be consistent with the presence of peripheral sensitization alone. More commonly, musculoskeletal disease is associated with symptoms and tenderness either adjacent to or removed from the site of tissue damage, reflecting the presence of more central change. Very intense or more widespread symptoms with diff-use pain and tenderness should alert the assessor to cortical sensitization, and prompt a search for personal or environ-mental factors likely to be playing a contributory role.

THE NEUROPHYSIOLOGICAL MECHANISMS UNDERLYING PERSISTENT MUSCULOSKELETAL PAIN

Peripheral nociceptors

Under normal conditions a specialized (nociceptive) pathway is responsible for the initial response to actual or potential bodily injury. The sequence involves three identifiable steps, beginning with *transduction* of noxious mechanical, thermal or chemical stimuli into electrical activity. The resultant *conduction* of axon potentials along the length of the nerve axon is followed by *transmission* across nerve synapses to secondary neurons in the spinal cord and higher centres.

All musculoskeletal tissues, with the probable exception of cartilage, receive an extensive sensory nerve supply. Encapsu-lated sensory receptors are associated with rapidly conducting A-β fibres, and for the most part are responsible for proprio-ception and related sensations. Small-diameter fibres, on the other hand, preferentially or exclusively respond to noxious stimuli and may be regarded as nociceptors. They have free nerve endings and include the thinly myelinated A-δ fibres and the unmyelinated C fibres. They are widely distributed in syno-vium, fibrous capsules, adipose tissues, ligaments, menisci and periosteum.[8]

Classically, only periosteal layers of bone were regarded as possessing an extensive nerve supply. Recent studies have revised this view by identifying the presence of small-diameter sensory fibres throughout all bone compartments, including bone marrow and mineralized bone.[9] This finding may have relevance to symptoms arising from fractures, bone tumours and conditions such as osteoarthritis where changes to sub-chondral bone are noted.

The receptive properties of nociceptors are determined by their expression of transducing ion-channel receptors. For the most part these are non-selective cation or sodium channels that are gated by temperature, chemical ligands and mechanical shearing forces.[10] Activation produces a flow of sodium and calcium ions into the nociceptor, resulting in an inward current that depolarizes the membrane. This, in turn, can lead to activation of voltage-gated sodium channels, which initiate a burst of action potentials reflecting the intensity and duration of the noxious stimulus.[10]

It is notable that within the joint and under normal conditions a high percentage of nociceptive neurons are non-responsive to mechanical or thermal stimuli in either the physiological or noxious range.[11] The terms 'sleeping' or 'silent' nociceptors were coined to describe these fibres, which only become active under pathological conditions as might be associated with, for example, synovitis.[12]

Peripheral sensitization

As is the case with all living tissues, the nociceptive pathway does not exist in isolation but is subject to modulation by factors both internal and external to the body. At a tissue level, substances present within the extracellular space act to augment or inhibit activity in peripheral nociceptors in a number of ways. Following acute injury some mediators, such as bradykinin, contribute to pain by directly activating nociceptors whereas others are generally considered to be sensitizing agents (Figure 3.3).

Prostaglandins, such as prostaglandin E_2, act to reduce the threshold for the activation of a number of receptors, including the heat-sensitive transient receptor potential V1 (TRPV1) channel and voltage-gated sodium ion channels.[13, 14] Mechan-isms of action include receptor-induced activation of adenyl cyclase, leading to increased levels of cyclic adenosine monophosphate (cAMP) and resultant activation of protein kinase A (PKA). Increased intracellular calcium activates protein kinase C (PKC), with both sets of kinases serving to phosphorylate additional target receptors and ion channels.[14, 15]

The functional consequences of enhanced receptor sensitivity are that nociceptors become spontaneously active or, more commonly, are activated by lower intensity stimuli than before. Within the joint, experimental application of prosta-glandin E_2 has been shown to sensitize nociceptors to

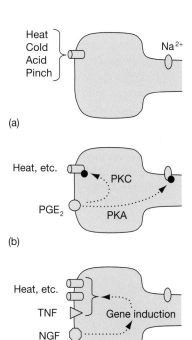

Figure 3.3. Contribution of peripheral nociceptors to pain. (a) Acute pain: noxious stimuli activate high-threshold ion channels, with resultant propagation of axon potentials. (b) Early-phase sensitization: mediators, including prostaglandin E_2, activate kinases to phosphorylate receptors/ion channels and lower the threshold for activation. (c) Late-phase sensitization: gene induction in response to growth factors resulting in changes to cell phenotype. (Adapted from Woolf.[10])

mechanical and other stimuli with a time course that matches the development of pain-related behaviour in awake animals.[16]

Other mediators, such as the endogenous opioids and cannabinoids, act at peripheral sites to reduce nociceptor activity. Opioid receptors have been demonstrated on the terminals of peripheral nerves, and local applications of opioid agonists reduce hyperalgesia in several experimental and clinical models.[17] Similarly, activation of the cannabinoid CB1 receptor is negatively coupled to adenylate cyclase and blocks the excitability of nociceptors, to reduce pain.[18]

Phosphorylation and other post-translational effects on existing receptors and ion channels are important in acute situations, whereas in disorders associated with persistent disease transcriptional upregulation of receptors and ion channels at a genomic level becomes more important. Although exact mechanisms have yet to be fully determined, various neurotrophin growth factors, including nerve growth factor (NGF), are believed to play a pivotal role by activating intracellular signalling pathways that include the mitogen-activated protein kinase p38.[10, 19]

In this manner, persistent inflammation or injury is associated with *phenotypic switching* and changes to the receptor profile and functional output of the cell. Increased expression of various receptors is apparent, including the TRPV1 and the bradykinin B1 receptor. There is also increased production and expression of the neuropeptides substance P and calcitonin gene related peptide, which play a role in modifying both central neuronal excitability and peripheral neurogenic inflammation.[5, 20] Finally, and possibly most dramatically of all, there is induction of novel receptors such as the tumour necrosis factor (TNF) receptor, which may serve to explain the antinociceptive effects of anti-TNF strategies in rheumatoid and other arthropathies.[21]

Nociception and the spinal dorsal horn

The grey matter of the spinal cord is divided into distinct laminae, or layers, on the basis of its neuronal architecture and functional activity.[22] Small-diameter fibres project to the more superficial laminae (I and II), whereas the larger diameter Aβ afferents terminate in the deeper laminae (primarily IV and V). Terminating nociceptor fibres synapse with second-order neurons, which are either projection neurons that relay encoded information to higher centres, or shorter interneurons with either excitatory or inhibitory properties.

The principal neurotransmitter for nociceptive neurons in the dorsal horn is the excitatory amino acid glutamate. Under basal conditions glutamate activates α-amino-5-hydroxy-3-methyl-4-isoxazole proprionic acid (AMPA) receptors on second-order neurons and serves as a mediator for transient (nociceptive) pain. This ion-channel receptor is selective mainly for sodium, with activation leading to sodium influx and the subsequent triggering of axon potentials.

Modulation of spinal processing is under tight control and occurs through both local and descending systems. One of the earliest indications for descending mechanisms came from observations that electrical stimulation of the periaqueductal grey (PAG) region of the rat brain produced potent analgesia.[23] This system contains so-called 'off-cells' and 'on-cells', which act

to suppress or facilitate spinal nociceptive responses, respectively.[24] It appears to be the basis of the fight or flight reaction to threatening stimuli.

Local or segmental mechanisms involve 'wide dynamic range' cells, which respond to input from both nociceptive and non-nociceptive fibres and receive inputs from relatively large areas.[25] They have complex receptive fields with two distinct regions. All encoded stimuli passing to the central region are excitatory, whereas encoded non-noxious stimuli from surrounding regions are inhibitory, which may explain the analgesic properties of counterirritants, acupuncture and transcutaneous nerve stimulation.

An extensive array of mediators has been identified within the dorsal horn (for reviews see Woolf[10] and Hunt and Mantyh[26]). Receptors for opioids, cannabinoids, γ-aminobutyric acid (GABA) and various calcium channels are present on the presynaptic terminals of primary nociceptors and serve to modulate glutamate release. Postsynaptic modulation also occurs via potassium and chloride channels, which respond to opioids and GABA and produce hyperpolarizing inhibitory potentials. Norepinephrine acting via alpha-2 adrenoceptors is an important facilitator of descending inhibition, whereas serotonin (5-hydroxytyptamine (5-HT)) acting via different 5-HT receptors can act to either inhibit or facilitate persistent pain states. This may explain why fear, depression and anger can enhance pain.

Spinal sensitization

The presence of enhanced central nociceptive processing in various musculoskeletal disorders has been confirmed using psychophysical techniques.[27, 28] Within the dorsal horn the cells become more responsive to nociceptive inputs as well as responding to inputs that had hitherto been suppressed. The clinical result is that injured tissues become more symptomatic and surrounding areas become tender and painful. Referred pain states may also occur.

In a similar fashion to that described for peripheral nociceptors, it is possible to discern acute and longer term mechanisms operating at a spinal level to produce these changes (Figure 3.4). Acute tissue injury results in the increased frequency and duration of axon potentials arriving in the dorsal horn. This triggers the release of various neuromodulators, including the neuropeptide substance P, from central nociceptive terminals and has the effect of functionally unmasking a second glutamate receptor on second-order neurons.[5] This *N*-methyl-D-aspartate (NMDA) receptor does not participate in responses to acute stimuli but is intimately involved in persistent neuroplastic and neuropathic pain states. It is a calcium-channel receptor, and activation results in the influx of calcium and the activation of calcium-dependent kinases, including PKC and Src.[29] As in the periphery, these kinases phosphorylate membrane-bound receptors and ion channels, which results in changes in cellular activity.

A change to gene regulation in second-order neurons becomes apparent in more persistent pain states. This may occur in response to neurotrophic factors released from primary

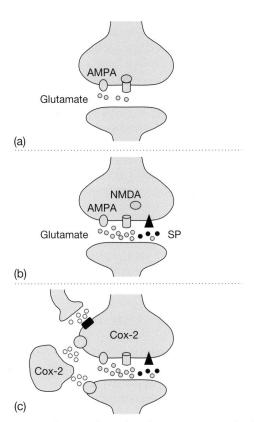

Figure 3.4. Contribution of spinal cord neurons to pain. (a) Acute pain: activation of the AMPA receptor by glutamate; the NMDA receptor is blocked. (b) Early-phase sensitization: activation of the NMDA receptor following removal of the magnesium ion block (mediated by substance P (SP) (●) acting on NK1 receptors (▲)). (c) Late-phase sensitization: gene induction with enhanced production of prostaglandins and other local mediators; modulation by descending facilitatory/inhibitory pathways.

nociceptor terminals or from surrounding non-neuronal cells (see below). Many of the changes mirror those observed in the dorsal root ganglia, suggesting common nociceptive mechanisms in both sets of neurons. Well-characterized changes in the expression of signalling molecules such as c-fos and neuromodulators such as dynorphin in response to peripheral tissue injury have been documented.[26]

Recent studies have highlighted the importance of non-neuronal glial cells as powerful modulators of nociceptive activity at a spinal level.[30] Activated glia produce cytokines such as interleukin-1 (IL-1) and interleukin-6 (IL-6), which in turn stimulate the release of mediators such as nitric oxide and growth factors. In particular, there is widespread upregulation of cyclo-oxygenase-2 (Cox-2) expression in both neuronal and non-neuronal tissue, with a parallel increase in prostaglandin levels, mostly PGE_2, in the cerebrospinal fluid (CSF).[31] A similar sensitizing effect on spinal neurons to that observed in the periphery has been reported.

Supraspinal mechanisms

Functionally, there appear to be two brain systems, each responsible for different aspects of perceived pain.[32] The lateral

pain system comprises the lateral thalamic nuclei and the somatosensory cortices. It is fast acting, and neurons are arranged in a somatotopically arranged fashion (i.e. the projections are arranged in a body map). It is now believed that the lateral system deals primarily with the sensory-discriminative aspects of pain, including the localization and identification of noxious stimuli.

The medial pain system is slower and non-somatotopic. Constituent neurons have large and often bilateral receptive fields, including multiple inputs from deep musculoskeletal structures. The medial system includes the medial thalamic nuclei, anterior cingulate and dorsolateral prefrontal cortices, and possibly structures concerned with the processing of fear, such as the amygdala. Deafferentation of the anterior cingulate gyrus does not abolish chronic pain but reduces its unpleasantness. These and other data have led to the suggestion that the medial pain system is concerned mainly with the motivational/affective components of the pain response.

Patterns of supraspinal activity

Studies using positron emission tomography (PET) and functional MRI (fMRI) have contributed to the current understanding of cerebral pain networks. In general, the same brain areas are activated during thermal- and pressure-induced pain in patients with chronic pain syndromes and in normal volunteers.[33] Subtle differences with respect to the patterns of response are detectable, however, with some pain states being associated with enhanced responses, whereas reduced responses are noted in others. For example, studies have shown increased correlation of catastrophizing with anterior cingulate activity in patients with fibromyalgia or chronic widespread pain.[34]

Accumulating experimental evidence and the failure of any single cortical lesion consistently to abolish pain suggests that there is no single or 'ultimate' pain centre. In keeping with other sensory modalities, such as vision, pain sensations appear to be processed in parallel networks or matrices distributed within cortical and subcortical structures.

THE RELEVANCE TO TREATMENT

Trends in analgesia

Tremendous progress has been made in the past few decades to define key processes underlying pain, but a substantial gap still remains between this accumulating knowledge and the development of effective pain therapy. At present, pain therapies provide moderate to good relief for less than one-third of patients with chronic pain.

It is salutary to remember that no new major class of analgesic agent was developed during the 20th century, apart from the extended role of tricyclic antidepressants as adjunct analgesics. League tables of analgesic efficacy continue to show the non-steroidal anti-inflammatory drugs (NSAIDs) as the most effective therapy for both acute and chronic pain (Figure 3.5).

The following sections are not intended to serve as a comprehensive review of available analgesics, as this is readily

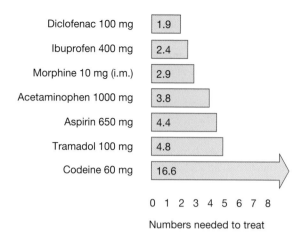

Figure 3.5. Oxford league table of commonly used analgesics in acute pain. Numbers needed to treat for 50% pain relief over 4–6 hours. No comparable data exist for analgesia for chronic pain. (Adapted from *Oxford League Table of Analgesics in Acute Pain*.[35])

available from other sources. Rather, the aim is to highlight mechanisms of action of the main analgesic drugs in current use and assess the potential for the development of novel therapies in the future.

Paracetamol (acetaminophen)

This effective, yet curiously enigmatic, drug continues to be one of the world's most commonly used medications. First used clinically in 1893, its mechanism of action remains uncertain. Currently it has no known endogenous binding sites and it lacks the ability of NSAIDs to inhibit peripheral Cox activity.[36] Claims have been made regarding inhibition of central Cox-2 activity (see below) or even the putative Cox-3 isoenzyme. Other potential mechanisms involve stimulation of descending inhibitory pathways or effects on NMDA receptor activity; however, these remain speculative at the present time.

Therapeutic guidelines for a number of musculoskeletal conditions recommend paracetamol as the first-line analgesic and it is undoubtedly effective in many conditions and across all age groups. A synergistic antinociceptive effect is noted when it is combined with various opioids, including codeine, tramadol and morphine.[37, 38] Available data suggest a less marked additive effect when administered in combination with NSAIDs.

Non-steroidal anti-inflammatory drugs

The principal anti-inflammatory and antinociceptive effects of NSAIDs have been linked to an inhibitory effect on Cox enzymes and a subsequent reduction in inflammatory prostaglandins such as PGE_2 and prostacyclin. Although the antinociceptive effect was traditionally felt to be acting primarily at a peripheral level, other more central actions for these drugs have been proposed in recent years.[39] This follows growing evidence that the anti-inflammatory and antinociceptive effects of NSAIDs are unrelated.

Poor penetration of NSAIDs into spinal and supraspinal structures has been cited to support claims for a purely peripheral site of antinociceptive action. However, penetration varies from drug to drug and is not totally dependent on obvious factors such as plasma binding or ionization. In fact, certain NSAIDs, such as ibuprofen or indomethacin, rapidly cross the blood–brain barrier, and CSF concentrations may exceed unbound plasma levels within a short space of time.[40] More direct evidence for a central antinociceptive NSAID effect is provided by experimental studies showing that intrathecal administration significantly reduces both CSF prostaglandin and long-term neuroplastic pain at doses that are inactive systemically.[41]

In general, the site of antinociceptive action seems to depend on the particular NSAID used, the site of drug delivery and the individual pharmacokinetic characteristics of the drug. The overall efficacy of NSAIDs coupled with questions regarding their cardiovascular safety has given new impetus to studies in this area and highlights the need for more targeted therapy.

Opioids

Alkaloid opioid compounds, initially derived from poppy seeds, have been used for several thousand years and remain the most potent antinociceptive agents in current clinical use. In addition to their antinociceptive actions, opioid peptides have profound effects on behaviours essential for survival, as well as on autonomic and immune responses. Concerns about their abuse potential and the high prevalence of other side-effects have limited the use of strong opioids in musculoskeletal disease, although combination therapy using weaker opioids is a popular therapeutic choice for many conditions.

Three subclasses of opioid receptors have been described, including the μ-, δ- and κ-opioid receptors. They are widely distributed in the supraspinal and spinal compartments of the central nervous system (CNS) and also expressed on the terminals of primary nociceptors. Agonists for the μ-receptor display the best antinociceptive activity, but also the highest abuse potential.

Some opioid-like agents, such as methadone and tramadol, have additional activity at non-opioid (NMDA, 5-HT and norepinephrine) receptors, which can prove useful in some situations. A synergistic interaction between opioids and NSAIDs is apparent, and this has also found widespread application in patients with persistent musculoskeletal pain.

Antidepressants

The antinociceptive action of antidepressants is independent of their effect on depression, and occurs at lower doses and after a shorter duration of treatment.[42] Tricyclic antidepressants (TCAs) have the best antinociceptive efficacy, although the mode of action remains uncertain. TCAs inhibit uptake of norepinephrine and 5-HT, block H_1 receptors and have anticholinergic effects, as well as blocking NMDA receptors and a number of sodium channels.

The main antinociceptive indication for TCAs is for neuropathic pain, although they have beneficial effects in patients with fibromyalgia as well as back pain. More modest effects have been noted in rheumatoid arthritis.[43] For the most part these agents remain useful as adjuvant therapy and are not considered front-line antinociceptive agents in most musculo-skeletal disorders.

Ion-channel blockade

The effectiveness of anticonvulsants, local anaesthetics and antiarrhythmic drugs in the treatment of neuropathic pain states probably reflects the fact that they are all sodium-channel blockers.[44] The identification of a specific (tetrodotoxin resistant) sodium channel solely on nociceptive neurons presents an attractive target for the development of drugs with the potential for less toxicity compared with existing agents, although this remains unrealized at the present time.

An alternative approach involves blockade of calcium channels. Gabapentin and pregabalin bind to calcium channels in various regions of the brain and spinal cord, and act as presynaptic inhibitors of the release of excitatory neurotransmitters. They are excreted exclusively by the kidneys and do not have pharmacokinetic interactions with other drugs, making them suitable for combination therapies. Studies have shown some benefit in patients with fibromyalgia, although in general their effectiveness in musculoskeletal pain remains unclear.[45]

Kinins and cytokinins

When injected into human skin, bradykinin causes an intense sensation of acute pain as a result of activation and/or sensitization of primary nociceptors. Bradykinin antagonists have potent antinociceptive activity in experimental arthritis and hold promise as novel analgesic agents.[46]

Cytokines released from immune cells as part of the inflammatory cascade, including IL-1, IL-8 and tumour necrosis factor α (TNF-α), are potent hyperalgesic agents owing to their ability to stimulate the production and release of other pro-inflammatory agents such as bradykinin. Direct effects on primary nociceptors during inflammatory states may also be clinically relevant. Agents that suppress the production or actions of either IL-1 or TNF-α have been shown to have potent analgesic activities in clinical trials in patients with rheumatoid arthritis, and ankylosing spondylitis in particular.[47]

Other therapies

At the spinal level the importance of NMDA and substance P receptors in the genesis of pain is now appreciated.[48] NMDA-receptor antagonists that are available for clinical use include ketamine and dextromethorphan, although the use of these drugs is limited by a lack of effectiveness at tolerated doses and psychomimetic adverse effects at higher doses.

α_2-Adrenoceptors modulate nociception at the level of the spinal cord. Agonists for this receptor have been shown to have antinociceptive properties, and clonidine has found clinical use as a combination analgesic with epidural opioids in cancer pain.[49] It is occasionally used in patients with chronic back pain, but has not been used extensively in other musculoskeletal conditions.

Cannabinoids have modest antinociceptive properties in patients with multiple sclerosis, but it remains unclear whether this class of drug will have wider applications for treating chronic pain.[18] Antagonists to cholecystokinin have also shown potential as antinociceptive agents but no clinical studies are as yet available.

SUMMARY

This chapter has stressed the importance of sensitization of nociceptive neurons at peripheral, spinal and supraspinal levels. Within each of these three cellular compartments sensitization has predictable consequences for nociceptive activity and pain perception. Appreciation of these mechanisms has led to better assessment methods and a more rational approach to the use of existing analgesics.

Key challenges remain. The characterization of the complex array of chemical mediators that underlie neural sensitization is an ongoing concern to both academics and the pharmaceutical

---

PRACTICE POINTS

- Three main classes of pain include: nociceptive pain, neuroplastic pain and neuropathic pain.

- The purpose of pain evaluation should be to: (1) define the anatomical source of pain, (2) define additional somatic and environmental factors contributing to pain, and (3) identify disability.

- Referred symptoms and signs reflect the presence of central sensitization, and treatment regimens should be tailored accordingly.

- The analgesic actions of NSAIDs are dissociated from their anti-inflammatory actions and reflect antinociceptive activities within the CNS as well as in the periphery.

- Consider the use of combination therapies with proven synergistic interactions to reduce overall toxicity (e.g. paracetamol + tramadol, NSAID + weak opioid).

- Manage the patient, not just the disease.

RESEARCH AGENDA

- To characterize mediators and growth factors contributing to neural plasticity in osteoarthritis and other so-called non-inflammatory disorders.

- To characterize the relative importance of peripheral versus central sensitization in the common symptomatic musculoskeletal diseases.

- To characterize individual risk factors associated with the development of chronic pain states.

- To develop clinically applicable techniques for identifying neural mechanisms in order to develop rational treatment strategies for chronic pain.

industry alike. Further identification of individual risk factors for the development of chronic pain remains a priority. Finally, much work remains to be done in overcoming outmoded dualistic concepts of pain and educating colleagues about the importance of neural plasticity in the genesis of chronic pain.

REFERENCES

1. Merskey H, Bogduk N (eds). *Classification of Chronic Pain*, 2nd edn. IASP Press, Seattle, WA, 1994.
2. Wagstaff S, Smith OV, Wood PHN. Verbal pain descriptors used by patients with arthritis. *Ann Rheum Dis* 1985; **44**: 262–265.
3. Farrell M, Gibson S, McMeeken J et al. Pain and hyperalgesia in osteoarthritis of the hands. *J Rheumatol* 2000; **27**: 441–447.
4. Creamer P, Lethbridge-Cejku M, Hochberg MC. Determinants of pain severity in knee osteoarthritis: effect of demographic and psychosocial variables using 3 pain measures. *J Rheumatol* 1999; **26**:1785–1792.
5. Kidd BL, Urban LA. Mechanisms of inflammatory pain. *Br J Anaesthes* 2001; **87**: 1–9.
6. Coderre TJ, Katz J, Vaccarino AL et al. Contribution of central neuroplasticity to pathological pain: review of clinical and experimental evidence. *Pain* 1993; **52**: 259–285.
7. Giesecke T, Gracely RH, Grant MA et al. Evidence of augmented central pain processing in idiopathic chronic low back pain. *Arthritis Rheum* 2004; **50**: 613–623.
8. Mapp PI, Kidd BL, Gibson SJ et al. Substance P, calcitonin-related peptide and C-flanking peptide of neuropeptide Y-immunoreactive fibres are present in normal synovium but depleted in patients with rheumatoid arthritis. *Neuroscience* 1990; **37**: 143–153.
9. Mach DB, Rogers SD, Sabino MC et al. Origins of skeletal pain: sensory and sympathetic innervation of the mouse femur. *Neuroscience* 2002; **113**: 155–166.
10. Woolf CJ. Pain: moving from symptom control toward mechanism-specific pharmacologic management. *Ann Intern Med* 2004; **16**: 441–451.
11. Grigg P, Schaible H-G, Schmidt RF. Mechanical sensitivity of group III and IV afferents from posterior articular nerve in normal and inflamed cat knee. *J Neurophysiol* 1986; **55**: 635–643.
12. Schaible H-G, Grubb BD. Afferent and spinal mechanisms of joint pain. *Pain* 1993; **55**: 5–54.
13. England S, Bevan SJ, Docherty RJ. Prostaglandin E_2 modulates the tetrodotoxin-resistant sodium current in neonatal rat dorsal root ganglion neurones via the cyclic AMP-protein kinase A cascade. *J Physiol* 1996; **495**: 429–440.
14. McCleskey EW, Gold MS. Ion channels of nociception. *Ann Rev Physiol* 1999; **61**: 835–856.
15. Numazaki M, Tominaga T, Toyooka H et al. Direct phosphorylation of capsaicin receptor VR1 by protein kinase Cepsilon and identification of two target serine residues. *J Biol Chem* 2002; **277**: 13375–13378.
16. Khasar SG, Ho T, Green PG et al. Comparison of prostaglandin E_1- and prostaglandin E_2-induced hyperalgesia in the rat. *Neuroscience* 1994; **62**: 345–350.
17. Stein C. Peripheral mechanisms of opioid analgesia. *Anesth Analg* 1993; **76**: 182–191.
18. Mackie K. Cannabinoid receptors as therapeutic targets. *Ann Rev Pharmacol Toxicol* 2006; **46**: 101–122.
19. Ji RR, Samad TA, Jin SX et al. p38 MAPK activation by NGF in primary sensory neurons after inflammation increases TRPV1 levels and maintains heat hyperalgesia. *Neuron* 2002; **36**: 57–68.
20. Kidd BL, Photiou A, Inglis JJ. The role of inflammatory mediators on nociception and pain in arthritis. *Novartis Found Symp* 2004; **260**: 122–133.
21. Inglis JJ, Nissim A, Lees DM et al. The differential contribution of tumour necrosis factor to thermal and mechanical hyperalgesia during chronic inflammation. *Arthritis Res Ther* 2005; **7**: R807–R816.
22. Rexed BA. Cytoarchitectonic atlas of the spinal cord in the cat. *J Comp Neurol* 1952; **96**: 415–495.
23. Reynolds DV. Surgery in the rat during electrical analgesia induced by focal brain stimulation. *Science* 1969; **164**: 444–445.
24. Heinricher MM, Morgan MM. Supraspinal mechanisms of opioid analgesia. In: Stein C (ed), *Opioids and Pain Control*. Cambridge University Press, Cambridge, 1999, pp. 46–69.
25. Fields HL. *Pain*. McGraw-Hill, New York, 1987.
26. Hunt SP, Mantyh PW. The molecular dynamics of pain control. *Nat Rev Neurosci* 2001; **2**: 83–91.
27. Bajaj P, Bajaj P, Graven-Nielsen T et al. Osteoarthritis and its association with muscle hyperalgesia: an experimental controlled study. *Pain* 2001; **93**: 107–114.
28. Morris VH, Cruwys SC, Kidd BL. Characterisation of capsaicin-induced mechanical hyperalgesia as a marker for altered nociceptive processing in patients with rheumatoid arthritis. *Pain* 1997; **71**: 179–186.
29. Woolf CJ, Salter MW. Neuronal plasticity: increasing the gain in pain. *Science* 2000; **288**: 1765–1769.
30. Watkins LR, Maier SF. Glia: a novel drug discovery target for clinical pain. *Nat Rev Drug Discov* 2003; **2**: 973–985.
31. Ghilardi JR, Svensson CI, Rogers SD et al. Constitutive spinal cyclooxygenase-2 participates in the initiation of tissue injury-induced hyperalgesia. *J Neurosci* 2004; **17**: 2727–2732
32. Jones AK, Kulkarni B, Derbyshire SW. Pain mechanisms and their disorders. *Br Med Bull* 2003; **65**: 83–93.
33. Gracely RH, Petzke F, Wolf JM et al. Functional magnetic resonance imaging evidence of augmented pain processing in fibromyalgia. *Arthritis Rheum* 2002; **46**: 1333–1343.
34. Gracely RH, Geisser ME, Giesecke T et al. Pain catastrophizing and neural responses to pain among persons with fibromyalgia. *Brain* 2004; **127**: 835–843.
35. Anon. *Oxford League Table of Analgesics in Acute Pain*. Available at: http://www.jr2.ox.ac.uk/bandolier/booth/painpag/Acutrev/Analgesics/Leagtab.html (accessed 29 August 2006).
36. Libert F, Bonnefont J, Bourinet E et al. Acetaminophen: a central analgesic drug that involves a spinaltropisetron-sensitive, non-5-HT(3) receptor-mediated effect. *Mol Pharmacol* 2004; **66**: 728–734.
37. Moore A, Collins S, Carroll D et al. Paracetamol with and without codeine in acute pain: a quantitative systematic review. *Pain* 1997; **70**: 193–201.
38. Schug SA, Sidebotham DA, McGuinnety M et al. Acetaminophen as an adjunct to morphine by patient-controlled analgesia in the management of acute postoperative pain. *Anesth Analg* 1998; **87**: 368–372.
39. McCormack K. Non-steroidal anti-inflammatory drugs and spinal nociceptive processing. *Pain* 1994; **59**: 9–43.
40. Bannwarth B, Demotes-Mainard F, Schaeverbeke T et al. Central analgesic effects of aspirin-like drugs. *Fundam Clin Pharmacol* 1995; **9**: 1–7.
41. Burian M, Geisslinger G. COX-dependent mechanisms involved in the antinociceptive action of NSAIDs at central and peripheral sites. *Pharmacol Ther* 2005; **107**: 139–154.
42. McQuay HJ, Moore RA. Antidepressants and chronic pain. *BMJ* 1997; **314**: 763–764.
43. Frank RG, Kashani JH, Parker JC et al. Antidepressant analgesia in rheumatoid arthritis. *Rheumatology* 1988; **15**: 1632–1638.
44. Tanelian DL, Brose WG. Neuropathic pain can be relieved by drugs that are use-dependent sodium channels blockers: lidocaine, carbamazepine, and mexiletine. *Anaesthesiology* 1991; **74**: 949–951.
45. Crofford LJ. Pharmaceutical treatment options for fibromyalgia. *Curr Rheumatol Rep* 2004; **6**: 274–280.
46. Sawynok J. Topical and peripherally acting analgesics. *Pharmacol Rev* 2003; **55**: 1–20.
47. Heiberg MS, Nordvag BY, Mikkelsen K et al. The comparative effectiveness of tumor necrosis factor-blocking agents in patients with rheumatoid arthritis and patients with ankylosing spondylitis: a six-month, longitudinal, observational, multicenter study. *Arthritis Rheum* 2005; **52**: 2506–2512.
48. Woolf CJ, Thompson SW. The induction and maintenance of central sensitization is dependent on *N*-methyl-D-aspartic acid receptor activation; implications for the treatment of post-injury pain hypersensitivity states. *Pain* 1991; **44**: 293–299.
49. Eisenach JC, Rauck RL, Buzzanell C et al. Epidural clonidine analgesia for intractable cancer pain. *Anaesthesiology* 1989; **71**: 647–652.

SECTION 3

Assessment

Chapter 4

Assessment of pain in patients with rheumatic diseases

Tuulikki Sokka

INTRODUCTION

The International Association for the Study of Pain describes pain as 'an unpleasant sensory and emotional experience associated with actual or potential tissue damage, or described in terms of such damage'.[1, 2] Pain is the most prominent symptom in most people with arthritis,[3–6] a common basis for primary care consultation[7–9] and a major basis of healthcare costs.[10] Nonetheless, quantitative information concerning pain, which is required to assess and document possible improvement, stabilization or worsening of pain over time, is rarely recorded in usual medical care. In a survey concerning US emergency department visits in 1999, 52% included no recorded information concerning the presenting level of pain.[11]

In acute medical situations, the primary setting of most medical education and training, quantitative assessment and recording of pain levels is not necessary. A patient with a fracture or myocardial infarction can easily provide critical information concerning pain status over the following few hours and days, without a need for quantitative data. Pain, as with other symptoms, is regarded as 'subjective', based on data obtained from the patient, and is viewed by the clinician largely as a clue to aid in assessing the critical 'objective' data obtained from physical examination, laboratory tests or imaging procedures. This view may be termed the 'traditional biomedical model',[12] which has been so successful in acute medical care that it is usually applied to chronic diseases as well.

At present chronic diseases are a very important problem in medical care. In the management of chronic disease the 'biomedical model' is not as successful in guiding diagnosis and management as in acute disease and has substantial limitations. For example, the most effective predictor of mortality in patients with rheumatoid arthritis (RA) is found in a patient questionnaire and the patient's level of formal education, rather than in data obtained from a physical examination, laboratory tests or radiography.[13–16] In the management of chronic rheumatic diseases it is virtually impossible to assess pain over long periods without quantitative data to estimate whether or not a patient has improved, is unchanged or is worse over months to years.

Pain is regarded as 'subjective,' being based on data obtained from the patient, in contrast to 'objective' data obtained from the laboratory, imaging and physical examination. However, quantitative data to estimate changes in levels of pain over long periods in patients with rheumatic diseases *cannot* be obtained from any source other than the patient. Efforts to assess pain through 'objective' external sources have not been as successful in providing reliable quantitative data as data derived from patients concerning their pain.

A clinical science of pain assessment using patient self-report questionnaires has been developed over the last few decades to facilitate the qualitative and quantitative assessment of pain status at any given time.[17–27] Despite limitations, which are intrinsic in any scientific measurement system, pain questionnaires have proven valuable in gaining new understanding of the mechanisms of the causation and control of pain. Furthermore, quantitative pain measures from patient questionnaires provide information to recognize whether or not patients improve or worsen over time, which is not available from any source other than the patient, as noted above.

Patient self-report questionnaires that include assessments of pain are required to evaluate the short-term efficacy and long-term effectiveness of therapies for all rheumatic conditions, including RA, osteoarthritis (OA) and fibromyalgia (FM). However, patient questionnaires remain largely a research tool, and are not widely used in routine clinical care. It is disappointing that most rheumatologists do not use patient questionnaires in routine clinical care and continue to expect the 'biomedical model' to characterize patient status most effectively through laboratory tests and imaging procedures. Nonetheless, many reports have documented the value of simple patient questionnaires in routine clinical care and suggested that use of these questionnaires would be of value in the infrastructure of routine rheumatology care.[28]

In this chapter, quantitative measures of pain are reviewed, with emphasis on patient self-report questionnaires. Results obtained using these questionnaires in RA, OA and FM are summarized. In addition, data that reveal significant associations between pain scores and objective physical examination, radiographic and laboratory data are summarized. The associations are, however, weaker than those with measures of functional and psychological status.

EARLY EFFORTS TO DEVELOP PHYSICAL QUANTITATIVE MEASURES OF PAIN TOLERANCE BY A HEALTH PROFESSIONAL

Early efforts to develop quantitative measures of pain sought to estimate pain threshold, tolerance, sensitivity and severity through 'objective' observation and report by a health professional. Some methods are described below:[29]

- *Dolorimeter.* A dolorimeter is an instrument that provides progressive pressure to a patient to indicate when they first experience pain and when pain becomes unbearable. Some types of dolorimeter have been used for many years to measure pain threshold, which is more accurately assessed than pain itself. The dolorimeter has proven of great value in research concerning pain thresholds and behaviours, but is not a useful clinical measure in clinical care.
- *Audiometer.* An audiometer is set at an arbitrary frequency and the patient is asked to turn the intensity dial until he or she identifies a point where the 'loudness of the sound matched the severity of the pain'. Three readings were made and the median taken as the pain score. However, a visual–analogue pain-scale score was found to be as effective as this procedure.[31]
- *Analgesic usage.* Beecher[30] estimated the severity of pain in terms of the analgesic dose required for pain relief. This method was used by anaesthesiologists.
- *Cold pressor method.* Patients are asked to immerse one hand in a lukewarm waterbath maintained at 35°C for 2 minutes and then transfer it to an ice waterbath maintained at 0°C. The patient is instructed to shout 'pain' when pain in the hand begins, to keep the hand in the ice water until pain becomes unbearable, and then to shout 'stop' and remove the hand. The 'pain' and 'stop' responses are timed separately for each hand.
- *Radiant heat method.* A dolorimeter is placed firmly against the forehead, and the pressure is gradually increased. Again, the patient shouts 'pain' on initial sensation, and 'stop' when pain becomes unbearable.
- *Electrical stimulation.* The patient places two fingers in saline beakers and electrical stimulation is increased gradually. Again, the patient shouts 'pain' when pain is felt and 'stop' when the stimulation is unbearable.

These methods have contributed to the understanding of pain mechanisms and behaviours, but are not sufficiently reliable, reproducible or practical for assessment of pain levels in clinical trials, other clinical research or routine clinical care.

Early researchers also attempted to distinguish 'organic' from 'behavioural' contributors to pain, as illustrated by the Emory Pain Estimate Model.[32] This model includes an estimation of four factors of tissue pathology (physical, neurological, radiological and laboratory) and four factors of pain behaviour (the McGill Pain Questionnaire, activity checklist, drug use rating scale and the Minnesota Multiphasic Personality Inventory (MMPI) profile (see below)). All eight measures are rated 0–10, with scores of 5 or more classified as 'high', and less than 5 as 'low'. These classifications led to the description of four classes of pain behaviour: (1) high pain behaviour and low organic pathology, characterized as 'pain amplifiers'; (2) low on both variables, characterized as 'pain verbalizers'; (3) high on both variables, classified as 'chronic sufferers'; and (4) high organic pathology and low pain behaviour, classified as 'pain reducers'. Higher ratings of impairment and disability were associated significantly with higher levels of physical pathology and pain behaviours, as might be expected. Again, this classification is of great interest in pain research, but is too complex and not necessarily reliable for use in clinical trials or the clinical care of patients with rheumatic diseases.

ASSESSMENT OF PAIN USING PATIENT QUESTIONNAIRES

The Minnesota Multiphasic Personality Inventory

The Minnesota Multiphasic Personality Inventory (MMPI)[33] is a patient self-report questionnaire. Although it is not strictly a pain questionnaire, it is included here as it was the first widely used patient questionnaire and has gained widespread acceptance over the last half century. The MMPI consists of 585 true/false statements, which are grouped into ten clinical scales and three validity scales. Patients with RA were described as having elevated scores on the hypochondriasis, depression and hysteria scales, findings which were interpreted initially as suggesting psychological difficulties associated with RA.[34, 35] However, the elevated scores were found to result in large part from the answers of 'false' to five statements: 'I am about as able to work as I ever was', 'I am in just as good physical health as most of my friends', 'During the past few years I have been well', 'I do not tire quickly' and 'I have few or no pains'.[36] Responses of 'false' may indicate tendencies to hypochondriasis, depression and hysteria in individuals who do not have a somatic disease, but in patients with RA such responses are an indicator of the somatic disease itself, rather than indicating psychological problems. The attribution of a psychological abnormality because of an incorrect interpretation of a questionnaire response is known as 'criterion contamination',[37] which has also been described in scales to assess depression in patients with RA, including the Beck Depression Inventory and the Center for Epidemiologic Studies Depression Scale (CES-D).[38] The phenomenon of criterion contamination illustrates the importance of careful interpretation of data from self-report questionnaires.

The McGill Pain Questionnaire

An early analytical approach to the assessment of pain was the McGill Pain Questionnaire.[17, 18] This questionnaire was developed from a study in which subjects with pain were asked to classify 102 words concerning pain, which had been obtained from the clinical literature. These words were categorized into three major classes:

1. sensory qualities – spatial, pressure, thermal and other properties
2. affective qualities – tension, fear and ordonomic properties
3. evaluative qualities – to describe intensity of pain.

Melzack and Torgerson[39] had asked groups of doctors, patients and students to assign an intensity value to each word, ranging from 'least' or 'mild' pain to 'worst' or 'excruciating' pain, to develop a pain questionnaire, which presented sensory, affective and evaluative words with an overall pain intensity recorded as a number from 1 to 5 (1, 'mild'; 2, 'discomforting'; 3, 'distressing'; 4, 'horrible'; 5, 'excruciating').

The complete McGill Pain Questionnaire[18] includes a pain diagram, which incorporates a figure of a human body on which the patient is asked to indicate locations of pain. A listing of 102 words in 20 categories is presented to the patient, who is asked to circle words to describe present pain. The questionnaire also includes queries concerning change of pain with time, and classification of pain intensity in the five categories noted above (mild, discomforting, distressing, horrible and excruciating). Early researchers disagreed on whether it was preferable that a research assistant read the instructions to the patient or self-report was used. There are advantages to each approach, and some patients need help to complete the questionnaire, but in general self-report by the patient is more reproducible and more easily administered. Four types of data obtained from the questionnaire (a mean pain rating index, an index based on ranked values of the words, the number of words chosen and the present pain intensity) were significantly correlated with one another.

The McGill Pain Questionnaire has provided a major advance in clinical research concerning pain. However, completion of the questionnaire requires 15–20 minutes, and even a short form[40] is not easily administered in a busy clinical setting. Simpler measures, such as a visual–analogue pain scale, appear to give information that is clinically as valuable, or more valuable, in considerably less time, and have become widely used in clinical research, clinical trials and clinical care.

Visual–analogue pain scales

The pain visual–analogue scale (VAS) was initially used in psychology by Freud and others in the early 1900s, and developed in rheumatology through a series of investigations by Huskisson et al. in the late 1970s.[19, 20, 41–44] These investigators described a variety of VASs, including vertical and horizontal scales, and scales with equally spaced lines with the indications of mild, moderate and severe pain. They pointed out that 'only the patient can measure [pain] severity',[41] and concluded that numbers should not be included and that supervision is helpful the first time a patient completes a VAS, but generally self-report is adequate thereafter.

The standard VAS is a 10 cm scale bordered on each side. At the '0' mark it says 'No pain at all' and at the '10' mark 'Pain as bad as it could be'. There are occasional distortions through photocopying and printing, and adjustments can be made so that the total score is 10.

Huskisson et al. recognized that the distribution of results was not normal, and non-parametric statistical methods were needed to analyse the results. They pointed out that 'It is usual to divide the scale at the end of the experiment into 20 parts', with support from the experimental finding that there were 21 noticeable differences between pain threshold and limits of tolerance, although later observers suggested that only seven different levels are distinguished by most patients.

Huskisson et al. also constructed VASs to assess pain relief from 'complete pain relief' to 'no pain relief.' They also pointed out that the alternative of a simple descriptive pain relief scale, using 'complete', 'moderate', 'slight' and 'no pain' relief, was possible, but much less sensitive than a VAS. A number of studies have established that data from self-report VASs are reproducible.[45, 46] In one study[46] an absolute VAS was found to be more reproducible than a comparative VAS.

With the development of optical scanning technology for automated computer entry of scores, VASs became presented in a format of 21 small boxes or circles for patients to assess their pain from 0–10 (or 100). Although no direct comparative studies have been performed to analyse automated optical scanning, results appear to have criterion validity. The visual–analogue pain scale has proven a great advance in the assessment of pain.

The Health Assessment Questionnaire (HAQ) and its derivatives: Modified Health Assessment Questionnaire (MHAQ), Clinical Health Assessment Questionnaire (CLINHAQ) and Multi-Dimensional Health Assessment Questionnaire (MDHAQ)

The HAQ was developed in the 1970s by Fries et al. and was published in *Arthritis and Rheumatism* in 1980.[21] This questionnaire provided a milestone in the development of a methodology using patient self-report to obtain information concerning functional disability, pain and global status. The HAQ includes VASs for pain, as well as global status, although its primary measurement is for functional disability. Functional status is assessed according to 20 activities of daily living (ADL), with response alternatives in four categories (0, 'without any difficulty'; 1, 'with some difficulty'; 2, 'with much difficulty'; 3, 'unable to do'), in addition to a VAS. The 20 ADL are grouped into eight categories (dressing, arising, eating, walking, bathing, reaching, gripping and performing errands) with two or three ADL each. In addition, there are queries concerning the use of aids and devices. The total score is the mean score derived from eight scores, one for each category. The score for each category is the highest score for two or three ADL within the category; in addition, a 1 is added to the score if the patient uses aids or devices for that category, so the final score is 0–3. The HAQ is presented on two sides of one page, and can be completed in 5 minutes in a waiting room. It has proven very easily accepted by patients, and has been widely used in clinical trials, clinical research and routine clinical care.

An initial modification of the HAQ was termed the Modified HAQ (MHAQ).[47] The MHAQ was developed to provide simplified scoring, and to allow the clinician to visualize an ADL score and VASs for pain and global status on one side of one page. The MHAQ includes eight ADL, one from the two or three of the eight categories of the HAQ. Scoring was simply the mean of the eight activities scored 0, 1, 2 or 3.

A further modification of the MHAQ involved the addition of five items to the eight included in the MHAQ, and this has been termed the Multi-Dimensional HAQ (MDHAQ).[48] The MDHAQ (Figure 4.1) includes ten ADL, with two additional physical ADL ('Are you able to walk 2 miles or 3 kilometres?' and 'Are you able to participate in sports and games as you would like?'). These items were included in recognition of the more effective rheumatology care since the mid-1980s, as about 25% of consecutive patients seen in a rheumatology clinic had normal MHAQ scores and 15% had normal HAQ scores, which are known as 'floor' effects. In addition, the MDHAQ includes queries concerning the psychological issues of sleep, anxiety and depression in the standard HAQ format, as well as VASs for pain, global status, fatigue and morning stiffness, all on one side of one page.[48, 49]

A different type of modification involved the development of the HAQ-II,[50] which provides even spacing of scoring intervals according to item response theory in Rasch analysis.[50]

All versions of the HAQ include a 10 cm visual–analogue pain scale. The more recent versions include a VAS with 21 small circles that has been adapted for automated optical scanning. This has not been formally studied compared with the standard VAS, but appears to function quite well in clinical research.

The Arthritis Impact Measurement Scales (AIMS)

The Arthritis Impact Measurement Scales (AIMS) was developed by Meenan et al.[22] to assess the physical, emotional and social well-being of individuals with arthritis. It comprises scores for nine categories (mobility, physical activity, social activity, social role, activities of daily living, pain, dexterity, anxiety and depression). Each score is based on four to six items with response alternatives on Likert-format scales. The pain category includes four questions: 'During the past month, how often have you had severe pain from your arthritis?', 'During the past month, how would you describe the arthritis pain you usually have?', 'During the past month, how long has your morning stiffness usually lasted from the time you wake up?' and 'During the past month, how often have you had pain in two or more joints at the same time?' The AIMS index has excellent psychometric validity and a reliability greater than the HAQ and its derivatives, and has been used in clinical trials to document the sensitivity of patient questionnaires to changes in clinical status. However, the HAQ and its derivatives are more easily completed by patients and more easily scored by health professionals in clinical trials and in routine care, and are considerably more widely used than the AIMS.

The Western Ontario McMaster (WOMAC) questionnaire

The WOMAC questionnaire was developed initially for use in OA clinical trials.[23, 24] The WOMAC consists of 24 items, five to assess pain, two to assess stiffness and 17 to assess physical function, based on a survey of 100 patients with primary OA of the hip and knee. The questions concerning pain include 'walking on flat surfaces', 'going up and down stairs', 'at night while in bed', 'sitting or lying' and 'standing upright'. It has been administered as a Likert scale with five or seven response options, and as a series of 10 cm VASs. The WOMAC has been extensively used in OA clinical trials throughout the world and is regarded as the gold standard for assessing OA of the lower limb.

The Nottingham Health Profile (NHP)

The NHP was introduced in the early 1980s as a generic health status questionnaire.[25] Generic health status questionnaires were developed for use in many types of disease, in contrast to the HAQ and AIMS, which were developed for use in patients with rheumatic diseases. The NHP is based on patient perceptions of health, to express how people feel when experiencing various states of ill health. The pain section of the NHP includes eight questions concerning pain with response alternatives 'yes' and 'no'. The scoring includes weighting of all 'yes' responses with a certain population-specific value, and adding the scores of individual questions together. The final score for each concept ranges from 0, indicating good health, to 100, which indicates poor situation.

The NHP has been used in clinical research, although it also has a floor effect (i.e. it captures only more severe ill health).[51] Furthermore, it is long and incorporates a complicated scoring system, and its use is unfeasible in most clinical trials and routine clinical care.

The Short-Form 36 (SF-36) questionnaire

A 36-item questionnaire called Short-Form 36 (SF-36), developed by Ware et al.,[26] was designed initially for use in health-policy surveys. The SF-36 assesses eight health concepts: physical activities, social activities, role activities, bodily pain, general mental health, role activities because of emotional problems, vitality and general health. The pain section includes two questions: 'How much bodily pain have you had during the past four weeks?' with response options 1–6 (1, none; 2, very mild; 3, mild; 4, moderate; 5, severe; 6, very severe), and 'During the past four weeks, how much did pain interfere with your normal work (including both work outside the home and housework)?' with response options 1–5 (1, not at all; 2, a little bit; 3, moderately; 4, quite a bit; 5, extremely).

The SF-36 is widely used and has documented validity in normal healthy populations and diverse patient groups. It is sensitive to changes in clinical status, and has a well-earned place in clinical trials. However, the scoring is complex, with recoding of the responses according to instructions on a scale of 0–100, where 100 indicates the best and 0 the worst health situation, and calculation of the mean value for the recoded responses. Therefore, the complicated scoring system renders the SF-36 unfeasible for use in routine clinical care.

Rheumatoid Arthritis Pain Scale (RAPS)

The RAPS was developed to measure pain in adult patients with RA.[27] The domains of RAPS include physiological, affective, sensory-discriminative and cognitive components, and consists of 24 items, which are scored using a seven-point Likert scale ranging from 0 ('never') to 6 ('always'), which is considered to represent a greater severity of pain. The RAPS, like the McGill Pain Questionnaire, clearly provides more information than a visual–analogue pain scale, and is useful in clinical research, although limited to specialized research settings.

THE USE OF PATIENT SELF-REPORT QUESTIONNAIRES IN ROUTINE CLINICAL CARE

As described above, several questionnaires have been developed to quantitate pain and disability in patients seen in rheumatology care. However, in usual clinical care and most clinical research a pain VAS score appears to capture as much information as more elaborate questionnaires designed to measure pain, and is often more sensitive to changes occurring in clinical trials and clinical care. The value of the longer questionnaires is well documented, but a VAS for pain appears to capture any information needed in a clinical study, including clinical trials.

In a busy clinic short questionnaires with simple scoring systems are the most feasible to be implemented as a part of routine care. The MDHAQ (see Figure 4.1) is a one-page, two-sided questionnaire that is completed by the patient as a self-report questionnaire in < 10 minutes in the waiting room and can be scored by a health professional in < 30 seconds.

It is important for the clinician to recognize the differences between research questionnaires, which may be very lengthy and require complex scoring systems, and a simple questionnaire designed to be used in routine clinical care.

PAIN IN RHEUMATOID ARTHRITIS

Pain is the major reason why patients with RA seek medical care,[3–6, 52] although these patients experience many other symptoms, such as joint swelling, tenderness, deformities and morning stiffness.

Patients with RA experience more pain compared with the general age- and sex-matched population.[53] Patients with RA are similar to people with widespread pain regarding pain intensity, emotional distress, sleep disturbances and overall satisfaction of life, whereas disability levels are higher in patients with RA.[54]

Having no joint pain is included in the American College of Rheumatology (ACR) remission criteria for RA.[55] On a 100 mm

VAS scale, < 10 mm has been interpreted as having no pain.[56] The 6th Outcome Measures in Rheumatology (OMERACT) conference suggested that a pain VAS score < 20 mm is an important cut-off for pain.[57] In a study including patients with inflammatory and degenerative rheumatic conditions, 75% of patients considered their status as 'acceptable' when their pain score was < 25 mm.[58] The estimated average level of pain was 20 mm on a 100 mm VAS in elderly general population.[59] Therefore, it appears that a score for pain of 10–25 mm on a 100 mm VAS in our elderly population may indicate that a real patient > 55 years old in a real clinic has an acceptable score for pain.

The course of pain follows the same pattern as other measures of disease activity in groups of patients with RA.[60] After the initial improvement the pain scores deteriorate over the ensuing years. However, Borg and Dawes[61] found that pain at the onset of the disease did not predict the pain level at 3 years, while in another study baseline pain in early disease was the only significant predictor of cumulative pain over a year.[62]

Changes in pain levels over 5 years or more have been reported in long-term follow-up studies done during the last decade[60, 63–71] (Table 4.1). Overall, improvement of pain over 5 years is more significant in patients with early disease, while improvement in pain is less pronounced in patients with longer disease duration at the onset of the follow-up.

Pain is the area of health in which most patients with RA would like to see improvement.[6, 52] Fries et al.[72, 73] showed that disease-modifying antirheumatic drugs (DMARDs) are the best drugs to relieve pain in RA in the long term. More frequent visits to rheumatologists were associated with greater improvements in pain and functional capacity over 1 year.[74] Several recent clinical trials of DMARDs have shown statistically significant improvements in pain over 6–24 months in treatment groups compared with groups that received control medications or placebo[75–92] (Table 4.2). Unfortunately, data concerning pain separately are not reported in all clinical trials, the results being presented as pooled indices such as ACR response criteria.

PAIN IN OSTEOARTHRITIS

Pain is the most important determinant of disability in patients with OA.[93–96] OA is traditionally considered as an inevitably progressive, degenerative disease process. With improved understanding, OA is now regarded as a collection of heterogeneous conditions with a dynamic course that also includes repair and periods of structural stability.[97–99]

Patients with OA may experience significant pain without much damage, but others have damage without much pain. It is not known whether pain is an early sign of the disease process in patients with OA, which should raise the alert to introduce preventive strategies in OA. Long-term follow-up studies are needed to answer the question of whether or not joint pain and stiffness reflect an ongoing disease process, and whether or not these symptoms predict structural abnormality.

Nevertheless, patients with OA seek help for pain. De Bock et al.[100] found a low association between a patient's perception

Multi-Dimensional Health Assessment Questionnaire (R698)

This questionnaire includes information not available from blood tests, X-rays, or any source other than you. Please try to answer each question, even if you do not think it is related to you at this time. <u>There are no right or wrong answers.</u> Please answer exactly as you think or feel. Thank you.

1. Please check (✓) the ONE best answer for your abilities at this time:
   OVER THE LAST WEEK, were you able to:

		Without **ANY** Difficulty	With **SOME** Difficulty	With **MUCH** Difficulty	UNABLE To Do
a.	Dress yourself, including tying shoelaces and doing buttons?	0	1	2	3
b.	Get in and out of bed?	0	1	2	3
c.	Lift a full cup or glass to your mouth?	0	1	2	3
d.	Walk outdoors on flat ground?	0	1	2	3
e.	Wash and dry your entire body?	0	1	2	3
f.	Bend down to pick up clothing from the floor?	0	1	2	3
g.	Turn regular faucets on and off?	0	1	2	3
h.	Get in and out of a car, bus, train, or airplane?	0	1	2	3
i.	Walk two miles?	0	1	2	3
j.	Participate in sports and games as you would like?	0	1	2	3
k.	Get a good night's sleep?	0	1.1	2.2	3.3
l.	Deal with feelings of anxiety or being nervous?	0	1.1	2.2	3.3
m.	Deal with feelings of depression or feeling blue?	0	1.1	2.2	3.3

2. How much pain have you had because of your condition OVER THE PAST WEEK? Please indicate below how severe your pain has been:

   NO PAIN ○○○○○○○○○○○○○○○○○○○○○ PAIN AS BAD AS IT COULD BE
   0 0.5 1.0 1.5 2.0 2.5 3.0 3.5 4.0 4.5 5.0 5.5 6.0 6.5 7.0 7.5 8.0 8.5 9.0 9.5 10

3. When you awakened in the morning OVER THE LAST WEEK, did you feel stiff? ☐ Yes ☐ No
   If 'No', please go to Item 4. If you answer '**Yes**', please write the number of minutes _____,
   or **hours** _____ until you are as limber as you will be for the day.

4. How much of a problem has UNUSUAL fatigue or tiredness been for you OVER THE PAST WEEK? Please indicate below:

   FATIGUE IS NO PROBLEM ○○○○○○○○○○○○○○○○○○○○○ FATIGUE IS A MAJOR PROBLEM
   0 0.5 1.0 1.5 2.0 2.5 3.0 3.5 4.0 4.5 5.0 5.5 6.0 6.5 7.0 7.5 8.0 8.5 9.0 9.5 10

5. How do you feel TODAY compared to ONE WEEK AGO? Please check (✓) only one.
   Much Better___(1),   Better___(2),   the Same___(3),   Worse___(4),   Much Worse___(5) than one week ago

6. Considering all the ways in which illness and health conditions may affect you at this time, please indicate below how you are doing:

   VERY WELL ○○○○○○○○○○○○○○○○○○○○○ VERY POORLY
   0 0.5 1.0 1.5 2.0 2.5 3.0 3.5 4.0 4.5 5.0 5.5 6.0 6.5 7.0 7.5 8.0 8.5 9.0 9.5 10

FOR OFFICE USE ONLY

FN ☐

1=0.33	16=5.33
2=0.67	17=5.67
3=1.00	18=6.00
4=1.33	19=6.33
5=1.67	20=6.67
6=2.00	21=7.00
7=2.33	22=7.33
8=2.67	23=7.67
9=3.00	24=8.00
10=3.33	25=8.33
11=3.67	26=8.67
12=4.00	27=9.00
13=4.33	28=9.33
14=4.67	29=9.67
15=5.00	30=10.0

PS ☐

PN ☐

AM ☐

FT ☐

CH ☐

GL ☐

Your Name _____   Today's Date _____   Time of Day _____ AM | PM
         First   Middle   Last

Street Address _____   City _____   State ____   Zip _____

Telephone (_____) _____   Social Security # _____   Date of Birth _____
      Area Code   Number   For Identification Purposes Only

SEX: ☐ Female   **ETHNIC** ☐ Asian ☐ Hispanic ☐ Other   MARITAL STATUS: ☐ Single   ☐ Married   ☐ Divorced
     ☐ Male   **GROUP:** ☐ Black ☐ White   ☐ Widowed   ☐ Separated

PLEASE TURN TO THE OTHER SIDE

Figure 4.1. Multidimensional Health Assessment Questionnaire for use in standard medical care (version 698). Reproduced, with permission, from Health Report Services, 210 La Vista Drive, Nashville, TN 37215, USA.

7. **Which of the following best describes you TODAY in your every day life? Please check (✓) only one:**

____ 1: I can do **everything** I want to do.
____ 2: I can do **most** of the things that I want to do, but have **some** limitations.
____ 3: I can do **some**, but not all, of the things I want to do, and I have **many** limitations.
____ 4: I can do **hardly any** of the things I want to do.

8. **Please place a check (✓) in the appropriate spot to indicate the amount of pain you are having today in each of the joint areas listed below:**

	None	Mild	Moderate	Severe		None	Mild	Moderate	Severe
LEFT FINGERS	____0	____1	____2	____3	RIGHT FINGERS	____0	____1	____2	____3
LEFT WRIST	____0	____1	____2	____3	RIGHT WRIST	____0	____1	____2	____3
LEFT ELBOW	____0	____1	____2	____3	RIGHT ELBOW	____0	____1	____2	____3
LEFT SHOULDER	____0	____1	____2	____3	RIGHT SHOULDER	____0	____1	____2	____3
LEFT HIP	____0	____1	____2	____3	RIGHT HIP	____0	____1	____2	____3
LEFT KNEE	____0	____1	____2	____3	RIGHT KNEE	____0	____1	____2	____3
LEFT ANKLE	____0	____1	____2	____3	RIGHT ANKLE	____0	____1	____2	____3
LEFT TOES	____0	____1	____2	____3	RIGHT TOES	____0	____1	____2	____3
NECK	____0	____1	____2	____3	BACK	____0	____1	____2	____3

9. **At this time are you?** (Please check (✓) all that apply.)

☐ Working full time   ☐ Retired   ☐ Student
☐ Working part time   ☐ Unemployed   ☐ Homemaker-full time   ☐ Disabled
☐ Other (describe): _____   **Now** your occupation is: _____

10. **How often do you aerobically exercise** (sweating, increased heary rate, shortness of breath) **for at least one-half hour (30 minutes)?** Please check (✓) only one.

☐ 3 or more times per week   ☐ 1–2 times per week   ☐ 1–2 times per month
☐ Do not exercise regularly   ☐ Cannot exercise due to disability/handicap

11. **How many years of school have you completed?** Please circle the number of years at school:

1   2   3   4   5   6   7   8   9   10   11   12   13   14   15   16   17   18   19   20

12. **Over the last 6 months have you had (please check (✓)):**

☐ No   ☐ Yes   An operation   ☐ No   ☐ Yes   Change(s) of arthritis drugs or other drugs
☐ No   ☐ Yes   Inpatient hospitalization   ☐ No   ☐ Yes   Change(s) of address
☐ No   ☐ Yes   A new illness   ☐ No   ☐ Yes   Change(s) of marital status
☐ No   ☐ Yes   An important new symptom   ☐ No   ☐ Yes   Change of job or work duties, quit work, retired
☐ No   ☐ Yes   Side effect(s) of any drug   ☐ No   ☐ Yes   Change of medical insurance, Medicare, etc.
☐ No   ☐ Yes   Cigarettes regularly   ☐ No   ☐ Yes   Change of primary care or other doctor

Please explian any "Yes" answer below. Also, please tell us about any other health, medical, stress-related, or any other matters that are affecting your life:

_____
_____
_____

WE ASK YOU FOR CONSENT TO REVIEW YOUR RECORDS FOR MEDICAL RESEARCH AND TO CONTACT YOU IN THE FUTURE. YOUR CARE WILL <u>NOT</u> BE AFFECTED IF YOU ANSWER "NO." I will allow my rheumatologist to release my medical record for medical research to designated investigators. I will allow these research investigators to send me similar questionnaires in the future, which I am not required to answer. I understand that all information will remain confidential with my physician and research associates only, and that I will not be identified in any manner in any research reports.

Please check (✓) in one box. Thank you!

☐ **YES**   ☐ **NO**   Signature _____   Date _____

THANK YOU FOR COMPLETING THIS QUESTIONNAIRE TO MONITOR YOUR MEDICAL SITUATION

Table 4.1. Pain in selected longitudinal observational studies over 5 years or more in patients with RA

Study	Mean disease duration at baseline (years)	Duration of follow-up (years)	Pain measure	Pain at baseline	Pain at evaluation	p for paired data
Egsmose et al. (1995)[63]	0.8 (all < 2)	5	VAS, scale 0–100	Early: 44 Delayed: 51	17 40	< 0.001 < 0.02
Eberhardt and Fex (1995)[64]	0.9 (all < 2)	5	VAS, scale 0–3	1.4	1.0	≤ 0.01
Lindqvist et al. (2002)[65]		10 (included 168 patients)	VAS, scale 0–3	1.2	1.2	NS
Mulherin et al. (1996)[66]	2.4 (range 0.2–12.0)	6	VAS, scale 0–100	47	32	< 0.005
Callahan et al. (1997)[67]	9.7	5	VAS, scale 0–100	52	47	NS
Munro et al. (1998)[68]	Range 0–2 Range 2–5 Range > 5	5	VAS, scale 0–3	1.7 1.8 1.9	1.1 1.5 1.5	< 0.01 0.313 0.039
Leirisalo-Repo et al. (1999)[60]	0.7 (all < 2)	8–9	VAS, scale 0–100	43	17	–
Uhlig et al. (2000)[69]	2.2 (all < 4)	5	AIMS, pain scale 0–10	4.6	4.7	0.12
Heiberg et al. (2005)[70] *	Disease duration was 13 years in patients with data at baseline, and 14 years in patients who were evaluated 7 years later		VAS, scale 0–100	46	36	Significant; p values not provided
Pincus et al. (2005)[71] †	Median disease duration was 7 years in patients included in the first evaluation (1985) and 9 years in the second evaluation (2000)		VAS, scale 0–100	52	49	0.38

AIMS, Arthritis Impact Measurement Scales; NS, not significant; VAS, visual–analogue scale for pain.

*Study was cross-sectional in part.

†Study was entirely cross-sectional.

of pain and the physician's assessment of pain in patients with OA. Therefore, it is reasonable to use patient questionnaires to document the amount of pain and disability in these patients, not only in clinical trials but also in routine clinical care.

In a clinical trial comparing two study drugs in OA,[101] differences in pain were seen according to the WOMAC scale as well as a VAS pain scale. The differences in the VAS pain scale were actually greater than those obtained with the WOMAC scale, suggesting that the VAS had a higher level of sensitivity to change in this clinical trial.

PAIN IN FIBROMYALGIA

FM is a condition characterized by widespread pain (involving all four quadrants of the body as well as the axial skeleton) and diffuse tenderness, without evidence of structural damage, such as seen in OA, or inflammation as seen in RA.

The aetiology and pathogenesis of pain in FM are unknown – the hypotheses consist of a variety of central and peripheral mechanisms. Nevertheless, the clinical measurements of pain in FM include the methods described previously. Recent reports

suggest that neuroimaging techniques may provide better understanding of the mechanism of pain in FM, in which no musculoskeletal damage can be identified, including PET and fMRI, which reveal a group of brain structures that are activated during painful conditions.[102–104] Gracely et al.[105] used fMRI in patients with FM and controls under two conditions: either the amount of the pain stimulus was the same, or the perception of pain was the same in patients and controls. If the pain stimulus was the same, the patients showed increased cerebral blood flow activation compared with the controls. However, when the pain perception was at the same level (i.e. the pain stimulus was greater in the controls to reach the same pain perception as the patients), the activation patterns were similar in patients and controls. Other studies that used the functional neuroimaging techniques showed that patients with FM had reduced blood flow in the thalami, caudate nuclei[106] and pontine tegmentum[107] at rest.

In patients with FM tissue damage is absent, but the experience of pain is present. It has been questioned whether functional imaging techniques can be used to differentiate 'real' pain from 'imagined' pain. However, pain is a subjective experience, and should not be equated with nociception, which is the excitation of nociceptors. Nociception may give rise to the experience of pain, but pain may arise in the absence of nociception. Nociception may also occur in the absence of pain. Therefore, the terms 'non-nociceptive pain' (e.g. neurogenic and psychogenic pain) and 'nociceptive pain' (e.g. inflammatory pain) need to be differentiated.

One approach to the recognition of higher scores for pain in FM with lower scores for functional disability was the observation that scores for pain were high relative to scores for functional disability on an MHAQ, with a mean of 1.6 in patients with non-inflammatory diffuse musculoskeletal pain, primarily FM, compared with a mean of 2.0 in patients with RA.[108] The pain VAS score was significantly higher in patients with FM (6.4) compared with that (5.2) in patients with RA. These observations were utilized in an analysis of 75 age- and sex-matched patients with RA compared with those with FM. Twenty of the 75 patients with FM, compared with no patients with RA, had a ratio greater than 5, while 50 (67%) of 75 patients with RA, compared to 21 (28%) with FM, had ratios of less than 3. These results were seen in patients with disease duration of less than 2 years, in whom the differential diagnosis might be most difficult. Receiver operator curve (ROC) data indicated that the observations compared favourably with laboratory tests in distinguishing patients with FM and RA.

Fibromyalgia pain is persistent; complete, sustained remission of pain is rare.[109] One study[110] concerning chronic widespread pain in the population indicated that subjects with widespread pain who were more than 50 years old and reported daytime tiredness and somatic symptoms initially were most likely to have chronic widespread pain 7 years later. In fact, 77% of the subjects who reported chronic widespread pain initially, reported chronic widespread pain also after 7 years.

In patients with an inflammatory condition, such as RA, pain is associated with measures of disease activity, and treating the underlying cause and reducing inflammatory activity also reduces pain. In FM no underlying cause for the pain has yet been identified and treatment of the pain has no target, unlike the inflammation in RA. Therefore, treatment of pain in FM is difficult. For example, Viitanen et al.[111] studied 20 female patients with FM in the course of a 3-week inpatient rehabilitation and compared with 20 female patients with RA. The pain intensity in the FM patients was found to be twice as high as that in patients with RA, and was reduced significantly more in patients with RA than in patients with FM. Indeed, there was little evidence for a significant decrease in pain in patients with FM. Although patients with FM were more depressed than patients with RA, a positive correlation between depression scores and pain scores was seen only in patients with RA.

ASSOCIATIONS OF PAIN AND OTHER MEASURES OF CLINICAL STATUS

Most 20th century medicine has derived from a biomedical model, a paradigm in which symptoms are thought to be explained by objective information from a physical examination,

radiography, imaging studies, laboratory tests and other high-technology procedures. This paradigm is expressed optimally in infectious diseases, where a test identifies a pathogen and a drug is used to treat the patient. It is less perfectly expressed in tests such as cardiography, serum glucose and rheumatoid factor tests, in which there is a strong probability of a diagnosis based on a positive finding in a test, but this is not an absolute correlation.

Analysis of scores for pain in RA indicate that there does exist a statistically significant correlation between pain scores and findings on radiography and the erythrocyte sedimentation rate (ESR), but the correlation coefficients (R) of < 0.3, indicate that less than 10% of the variation in pain scores can be explained by the variation in radiographic scores or laboratory tests. Some studies have shown a slightly stronger association between pain scores and joint swelling and tenderness, with values of R of 0.4–0.6 indicating an explanation of the 15–35% variation in these measures by variation in pain scores. However, the strongest associations between pain scores and other variables in RA are seen with scores for functional status, as well as scores for the psychological constructs of anxiety, depression, helplessness and lack of self-efficacy. Selected studies with correlation coefficients of pain with other measures of disease are reviewed in more detail in Table 4.3.[64, 112–120]

Structural changes such as cartilage loss, periarticular bone growth, osteophyte formation and sclerosis are typical in OA. However, the clinical evaluation of OA is confounded by the discrepancy between the extent of structural damage and the severity of symptoms, including joint pain, use-related stiffness and disability.[121–123] A population-based study of OA derived from the US National Health and Nutrition Examination Survey (NHANES1)[124] indicated that 53% of individuals who had radiographic findings of stage 3–4 OA according to the Kellgren–Lawrence Scale did not report any knee pain. Conversely, about 85% of people who reported significant knee pain did not have significant radiographic abnormalities. Clearly a higher proportion of the patients who come to clinical attention because of pain have radiographic abnormalities, but the correlation is far from perfect.

The dissociation of pain scores and objective findings becomes most apparent in FM, which is almost defined as having severe pain in the absence of evidence of inflammatory activity or structural damage. Indeed, the high ratio of pain scores to functional disability scores can be used as a diagnostic clue to the presence of FM.[108]

These observations suggest quite definitively that scores for pain are not correlated one on one with objective data. The most reproducible data contain pain as derived from the patient rather than from the early efforts to measure pain through objective measures.

SUMMARY

Pain is a personal experience. Therefore, information about the pain can be obtained from the patient only. Several self-report questionnaires have been developed, all of which are well-

Table 4.2. Pain (on a 0–100 mm VAS for pain) in selected clinical trials in RA

Study	Mean disease duration (years)	Duration of study (months)	Primary outcome measure	Baseline pain VAS		Outcome pain VAS		p for treatment effect	Therapy
				Treatment group	Control/ placebo	Treatment group	Control/ placebo		
Tugwell et al. (1995)[75]	9–11	6	SJC	41	45	29	42	0.04	CYA vs placebo in patients with partial response to MTX
O'Dell et al. (1996)[76]	6–10	24	Paulus50	60	60	20	30	0.02	MTX + SSZ + HCQ vs MTX
Boers et al. (1997)[77]	Median duration 4 months	12	Pooled index	55	54	32	29	0.66	MTX + SSZ + HCQ vs SSZ
Möttönen et al. (1999)[78]	All < 2	24	Remission	Not reported		Not reported			MTX + SSZ + HCQ vs single
Weinblatt et al. (1999)[79]	13	12	ACR20	Not reported		Not reported			Leflunomide vs placebo in patients with partial response to MTX
Smolen et al. (1999)[80]	6–8	6	TJC, SJC, Doctor global, Patient global	63	Placebo: 59 SSZ: 55	36	Placebo: 50 SSZ: 35	0.0001	Leflunomide vs SSZ vs placebo
US301 Strand et al. (1999)[81,82]	7	12	ACR20	59	64	37	60	≤ 0.001	Leflunomide vs placebo
US301 Cohen et al. (2001)[83]	7	24	ACR20	55	53	22	29	≤ 0.05	Leflunomide vs MTX
ATTRACT Maini et al. (1999)[84]	7–9	7	Descriptive	66–70	67	31–38	59	NA	Infliximab vs placebo in patients with partial response to MTX

Study		Weeks	Outcome						Comparison
ATTRACT Lipsky et al. (2000)[85]	7–9	12	ACR20	Not reported					Infliximab vs placebo in patients with partial response to MTX
ATTRACT St. Clair et al. (2002)[86]	7–9	24	ACR20	Not reported					Infliximab vs placebo in patients with partial response to MTX
Weinblatt et al. (1999)[87]	13.6	6	ACR20	50	56	18	44	0.001	Etanercept vs placebo in patients with partial response to MTX
ERA Bathon et al. (2000)[88]	All < 3	12	ACR20/50/70	Not reported					Etanercept vs MTX
ERA Genovese et al. (2002)[89]	All < 3	24	ACR20/50/70	Not reported					Etanercept vs MTX
Keystone et al. (2004)[90]	8–11	2	ACR20	50 mg: 53 / 25 mg: 57		50 mg: 39 / 25 mg: 42	53	NA	Etanercept vs placebo
ARMADA Weinblatt et al. (2003)[91]	11–13	6	ACR20	80 mg: 55 / 40 mg: 53 / 20 mg: 55		80 mg: 27 / 40 mg: 28 / 20 mg: 30	49	< 0.001	Adalimumab vs placebo in patients with partial response to MTX
Keystone et al. (2004)[92]	11	12	ACR20, HAQ, Radiographic progression	40 mg: 56 / 20 mg: 55		40 mg: 27 / 20 mg: 28	45	NA	Adalimumab vs placebo in patients with partial response to MTX

ACR20/50/70, American College of Rheumatology response criteria for rheumatoid arthritis; ATTRACT, Anti-Tumor Necrosis Factor Trial in Rheumatoid Arthritis with Concomitant Therapy; CYA, cyclosporin A; ERA, Early Rheumatoid Arthritis; HAQ, Health Assessment Questionnaire; HCQ, hydroxychloroquine; MTX, methotrexate; NA, not available; SJC, swollen joint count; SSZ, sulfasalazine; TJC, tender joint count; VAS, visual–analogue scale.

Table 4.3. Correlation coefficients between pain and other measures in RA

Study	Pain measure	No. of patients	Correlation coefficients between pain and other measures										
			Age	Disease duration	Education	HAQ/MHAQ	Patient global	Disease activity, pooled	ESR	SJC	TJC	AM	x-Rays
Callahan et al. (1987)[112]	VAS	385	−0.06	0.17	−0.14	0.55	0.53	–	0.24	0.33	0.34	0.24	–
Hagglund et al. (1989)[113]	AIMS pain scale	53	–	–	–	–	–	–	0.14	0.45	–	–	–
Serbo and Jajic (1991)[114]	VAS	61	–	–	–	0.52	–	–	–	–	–	–	–
Stenström et al. (1992)[115]	VAS, activity-induced pain	69	0.08	0.12	–	0.55	–	–	0.06	0.04	0.66	–	0.21
Hakala et al. (1994)[116]	VAS	103	–	–	–	0.36	–	–	–	–	–	–	–
Smedstad et al. (1995)[117]	VAS	238	–	–	–	–	–	–	–	–	0.06	–	–
Eberhardt and Fex (1995)[64]	VAS	67 (baseline)	–	–	–	0.44	–	–	–	–	–	–	–
		67 (at 5 years)	–	–	–	0.59	–	–	–	–	–	–	–
Rojkovich and Gibson (1998)[118]	VAS	Daytime movement: 251	0.14	0.16	–	–	–	–	0.17	0.03	0.25	–	0.09
		Daytime rest: 232	0.19	0.02	–	–	–	–	0.18	0.03	0.25	–	0.16
		Nocturnal: 181	0.02	−0.13	–	–	–	–	0.25	0.21	0.36	–	0.08
Sokka et al. (2000)[119]	VAS	141	–	–	–	0.65	–	–	–	–	–	–	0.01
Sarzi-Puttini et al. (2002)[120]	VAS	105	0.04	0.07	–	0.42	0.57	–	0.38	0.05	0.04	0.43	0.06

–, Not available; AIMS, Arthritis Impact Measurement Scales; AM, morning stiffness; ESR, erythrocyte sedimentation rate; HAQ, Health Assessment Questionnaire; MHAQ, Modified Health Assessment Questionnaire; SJC, swollen joint count; TJC, tender joint count; VAS, visual–analogue scale.

PRACTICE POINTS

- Pain is the most prominent symptom in people with musculoskeletal disorders, and the most common reason to seek medical help, but is rarely recorded in usual medical care.

- Since pain is a personal experience estimated changes in levels of pain over long periods in patients with rheumatic diseases *cannot* be obtained from any source other than the patient.

- Several self-report questionnaires have been developed to measure pain and disability, and are well-documented tools for use in clinical trials.

- Short questionnaires with no complicated scoring systems are most feasible to be implemented as a part of routine care.

- The MDHAQ is a one-page, two-sided questionnaire that includes a pain VAS. It is completed by the patient as a self-report questionnaire in < 10 minutes in the waiting room and can be scored by a health professional in < 30 seconds.

Rheumatoid arthritis

- Evaluation of pain as a part of clinical monitoring is recommended.

- Results of randomized controlled trials are too often presented as pooled data; data concerning separate measures such as pain should be presented also.

Osteoarthritis

- Understanding of OA has improved over the years.

- Discrepancy of pain and structural damage is marked; in early disease pain might serve as a sign to start preventive strategies of OA.

- Visual analogue scale for pain is a simple and satisfactory measure in a clinic to monitor pain along with other measures included in the MDHAQ.

Fibromyalgia

- Fibromyalgic pain is rather persistent. More research is needed to get a better understanding of pain in patients with FM.

RESEARCH AGENDA

Rheumatoid arthritis

- Support for long-term observational databases of patients with RA is needed in order to document effective long-term therapies in routine clinical use, especially at this time when new treatment modalities are available.

Osteoarthritis

- Discrepancy of pain and structural damage is not completely understood in patients with OA. Long-term follow-up studies are needed to determine whether or not joint pain and stiffness reflect an ongoing disease process, and whether or not these symptoms predict structural abnormality.

Fibromyalgia

- More research is needed for a better understanding of the underlying cause of pain in patients with FM.

REFERENCES

1. Merskey H. Pain terms: a list with definitions and notes on usage recommended by the IASP Subcommittee on Taxonomy. *Pain* 1979; **6**: 249–252.
2. IASP Task Force on Taxonomy. *Classification of Chronic Pain: Descriptions of Chronic Pain Syndromes and Definitions of Pain Terms*, 2nd edn. IASP Press, Seattle, WA, 1994.
3. Gibson T, Clark B. Use of simple analgesics in rheumatoid arthritis. *Ann Rheum Dis* 1985; **44**: 27–29.
4. McKenna F, Wright V. Pain and rheumatoid arthritis [Letter]. *Ann Rheum Dis* 1985; **44**: 805.
5. Kazis LE, Meenan RF, Anderson JJ. Pain in the rheumatic diseases: investigation of a key health status component. *Arthritis Rheum* 1983; **26**: 1017–1022.
6. Anderson KO, Bradley LA, Turner RA et al. Pain behavior of rheumatoid arthritis patients enrolled in experimental drug trials. *Arthritis Care Res* 1994; **7**: 64–68.
7. Rekola KE, Keinanen-Kiukaanniemi K, Takala J. Use of primary health services in sparsely populated country districts by patients with musculoskeletal symptoms: consultations with a physician. *J Epidemiol Commun Health* 1993; **47**: 153–157.
8. Mantyselka P, Kumpusalo E, Ahonen R et al. Pain as a reason to visit the doctor: a study in Finnish primary health care. *Pain* 2001; **89**: 175–180.
9. Uhlig T, Hagen KB, Kvien TK. Why do patients with chronic musculoskeletal disorders consult their primary care physicians? *Curr Opin Rheumatol* 2002; **14**: 104–108.
10. Crook J, Rideout E, Browne G. The prevalence of pain complaints in a general population. *Pain* 1984; **18**: 229–314.
11. McLean SA, Maio RF, Domeier RM. The epidemiology of pain in the prehospital setting. *Prehosp Emerg Care* 2002; **6**: 402–405.
12. Engel GL. The need for a new medical model: a challenge for biomedicine. *Science* 1977; **196**: 129–136.
13. Pincus T, Callahan LF, Sale WG et al. Severe functional declines, work disability, and increased mortality in seventy-five rheumatoid arthritis patients studied over nine years. *Arthritis Rheum* 1984; **27**: 864–872.
14. Pincus T, Callahan LF. Formal education as a marker for increased mortality and morbidity in rheumatoid arthritis. *J Chronic Dis* 1985; **38**: 973–984.
15. Pincus T, Brooks RH, Callahan LF. Prediction of long-term mortality in patients with rheumatoid arthritis according to simple questionnaire and joint count measures. *Ann Intern Med* 1994; **120**: 26–34.
16. Pincus T, Callahan LF. Associations of low formal education level and poor health status: behavioral, in addition to demographic and medical, explanations? *J Clin Epidemiol* 1994; **47**: 355–361.

documented tools for research purposes. However, in a busy rheumatology clinic the use of large questionnaires is not feasible. In routine clinical care a questionnaire should be easy to complete and easy to score, such as a pain VAS. It is recommended that quantitative assessment of pain be included at each visit in routine rheumatology care, along with assessment of functional disability, global status and other patient variables, using a patient self-report questionnaire such as the one-page, two-sided MDHAQ. This questionnaire provides clinically useful information to the doctor in treating patients with rheumatic conditions.

17. Melzack R. The McGill Pain Questionnaire: major properties and scoring methods. *Pain* 1975; **1**: 277–299.

18. Melzack R. The McGill pain questionnaire. In: Melzack R (ed.), *Pain Measurement and Assessment*. Raven Press, New York, 1983, pp. 33–37.

19. Huskisson EC. Measurement of pain. *Lancet* 1974; ii:1127–1131.

20. Huskisson EC. Assessment for clinical trials. *Clin Rheum Dis* 1976; **2**: 37–49.

21. Fries JF, Spitz P, Kraines RG et al. Measurement of patient outcome in arthritis. *Arthritis Rheum* 1980; **23**: 137–145.

22. Meenan RF, Gertman PM, Mason JH. Measuring health status in arthritis: the arthritis impact measurement scales. *Arthritis Rheum* 1980; **23**: 146–152.

23. Bellamy N, Buchanan WW, Goldsmith CH et al. Validation study of WOMAC: a health status instrument for measuring clinically important patient relevant outcomes to antirheumatic drug therapy in patients with osteoarthritis of the hip or knee. *J Rheumatol* 1988; **15**: 1833–1840.

24. Bellamy N. Pain assessment in osteoarthritis: experience with the WOMAC osteoarthritis index. *Semin Arthritis Rheum* 1989; **18**(Suppl 2): 14–17.

25. Hunt SM, McEwen J, McKenna SP. Measuring health status: a new tool for clinicians and epidemiologists. *J R Coll Gen Pract* 1985; **35**: 185–188.

26. Ware JE Jr, Sherbourne CD. The MOS 36-item short-form health survey (SF-36): I. Conceptual framework and item selection. *Med Care* 1992; **30**: 473–481.

27. Anderson DL. Development of an instrument to measure pain in rheumatoid arthritis: Rheumatoid Arthritis Pain Scale (RAPS). *Arthritis Care Res* 2001; **45**: 317–323.

28. Pincus T, Wolfe F. An infrastructure of patient questionnaires at each rheumatology visit: improving efficiency and documenting care. *J Rheumatol* 2000; **27**: 2727–2730.

29. Wolfe BB. Factor analysis of human pain responses: pain endurance as a specific pain factor. *J Abnorm Psychol* 1971; **78**: 292–298.

30. Beecher HK. A method for quantifying the intensity of pain. *Science* 1953; **118**: 322–324.

31. Woodforde JM, Merskey H. Some relationships between subjective measures of pain. *J Psychosom Res* 1972; **16**: 173–178.

32. Brena SF, Koch DL. A 'pain estimate' model for quantification and classification of chronic pain states. *Anesth Rev* 1975; **2**: 8–13.

33. McKinley JC, Hathaway SR. The identification and measurement of the psychoneuroses in medical practice: the Minnesota Multiphasic Personality Inventory. *JAMA* 1943; **122**: 161–167.

34. Moos RH, Solomon GF. Minnesota Multiphasic Personality Inventory response patterns in patients with rheumatoid arthritis. *J Psychosom Res* 1964; **8**: 17–28.

35. Liang MH, Rogers M, Larson M et al. The psychosocial impact of systemic lupus erythematosus and rheumatoid arthritis. *Arthritis Rheum* 1984; **27**: 13–19.

36. Pincus T, Callahan LF, Bradley LA et al. Elevated MMPI scores for hypochondriasis, depression, and hysteria in patients with rheumatoid arthritis reflect disease rather than psychological status. *Arthritis Rheum* 1986; **29**: 1456–1466.

37. Pincus T, Callahan LF. Depression scales in rheumatoid arthritis: criterion contamination in interpretation of patient responses. *Patient Educ Counsel* 1993; **20**: 133–143.

38. Callahan LF, Kaplan MR, Pincus T. The Beck Depression Inventory, Center for Epidemiological Studies Depression Scale (CES-D), and General Well-being Schedule Depression Subscale in rheumatoid arthritis: criterion contamination of responses. *Arthritis Care Res* 1991; **4**: 3–11.

39. Melzack R, Torgerson WS. On the language of pain. *Anesthesiology* 1971; **34**: 50–59.

40. Melzack R. The short-form McGill Pain Questionnaire. *Pain* 1987; **30**: 191–197.

41. Scott J, Huskisson EC. Graphic representation of pain. *Pain* 1976; **2**: 175–184.

42. Scott J, Huskisson EC. Vertical or horizontal visual analogue scales. *Ann Rheum Dis* 1979; **38**: 560.

43. Huskisson EC. Measurement of pain. *J Rheumatol* 1982; **9**: 768–769.

44. Huskisson EC. Visual analogue scales. In: Melzack R (ed.), *Pain Measurement and Assessment*. Raven Press, New York, 1983, pp. 33–37.

45. Dixon JS, Bird HA. Reproducibility along a 10 cm vertical visual analogue scale. *Ann Rheum Dis* 1981; **40**: 87–89.

46. Carlsson AM. Assessment of chronic pain. I. Aspects of the reliability and validity of the visual analogue scale. *Pain* 1983; **16**: 87–101.

47. Pincus T, Summey JA, Soraci SA Jr et al. Assessment of patient satisfaction in activities of daily living using a modified Stanford Health Assessment Questionnaire. *Arthritis Rheum* 1983; **26**: 1346–1353.

48. Pincus T, Swearingen C, Wolfe F. Toward a Multidimensional Health Assessment Questionnaire (MDHAQ): assessment of advanced activities of daily living and psychological status in the patient friendly health assessment questionnaire format. *Arthritis Rheum* 1999; **42**: 2220–2230.

49. Pincus T, Sokka T, Kautiainen H. Further development of a physical function scale on a MDHAQ for standard care of patients with rheumatic diseases. *J Rheumatol* 2005; **32**: 1432–1439. Erratum: *J Rheumatol* 2005; **32**: 2280

50. Wolfe F, Michaud K, Pincus T. Development and validation of the health Assessment Questionnaire II: a revised version of the Health Assessment Questionnaire. *Arthritis Rheum* 2004; **50**: 3296–3305.

51. Carr AJ, Thompson PW, Kirwan JR. Quality of life measures. *Br J Rheumatol* 1996; **35**: 275–281.

52. Heiberg T, Kvien TK. Preferences for improved health examined in 1,024 patients with rheumatoid arthritis: pain has highest priority. *Arthritis Rheum* 2002; **47**: 391–397.

53. Sokka T, Krishnan E, Häkkinen A et al. Functional disability in rheumatoid arthritis patients compared with a community population in Finland. *Arthritis Rheum* 2003; **48**: 59–63.

54. Hagen KB, Kvien TK, Bjørndal A. Musculoskeletal pain and quality of life in patients with noninflammatory joint pain compared to rheumatoid arthritis: a population survey. *J Rheumatol* 1997; **24**: 1703–1709.

55. Pinals RS, Masi AT, Larsen RA et al. Preliminary criteria for clinical remission in rheumatoid arthritis. *Arthritis Rheum* 1981; **24**: 1308–1315.

56. Sokka T, Pincus T. Most patients receiving routine care for rheumatoid arthritis in 2001 did not meet inclusion criteria for most recent clinical trials or American College of Rheumatology criteria for remission. *J Rheumatol* 2003; **30**: 1138–1146.

57. Wells G, Anderson J, Boers M et al. MCID/Low Disease Activity State Workshop: summary, recommendations, and research agenda. *J Rheumatol* 2003; **30**: 1115–1118.

58. Falgarone G, Zerkak D, Bauer C et al. How to define a Minimal Clinically Individual State (MCIS) with pain VAS in daily practice for patients suffering from musculoskeletal disorders. *Clin Exp Rheumatol* 2005; **23**: 235–238.

59. Krishnan E, Hakkinien A, Sokka T et al. Impact of age and comorbidities on the criteria for remission and response in rheumatoid arthritis. *Ann Rheum Dis* 2005; **64**: 1350–1352.

60. Leirisalo-Repo M, Paimela L, Peltomaa R et al. Functional and radiological outcome in patients with early RA – a longitudinal observational study. *Arthritis Rheum* 1999; **42**: S130.

61. Borg AA, Dawes PT. Measures of pain and disease activity in rheumatoid arthritis. *Br J Rheumatol* 1993; **32**: 1028–1029.

62. van der Heide A, Jacobs JW, Haanen HC et al. Is it possible to predict the first year extent of pain and disability for patients with rheumatoid arthritis? *J Rheumatol* 1995; **22**: 1466–1470.

63. Egsmose C, Lund B, Borg G et al. Patients with rheumatoid arthritis benefit from early 2nd line therapy: 5 year followup of a prospective double blind placebo controlled study. *J Rheumatol* 1995; **22**: 2208–2213.

64. Eberhardt KB, Fex E. Functional impairment and disability in early rheumatoid arthritis – development over 5 years. *J Rheumatol* 1995; **22**: 1037–1042.

65. Lindqvist E, Saxne T, Geborek P et al. Ten year outcome in a cohort of patients with early rheumatoid arthritis: health status, disease process, and damage. *Ann Rheum Dis* 2002; **61**: 1055–1059.

66. Mulherin D, Fitzgerald O, Bresnihan B. Clinical improvement and radiological deterioration in rheumatoid arthritis: evidence that pathogenesis of synovial inflammation and articular erosion may differ. *Br J Rheumatol* 1996; **35**: 1263–1268.

67. Callahan LF, Pincus T, Huston JW et al. Measures of activity and damage in rheumatoid arthritis: depiction of changes and prediction of mortality over five years. *Arthritis Care Res* 1997; **10**: 381–394.

68. Munro R, Hampson R, McEntegart A et al. Improved functional outcome in patients with early rheumatoid arthritis treated with intramuscular gold: results of a five year prospective study. *Ann Rheum Dis* 1998; **57**: 88–93.

69. Uhlig T, Smedstad LM, Vaglum P, Moum T, Gerard N, Kvien TK. The course of rheumatoid arthritis and predictors of psychological, physical and radiographic outcome after 5 years of follow-up. *Rheumatology* 2000; **39**: 732–741.

70. Heiberg T, Finset A, Uhlig T et al. Seven year changes in health status and priorities for improvement of health in patients with rheumatoid arthritis. *Ann Rheum Dis* 2005; **64**: 191–195.

71. Pincus T, Sokka T, Kautiainen H. Patients seen for standard rheumatoid arthritis care have significantly better articular, radiographic, laboratory, and functional status in 2000 than in 1985. *Arthritis Rheum* 2005; **52**: 1009–1019.

72. Fries JF, Spitz PW, Mitchell DM et al. Impact of specific therapy upon rheumatoid arthritis. *Arthritis Rheum* 1986; **29**: 620–627.

73. Fries JF. Reevaluating the therapeutic approach to rheumatoid arthritis: the 'sawtooth' strategy. *J Rheumatol* 1990; **17**(Suppl 22):12–15.

74. Ward MM. Rheumatology visit frequency and changes in functional disability and pain in patients with rheumatoid arthritis. *J Rheumatol* 1997; **24**: 35–42.

75. Tugwell P, Pincus T, Yocum D et al. Combination therapy with cyclosporine and methotrexate in severe rheumatoid arthritis. *N Engl J Med* 1995; **333**: 137–141.

76. O'Dell JR, Haire CE, Erikson N et al. Treatment of rheumatoid arthritis with methotrexate alone, sulfasalazine and hydroxychloroquine, or a combination of all three medications. *N Engl J Med* 1996; **334**: 1287–1291.

77. Boers M, Verhoeven AC, Markusse HM et al. Randomised comparison of combined step-down prednisolone, methotrexate and sulphasalazine with sulphasalazine alone in early rheumatoid arthritis. *Lancet* 1997; **350**: 309–318.

78. Möttönen T, Hannonen P, Leirisalo-Repo M et al. Comparison of combination therapy with single-drug therapy in early rheumatoid arthritis: a randomised trial. FIN-RACo trial group. *Lancet* 1999; **353**: 1568–1573.

79. Weinblatt ME, Kremer JM, Bankhurst AD et al. A trial of etanercept, a recombinant tumor necrosis factor receptor: Fc fusion protein, in patients with rheumatoid arthritis receiving methotrexate. *N Engl J Med* 1999; **340**: 253–259.

80. Smolen JS, Kalden JR, Scott DL et al. Efficacy and safety of leflunomide compared with placebo and sulphasalazine in active rheumatoid arthritis: a double-blind, randomised, multicentre trial. *Lancet* 1999; **353**: 259–266.

81. Strand V, Tugwell P, Bombardier C et al. Function and health-related quality of life: results from a randomized controlled trial of leflunomide versus methotrexate or placebo in patients with active rheumatoid arthritis. *Arthritis Rheum* 1999; **42**: 1870–1878.

82. Strand V, Cohen S, Schiff M et al. Treatment of active rheumatoid arthritis with leflunomide compared with placebo and methotrexate. *Arch Intern Med* 1999; **159**: 2542–2550.

83. Cohen S, Cannon GW, Schiff M et al. Two-year, blinded, randomized, controlled trial of treatment of active rheumatoid arthritis with leflunomide compared with methotrexate. Utilization of leflunomide in the Treatment of Rheumatoid Arthritis Trial Investigator Group. *Arthritis Rheum* 2001; **44**: 1984–1992.

84. Maini R, St Clair EW, Breedveld F et al. Infliximab (chimeric anti-tumour necrosis factor alpha monoclonal antibody) versus placebo in rheumatoid arthritis patients receiving concomitant methotrexate: a randomized phase III trial. *Lancet* 1999; **354**: 1932–1939.

85. Lipsky PE, van der Heijde DMFM, St Clair EW et al. Infliximab and methotrexate in the treatment of rheumatoid arthritis. *N Engl J Med* 2000; **343**: 1594–1602.

86. St Clair EW, Wagner CL, Fasanmade AA et al. The relationship of serum infliximab concentrations to clinical improvement in rheumatoid arthritis: results from ATTRACT, a multicenter, randomized, double-blind, placebo-controlled trial. *Arthritis Rheum* 2002; **46**: 1451–1459.

87. Weinblatt ME, Kremer JM, Coblyn JS et al. Pharmacokinetics, safety, and efficacy of combination treatment with methotrexate and leflunomide in patients with active rheumatoid arthritis. *Arthritis Rheum* 1999; **42**: 1322–1328.

88. Bathon JM, Martin RW, Fleischmann RM et al. A comparison of etanercept and methotrexate in patients with early rheumatoid arthritis. *N Engl J Med* 2000; **343**: 1586–1593.

89. Genovese MC, Bathon JM, Martin RW et al. Etanercept versus methotrexate in patients with early rheumatoid arthritis: two-year radiographic and clinical outcomes. *Arthritis Rheum* 2002; **46**: 1443–1450.

90. Keystone EC, Schiff MH, Kremer JM et al. Once-weekly administration of 50 mg etanercept in patients with active rheumatoid arthritis. Results of a multicenter, randomized, double-blind, placebo-controlled trial. *Arthritis Rheum* 2004; **50**: 353–363.

91. Weinblatt ME, Keystone EC, Furst DE et al. Adalimumab, a fully human anti-tumor necrosis factor a monoclonal antibody, for the treatment of rheumatoid arthritis in patients taking concomitant methotrexate: the ARMADA trial. *Arthritis Rheum* 2003; **48**: 35–45.

92. Keystone EC, Kavanaugh AF, Sharp JT et al. Radiographic, clinical and functional outcomes of treatment with adalimumab (a human anti-tumor necrosis factor monoclonal antibody) in patients with active rheumatoid arthritis receiving concomitant methotrexate therapy: a randomized, placebo-controlled, 52-week trial. *Arthritis Rheum* 2004; **50**: 1400–1411.

93. Salaffi F, Cavalieri F, Nolli M et al. Analysis of disability in knee osteoarthritis. Relationship with age and psychological variables but not with radiographic score. *J Rheumatol* 1991; **18**: 1581–1586.

94. Jordan J, Luta G, Renner J et al. Knee pain and knee osteoarthritis severity in self-reported task specific disability: the Johnston County Osteoarthritis Project. *J Rheumatol* 1997; **24**: 1344–1349.

95. van Baar ME, Dekker J, Lemmens JAM et al. Pain and disability in patients with osteoarthritis of hip or knee: the relationship with articular, kinesiological, and psychological characteristics. *J Rheumatol* 1998; **25**: 125–133.

96. Creamer P, Lethbridge-Cejku M, Hochberg MC. Determinants of pain severity in knee osteoarthritis: effect of demographic and psychosocial variables using 3 pain measures. *J Rheumatol* 1999; **26**: 1785–1792.

97. Spector TD, Dacre JE, Harris PA et al. Radiological progression of

osteoarthritis: an 11 year follow up study of the knee. *Ann Rheum Dis* 1992; **51**: 1107–1110.

98. Felson DT, Zhang Y, Hannan MT et al. The incidence and natural history of knee osteoarthritis in the elderly. The Framingham Osteoarthritis Study. *Arthritis Rheum* 1995; **38**: 1500–1505.

99. Peat G, Croft P, Hay E. Clinical assessment of the osteoarthritis patient. *Best Practice Res Clin Rheumatol* 2001; **15**: 527–544.

100. de Bock GH, van Marwijk HWJ, Kaptein AA et al. Osteoarthritis pain assessment in family practice. *Arthritis Care Res* 1994; **7**: 40–45.

101. Pincus T, Koch GG, Sokka T et al. A randomized, double-blind, crossover clinical trial of diclofenac plus misoprostol versus acetaminophen in patients with osteoarthritis of the hip or knee. *Arthritis Rheum* 2001; **44**: 1587–1598.

102. Derbyshire SWG. Imaging the brain in pain. *Am Pain Soc* 1999; **9**: 7–8.

103. Jones AK, Brown WD, Friston KJ et al. Cortical and subcortical localization of response to pain in man using positron emission tomography. *Proc R Soc London, Ser B* 1991; **244**: 39–44.

104. Casey KL. Match and mismatch: identifying the neuronal determinants of pain. *Ann Intern Med* 1996; **124**: 995–998.

105. Gracely RH, Petzke F, Wolf JM et al. Functional magnetic resonance imaging evidence of augmented pain processing in fibromyalgia. *Arthritis Rheum* 2002; **46**: 1333–1343.

106. Mountz JD, Zhou T, Chen J. Use of sensitive assays to detect soluble Fas in patients with systemic lupus erythematosus: comment on the article by Knipping et al. and the article by Goel at al. [letter]. *Arthritis Rheum* 1996; **39**: 1611–1612.

107. Kwiatek R, Barnden L, Tedman R et al. Regional cerebral blood flow in fibromyalgia: single-photon-emission computed tomography evidence of reduction in the pontine tegmentum and thalami. *Arthritis Rheum* 2000; **43**: 2823–2833.

108. Callahan LF, Pincus T. The P-VAS/D-ADL ratio: a clue from a self-report questionnaire to distinguish rheumatoid arthritis from noninflammatory diffuse musculoskeletal pain. *Arthritis Rheum* 1990; **33**: 1317–1322.

109. Forseth KKO, Gran JT. Management of fibromyalgia: what are the best treatment choices? *Drugs* 2002; **62**: 577–592.

110. Papageorgiou AC, Silman AJ, Macfarlane GJ. Chronic widespread pain in the population: a seven year follow up study. *Ann Rheum Dis* 2002; **61**: 1071–1074.

111. Viitanen JV, Kautiainen H, Isomäki H. Pain intensity in patients with fibromyalgia and rheumatoid arthritis. *Scand J Rheumatol* 1993; **22**: 131–135.

112. Callahan LF, Brooks RH, Summey JA et al. Quantitative pain assessment for routine care of rheumatoid arthritis patients, using a pain scale based on activities of daily living and a visual analogue pain scale. *Arthritis Rheum* 1987; **30**: 630–636.

113. Hagglund KJ, Haley WE, Reveille JD et al. Predicting individual differences in pain and functional impairment among patients with rheumatoid arthritis. *Arthritis Rheum* 1989; **32**: 851–858.

114. Serbo B, Jajic I. Relationship of the functional status, duration of the disease and pain intensity and some psychological variables in patients with rheumatoid arthritis. *Clin Rheumatol* 1991; **10**: 19–22.

115. Stenström CH, Lindell B, Swanberg P et al. Activity-induced pain in rheumatoid arthritis functional class II and its relations with demographic, medical, functional, psychosocial, and work variables. *Arthritis Care Res* 1992; **5**: 42–48.

116. Hakala M, Nieminen P, Manelius J. Joint impairment is strongly correlated with disability measured by self-report questionnaires. Functional status assessment of individuals with rheumatoid arthritis in a population based series. *J Rheumatol* 1994; **21**: 64–69.

117. Smedstad LM, Vaglum P, Kvien TK et al. The relationship between self-reported pain and sociodemographic variables, anxiety, and depressive symptoms in rheumatoid arthritis. *J Rheumatol* 1995; **22**: 514–520.

118. Rojkovich B, Gibson T. Day and night pain measurement in rheumatoid arthritis. *Ann Rheum Dis* 1998; **57**: 434–436.

119. Sokka T, Kankainen A, Hannonen P. Scores for functional disability in patients with rheumatoid arthritis are correlated at higher levels with pain scores than with radiographic scores. *Arthritis Rheum* 2000; **43**: 386–389.

120. Sarzi-Puttini P, Fiorini T, Panni B et al. Correlation of the score for subjective pain with physical disability, clinical and radiographic scores in recent onset rheumatoid arthritis. *BMC Musculoskelet Disord* 2002; **3**: 18.

121. Odding E, Valkenburg HA, Algra D et al. Associations of radiological osteoarthritis of the hip and knee with locomotor disability in the Rotterdam Study. *Ann Rheum Dis* 1998; **57**: 203–208.

122. Dieppe PA, Cushnaghan J, Shepstone L. The Bristol 'OA500' study: progression of osteoarthritis (OA) over 3 years and the relationship between clinical and radiographic changes at the knee joint. *Osteoarthritis Cartilage* 1997; **5**: 87–97.

123. Creamer P, Lethbridge-Cejku M, Hochberg MC. Factors associated with functional impairment in symptomatic knee osteoarthritis. *Rheumatology* 2000; **39**: 490–496.

124. Hannan MT, Felson DT, Pincus T. Analysis of the discordance between radiographic changes and knee pain in osteoarthritis of the knee. *J Rheumatol* 2000; **27**: 1513–1517.

Chapter 5
Assessment of neuropathic pain

Ellen Jørum

INTRODUCTION

The prevalence of chronic pain is largely unknown, but is greater than was previously thought. Few epidemiological studies are available. A large European study involving 46,394 persons from 16 countries, has shown a prevalence of chronic pain lasting more than 6 months of 19%.[1] Other European studies have reported a prevalence of chronic pain of between 11% and 55%,[2] but this includes all forms of chronic pain, not just neuropathic pain. The prevalence of neuropathic pain is unclear. A prevalence of 28% in multiple sclerosis has been shown,[3] 66% following spinal cord injuries[4] and 8% following stroke.[5] In the USA it is estimated that more than 3 million patients suffer from painful diabetic neuropathy and 1 million from postherpetic neuralgia.[6]

Neuropathic pain conditions are underdiagnosed and consequently many patients do not receive proper treatment. Those that do receive treatment are often treated with traditional, weak and medium-strong pain-relieving medication, which has no documented effect in neuropathic pain, and not with drugs that are documented as effective, such as antiepileptic agents and amitriptyline.[6]

DIFFERENT TYPES OF PAIN

Pain conditions may be categorized in many ways. A common classification of pain is:

- Nociceptive pain, which results from activation of nociceptors (either normal or sensitized). Examples include muscle pain, pain due to skin lesions or pain arising from other peripheral tissues.
- Neuropathic pain.
- Psychogenic pain.

This chapter deals only with neuropathic pain, which is defined as 'pain initiated or caused by a primary lesion or dysfunction in the nervous system'.[7] The term 'dysfunction' was originally used in order to include trigeminal neuralgia as a neuropathic pain condition, but was later often used to explain central sensitization (this is described further below, see under 'Mechanisms of neuropathic pain'). Almost all forms of pain (including nociceptive pain) may involve central sensitization and may therefore wrongly be called neuropathic. It is suggested that the word 'dysfunction' is omitted from the definition of neuropathic pain.[6, 8]

CAUSES OF NEUROPATHIC PAIN

Some common causes of neuropathic pain are listed in Box 5.1. In general, any lesion of the nervous system, but in particular lesions affecting the sensory nerve fibres and pathways (particularly small nerve fibres), may produce neuropathic pain.

CLINICAL PRESENTATION

Neuropathic pain is characterized by the following possible types of pain:

Box 5.1. Examples of causes of neuropathic pain

Neuropathic pain of peripheral origin
- Entrapment of peripheral nerves (e.g. carpal tunnel)
- Injuries of peripheral nerves (trauma, accident, surgery)
- Infections of nervous tissue (e.g. postherpetic neuralgia)
- Painful neuropathies (e.g. painful diabetic neuropathy)
- Complex regional pain syndrome (CRPS) type 2, previously called causalgia

Neuropathic pain of central origin
- Pain following spinal cord injuries
- Pain in multiple sclerosis
- Pain following cerebral infarcts

- *Spontaneous persistent (stimulus-independent) pain* is for most patients the most troublesome type of pain. It is described variously as burning, aching, throbbing, sore or cutting. All these pain descriptors are encountered in descriptions of other types of pain, for example nociceptive pain.[9] It is not possible therefore to depend on the description and character of the pain alone when making a diagnosis of neuropathic pain. The pain may be deep and/or superficial. The intensity of the pain may vary spontaneously, but will in general increase during and following physical exercise, and with exposure to cold.
- *Spontaneous paroxysmal pain* or shock-like pain of short duration (often seconds) radiating from the painful area and with a large variation in frequency (from none to several times per day).
- *Evoked (stimulus-dependent) pain* may be evoked by stimuli such as light touch or cold, or less frequently heat, applied to the skin. The patient reports that it is painful to dress in the morning and that it hurts to keep the painful extremity or other body area under the bedcover during the night and when someone accidentally touches them.

CLINICAL EVALUATION

The most important part of an assessment of neuropathic pain is a thorough interview of the patient, with special emphasis on spontaneous, persistent and paroxysmal pain, as well as evoked pain. It is recommended that patients mark their different forms of pain on body charts. The description or descriptions of the different forms of pain, as well as the events that may provoke or worsen the pain, must be clarified. Pain intensity may be evaluated using a large number of scales, of which the visual–analogue scale is the simplest. The presence of spontaneous persistent and paroxysmal pain as well as evoked pain suggests neuropathic pain, but this occurrence is not sufficient for the diagnosis to be made.

The next step in the evaluation of the patient is a clinical neurological examination of the patient. The purpose is to locate the site of the lesion within the peripheral or central nervous system (CNS). It is often necessary to refer the patient for supplementary investigations such as electromyography (EMG) or neurography to obtain objective documentation of peripheral nerve damage, or for a computed tomography (CT) or magnetic resonance imaging (MRI) scan to document lesions within the CNS. It is important to be aware that neuropathic pain may be caused by a neurological disease, such as multiple sclerosis, so that a thorough clinical neurological examination, including testing of movement and reflexes, is essential. Referral to a neurologist is often necessary, but all doctors should be able to perform a simple neurological examination.

Neuropathic pain is almost always characterized by alterations in sensation, so it is important to focus in particular on the sensory examination. Sensory changes may include hypo- or hyperalgesia, hypo- or hyperaesthesia, as well as qualitative, spatial or temporal alterations. The aim of investigations is to examine whether the sensory changes are related to a lesion of a specific nerve or nerve root or to a central lesion. Sophisticated equipment is usually unnecessary. Most doctors have cotton swabs or a light brush and needles available. It is, however, important to be aware that the use of cotton may often evoke pain (allodynia to light touch), thus masking possible reduced sensation to light touch. The sense of light touch may be tested more elaborately by means of nylon filaments (von Frey). These are composed of a series of filaments of varying thickness, calibrated according to the force required to make them bend. The hairs primarily stimulate the rapidly adapting cutaneous receptors when hairs with low bending pressures are applied to the skin.

Cotton or a brush lightly applied to the skin may also be used to determine an area of allodynia to light touch. Allodynia is defined as pain due to a stimulus that does not normally provoke pain.[7] The sensation of sharp pain is often reduced in patients with neuropathic pain, but by using a needle or other sharp object the following phenomenon will often be encountered: the sensation of pin-prick may be reduced, but at the same time the patient reports an unpleasant after-sensation, which radiates from the site of stimulation – this is pin-prick hyperalgesia. Hyperalgesia is defined as an increased response to a stimulus that is normally painful.[7]

In most neuropathic pain states the lesion involves the small-fibre systems, either the small nerve fibres in a peripheral nerve or their central projections in the spinothalamic tract. Sensory testing of small nerve fibre function is, therefore, of special importance. In general practice, equipment available for small-fibre testing will be limited. Apart from pin-prick (a test of A-δ fibres), thermal sensation is also important. A cool object, such as a tuning fork or a tube of cold water, is an easy way to detect reduced sensation to cold. A difference of one side from the other in the case of unilateral involvement or improved cold sensation in proximal parts of the extremities in a polyneuropathy may confirm the involvement of small A-δ nerve fibres.

In hospital departments (neurological units, pain clinics, clinical neurophysiology laboratories) more sophisticated equipment is available. An easy way to determine reduced sensitivity to cold and warmth is the use of thermo-rolls, which are metal rolls adjusted to temperatures of 25°C for cool and 40°C for warmth. These are rolled over the patient's skin. Detailed information about thermal sensation may be obtained by the quantitative determination of thermal thresholds, such as heat and heat pain (C-fibres), cool (A-δ fibres) and cold pain (A-δ and C fibres). A detailed description of the method is given elsewhere.[10] All quantitative sensory testing requires that the patient be awake and fully capable of cooperating during the examination. It is not easy to test children.

The test results must be regarded as semi-objective. It is also important to be aware that determinations of thermal threshold are less sensitive than other tests of peripheral small fibre function, such as skin biopsies and the quantitative sudomotor axon reflex test (QSART).[11] The advantage of the thermal threshold determination is that it is non-invasive and easy to perform. The interpretation of the results is not always simple, however, and it is of utmost importance to stress that the results must be correlated with the clinical symptoms and findings in the patient in order to avoid incorrect conclusions. It is also important to remember that thermal testing measures the function of the small nerve fibre systems from the periphery to the cerebral cortex. The level of the lesion cannot be determined by this test procedure alone.

Autonomic dysfunction

In an evaluation of a possible complex regional pain syndrome (CRPS type 1 and 2), assessment of autonomic dysfunction is of great value. Oedema is a frequent finding, but may be intermittent and not always present at the time of examination. Discoloration of the skin (red/blue) may be present, and increased or reduced sweating. The latter may be measured objectively using the QSART.[11, 12] The patient often complains that the affected extremity is colder than the normal side, reflecting disturbed circulation. The latter may be documented objectively by measuring the skin temperature; a difference between the right or left of 1°C or more is significant. Trophic changes of skin are seen as thin, glossy skin, and trophic changes of nails are reported as slower growth than on the affected side.

Central sensitization

Most neuropathic pain states are characterized by signs of central sensitization, making an assessment of these phenomena important. It is recommended that the presence of allodynia to light touch, and its distribution, is assessed by the use of cotton wool or a brush lightly applied to the skin. The presence of hyperalgesia to punctate stimuli is detected with von Frey hairs, or in general practice with a sharp object (e.g. a needle). The areas affected may be marked on body charts. The area of punctate hyperalgesia will in general be larger than the area of allodynia to light touch. The presence of allodynia and/or hyperalgesia is suggestive of neuropathic pain, but is not diagnostic, as these may occur also in nociceptive pain.

Abnormal temporal summation (due to central sensitization) is tested by repetitive stimulation of a painful area by a thick von Frey hair at a frequency of 3/second over several seconds. In patients with neuropathic pain, an intense and sudden pain may appear after a latency of a few seconds, often radiating from the site of stimulation and with an unpleasant after-sensation.

Supplementary investigations

When a peripheral nerve injury is suspected, EMG/neurography is recommended as an objective measurement of the extent and level of involvement and as an evaluation of the prognosis. It is important to be aware that routine neurography will assess only the function of the large myelinated nerve fibres, i.e. motor nerve fibres in a motor nerve fascicle, and the large, myelinated nerve fibres mediating impulses of light touch, vibration and pressure in a sensory nerve fascicle. Involvement of the small nerve fibres is frequent in patients with neuropathic pain but is not detected using EMG or neurography. Because small-fibre dysfunction may be the only finding in some patients with neuropathic pain of peripheral origin (e.g. small-fibre neuropathies), it may be argued that there is no indication for EMG and neurography. The present author disagrees, because results of EMG and neurography will, in the case of large fibres being involved, contribute to an understanding of the extent of the lesion as well as giving an insight into the prognosis. It is important, however, to be aware of the limitations.

In routine neurophysiological practice, sensory evoked potentials are derived from peripheral electrical stimulation, which projects to the dorsal columns and hence assesses the neural transmission of such sensory qualities as light touch, vibration and pressure. On the other hand, sensory evoked potentials following laser stimulation relate to pain and nociceptive impulses projected in the spinothalamic tract,[13] but this method is only available in a few laboratories.

CT and MRI investigations are important in order to visualize lesions in the CNS.

MECHANISMS OF NEUROPATHIC PAIN

The neurophysiological mechanisms of neuropathic pain are complex and most are still unknown. Both peripheral and central mechanisms may be involved in spontaneous persistent and paroxysmal pain following a peripheral nerve lesion. From animal experiments, both ectopic discharges in injured axons and abnormal, ephaptic contact between nerve fibres have been demonstrated.[14] There are relatively few studies from recordings in humans. Sensitization of originally mechanical- and heat-insensitive C-fibres has been demonstrated in patients with chronic pain.[15] Spontaneous activity and abnormal ephaptic coupling between afferent C-fibres has been seen in patients with neuropathic pain (R. Schmidt, K. Ørstavik, M. Schmelz, M. Hilliges, C. Weidner, B. Namer, E. Jørum, H. Handwerker and E. Torebjörk, personal communication, 2005). Of relevance to sympathetically mediated pain is abnormal coupling between afferent and efferent sympathetic C-fibres and the activation of insensitive C-fibres by catecholamines.[16]

Microneurography is an invasive, technically difficult method that is not available for routine investigations. There are no other routine methods that identify the different possible mechanisms in individual axons. This limits a mechanism-based classification in the individual patient.[17] We know, however, that most neuropathic pain conditions involve lesions of small nerve fibres (see above). It is possible to confirm a lesion of these nerve fibres objectively, but not to define the mechanism in more detail.

Mechanisms of evoked pain are to some extent better understood. It is well documented that some forms of evoked pain, such as allodynia to light touch and punctate hyperalgesia, are caused by central sensitization of dorsal horn neurons following an excessive barrage of pain impulses arriving in the spinal cord.[18] In the patient this produces hypersensitivity to tactile stimuli and can be detected clinically by the presence of allodynia to light touch and hyperalgesia to punctate stimuli. The major problem is that both allodynia to light touch and punctate hyperalgesia may be secondary to nociceptive pain; for

PRACTICE POINTS

- A thorough clinical examination is essential for the diagnosis of neuropathic pain.

- Neuropathic pain is usually characterized by the presence of spontaneous (constant and/or paroxysmal) pain as well as evoked pain.

- A clinical neurological examination is necessary for the evaluation of the level of injury.

- Neuropathic pain is almost always characterized by sensory abnormalities.

example, muscle pain and visceral pain referred to the skin and associated with cutaneous sensory abnormalities. The presence of evoked pain will often indicate neuropathic pain, but is not diagnostic for neuropathic pain.

SUMMARY

Neuropathic pain is defined as pain initiated or caused by a primary lesion in or dysfunction of the nervous system. The term 'dysfunction' is not clearly defined and is probably best omitted. The prevalence of neuropathic pain is unknown, but a few detailed studies show that it is more common than was previously assumed. It is underdiagnosed and consequently is not properly treated. Some common causes of neuropathic pain are entrapment and injuries of peripheral nerves, painful neuropathies, infections involving the nervous system (e.g. postherpetic neuralgia), spinal cord injuries, multiple sclerosis and cerebral infarcts. Evaluation of neuropathic pain is based on a thorough clinical examination, which must include detailed

RESEARCH AGENDA

- Since many of the mechanisms involved in neuropathic pain are still unclear, the major research agenda is further to explore and study the putative mechanisms.

- To develop appropriate clinical tests for the identification of the mechanisms involved in the individual patient with neuropathic pain.

questioning about different types of pain. Both spontaneous (persistent and paroxysmal) and evoked pain may occur. The persistent pain may be described using a large number of adjectives, such as burning, aching, throbbing, sore or cutting, but there is no pain descriptor that is diagnostic for neuropathic pain. Pain is usually evoked by lightly touching the skin or by exposure to cold. A clinical neurological examination is necessary in the evaluation of the level of injury, with EMG and neurography for peripheral nerve lesions and CT or MRI for central lesions. Neuropathic pain is almost always characterized by changes in sensation, usually involving the small-fibre system (peripheral nerve fibres or central projections). It is essential to examine for sensory dysfunction.

REFERENCES

1. Breivik H, Collett B, Ventafridda V et al. Survey of chronic pain in Europe: prevalence, impact on daily life and treatment. *Eur J Pain* 2006; **10**: 287–333.
2. Harstall C, Ospina M. How prevalent is chronic pain? *Pain: Clin Update* 2003; **11**: 1–4.
3. Österberg A, Boivie J, Thuomas KÅ. Central pain in multiple sclerosis – prevalence and clinical characteristics. *Eur J Pain* 2005; **9**: 531–542.
4. Siddall PJ, Yezierski RP, Loeser PD. Pain following spinal cord injury: clinical features, prevalence and taxonomy. *Tech Corner IASP News* 2000; 2000–2003.
5. Andersen G. Incidence of central post-stroke pain. *Pain* 1995; **61**: 187–193.
6. Dworkin RH, Backonja M, Rowbotham MC et al. Advances in neuropathic pain. *Arch Neurol* 2003; **60**: 1524–1534.
7. Merskey H, Bogduk N. *Classification of Chronic Pain*. IASP Press, New York, 1994.
8. Gruccu G, Anand P, Attal N et al. EFNS guidelines on neuropathic pain assessment. *Eur J Neurol* 2004; **11**: 153–162.
9. Rasmussen PV, Sindrup SH, Jensen TS et al. Symptoms and signs in patients with suspected neuropathic pain. *Pain* 2004; **110**: 461–469.
10. Jørum E, Arendt-Nielsen L. Sensory testing and clinical neurophysiology. In: Breivik H, Campell W, Eccleston C (eds), *Clinical Pain Management – Practical Applications and Procedures*. Arnold, London, 2002, pp. 27–38.
11. Low P. Evaluation of sudomotor function. *Clin Neurophysiol* 2004; **115**: 1506–1513.
12. Sandroni P, Low PA, Ferrer T et al. Complex regional pain syndrome (CRPS 1): prospective study and laboratory evaluation. *Clin J Pain* 1998; **14**: 282–289.
13. Arendt-Nielsen L. First pain related evoked potentials to argon laser stimuli – recording and quantification. *Neurol Neurosurg Psychiatry* 1990; **53**: 398–404.
14. Devor M. The pathophysiology of damaged peripheral nerves. In: Wall PD, Melxack R (eds) *Textbook of Pain*, 3rd edn. Churchill Livingstone, Edinburgh, 1994, pp. 79–100.
15. Ørstavik K, Weidner C, Schmidt R et al. Pathological C-fibres in patients with a chronic painful condition. *Brain* 2003; **126**: 567–578.
16. Jørum E, Ørstavik K, Schmidt R, Namer B, Carr RW, Kvarstein G, Hilliges M, Handwerker H, Torebjörk E, Schmelz M. Cathecholamine-induced excitation of nociceptors in sympathetically maintained pain. *Pain* 2006; in press.
17. Woolf C, Bennett GJ, Doherty M et al. Towards a mechanism-based classification of pain. *Pain* 1998; **77**: 227–229.
18. Woolf CJ, King AE. Dynamic alterations in the cutaneous mechanosensitive receptive fields of dorsal horn neurons in the rat spinal cord. *J Neurosci* 1990; **10**: 2717–2726.

Chapter 6
Diagnostic nerve blocks in chronic pain

Nikolai Bogduk

INTRODUCTION

Local anaesthetics are unique drugs. Whereas opioids and other drugs are capable of relieving pain to greater or lesser extents, local anaesthetics are the only drugs that can stop pain completely. Because of this property, local anaesthetics have been used extensively to provide regional or spinal anaesthesia for surgical procedures and childbirth. Their limited duration of action, however, has precluded local anaesthetics from being used as a long-term therapeutic agent for persistent pain. Nevertheless, local anaesthetics have found a particular niche in the management of certain chronic pain problems.

When the source of pain needs to be known, but cannot be determined by other means, such as physical examination or medical imaging, either the source or its nerve supply can be determined by performing diagnostic blocks of the suspected structure. In formal terms, a diagnostic block is the deliberate administration of a local anaesthetic in order to relieve pain temporarily with the express purpose of obtaining diagnostic information.

Diagnostic blocks have been used to study a variety of pain conditions. Some applications have survived unchallenged because they constitute traditional practices in anaesthesiology. More recent and innovative applications have had to survive close scrutiny, and have not been widely accepted despite the data that validates them.

MECHANISMS

The mechanism of action of local anaesthetics is complex, and differs according to the agent used and the state of the nerve being blocked. Local anaesthetics act on sodium channels to prevent or impede sodium flux, but their binding and duration of action depends on whether the channels are resting, open, closed or inactivated.[1, 2] In turn, these states of the channels depend on whether the membrane is being depolarized and the frequency of depolarization. In nerves that are actively conducting, local anaesthetics have a greater affinity for the channel than they have in resting nerves.

This difference in affinity underlies certain quantitative properties of local anaesthetics that pertain to the interpretation of diagnostic blocks. The duration of action of local anaesthetics has been determined by observation in subjects who were not experiencing ongoing or chronic pain. What was tested was cutaneous anaesthesia in patients undergoing minor surgical procedures or during childbirth. Accurate figures are difficult to ascertain because some investigators added adrenalin to the local anaesthetic, whereas others did not. Nevertheless, representative figures for lignocaine would be mean duration of 2–4 hours, with a standard deviation of 1–3 hours.[3–6] A duration of up to 7 hours is not unusual, and periods longer than 10 hours have been reported.[4] For bupivacaine, a mean duration of 4–8 hours with a standard deviation of 2–3 hours would be representative.[3–6] Periods of anaesthesia up to 12 hours are not unusual.

These figures should be understood to apply to individuals about to experience pain. They may not, and do not necessarily, apply to patients with persistent or chronic pain. Indeed, patients with neuropathic pain often exhibit extraordinarily prolonged responses to lignocaine,[7] probably because the agent is able to bind strongly and persistently to open and changing sodium channels. What the 'normal' duration of action of local anaesthetics is in patients with chronic pain has not been determined.

PRINCIPLES

The technical aspects of diagnostic blocks are important. Blocks should be performed with minimum discomfort to the patient. They should be performed adroitly, with as few as possible adjustments and readjustments of the needle used to deliver the local anaesthetic. For this reason, some practitioners measure and pride themselves on how quickly and slickly they can perform a block. However, expertise does not rest with the technical execution of the procedure alone but also on the interpretation of the patient's response.

Although diagnostic blocks may be performed in the same technical manner as blocks performed to provide regional anaesthesia, diagnostic blocks are performed in a different context. They are performed not to achieve an effect, such as numbness, but to determine if the patient's pain is relieved as a result of selectively blocking a particular structure. The quality of the block, therefore, depends on two factors: the accuracy of the block and the credibility of the response.

Accuracy

The inference to be drawn from a diagnostic block is that anaesthetizing a particular structure is what is responsible for the response. For this inference to be valid, the block must be target specific. Consequently, it must be shown that a diagnostic block accurately anaesthetizes the target structure and does not inadvertently anaesthetize some other structure that might be responsible for the patient's pain. This criterion requires not only the accurate delivery of a needle onto or into the target structure, but also the subsequent injection of a minimal volume of local anaesthetic. If volumes are too great the agent will spread to adjacent structures, and the investigator cannot be certain that the resultant effect is not due to anaesthetization of those adjacent structures.

Some practitioners might feel insecure about injecting small volumes, fearing that if they use too little of an agent they might fail to anaesthetize the target structure adequately. Accordingly, they use larger volumes just to be certain that the target structure is 'covered'. This form of overkill might be acceptable for inducing regional anaesthesia for a surgical procedure, but is inappropriate for the conduct of a diagnostic block. For a diagnostic block the obligation is not to secure anaesthesia at all costs but to ensure that the block is target specific. Operators should understand that little of the injected agent remains at the site of injection when large volumes are injected. As greater volumes are injected they disperse away from the target structure. Greater volumes, therefore, increase the risk of compromising the specificity of the block. Consequently, target specificity is always subject to an inescapable tension between injecting too little (and incurring a false-negative response) and injecting too much (and incurring a false-positive response). Operators might need to accept a small risk of false-negative results instead of habitually using large volumes and incurring too many false-positive results.

Where an agent is injected, and how far it spreads, can be determined by performing the diagnostic block under fluoroscopic control with a test dose of contrast medium. This demonstrates where the injection went and, more particularly, where it did not go. This facility has not been used for the more traditional and conventional diagnostic blocks in anaesthetic practice. Instead, practitioners have been taught to rely on anatomical

acumen to locate the target structure and to anaesthetize it selectively.

While this may be acceptable for blocks of peripheral and superficial nerves, the location of which is well known, and which do not lie near other significant structures, it is progressively less acceptable for deeper and more central structures. Not only are deeper structures harder to pinpoint in three dimensions, needles used to access them can stray from the desired course as they encounter resistance from intervening tissues. Accordingly, radiographic controls are effectively mandatory for deep targets. Without imaging to document accurate injection, an operator cannot be certain that their block has been target specific. Confidence in one's technique is not a substitute for objective evidence of accuracy.

Controls

There are no objective tests for the presence of pain or for its relief. Investigators rely only on what the patient reports. But patients can report relief of pain for reasons other than the effect of a local anaesthetic injected during a diagnostic block. They may have an expectation that the block will relieve their pain, particularly if they have been coached or instructed to expect a positive response. Unprompted, they might want the response to be positive so that they qualify for the resultant treatment that promises to relieve their pain permanently. Mischievous patients with medico-legal claims might choose to report relief in order to vindicate their claim.

Because of these extraneous, confounding factors, a positive response to a block cannot be summarily attributed to the effect of the local anaesthetic injected. Some form of control is necessary if the response is to be valid, and for the interpretation of the response to be correct.

The ultimate form of control is a placebo control, in which an inactive agent is injected to test for spurious responses. However, for two reasons, placebos cannot be administered in an arbitrary manner. In the first instance, administering a placebo on a single-blind basis is considered unethical in some jurisdictions. Patients would need to be informed that they might receive an inactive agent. Under those conditions, it transpires that if placebos are to be used, at least three injections are required.

The first injection must be an active agent, in order to provide prima facie information that anaesthetizing the target structure does, in fact, relieve the patient's pain. There is no point wasting resources and effort testing with a placebo a structure that is not involved in the patient's pain. The second injection cannot routinely be the placebo, for mischievous patients would know that the second injection is always the 'dummy'. In order to retain the effects of chance, the second injection must be randomized to be either an active or inactive agent. A third injection is required to administer the complementary agent. Under those conditions, a genuine response is one in which the patient reports complete relief of pain on each occasion that a local anaesthetic was used and no relief when the placebo was used. The validity of the response is made more secure if the injections are performed under double-blind conditions, so that the operator does not subconsciously communicate cues as to what to expect.

Whereas the triple block, placebo paradigm satisfies scientific rigour, it is not readily implemented in clinical practice. It involves multiple procedures and additional costs. An alternative paradigm is available. In textbooks of pain medicine, eminent authorities have advocated comparative local anaesthetic blocks in order to guard against placebo responses.[8–12] These involve administering a particular agent on the occasion of the first block, but using a different agent on a second occasion. The agents advocated are lignocaine and bupivacaine. The paradigm maintains that a genuine patient will report short-lasting relief when lignocaine is used and long-lasting relief when bupivacaine is used.

An important consideration for the interpretation of responses to comparative blocks is that it is not the absolute duration of relief that is important but the relative duration. In some individuals lignocaine lasts longer than does bupivacaine in other individuals. It is not a matter that the typical duration of action of lignocaine is 2 hours and that of bupivacaine is 4 hours. Lignocaine can last as long as 7 hours in some individuals, and bupivacaine as little as 1 hour in others. However, it has been shown that in the one individual, when both agents are injected simultaneously into symmetrical sites, bupivacaine consistently outlasts lignocaine.[5, 6] Therefore, the essential criterion for a positive response to comparative blocks is that the effect of bupivacaine is longer than that of lignocaine.

The comparative block paradigm was promoted on theoretical grounds, capitalizing on the known difference in duration of action of lignocaine and bupivacaine; but when promoted it had not been tested empirically. For more conventional diagnostic blocks it has still not been tested, but it has been tested in two ways in the context of diagnostic blocks of the medial branches of the cervical dorsal rami.

In one study, Barnsley et al.[13] administered lignocaine and bupivacaine on separate occasions under double-blind conditions. They considered true-positive responses to be ones in which the patients reported longer lasting relief of their pain when bupivacaine was used than when lignocaine was used. To establish the validity of the response they used a statistical test involving the binomial distribution. They found that the chances that the patients had guessed the correct agents were less than 2 in 10,000, on which grounds they concluded that the comparative block paradigm was valid.

Another study used a more conventional strategy. Lord et al.[14] subjected patients to triple blocks under double-blind conditions, using lignocaine, bupivacaine and normal saline in a randomized manner. They compared the diagnostic decision that would have been made on the basis of the responses to the two local anaesthetics alone, with the decision based on the response to normal saline. True responses were considered to be ones in which pain was relieved on each occasion when a local anaesthetic was used but not relieved when normal saline was used. False responses were ones in which pain was relieved when normal saline was injected. Contingency tables revealed that comparative blocks had a specificity of 88%. This means that

among patients with a positive response to comparative blocks, there is only a 12% chance that it is due to a placebo effect.

On the other hand, the sensitivity of comparative blocks was only 54%.[14] This means that, when strictly applied, the criteria for a positive response do not detect all patients with a genuine response. These criteria exclude some patients who do not respond to placebo blocks, but who experience paradoxically longer lasting relief following lignocaine than with bupivacaine. This type of response may be due to the different duration of action of lignocaine on open sodium channels in patients with ongoing pain. Consequently, failure to satisfy the comparative block criterion does not necessarily mean that the patient has reported a placebo response. Indeed, some 65% of patients who report discordant responses to lignocaine and bupivacaine do not respond to placebo blocks.[14]

Accordingly, the strength of comparative blocks lies not in detecting placebo responders, but in identifying true responses. If a patient has longer lasting relief with bupivacaine the investigator can be 88% certain that the response is true. If the criteria are relaxed to accept complete relief of pain irrespective of which agent lasted longer, the investigator can be 65% certain that the response is true.

Which type of control an investigator chooses to use, and which criteria should be used to assess comparative blocks, is a matter of preference depending on the circumstances. If an investigator wants to be or needs to be absolutely certain, placebo-controlled, triple blocks should be used. If a certainty of 88% is enough, comparative blocks with strict criteria can be used. If, on the other hand, the investigator can tolerate a false-positive rate of 35%, comparative blocks with relaxed criteria will suffice.

Cost-effectiveness

Controlled diagnostic blocks have scientific appeal in that they ensure the validity of the diagnostic inferences drawn about the response to blocks. However, they are not appealing logistically or financially.

Some practitioners seem reluctant to implement controls, preferring instead to rely just on the response to a single block. Such practice, however, ignores the prevalence of false-positive responses. It assumes that all positive responses are true responses, whereas the experimental data reveal that this is not the case. Single blocks are not valid. To shun controls for logistic reasons, therefore, is tantamount to shunning validity.

Some insurers are reluctant to pay for repeat blocks, which are necessary if controls are to be implemented. They seem not to understand or appreciate the virtue of validating the responses. They prefer to believe and accept the responses to single blocks, in the interests of keeping costs low.

A theoretical study has provided a model for assessing the cost-effectiveness of controlled diagnostic blocks.[15] This study showed that controlled blocks were effective, provided that the cost of treatment (or other subsequent costs) exceeded the cost of a block by a certain ratio. That ratio differed according to the nature of the condition being investigated and the prevalence of that condition.

The study showed that, under certain systems of reimbursement, in which the costs of treatment substantially outweighed the cost of blocks, controlled diagnostic blocks (and even placebo-controlled, triple blocks) were cost-effective. They succeeded in minimizing the number of patients with false-positive responses to an initial block who would go on to treatment that was destined to fail. Under other systems of reimbursement, however, the study found that the cost difference between blocks and treatment was too small, and controlled blocks were not cost-effective. This arose particularly in the USA, where facility fees dwarf physicians' fees, and render undertaking controls cost-ineffective. In effect, fee structures can inhibit proper intellectual practice, and render it more economical to have patients with an incorrect diagnosis undergo and fail treatment, instead of getting an accurate diagnosis in the first instance.

This irony should not constitute grounds for not using controlled blocks. It is a short-sighted argument that looks only at the immediate costs of investigation. It ignores the secondary costs of thousands of patients who become disaffected when treatment fails, and who continue to seek care. It ignores the fact that physicians skilled at performing blocks are wasting intellectual resources and time performing treatments that will fail, instead of directing those resources to actually helping patients. Even more shocking is patients receiving compensation settlements on the basis of single blocks, the result of which might be false.

NEUROPATHIC PAIN

Diagnostic blocks are sometimes used to study neuropathic pain, both in a research setting and in conventional practice. Injured nerves can be blocked at the site of injury or proximal to the site of injury, in order to determine if symptoms are generated by traffic along that nerve from the site of injury. Often they are not, and the block is negative. In that event, the block reveals that symptoms are mediated by some other nerve, or by more central mechanisms. In some instances, blocks of adjacent or overlapping nerves may relieve certain symptoms. This reveals that those nerves, rather than the injured nerve, are responsible for the symptoms.

When used in this way diagnostic blocks serve not so much to formulate a particular diagnosis but to elaborate the source and mechanisms of particular symptoms. The actual diagnosis of neuropathic pain is already apparent from the history and clinical examination. What is of interest is which nerves are mediating particular symptoms or signs.

Diagnostic blocks used for such purposes have been assumed to be valid. It is assumed that the local anaesthetic used actually blocks the target nerve (and no other relevant structure), and that the response is due to the action of the local anaesthetic. Controls have typically not been used, or called for. This lack of rigour is tolerated because the condition being studied is usually not controversial. The same concession does not apply for other diagnostic blocks. However, lessons learned from other conditions suggest that perhaps even conventional peripheral nerve blocks should be subjected to controls, when relief of pain is the cardinal outcome measure, and if that relief predicates a subsequent treatment.

SYMPATHETIC BLOCKS

Blocks of the sympathetic nervous system have traditionally been used to implicate the sympathetic nervous system in the production of pain in complex regional pain syndromes. They are used either to diagnose sympathetically maintained pain, to predict the response to sympathectomy, or both.

Some experts advocate that sympathetic blocks[16] should be performed under fluoroscopic guidance in order to ensure accuracy and safety of these blocks. Others, however, are satisfied to use traditional, blind techniques that rely on surface markings, palpation, and angle and depth of insertion,[12] with fluoroscopy being reserved for neurolytic blocks.[17] This latter type of practice has been criticized – the large volumes injected spread to anaesthetize structures other than the target nerve, thereby compromising the specificity of the block.[18] Others have observed that, in practice, only a minority of sympathetic blocks satisfy the requirements for a valid block.[19]

A more serious concern about sympathetic blocks is the lack of pharmacological controls. Since sympathetic blocks are traditional anaesthetic procedures they have usually been exempt from controls. Indeed, textbooks that describe and advocate these procedures conspicuously do not mention the need for controls.[12, 16] Even authors who demand controls for other blocks do not require them for sympathetic blocks.[20] Although lumbar sympathetic blocks have not been studied in this regard, sobering data have emerged concerning stellate ganglion blocks.

Price et al.[21] performed stellate ganglion blocks on patients with complex regional pain syndromes of the upper limb, using either a local anaesthetic or normal saline. Strikingly, they found that normal saline was virtually as effective as local anaesthetic in relieving pain and other features. Indeed, there was no significant difference in the incidence of positive responses, or the degree of pain relief, when the two agents were compared. Where the agents differed, however, was in the duration of effect. On average, symptoms returned within 12 hours when the patients received normal saline, but over 3–5 days when they received a local anaesthetic. However, while there were statistically significant differences in mean durations of effect, some patients treated with normal saline had responses that lasted 1–3 days, while some patients treated with local anaesthetic had responses for only 1 day.

These results warn that the effects seen immediately after sympathetic blocks, or even on the following day or two, cannot be summarily attributed to the action of local anaesthetic. The same effects appear if normal saline is used. Therefore, relief of pain or other features cannot be attributed to having anaesthetized sympathetic nerves. For sympathetic blocks to be valid, controls are essential, in case a response due to non-specific effects is misattributed to the action of the local anaesthetic. Failure to do so risks interventions such as sympathectomy being undertaken in patients who will not respond to the intervention.

MEDIAL BRANCH BLOCKS

The zygapophysial joints are a possible source of spinal pain, both in the cervical region and in the lumbar region, but there are no clinical or imaging features by which zygapophysial joint pain can be diagnosed.[22–28] The only means of diagnosing pain stemming from these joints are blocks of the nerves that innervate them: the medial branches of the dorsal rami.

Medial branch blocks have not met with universal approval and acceptance. Indeed, they have attracted stern resistance and criticism from some authorities.[20, 29] Yet, in some instances such criticism occurs in chapters in books[20] but the succeeding chapter endorses and advocates these blocks.[30] A thorough consideration of the literature reveals that, despite the criticism, these blocks are ironically the most extensively tested and best validated of all diagnostic blocks in pain medicine. Their faults are only that they did not arise from within the mainstream and that they pertain to patients with conditions that are subject to litigation; both of which features seem to incite resentment.

Principles

The medial branches of the dorsal rami of the spinal nerves assume constant anatomical relationships to bone. This allows their location to be identified under fluoroscopy, so that the nerve can be blocked accurately and selectively.[31, 32]

If stated strictly, the objective of a medial branch block is to determine whether or not a particular medial branch mediates the patient's pain. This is achieved by selectively anaesthetizing the selected nerve. In practice, however, the prevailing concept is that medial branch blocks test for pain stemming from a particular zygapophysial joint. Under those conditions, each of the two nerves that supply the target joint need to be anaesthetized. Medial branches can be anaesthetized with as little as 0.3 mL of local anaesthetic. Larger volumes are not required.

For medial branch blocks to be valid, they must satisfy the criteria for face validity and for construct validity. It should be shown that: medial branch blocks do block the target nerve and no other significant structure; that they do relieve zygapophysial joint pain; and that they do distinguish between pain arising from the target joint and pain from other sources. Moreover, they should have predictive validity, alias therapeutic utility – a positive block should lead to successful therapy. To various extents and in various ways these criteria have been tested and satisfied both for lumbar medial branch blocks and for cervical medial branch blocks.

Lumbar medial branch blocks

Studies in normal volunteers have shown that lumbar medial branch blocks protect subjects from experimentally induced zygapophysial joint pain.[33] Studies have also shown that material injected onto the lumbar medial branches does not spread to adjacent structures, which if anaesthetized might relieve a patient's pain.[34] If the correct target points are used and if small volumes are injected (< 0.5 mL), injectate does not spread into the epidural space, does not spread to other medial branches and does not infiltrate the back muscles indiscriminately. On these grounds, lumbar medial branch blocks have consummate face validity and target specificity. There is, however, an 8% chance of the injection being made into the vena commitans of the medial branch.[33] While venous uptake of < 0.5 mL of local anaesthetic does not constitute a complication, it does give rise to a risk of a false-negative response. For this reason, proponents advocate checking the injection with a preliminary injection of contrast medium in order to test for venous uptake.

Single blocks of lumbar medial branches have a false-positive rate of 25–41%.[22, 23, 35] This means that if the prevalence of lumbar zygapophysial joint pain is 15% (see below), for every three blocks that appear to be positive, two will be false-positive. If the prevalence is 5%, five out of every six blocks will be false-positive. Such yields of false-positive results are unacceptable and indicate that a valid diagnosis cannot be made using a single diagnostic block.

The validity of medial branch blocks is secured by performing controlled blocks in each and every patient. In principle, these could be placebo-controlled, triple blocks. In practice, comparative local anaesthetic blocks are likely to be more palatable.

Lumbar medial branch blocks have diagnostic utility. When performed under controlled conditions they serve to identify patients whose pain stems from the lumbar zygapophysial joints. Establishing such a diagnosis serves to save the patient from continuing and futile pursuit of a diagnosis by other means. Several studies have estimated the prevalence of zygapophysial joint pain in patients with chronic back pain. Among injured workers, with a median age of 38 years, the prevalence was found to be 15% (95% confidence interval (CI) 10–20%).[24] In an older population, without a history of trauma, the prevalence was found to be 40% (95% CI 27–53%).[25] A similar prevalence (45%; 95% CI 39–54%) was found in a heterogeneous population attending a pain clinic.[22]

These figures, however, probably overestimate the actual prevalence of lumbar zygapophysial joint pain, because they are based on a criterion standard of at least 50% relief of pain, not complete relief of pain. This criterion is specious. Proponents contend that 50% relief implies that the joint blocked is only one of two or more sources of pain. However, no one has ever demonstrated what those other sources are. Formal studies have shown that zygapophysial joint pain occurs concurrently with either discogenic pain or sacroiliac joint pain in fewer than 3% of cases.[36, 37] So these other structures cannot be the elusive, other source of pain in patients who obtain partial relief from lumbar medial branch blocks. A more demanding interpretation is that 50% relief amounts to no more than an indeterminate response, or even a placebo response.

When studies have used complete relief of pain as the criterion standard, the prevalence of lumbar zygapophysial joint pain drops to only about 5%, in a general population.[38, 39] If the standard is relaxed to 90% relief, a prevalence of 32% has been reported in an elderly population.[25]

For those patients in whom controlled, lumbar medial branch blocks are positive, treatment is available in the form of percutaneous radiofrequency neurotomy. This procedure has been shown not be a placebo,[40] and can provide lasting results in properly selected patients, provided that the operation is performed meticulously.[41] Some 80% of patients can expect at least 60% relief of their pain, lasting for at least 12 months; and 60% of patients can expect at least 80% relief of their pain for at least 12 months.[41]

Cervical medial branch blocks

Studies have shown that cervical medial branch blocks are target specific. Solutions injected at the correct target point do not spread to the epidural space; they do not anaesthetize spinal nerves or ventral rami; they do not spread to other medial branches; and they do not infiltrate the posterior neck muscles indiscriminately.[42] Much of the solution injected remains pooled at the target site, under the tendon of the semispinalis capitis, and any excess solution spreads away from this point in the cleavage plane deep to the semispinalis and superficial to the multifidus. Cervical medial branch blocks, therefore, satisfy the criteria for face validity.

Single blocks of the cervical medial branches are liable to false-positive responses. Some 27% of positive responses to an initial block prove to be false-positive upon subsequent testing.[43] The validity of cervical medial branch blocks is secured by performing controlled blocks in each and every case.[13, 14]

Cervical medial branch blocks have enormous diagnostic utility. Several studies have now shown that cervical zygapophysial joint pain is a very common basis, if not the single most common basis, for chronic neck pain after whiplash injury. In three studies using a criterion of complete relief of pain the prevalence estimates were 54% (95% CI 40–68%),[44] 60% (95% CI 46–73%)[45] and 36% (95% CI 27–45%).[46] In drivers who sustain a whiplash injury at high impact speeds, the prevalence has been found to be 74% (95% CI 65–83%).[47] No diagnosis of cervical zygapophysial joint pain can be made other than by medial branch blocks. Not using blocks denies a valid diagnosis in some 60% of patients. Perhaps of greater significance is the fact that double-blind controlled blocks can be used to establish a diagnosis in patients with an insurance claim, but who are suspected, if not accused, of malingering.[48] Controlled blocks can establish that they really do suffer pain.

Cervical medial branch blocks have therapeutic utility. Patients with a positive response to controlled blocks become eligible for percutaneous radiofrequency neurotomy. This is the only treatment for chronic neck pain that has been validated in a randomized, double-blind, controlled trial, and it is the only treatment that has been shown to be capable of totally eliminating neck pain and eliminating psychological distress secondary to that pain.[49] The effects are long lasting, and can be reinstated by repeating the procedure if the pain recurs.[50] The results are not influenced by litigation status. Patients with a legal claim respond just as well as those who have settled their claim.[50, 51]

With respect to predictive utility, the outcomes from radiofrequency neurotomy are the same regardless of what type of control block is used. Patients respond equally well if they are positive to placebo-controlled blocks or to comparative blocks. For practical purposes, therefore, comparative blocks seem to be sufficient to screen patients for cervical medial branch neurotomy.

DIAGNOSTIC EPIDURALS

In 1985, Cherry et al.[52] introduced a novel form of diagnostic epidural block. It was designed to serve as a screening test to distinguish nociceptive pain from non-nociceptive and, ostensibly, central pain. The protocol required administering normal saline and fentanyl through an epidural catheter, at 20 minute intervals, followed by intravenous naloxone, and then epidural lignocaine.

Depending on the nature of the responses, inferences could be drawn about the nature of the patient's pain. A patient with nociceptive pain would have no response to each of the injections of normal saline, but would obtain relief from fentanyl, which would be reversed by naloxone, and reinstated by lignocaine. Spurious responses, not conforming to this pattern, suggest factors other than nociception to be the basis for the complaint of pain.

Cherry et al.[52] proposed that diagnostic epidurals could be used to identify patients who had a genuine, peripheral source of pain, but which was not evident on conventional investigations. A positive response could be used to justify a more concerted investigation of the patient's possible source of pain. In contrast, a spurious response would constitute grounds for not pursuing a physical source of pain.

The same workers[52] illustrated the application of their protocol with a few case studies, but no systematic studies of this procedure, and no validation studies have subsequently been reported. This is perhaps unfortunate. In principle, diagnostic epidurals hold promise as a screening test before any more specific diagnostic blocks are undertaken, particularly in the context of controversial spinal pain. If diagnostic epidurals were to be shown to be valid for nociceptive pain, they could be applied to identify those patients in whom further, and perhaps intensive, investigation with diagnostic blocks was justified, and those patients in whom further blocks were not justified. Such a screening test would improve the efficiency of diagnostic blocks by screening out patients who are not likely to respond or who are likely to have spurious results.

INTRA-ARTICULAR BLOCKS

Some joints cannot be anaesthetized by blocking the nerves that supply them, because the nerves are inaccessible or cannot be selectively anaesthetized. Those joints, however, can be blocked with intra-articular injections of local anaesthetic.

Although local anaesthetics are commonly injected into large joints of the limb, such as the shoulder, hip and knee, these injections are typically performed for therapeutic purposes. They are not employed as a diagnostic tool because, by convention, there is no doubt that the target joint is the source of pain. An intriguing study on the knee, however, has cast doubt on the probity of this confidence.[53] Twenty patients were randomized to receive an intra-articular injection of bupivacaine or normal saline. The group results showed that significant reductions in pain occurred only in the local anaesthetic group.[53] However, two features emerged from within each group. Only five of the ten patients who received local anaesthetic obtained complete relief of pain. Two had no change, and two had only partial relief. This suggests that in some patients believed to have joint pain the pain does not arise from within the joint. In the placebo group, two patients reported dramatic relief of pain, from 30 to 3, and from 72 to 10, on a 100-point visual–analogue scale. At 24 hours after injection four patients each in the local anaesthetic group and the placebo group reported their pain to be better or much better. These outcomes warn of the need to control for possible placebo responses, even with intra-articular blocks.

Intra-articular blocks of the lumbar or cervical zygapophysial joints are sometimes, if not often, used as a diagnostic test of pain from these joints. The validity of these blocks, however, has not been tested and established in the same manner as have medial branch blocks of the same structures. For that reason, the test of choice for zygapophysial joint pain must be medial branch blocks.

Two types of control have been used to pinpoint pain stemming from the sacroiliac joint. In one study, anatomical controls were used, in that patients underwent zygapophysial joint blocks, under single-blind conditions, prior to undergoing sacroiliac joint blocks.[37] The patients had no response to the zygapophysial joint blocks but positive responses to intra-articular blocks of the sacroiliac joint. This study established a prevalence of 13% (95% CI 6–20%) for sacroiliac joint pain among patients with chronic low back pain.[37] The other study used comparative local anaesthetic blocks, administered intra-articularly.[54] It found a prevalence of 20%.

DISCUSSION

Virtually any nerve in the body can be blocked. Therefore, a chapter on diagnostic blocks could list a litany of different procedures defined by the target nerve. Indeed, this is what many textbook chapters on blocks do. However, such chapters typically focus on how and when to perform the blocks. They seldom consider the validity and utility of the block.

In the present chapter, the emphasis has been on medial branch blocks, but not because these are the only blocks in pain medicine, or the most important blocks, but because they have been the most comprehensively studied and validated blocks. Despite being a relatively recent innovation they set the benchmark of standards for diagnostic blocks.

Research has shown that medial branch blocks are target specific and have face validity. They have construct validity, but only when they are performed under controlled conditions. Single blocks are not valid because they suffer too high a rate of false-positive results. Controlled blocks are mandatory. This is not a rule for academics or restricted to research studies. If

practitioners in conventional practice are not performing medial branch blocks under controlled conditions, they are not practising valid procedures. The responses they encounter will be confounded by a high incidence of false-positive responses.

These same principles should apply to all diagnostic blocks in pain medicine, be they sympathetic blocks, blocks of branches of the trigeminal nerve, blocks of intercostal or abdominal nerves, or blocks of other peripheral nerves. Unless blocks are controlled the risk arises of the response being false-positive, and the diagnosis being wrong. The utility and validity of diagnostic blocks in pain medicine lie not in the fast and clever execution of the block but in the quality of the information obtained. For that, controls are imperative.

SUMMARY

- Diagnostic blocks are performed in a different context and for a different purpose from that of regional anaesthetic blocks.

PRACTICE POINTS

- Diagnostic blocks are not equivalent to providing regional anaesthesia.
- Diagnostic blocks are performed to obtain information, and are therefore subject to different considerations from those that apply to regional anaesthesia.
- Diagnostic blocks are subject to false-positive responses.
- In order to be valid, diagnostic blocks must be target-specific and must be controlled.
- Fluoroscopy and contrast medium can be used to determine the accuracy of a diagnostic block.
- In order to control for false-positive responses, diagnostic blocks should be performed using placebo controls or comparative local anaesthetic blocks.
- Some systems of reimbursement inhibit good practice by not paying for controlled blocks.
- Although apparently cost-effective in the short-term for individual cases, not using controlled blocks is wasteful of resources at large, and in the long-term.
- The symptoms of complex regional pain syndromes can be relieved equally well by normal saline as by lignocaine.
- In light of the above point, practitioners should not be satisfied that an uncontrolled sympathetic block is diagnostic of sympathetic-mediated symptoms.
- In order to be valid, all sympathetic blocks should be controlled.
- Of all diagnostic blocks, medial branch blocks have been the most comprehensively studied.
- Medial branch blocks have been shown to have face validity, construct validity, diagnostic utility and therapeutic utility.

- Diagnostic blocks are performed to obtain diagnostic information about a patient's pain or other symptoms.
- For diagnostic blocks to be valid, they must be accurate and target specific, and be performed under controlled conditions.
- Studies have shown that uncontrolled blocks are associated with unacceptably high rates of false-positive responses.
- Even the effects of sympathetic blocks may be false-positive.
- Medial branch blocks of the cervical and lumbar dorsal rami have been extensively validated, and serve as a model for how other blocks should be validated.
- Diagnostic epidural blocks with opioids have the potential to serve as a screening test for nociceptive pain of unknown origin, but need to be validated.
- When nerve blocks are not possible for certain joints, intra-articular blocks can be used, but should be subjected to controls.

RESEARCH AGENDA

- The validity of comparative blocks needs to be assessed for blocks other than medial branch blocks.
- The validity of lumbar sympathetic blocks should be tested against controlled blocks.
- There is a pressing need for diagnostic epidural blocks with opioids to be validated as a screening test for nociceptive pain.

REFERENCES

1. Strichartz GR. Neural physiology and local anesthetic action. In: Cousins MJ, Bridenbaugh PO (eds), *Neural Blockade in Clinical Anesthesia and Management of Pain*, 2nd edn. JB Lippincott, Philadelphia, PA, 1988, pp. 25–45.
2. Butterworth JF, Strichartz GR. Molecular mechanisms of local anesthesia: a review. *Anesthesiology* 1990; **72**: 711–734.
3. Rubin AP, Lawson DIF. A controlled trial of bupivacaine: a comparison with lignocaine. *Anaesthesia* 1968; **23**: 327–331.
4. Watt MJ, Ross DM, Atkinson RS. A double blind trial of bupivacaine and lignocaine. *Anaesthesia* 1968; **23**: 331–337.
5. Moore DC, Bridenbaugh LD, Bridenbaugh PO et al. Bupivacaine for peripheral nerve block: a comparison with mepivacaine, lidocaine, and tetracaine. *Anesthesiology* 1970; **32**: 460–463.
6. Moore DC, Bridenbaugh LD, Bridenbaugh PO et al. Bupivacaine: a review of 2,077 cases. *JAMA* 1970; **214**: 713–718.
7. Arner S, Lindblom U, Meyerson BA et al. Prolonged relief of neuralgia after regional anaesthetic blocks. A call for further experimental and systematic clinical studies. *Pain* 1990; **43**: 287–297.
8. Bonica JJ. Local anesthesia and regional blocks. In: Wall PD, Melzack R (eds), *Textbook of Pain*, 2nd edn. Churchill Livingston, Edinburgh, 1989, pp. 724–743.
9. Bonica JJ, Buckley FP. Regional analgesia with local anesthetics. In: Bonica JJ (ed.), *The Management of Pain*, vol. II. Lea and Febiger, Philadelphia, PA, 1990, pp. 1883–1966.
10. Boas RA. Nerve blocks in the diagnosis of low back pain. *Neurosurg Clin North Am* 1991; **2**: 807–816.
11. Bonica JJ, Butler SH. Local anaesthesia and regional blocks. In: Wall PD, Melzack R (eds), *Textbook of Pain*, 3rd edn. Churchill Livingstone, Edinburgh, 1994, pp. 997–1023.
12. Buckley FP. Regional anesthesia with local anesthetics. In: Loeser JD (ed.), *Bonica's Management of Pain*, 3rd edn. Lippincott Williams & Wilkins, Philadelphia, PA, 2001, pp. 1893–1952.
13. Barnsley L, Lord S, Bogduk N. Comparative local anaesthetic blocks in the diagnosis of cervical zygapophysial joints pain. *Pain* 1993; **55**: 99–106.
14. Lord SM, Barnsley L, Bogduk N. The utility of comparative local anaesthetic blocks versus placebo-controlled blocks for the diagnosis of cervical zygapophysial joint pain. *Clin J Pain* 1995; **11**: 208–213.
15. Bogduk N, Holmes S. Controlled zygapophysial joint blocks: the travesty of cost-effectiveness. *Pain Med* 2000, **1**: 25–34.
16. Hanningto-Kiff JG. Sympathetic nerve blocks in painful limb disorders. In: Wall PD, Melzack R (eds), *Textbook of Pain*, 3rd edn. Churchill Livingstone, Edinburgh, 1994, pp. 1035–1052.
17. Butler SH, Charlton JE. Neurolytic blockade and hypophysectomy. In: Loeser JD (ed.), *Bonica's Management of Pain*, 3rd edn. Lippincott Williams & Wilkins, Philadelphia, PA, 2001, pp. 1967–2010.
18. Haddox JD. A call for clarity. In: Campbell JN (ed.), *Pain 1996. An Updated Review. Refresher Course Syllabus*. IASP Press, Seattle, WA, 1996, pp. 97–99.
19. Malmquist ELA, Bengtssom M, Sorensen J. Efficacy of stellate ganglion block: a clinical study with bupivacaine. *Regional Anesth* 1992; **17**: 340–347.
20. Hogan QH, Abram SE. Diagnostic and prognostic neural blockade. In: Cousins MJ, Bridenbaugh PO (eds), *Neural Blockade in Clinical Anesthesia and Management of Pain*, 3rd edn. Lippincott-Raven, Philadelphia, 1998, pp. 937–977.
21. Price DD, Long S, Wilsey B et al. Analysis of peak magnitude and duration of analgesia produced by local anesthetics injected into sympathetic ganglion of complex regional pain syndrome patients. *Clin J Pain* 1998; **14**: 216–226.
22. Manchikanti L, Pampati V, Fellows B et al. Prevalence of lumbar facet joint pain in chronic low back pain. *Pain Physician* 1999; **2**: 59–64.
23. Manchikanti L, Pampati V, Fellows B et al. The diagnostic validity and therapeutic value of lumbar facet joint nerve blocks with or without adjuvant agents. *Curr Rev Pain* 2000; **4**: 337–344.
24. Schwarzer AC, Aprill CN, Derby R et al. Clinical features of patients with pain stemming from the lumbar zygapophysial joints. Is the lumbar facet syndrome a clinical entity? *Spine* 1994; **19**: 1132–1137.
25. Schwarzer AC, Wang S, Bogduk N et al. Prevalence and clinical features of lumbar zygapophysial joint pain: a study in an Australian population with chronic low back pain. *Ann Rheum Dis* 1995; **54**: 100–106.
26. Schwarzer AC, Derby R, Aprill CN et al. Pain from the lumbar zygapophysial joints: a test of two models. *J Spinal Dis* 1994; **7**: 331–336.
27. Manchikanti L, Pampati V, Fellows B et al. The inability of the clinical picture to characterize pain from facet joints. *Pain Physician* 2000; **3**: 158–166.
28. Schwarzer AC, Wang S, O'Driscoll D et al. The ability of computed tomography to identify a painful zygapophysial joint in patients with chronic low back pain. *Spine* 1995; **20**: 907–912.
29. Hogan QH, Abrams SE. Neural blockade for diagnosis and prognosis: a review. *Anesthesiology* 1997; **86**: 216–241.
30. Manning DC, Rowlingson JC. Back pain and the role of neural blockade. In: Cousins MJ, Bridenbaugh PO (eds), *Neural Blockade in Clinical Anesthesia and Management of Pain*, 3rd edn. Lippincott-Raven, Philadelphia, 1998, pp. 879–914.
31. Bogduk N, Wilson AS, Tynan W. The human lumbar dorsal rami. *J Anat* 1982; **134**: 383–397.
32. Bogduk N. The clinical anatomy of the cervical dorsal rami. *Spine* 1982; **7**: 319–330.
33. Kaplan M, Dreyfuss P, Halbrook B et al. The ability of lumbar medial branch blocks to anesthetize the zygapophysial joint. *Spine* 1998; **23**: 1847–1852.
34. Dreyfuss P, Schwarzer AC, Lau P et al. Specificity of lumbar medial branch and L5 dorsal ramus blocks: a computed tomographic study. *Spine* 1997; **22**: 895–902.
35. Schwarzer AC, Aprill CN, Derby R et al. The false-positive rate of uncontrolled diagnostic blocks of the lumbar zygapophysial joints. *Pain* 1994; **58**: 195–200.
36. Schwarzer AC, Aprill CN, Derby R et al. The prevalence and clinical features of internal disc disruption in patients with chronic low back pain. *Spine* 1995; **20**: 1878–1883.
37. Schwarzer AC, Aprill CN, Bogduk N. The sacroiliac joint in chronic low back pain. *Spine* 1995; **20**: 31–37.
38. Carette S, Marcoux S, Truchon R et al. A controlled trial of corticosteroid injections into facet joints for chronic low back pain. *N Engl J Med* 1991; **325**: 1002–1007.
39. Jackson RP, Jacobs RR, Montesano PX. Facet joint injection in low back pain. A prospective study. *Spine* 1988; **13**: 966–971.
40. van Kleef M, Barendse GAM, Kessels A et al. Randomized trial of radiofrequency lumbar facet denervation for chronic low back pain. *Spine* 1999; **24**: 1937–1942.

41. Dreyfuss P, Halbrook B, Pauza K et al. Efficacy and validity of radiofrequency neurotomy for chronic lumbar zygapophysial joint pain. *Spine* 2000; **25**: 1270–1277

42. Barnsley L, Bogduk N. Medial branch blocks are specific for the diagnosis of cervical zygapophysial joint pain. *Region Anesth* 1993; **18**: 343–350.

43. Barnsley L, Lord S, Wallis B et al. False-positive rates of cervical zygapophysial joint blocks. *Clin J Pain* 1993; **9**: 124–130.

44. Barnsley L, Lord SM, Wallis BJ et al. The prevalence of chronic cervical zygapophysial joint pain after whiplash. *Spine* 1995; **20**: 20–26.

45. Lord S, Barnsley L, Wallis BJ et al. Chronic cervical zygapohysial joint pain after whiplash: a placebo-controlled prevalence study. *Spine* 1996; **21**: 1737–1745.

46. Speldewinde GC, Bashford GM, Davidson IR. Diagnostic cervical zygapophysial joint blocks for chronic cervical pain. *Med J Aust* 2001; **174**: 174–176.

47. Gibson T, Bogduk N, Macpherson J et al. Crash characteristics of whiplash associated chronic neck pain. *J Musculoskelet Pain* 2000; **8**: 87–95.

48. Bogduk N. Diagnostic blocks. A truth serum for malingering. *Clin J Pain* 2004; **20**: 409–414.

49. Lord SM, Barnsley L, Wallis BJ et al. Percutaneous radio-frequency neurotomy for chronic cervical zygapophysial-joint pain. *N Engl J Med* 1996; **335**: 1721–1726.

50. McDonald G, Lord SM, Bogduk N. Long-term follow-up of cervical radio-frequency neurotomy for chronic neck pain. *Neurosurgery* 1999; **45**: 61–68.

51. Sapir D, Gorup JM. Radiofrequency medial branch neurotomy in litigant and nonlitigant patients with cervical whiplash. *Spine* 2001; **26**: E268–E273.

52. Cherry DA, Gourlay GK, McLachlan M et al. Diagnostic epidural opioid blockade and chronic pain: preliminary report. *Pain* 1985; **21**: 143–152.

53. Creamer P, Hunt M, Dieppe P. Pain mechanisms in osteoarthritis of the knee. Effect of intra-articular anesthetic. *J Rheumatol* 1996; **23**: 1031–1036.

54. Maigne JY, Aivaliklis A, Pfefer F. Results of sacroiliac joint double block and value of sacroiliac pain provocation tests in 54 patients with low-back pain. *Spine* 1996; **21**: 1889–1892.

SECTION 4

Spinal pain

Chapter 7
Neck pain

Robert Ferrari and Anthony S. Russell

INTRODUCTION

The problem with neck pain is that it does not end there. Neck pain, especially chronic neck pain, is often accompanied by a host of other symptoms the association of which is difficult to explain on a physiological basis alone. Neck pain is often just one feature of the nebulous syndromes such as chronic whiplash, myofascial pain syndrome, fibromyalgia and cervicobrachial syndrome. Chronic neck pain also brings with it the spectre of litigation (e.g. whiplash issues) and disability claims. In addition, there is a tendency for overinvestigation and overtreatment, often as a result of the level of a patient's distress at the failure of the medical community to provide helpful answers.

In this chapter we deal with the fact that the epidemiology of neck pain clearly indicates this to be a major health and economic burden, but the traditional diagnostic approach based on history, physical examination and investigations provides little solution for most patients. We argue that much of this endemic musculoskeletal problem is fostered by psychosocial factors, including personality traits, social status (or lack thereof), iatrogenic and legal factors, and an excessive reliance on the 'injury or disease' model. The reader is referred to the review by Bogduk[1] for a discussion of and the approach to neck pain in general. In addition to providing an update to this review, we focus here on certain aspects that deal more with how the current medical approach to neck pain, and whiplash in particular, is unhelpful and requires a reevaluation in favour of a new paradigm.

DEFINITION AND AETIOLOGY

Neck pain is generally defined as stiffness and/or pain felt dorsally in the cervical region somewhere between the occipital condyles and the C7 vertebral prominence. Neck pain, however, is often accompanied by pain in the occiput (a headache), the upper thoracic region and the jaws. Clinically, it is recognized

that even in subjects with no evidence of nerve-root irritation or compression, neck pain may be associated with pain referred along myotomal patterns to the anterior chest, arm and dorsal spine regions. The neurological examination would, of course, be normal.

The less common causes of neck pain include tumours, systemic arthropathy (e.g. rheumatoid arthritis, ankylosing spondylitis), infections, thyroid disorders, oesophageal obstruction or reflux disease. In addition, the neck is a site for referred pain from cardiac, gastric and diaphragmatic disease processes. Yet, perhaps 95% of neck pain patients will receive a more benign diagnosis (e.g. neck sprain, mechanical neck pain, muscular neck pain, myofascial pain syndrome, postural neck pain). These latter diagnoses are both a blessing and a curse for the patient. While they reflect a benign aspect in terms of mortality, the vagueness of the diagnosis often leaves the patient searching for a more definitive pathological understanding of their pain, and they soon encounter many who are willing to creatively ascribe the pain to facet joint and other subluxations, trigger points and muscle bands, chronic musculoligamentous injury, etc. The non-specificity of most neck pain is fodder for the imaginative therapist to produce a remarkable array of unprovable and untestable explanations.

The most remarkable aspects of the aetiology of neck pain, acute as well as chronic, are how seldom we know or can tell the patient we have identified the source of pain. The corollary is how often obvious pathology exists in entirely asymptomatic patients. A population-based best estimate of the outcome of acute neck pain is that at least 80% of all acute neck pain resolves within days to weeks.[2-4] Even though we believe that there should be a structural cause for neck pain that lasts for a short period like this, we can seldom identify a source. In chronic neck pain, i.e. that lasting at least 6 weeks, we again do not know the structural basis in most cases. When pain is referred to the neck from other sites (i.e. myocardial ischaemia), although we have a general theory of this referral pattern from an anatomical understanding of nerve-root embryology, we do not know why some patients with myocardial ischaemia have neck pain and others do not. Finally, we know from clinical experience and radiological studies, for example, that patients with rheumatoid arthritis can have extensive inflammatory destruction of the atlantoaxial structure but have no symptoms at all. In other studies (see below) individuals may have large osteophytes and marked degenerative changes, again with no symptoms.

EPIDEMIOLOGY AND RISK FACTORS

Chronic neck pain is perhaps second only to chronic low back pain as the most common musculoskeletal disorder associated with injury and disability claims, both in the workplace and after motor-vehicle collisions. At any given time, approximately 10% of the population reports having neck pain on at least 7 days per month, and neck pain (of unspecified duration) occurs in at least 80% of the population at some time,[2–4] with a 20–30% annual incidence of acute neck pain in population-based studies.[5–7] These figures hold for a number of different countries,[8, 9] although there are limited data that neck pain may be less common in Asia.[10]

Linton[11] examined studies dealing with psychosocial risk factors in acute neck and back pain. Factors cited include preceding stressful life events or depression. Depressive symptoms have been shown to be associated with the onset of an episode of neck or back pain.[12] Moreover, those with high levels of depressive symptoms are at a four-fold increased risk of troublesome neck and low back pain. It is not clear why these associations evolve. Perhaps psychological distress causes individuals to notice, amplify and focus on life's ordinary and minor aches and pains, or maybe psychological distress can manifest itself as spinal pain. Independent risk factors for incident neck pain also include poor general health at baseline, female gender, obesity, a previous history of neck injury or of concomitant pain elsewhere, and higher numbers of children.[2, 5, 6, 13] These are, interestingly, the same risk factors for other regional musculoskeletal pain disorders.[2]

Other risk factors for incident neck pain that have a more 'mechanical' or 'occupational' flavour include duration of sitting, duration of twisting and bending the trunk in working postures.[14] Studies thus far, however, have failed to find neck flexion, neck extension, neck rotation, arm force and posture, hand–arm vibration, workplace design or sports/exercise to be risk factors for incident neck pain.[15] There has been only one prospective study to assess the relationship between work-related psychosocial factors and incident neck pain, with appropriate adjustment for both work-related and non-work-related physical factors and individual characteristics. This study, reported recently by Ariens and coworkers,[16] indicates that high quantitative job demands (e.g. working under time pressure or working to deadlines) and low coworker support are independent risk factors for neck pain. Not surprisingly, given the relatively few physical risk factors for acute neck pain, many mechanical interventions studied for the prevention of neck

pain in the workplace have failed to demonstrate any benefit, except for exercises, which modestly reduce the future incidence of neck pain and work absenteeism.[17] Similarly, attempting to prevent acute neck pain after motor-vehicle collisions by the introduction of head restraints has not appeared to slow the increasing numbers of whiplash injuries being reported. Neck pain thus remains costly, a common cause of disability, and responsible for a significant proportion of work absenteeism and lost productivity.[2]

However, various studies have shown that not everyone with neck (or back) pain seeks healthcare, and those individuals who thereby become 'patients' are a self-selected subgroup. There is a wide array of independent predictors of who will seek a healthcare provider.[18–20] Cote et al.,[18] for example, studied approximately 800 subjects from a population-based sample in Saskatchewan, Canada, these subjects having experienced neck or back pain in the preceding 4 weeks. They found that approximately 25% of subjects sought some form of healthcare provider. While it is encouraging that 75% were not attending a healthcare provider, the fact that spinal pain is so common means that the 25% who do so will still account for a large healthcare expenditure for the treatment of neck pain. As expected, various factors such as neck pain severity and duration, and the presence of comorbidities were predictors of who sought healthcare. Cote et al. further found, however, that even if one controls for pain severity, pain duration, socio-economic status, comorbidities and various other factors known to modify healthcare seeking (i.e. medicalization), spinal pain that occurred in the setting of a traffic collision or that was attributed to an occupational factor was more likely to lead to medicalization than when it occurred in other settings (usually without an 'external' attributable cause). This suggests that, all else being equal in terms of the subject characteristics and the neck pain characteristics, the subject's impression of the need to attend a healthcare provider is modified by his or her own attribution of cause and effect. This might be a personal response stemming from the individual, but may also be directed by employers and 'on-the-scene' attendants (in the case of a traffic collision). Whether this response pattern varies from one culture to another has not been well studied, although there is evidence that race itself is a factor that predicts healthcare seeking, even within a given society.[19, 20]

Most individuals have short-lived episodes of neck pain, and therefore the challenge in understanding the transition from acute to chronic pain is to identify at an early stage distinguishing risk factors that predict this progression. Linton's review[11] and Carroll et al. more recent prospective, population-based study[12] provide strong evidence that this transition could be independently predicted by concurrent psychosocial factors. Linton suggested, on the basis of convincing data, that passive coping strategies, fear-avoidance behaviours and catastrophizing are predictors of persistent pain and disability. It is our clinical experience that the medical community usually fails either to assess or subsequently manage the psychosocial events and dysfunctions that patients bring to their physicians, perhaps because they are 'masked', or presented only in terms of the

PHYSICAL SYMPTOMS AND SIGNS

pain. According to available evidence, these psychosocial problems do not go away, but are simply repackaged as part of the chronic pain syndrome.

The traditional medical model involves searching for underlying tissue pathology, and is based on an analysis of the history, physical examination and investigations. No studies have examined the specificity or sensitivity of various symptoms or signs for differing diagnoses in neck pain patients. An attempt has been made using 'red flags' in patients with low back pain. Even here they have poor specificity, and no similar factors have been studied for neck pain. Nor are there studies, therefore, that can tell the clinician how well a given symptom or sign or combination thereof separates more benign causes from more serious ones (i.e. muscular pain versus malignancy). Nevertheless, clinical experience has taught us that patients with predominantly nocturnal neck pain, or neck pain associated with any of night sweats, fevers, weight loss, swallowing difficulties or voice hoarseness appear more likely to have a specific identifiable disease as the cause of the pain. Investigations are probably useful in these patients, even with a paucity of any significant physical findings. Among physical examination findings in neck pain patients the detection of any region of swelling, or the observation of clear and objective neurological findings such as an absent reflex, hyperreflexia with extensor plantar responses, muscle wasting or weakness, or sensory loss of a clear dermatomal distribution are also likely to yield a structural cause upon investigation. The specificity and sensitivity of range of motion has not been studied, but remains a sign that can be modified by the subjective factors such as pain sensation, and we would regard it as unhelpful. When neck pain is part of a more systemic disease, such as rheumatoid arthritis or ankylosing spondylitis, the diagnosis is seldom difficult.

However, the dilemma for physicians is that most cases of neck pain lack any of the features that point to a specific pathology. The most common symptoms in neck pain patients both in primary care and tertiary care centres are expressed with a report of pain intensity, pain location and character (dull, sharp, constant, intermittent, etc.), radiating or referred pain, and numbness or sensory changes. Physical examination in most neck pain patients is positive only for reduced range of active motion and tenderness on palpation. In a systematic review of the literature concerning the reliability of spinal palpation for diagnosis of neck pain, Seffinger et al.[21] concluded that so-called soft-tissue paraspinal palpatory diagnostic tests are not reliable. Despite this, these tests are in common use and touted by clinical practitioners as having importance.

Contrary to many other medical disorders, we do not know what, if any, structural factors or tissue pathology causes most cases of neck pain. The medical model here fails in its traditional approach – we cannot as readily 'fix' what we cannot identify pathologically. Instead, the illness is largely subjective in nature, and associated symptoms, especially in patients with chronic neck pain, are usually equally vague, including arm fatigue, headache, dizziness, generalized weakness and tingling. There are, of course, many healthcare providers who appear to be able to convincingly explain to patients the specific anatomical abnormality underlying their symptoms. This might provide a degree of short-term reassurance to a patient, especially one who is destined for a rapid, spontaneous improvement. Until this has been demonstrated, however, we believe this approach is dishonest and is clearly not 'evidence based'. Indeed, it is this widespread set of symptoms so commonly seen in whiplash patients that has led us to suggest whiplash should be regarded as a general illness, and that a search for a specific cervical lesion would be wasted effort and obviously illusory if positive.[22]

History-taking may help to identify prognostic factors that encourage other treatment approaches or closer follow-up of the acute neck pain patient. Borghouts et al.[23] reviewed various studies of the clinical course, and prognostic factors of the non-specific forms of neck pain physicians encounter most. They found the available studies to be small and of generally poor quality, yet they did report that the pain characteristics of local versus radiating did not predict long-term outcome. A higher intensity of pain and a history of previous neck pain were more likely to be associated with a chronic course. Still, this was as much as could be concluded from the available studies. In chronic pain in general, the tender-point count, beloved by fibromyalgia diagnosticians, is an indicator of emotional distress rather than diagnostic specificity or pathology,[24] and it correlates with fatigue and depression independently of the presence or absence of pain.[25] In chronic neck pain patients specifically, 'state anxiety' (i.e. not an anxiety state, but anxiety that comes on with the starting of some undertaking) is a predictor of tender-point count independently of pain severity and duration.[26, 27] This may explain, for example, why in one study more tender points were seen in whiplash patients (without fracture) versus leg fracture patients, despite the fact that leg fracture patients suffer more extensive tissue damage than whiplash patients.[28, 29]

The prognostic factors in whiplash patients have also been reviewed. Cote et al.[30] analysed all outcome studies done before 2001 and synthesized the information from all the prognostic studies concerning whiplash patients. They found that studies consistently revealed age greater than 40 years, female gender, more intense baseline neck or back pain, more intense baseline headache, the presence of baseline radicular signs and symptoms, and the presence of depressive or other significant emotional distress symptoms within the early weeks after injury to be associated with a worse outcome. These factors are prognostic in both a tort and no-fault system, quite apart from the effect the tort system itself has on prognosis.[31] What is of equal significance, however, is the many factors that were carefully studied, especially in thousands of patients in Saskatchewan, that did not predict outcome. Although early (pre-1995) studies had suggested that factors such as head position at the time of collision, initial x-ray findings, the direction of impact and the amount of vehicle damage were prognostic, subsequent larger and better designed studies have not affirmed these findings, and have even contradicted them.[30, 31] In Saskatchewan (Canada) claimants, for example, whether a collision was a rear, frontal or side impact had no bearing on outcome, neither did seat-belt or head-restraint use or position of the head restraint, general health before the collision, previous whiplash injury or symptoms before collision. Many current beliefs about prognostic factors are held based on pre-1995 studies, but these studies were very small, and with a highly selected group of subjects and inadequate data collection for confounders. Studies done since 2001, conducted in Australia[32] and The Netherlands,[33] have also confirmed the prognostic importance. of female gender, high initial neck pain and higher levels of initial psychological distress, suggesting that these are fairly universal factors. Why female gender should portend a worse prognosis is unclear. It may be related to physical stature, or to different psychological responses to injury.

Coping style may be an important prognostic factor for neck pain in general, and in whiplash, as well, and there exist simple, brief questionnaires to assess this in clinical practice.[34] The chronic pain literature, especially that which focuses on neck and back pain, contains considerable research that attempts to discern why patients with similar pain levels can have such divergent outcomes, some seeming to recover from acute pain within days to weeks, and others developing chronic pain and disability. That is, while high levels of initial pain in whiplash patients predict a poorer outcome, not all patients with high levels of initial pain develop chronic pain. Studies suggest that, irrespective of pain levels, it is more important how the person copes with pain. Research with neck and back pain patients (see the review of this research by Carroll et al.[35]) has considered chiefly two types of coping style: active and passive. Active coping refers to those coping strategies that involve taking responsibility for pain management and include attempts to control the pain or to function in spite of pain. Passive coping refers to strategies that involve giving responsibility for pain management to an outside source or allowing other areas of life to be adversely affected by pain. Previous research has assessed the factors associated with active and passive coping in isolation. Passive coping is generally found to be associated with increased severity of depression, higher levels of activity limitation and helplessness.[35] Active coping has been found to be associated with less severe depression, increased activity level and less functional impairment, but to be unrelated to pain severity. It is intuitively apparent that higher pain levels will stress any coping style, all the more so if the coping mechanisms are limited, but it has been found that many people use combinations of active and passive coping, and that for any pain level the higher the passive coping usage the worse the outcome.

Using markers of coping styles, Carroll et al.[35] further showed that the development of disabling neck/low back pain was strongly associated with the high use of passive coping strategies, regardless of levels of active coping. That is, even if a person is staying busy or active, and engaging in physical exercise, the concomitant tendency to hold passive strategies such as relying heavily on pain medications, frequently focusing on and discussing their pain with others, and cancelling social activities negates the beneficial effects of the active coping.

Passive coping is hazardous to the outcome. Recent research with whiplash patients confirms the relevance of coping styles to recovery,[36] although more research is needed.

Besides historical (and prognostic) factors to consider, there is additional research that has been directed at signs on physical examination that may be markers for chronicity, and which may provide a useful measure to the clinician in deciding when a more in-depth analysis of psychosocial factors is warranted. Just as there are so-called non-organic or behavioural (Waddell) signs in low back pain, research has begun to develop a framework for similar signs in neck pain. Sobel et al.[37] have suggested that these might include superficial tenderness, rotation less than 50% to the left and right, regional sensory disturbances (not conforming to a dermatomal, nerve root or peripheral nerve distribution), jerky, give-way weakness in the arms and overreaction (stiff or rigid movements, rubbing the affected area, clutching or grabbing the area, grimacing, sighing). While these have been tested for interrater variability, they have yet to be tested in the way behavioural signs for low back pain have been studied, showing them to be useful to detect the effects of underlying psychological distress (correlation with psychometric measures), and as predictors of poor surgical and rehabilitation outcomes in the absence of psychological intervention. In low back pain these signs have also been of value in deciding when it is useful to introduce psychological intervention during rehabilitation, with an effectiveness such that after inclusion of such therapy the non-organic signs no longer predict adverse outcomes.[38, 39] There are important caveats, however, to these signs. First, while they may obviously suggest a malingerer, who wrongly thinks they are making a more convincing impression on the examiner, these signs are found even in individuals with known physical pathology. Their presence reflects not the absence of organicity (thus, 'behavioural' signs is a better term than 'non-organic'), but rather that the severity of symptoms, disability and behaviour cannot be explained alone on the basis of physical pathology. Thus, anxiety, depression and a tendency to focus on a symptom will amplify the pain response, and affect the behaviour during examination in ways that physical pathology will not.

In summary, in most neck pain patients the history and physical examination will not lead to a specific pathological diagnosis, but will perhaps allow the clinician to reassure the patient that more serious causes of neck pain are not evident. Given that pain intensity is a predictor of a higher likelihood of chronicity, this together with consideration of behavioural signs may at least help the clinician identify early the patient that needs a much more intensive discussion of their concerns about their neck pain, what they have heard, what they fear, and why they need to understand and be reassured of the benign nature of their condition. High tender-point counts are a marker for distress, and concomitant psychosocial stressors or attribution issues may explain why the patient has brought their neck pain to a physician on this occasion. The patient's life circumstances and concerns need to be explored in such cases, as otherwise they simply resurface in the development of chronic pain.

DIAGNOSIS AND RADIOLOGICAL ASSESSMENT

It is worth emphasizing here the rather disappointing fact that the myriad of imaging techniques available to physicians provide little or no diagnostic assistance in most neck pain patients. Radiological investigation seems pertinent when a patient presents with neck pain and any of weight loss, dysphagia, neck lumps, nocturnal pain only, or physical examination findings suggestive of radiculopathy (loss of reflexes, objective motor weakness, dermatomal-pattern sensory loss), but most neck pain patients lack these symptoms. In cases of trauma, an x-ray is often used to look for fracture. A recent study suggests a 'neck rule' for ordering x-rays in those with neck pain following trauma. Hoffman et al.[40] studied over 30,000 cases of blunt trauma to the neck (i.e. no penetrating injury) of various causes, but mainly following motor-vehicle collisions. They developed a decision instrument that requires patients to meet five criteria in order to be classified as having a low probability of injury: no midline cervical tenderness, no focal neurological deficit, normal alertness, no intoxication and no painful, distracting injury (another injury that was painful enough it might distract the patient from noticing the severity of their neck tenderness). With this decision rule, eight of 818 patients with bony injury were missed, and only two of these eight were considered to have clinically significant injuries (i.e. those with potential for complications). Another prospective study, by Stiell et al.,[41] in nine Canadian emergency departments evaluated decision rules for x-rays in patients with trauma. None of 1812 patients who had been involved in a simple rear-end collision were found to have evidence on x-ray of cervical spine injury. Despite the apparent usefulness of these criteria sets, concerns have been raised that to be the physician who misses these few cases of relevant injury is hazardous in the current medico-legal environment. Thus, many physicians will order neck x-rays despite this rule. While this may be a problem from an economic standpoint, we feel the greater problem with x-rays is the wrongful attribution of significance to otherwise benign findings.

The temptation to attribute a patient's pain to those radiological findings that are seen (e.g. degenerative changes) has long been present because it is difficult to understand why they should *not* be a cause of pain. The term 'degenerative disc disease', coined in the 1940s, continues to be the peg on which the chronic neck pain syndrome is hung by some physicians, although it is patently clear that once studies control for age, there is no independent correlation between symptoms and any such sample of disc findings, regardless of how they are detected (x-ray, discography, computed tomography (CT) scan, magnetic resonance imaging (MRI)). The history of these studies is reviewed in detail elsewhere.[42] Even findings of disc protrusion (without nerve root or spinal cord compression), spinal stenosis and small degrees of subluxation of one vertebra, or angulations of one in respect to adjacent ones, have no predictive value for the presence of neck pain, and are just as frequently found in asymptomatic subjects. On the other hand, where there is a good clinical reason to suspect a specific root

lesion (based on the neurological examination), CT or MRI may provide necessary preoperative anatomical confirmation. Yet, the notion that degenerative disc disease or cervical osteoarthritis is specifically associated with neck pain remains a myth propagated to this day.[43]

The problem with continuing to tell patients that their pain arises from degenerative change or osteoarthritis of the spine is that (a) it is untrue and (b) we believe it immediately gives the patient the impression that they have a chronic, unrelenting and probably untreatable cause of pain, much like osteoarthritis in knees or hips. Given the risk that the patient may respond to this diagnosis by withdrawing from activities (something that may make sense to an arthritis patient), developing anxiety, keeping pain diaries and seeking many different forms of 'cure', the chance of harming the patient by attributing their pain to the radiological findings should be too much of a concern for physicians to do it so lightly. Patients should be told that they would have their neck pain regardless of what their x-rays look like, and that they would (and did) have degenerative changes ('arthritis of the spine') even without pain. This series of explanations, while they do not give the patient what they often crave – a clear diagnosis – also contribute to iatrogenic effects that might otherwise lead acute neck pain to become chronic neck pain.

Providing evidence that x-rays do not help in diagnosis, Johnson and Lucas[44] undertook an evaluation of the value of screening cervical spine x-rays in patients with non-traumatic neck pain. They found that 54% of 470 patients had x-rays read as degenerative changes, 35% were read as normal, 8.5% were read as consistent with muscle spasm, and the remainder were read as having anatomical or congenital variants or old compression fractures. The x-rays led to no diagnoses, such as acute fracture, dislocation or neoplasm, that would have placed the patient at jeopardy had the x-ray not been done. Furthermore, Borghouts et al.[23] found that radiological findings of disc and joint degeneration in the cervical spine did not predict the outcome of acute neck pain, so the physician cannot even use them for prognosis.

Finally, in the case of acute whiplash injury, a common consideration for ordering an x-ray in patients with neck pain, radiological studies (including MRI) are of no value in the acute or chronic setting, other than in excluding a fracture or dislocation, or for confirming the mechanism for nerve-root compression in the small minority of patients with grade 3 or 4 whiplash-associated disorder. The limited value of radiological procedures in whiplash patients has also been dealt with in detail elsewhere.[45]

TREATMENT

Acute neck pain

Despite the fact that only 25% of acute neck pain may lead to healthcare seeking,[4] and only a percentage of these patients will develop chronic pain, this percentage accounts for disproportionately higher costs. Thus, for example, the Quebec Task Force on Whiplash-Associated Disorders found that 12% of whiplash patients in Quebec remained in chronic pain 1 year after their collision. Yet, these 12% accounted for 47% of costs of all whiplash injuries in terms of treatment and lost wages.[46] Thus, treatments that prevent the progression from acute to chronic pain are highly desirable.

Most studies on the treatment of acute neck pain have dealt with whiplash patients. In 1995 the Quebec Task Force on Whiplash-Associated Disorders reviewed the studies on the treatment of acute whiplash patients done up to 1994.[47] The conclusions from that review, and a similar review by Kjellman et al.[48] for the same time period (although the latter included foreign-language studies), emphasize the paucity of good-quality studies. Still, from the available data it is clear that therapy prescriptions that have an exercise component (active therapy) are superior to those that do not (i.e. those relying on passive therapy modalities such as ultrasound, manipulation, massage, heat, transcutaneous electrical nerve stimulation (TENS) and laser). Shown not to be efficacious by controlled study are electromagnetic therapy, traction, collars, TENS, ultrasound, spray and stretch, local corticosteroid injections, trigger-point injections and laser therapy.[47] The Quebec Task Force found evidence for the effectiveness of manipulation/chiropractic therapy in acute neck pain to be equivocal, as study design either reflected significantly different baseline characteristics in cohorts, or some studies failed to find a therapeutic effect. Because of the mixed prescriptions of multiple passive modalities and multiple exercises in some studies, it is not clear whether exercise is better because it is effective, or because passive therapy is harmful, or both. It is also not clear what aspect or type of exercise therapy is more effective.

Since 1994 there have been a few more studies of the treatment of acute neck pain. The results of these have been summarized by Peeters et al.,[49] and again indicate that exercise therapies are superior to passive modalities and that 'rest makes rusty', a view supported in a subsequent updated review.[50] One of the most impressive studies in acute whiplash patients was that by Borchgrevink et al.[51] in Norway, where the therapeutic advice to 'act-as-usual' was compared with not having that advice, in a randomized group of 241 neck pain patients whose onset of pain was within 24 hours of a motor-vehicle collision, and who had no signs or radiological findings to suggest neurological injury or fracture. All patients received instructions for self-training of the neck (neck school) and a 5-day prescription for a non-steroidal anti-inflammatory drug (NSAID). One group was instructed to act as usual and received no sick leave or collar. Patients in the immobilization group received 14 days of sick leave and a soft collar. At 6 months after the collision the 'act as usual' group had a better outcome on several variables, including pain, concentration and memory. The study is impressive because the difference between the two groups was simply advice with no sick leave and no collar, versus no advice and both sick leave and a collar. The extent to which it was the advice that was beneficial versus the collar being harmful is, however, not known, yet the outcome in the 'act as usual' group was better than is typically reported in most studies, suggesting some definite benefit from that advice. The effect of an intervention to not give sick leave and to tell the patient to act as usual points to the importance of modifying behaviour in preventing the transition from acute to chronic neck pain. More studies of this type are needed.

In patients with acute low back pain, an explanatory, reassuring booklet ('the back book') has been shown to be a useful therapeutic addition.[52] A similar book, 'the whiplash book', has been shown to alter beliefs about whiplash injury in traumatized and non-traumatized subjects,[53] although studies have yet to test its effectiveness on recovery from acute whiplash injury. A recent study tested the effectiveness of a summarized version of this booklet, with evidence-based advice provided through ten statements of 'DOs' and 'DON'Ts'.[54] Given to patients in the emergency-room setting, however, this simple pamphlet did not affect recovery rates from acute whiplash. It may be that the material was not robust enough to produce an effect, or that educational materials are more likely to have effectiveness in the general-practitioner/family-physician setting where there may be opportunity to review and reinforce the educational message being provided. Studies in the primary-care setting are thus needed.

Chronic neck pain

The studies evaluating treatments for chronic neck pain suffer from being few in number, having very mixed populations, and providing limited clinical information about the patients, as well as having widely varying inclusion and exclusion criteria. The review by Kjellman et al.[48] of studies done up to 1995 reveals that for chronic neck pain of varying duration (from 3 months to more than 2 years), only five of 27 randomized clinical trials of treatment of chronic neck pain had follow-ups to 6 months or more, and four of these five studies found negative outcomes for the treatment intervention. Still, exercise programmes appeared to have the larger benefit.

Exercise therapy

The first trial of multidisciplinary (exercise, occupational therapy and behavioural intervention) treatment for chronic whiplash was conducted by Vendrig et al.[55] They conducted an uncontrolled trial of exercise in which the subjects were diagnosed as having chronic whiplash and had been off work for at least 6 months. A total of 26 subjects underwent a 4 week exercise rehabilitation programme, with educational efforts designed to abolish inappropriate pain behaviour and to restore fitness. Group sessions involved discussion of deeply rooted beliefs regarding symptoms and disability. These subjects had high levels of pain and distress when entering the programme. At 6 months' follow-up 96% lacked indications of psychological distress and 46% were pain-free. Even the group with persisting symptoms had a 50% reduction in their severity. The result was a complete-return-to-work rate of 65% and a return-to-work (partial or complete) rate of 92% at 6 months' follow-up. During the follow-up phase of 6 months, less than 20% of subjects sought any other care. Although these results are most impressive, there was no parallel, untreated control group for comparison. Another recent study of chronic neck pain, but this time not specifying whether collision victims were included, compared exercise and adding spinal manipulation to exercise.[56] The addition of spinal manipulation was not beneficial, and exercise therapy alone was better than spinal manipulation alone in various outcome measures. Indeed, it appears that whenever there seems to be an effect of mobilization/manipulation techniques in chronic neck pain, it is only if exercise is included in the treatment.[57] Taimela et al.[58] compared 24 sessions of proprioceptive exercise and behavioural support to a neck lecture and two sessions of instructions for home exercises; a further control group was given only a recommendation to exercise and one lecture on neck care. The subjects were recruited from occupational healthcare systems, and were diagnosed as having 'non-specific chronic neck pain'. The study was small, with about 25 patients in each group, and although the self-experienced benefit rating from each of the groups was highest in the group with the 24 sessions of supervised exercise therapy and lowest in the group simply given a recommendation to exercise, no change was noted in objective measures, and all groups experienced some improvement. Similar results have recently been obtained by Chiu et al.[59]

Thus, there is still a lack of large, randomized controlled trials of treatment of chronic neck pain. The most optimistic approach seems to be that which includes changing illness behaviour. Indeed, the exact form of the exercise component may be less relevant. Waling et al.[60] showed, in a group of 103 women with chronic neck pain, that three very different exercise approaches (strength, endurance and coordination) led to similar outcomes in pain reduction, leading the authors to conclude that the type of exercise is less important than the fact that the patient is exercising.

Cognitive therapy

There is a lack of studies to address the benefits of cognitive therapy in chronic neck pain patients, although there does appear to be some benefit in conditions such as chronic low back pain and fibromyalgia. While this may be worth studying in chronic neck pain, this is an expensive form of therapy with high personnel demands. In a sense, exercise therapy may be the 'behavioural' component of cognitive–behavioural therapy, but formal cognitive approaches remain uninvestigated for chronic neck pain.

Radiofrequency neurotomy

After utilizing placebo control and then comparative anaesthetic responses in a small, poorly defined group of subjects, Lord et al.[61] were able to screen patients to find 24 that had relief of pain with diagnostic blocks of the nerve supply to specific cervical facet joints. These 24 subjects were then randomized to receive either radiofrequency neurotomy of the nerve supply to the affected facet joint or a sham procedure (12 patients in each group). A total of six subjects in the control group and three in the treatment group failed to have benefit from the procedure. At 27 weeks only one control subject had persistent relief of pain after the procedure, compared with seven of the 12 subjects in the active treatment arm. The problem is that ten of the 12 control subjects were in litigation, compared with only four in the treatment group. If litigation status has any substantial effect on response to therapy, this is a significant confounding variable, especially in a small study where confounders cannot be readily discounted. In a larger, but uncontrolled study, Sapir and Gorup[62] treated 46 subjects with radiofrequency neurotomy for so-called 'facet joint pain', and 2 weeks after the procedure the majority of subjects had a 50% reduction or more in neck pain. Of course, without a control group the level of true effectiveness of the procedure itself is difficult to interpret. And that is the extent of trials of radiofrequency neurotomy for neck pain. The lack of sufficient data limits the clinician's ability to recommend this invasive procedure. There has only been one placebo-controlled trial to date, and that had a major confounder in the control group.[63]

Bugs and drugs

Botulinum toxin A has had many applications, and one of the more recent to be studied is its use in the treatment of chronic neck pain. Wheeler et al.[64] have reported a placebo-controlled study of 50 subjects with neck pain of at least 3 months' duration, about half of whom related their neck pain to motor-vehicle collisions. One randomized group received botulinum toxin A by injection into cervical muscles, while the control group received saline injections. Both groups showed significant improvement at various follow-up times over 4 months, the authors thus concluding that given as a single set of injections, the toxin was not beneficial for chronic neck pain.

As whiplash patients often report sleep disorder, a placebo-controlled trial of melatonin for subjects found to have delayed melatonin secretion onset has been completed.[65] A total of 80 patients with chronic neck pain of, on average, about 2 years' duration, were randomized to receive either melatonin tablets or placebo daily for 4 weeks. After 4 weeks, although the melatonin secretion onset time had changed, there was no clinical effect on subject's reported quality of health as measured using the Short Form 36 (SF-36), nor any effect on cognitive test results, but those in the treatment group fell asleep earlier and woke up earlier.

Summary

Although the general impression of therapy for either acute or chronic neck pain is that 'rest makes rusty' and exercise is better than other prescribed therapies, it is clear that unproven therapies are still frequently prescribed. As such, the medical community needs to revise its approach. Although there have not been enough studies to convince physicians and society in general that exercise and less, rather than more, therapy is the best approach, the traditional approach thus far of 'healing an injury or a disease' is failing us. As such, the philosophy must change.

PARADIGM SHIFT

One way to change our approach is to look at the factors known to affect the outcome from acute neck pain, and study and utilize an approach that directly addresses those very factors.

Previous neck pain episodes, for example, have an effect as a poor prognostic factor for the outcome (development of chronicity) in future neck pain episodes. This is either for some physical reason, or it is due to the effect that previous experience has on future illness behaviour, or both. It may be tempting, even for physicians, to assume there is an underlying physical basis to explain why previous neck pain episodes affect the outcome of future, distinct (in time) episodes. If there is a physical explanation, however, it is one about which we have no knowledge, and it cannot direct us toward a helpful therapeutic approach. If, however, illness behaviour with future pain episodes is in part affected by a person's past experience, then it seems intuitively correct that asking patients about their previous experiences and about the choices they made (whether to rest from normal activities and work, to wear a collar, to avoid exercise therapies and use passive therapies, to rely on medications primarily) is paramount in developing a change in this pattern of illness behaviour. That is something that can be done without needing an anatomical diagnosis for the neck pain. Patients may legitimately believe that all the previous therapy approaches were valid given that they were prescribed by someone as if they were meant to work. It should not be surprising to clinicians that patients not only follow their advice when given, but that they will do so again, unless given reason to do otherwise. Studies of the whiplash syndrome show that rest is harmful, while 'acting as usual' is helpful. Collars are harmful, as are passive therapies versus active therapies. Patients need to be told all this, so that they can 'buy in' to the reason why the current neck pain episode need not follow the same pattern of previous episodes and, indeed, that previous episodes, because they were dealt with so differently, can be deemed irrelevant to what will happen with this current neck pain episode.

A high intensity of acute neck pain is also a negative prognostic factor. But we do not have any evidence that this is because of more severe pathology. So we should not tell patients that. We do have research that shows that how a symptom is perceived can be largely influenced by factors that generate symptom amplification, such as viewing a symptom as having a more serious cause, excessive attention to symptoms by others, a pain diary and any anxiety state. Although this has not been tested directly in the therapy for acute neck pain, the fact that advice to 'act as usual' (as if the neck pain was benign in origin) leads to a better outcome suggests that how the patient views their pain and how they respond to it can be altered. Preliminary studies with 'the whiplash book' support this notion.[53] As mentioned above, Vendrig et al.[55] examined the effect of advice that specifically challenges patients' views of the seriousness of their pain and of the need to modify activities (mainly withdrawal from activities according to pain levels). This study found a high rate of success (return to work and normal function) in a group of patients who had been totally disabled with high pain levels for more than 6 months. The authors admit that the patients have to be willing to consider and act on this advice, but that is the whole point: the choices patients make have an effect on their outcome.

Beyond this, we need to ask ourselves why neck pain in the occupational and motor-vehicle-collision setting is viewed, as Cote et al.[4] found, as a more necessary reason to seek healthcare than other neck pain. We thus need to concentrate, in addition, on more system-wide, cultural factors that influence this behaviour. A social marketing campaign for low back pain was shown by Buchbinder et al.[66] to affect both practitioner attitudes to treating low back pain and public attitudes about how to respond to acute low back pain, and to reduce disability and costs associated with work-related low back pain.

Adding to this approach, one must at some point ask 'Why has this person developed this behaviour now?' People have pain episodes during many phases of their life. What causes them to behave differently on this occasion? A study reported recently by van der Windt et al.[67] indicates that general psychological well-being (or lack of) rather than specific somatic symptoms predicts healthcare seeking. Often, one can find a series of life stressors predating the illness, or an associated detrimental event (e.g. engaging in litigation) that is magnifying the abnormal behaviour in the first place. In the setting of a motor-vehicle collision, as well, fear may start when the patient, in a state of near panic after the collision, is taken out of the car by paramedics, given a hard collar, placed on a spine board and taken off to the hospital with sirens blaring. Even when the injured party feels well, the police are instructed to ask about neck pain, and suggest a medical visit immediately if there are any symptoms. These are considered important or necessary responses from the paramedics and police, but they never-

PRACTICE POINTS

- Most people with acute neck pain do not seek medical attention, but those who do account for significant healthcare costs, second (amongst musculoskeletal disorders) probably only to low back pain in this regard.

- Those who seek care for acute neck pain are more likely to have experienced their pain at work or after a motor-vehicle collision, and are more likely to have a poor psychological well-being.

- Most patients with neck pain will not be given a precise structural or pathological diagnosis, but their condition will instead be labelled as soft-tissue injury, whiplash injury, soft-tissue rheumatism, myofascial pain, mechanical neck pain, etc.

- Reviewing a patient's past experience with neck pain (trying to understand how they approached treatment previously) and their current habits of pain diaries, or attending multiple therapists, may be important in providing the education and reassurance needed to alter past illness behaviours.

- Do not tell patients that the finding of disc degeneration on x-ray is relevant to their pain. It has nothing to do with their pain, is normal for them and does not predict their outcome.

- Rest makes rusty.

theless do magnify the emotional impact of the event. Although the patient may be reluctant to pursue these issues, if the physician is first clear with the patient that the symptoms are legitimate, and have various physical sources, then the psychological sources of symptoms may also be accepted as part of the clinical picture to be dealt with. The bottom line is that neck pain does not end there. Physicians need to appreciate that most individuals with neck pain do not attend a physician, so those who do are different in some way. Also, those who attend physicians do so in part because this particular occasion of neck pain is either associated with a 'special event' (e.g. a motor-vehicle collision), or because the patient's current psychological well-being is poor, and this is what really makes them seek our help.

When the mind suffers ... the body cries out.
(Cardinal Lumberto to Don Michael Coleone in *Godfather III*)

RESEARCH AGENDA

- More research is needed to address the variance in outcome for acute neck pain that can be accounted for by factors such as anxiety, expectation of chronicity (symptom expectation) and pain diaries (symptom amplification).

- More studies are needed to test interventions that alter illness behaviours or habits, such as advice to avoid pain diaries, to not withdraw from activities and to exercise despite initial discomfort and fears, not viewing hurt the same as harm.

- Studies of public health campaigns to reduce chronic pain and disability from neck pain are warranted.

REFERENCES

1. Bogduk N. The neck. *Bailliere's Clin Rheumatol* 1999; **13**: 261–285.
2. Makela M, Heliovaara M, Sievers K et al. Prevalence, determinants, and consequences of chronic neck pain in Finland. *Am J Epidemiol* 1991: **134**: 1356–1367.
3. Bovim G, Schrader H, Sand T. Neck pain in the general population. *Spine* 1994; **19**: 1307–1309.
4. Cote P, Cassidy JD, Carroll L. The Saskatchewan Health and Back Pain Survey: the prevalence of neck pain and related disability in Saskatchewan adults. *Spine* 1998; **23**: 1689–1698.
5. Croft PR, Lewis M, Papageorgiou AC et al. Risk factors for neck pain: a longitudinal study in the general population. *Pain* 2001; **93**: 317–325.
6. Leclerc A, Niedhammer I, Landre MF et al. One-year predictive factors for various aspects of neck disorders. *Spine* 1999; **24**: 1455–1462.
7. Cote P, Cassidy JD, Carroll LJ et al. The annual incidence and course of neck pain in the general population: a population-based cohort study. *Pain* 2004; **112**: 267–273.
8. Guez M, Hildingsson C, Nilsson M et al. The prevalence of neck pain: a population-based study from northern Sweden. *Acta Orthop Scand* 2002; **73**: 455–459.
9. Bot SD, van der Waal JM, Terwee CB et al. Incidence and prevalence of complaints of the neck and upper extremity in general practice. *Ann Rheum Dis* 2005; **64**: 118–23.
10. Lau EMC, Sham A, Wong KC. The prevalence of and risk factors for neck pain in Hong Kong Chinese. *J Public Health Med* 1996; **18**: 396–399.
11. Linton S. A review of psychological risk factors in back and neck pain. *Spine* 2000; **25**: 1148–1156.
12. Carroll LJ, Cassidy JD, Cote P. Depression as a risk factor for onset of an episode of troublesome neck and low back pain. *Pain* 2004; **107**: 134–139.
13. Fredrikson K, Alfredsson L, Koster M et al. Risk factors for neck and upper limb disorders: results from 24 years of follow-up. *Occup Environ Med* 1999; **56**: 59–66.
14. Krause N, Ragland DR, Grenier BA et al. Physical workload and ergonomic factors associated with prevalence of back and neck pain in urban transit operators. *Spine* 1997; **22**: 2117–2127.
15. Ariens GAM, van Mechelen W, Bongers P et al. Physical risk factors for neck pain. *Scand J Work Environ Health* 2000; **26**: 7–19.
16. Ariens GAM, Bongers PM, Hoogenddoorn WE et al. High quantitative job demands and low coworker support as risk factors for neck pain. *Spine* 2001; **26**: 1896–1903.
17. Linton SJ, van Tulder MW. Preventative interventions for back and neck pain problems. *Spine* 2001; **26**: 778–787.
18. Cote P, Cassidy JD, Carroll L. The treatment of neck and low back pain. who seeks care? Who goes where? *Med Care* 2001; **39**: 956–967.
19. Carey TS, Evans AT, Hadler NM et al. Acute severe low back pain. A population-based study of prevalence and care-seeking. *Spine* 1996; **21**: 339–344.
20. Hurwitz EL, Morgenstern H. The effect of comorbidity on care seeking for back problems in the United States. *Ann Epidemiol* 1999; **9**: 262–270.
21. Seffinger MA, Najm WI, Mishra SI et al. Reliability of spinal palpation for diagnosis of back and neck pain: a systematic review of the literature. *Spine* 2004; **29**: E413–E425.
22. Ferrari R, Russell AS, Carroll LJ et al. A re-examination of the whiplash-associated disorders (WAD) as a systemic illness. *Ann Rheum Dis* 2005; **64**:1337–1342..
23. Borghouts JAJ, Koes BW, Bouter LM. The clinical course and prognostic factors of non-specific neck pain: a systematic review. *Pain* 1998; **77**: 1–3.
24. Wolfe F. The relation between tender points and fibromyalgia symptom variables: evidence that fibromyalgia is not a discrete disorder in the clinic. *Ann Rheum Dis* 1997; **56**: 268–271.
25. Croft P, Schollum J, Silman A. Population study of tender point counts and pain as evidence of fibromyalgia. *BMJ* 1994; **309**: 696–699.
26. McBeth J, Macfarlane GJ, Benjamin S et al. The association between tender points, psychological distress, and adverse childhood experiences: a community-based study. *Arthritis Rheum* 1999; **42**: 1397–1404.
27. Dyrehag LE, Widerström-Noga EG, Carlsson SG et al. Relations between self-rated musculoskeletal symptoms and signs and psychological distress in chronic neck and shoulder pain. *Scand J Rheum Med* 1998; **30**: 235–242.
28. Buskila D, Neumann L, Vaisberg G et al. Increased rates of fibromyalgia following cervical spine injury. A controlled study of 161 cases of traumatic injury. *Arthritis Rheum* 1997; **40**: 446–452.
29. Ferrari R, Russell AS. Neck injury and chronic pain syndromes: comment on article by Buskila et al. *Arthritis Rheum* 1998; **41**: 758–759.
30. Cote P, Cassidy JD, Carroll L et al. A systematic review of the prognosis of acute whiplash and a new conceptual framework to synthesize the literature. *Spine* 2001; **26**: E445–E458.
31. Cassidy JD, Carroll L, Cote P et al. Effect of eliminating compensation for pain and suffering on the outcome of insurance claims for whiplash injury. *N Engl J Med* 2000; **342**: 1179–1186.
32. Gun RT, Osti OL, O'Riordan A et al. Risk factors for prolonged disability after whiplash injury: a prospective study. *Spine* 2005; **30**: 386–391.
33. Hendriks EJ, Scholten-Peeters GG, van der Windt DA et al. Prognostic factors for poor recovery in acute whiplash patients. *Pain* 2005; **114**: 408–416.
34. Brown GK, Nicassio PM. Development of a questionnaire for the assessment of active and passive coping strategies in chronic pain patients. *Pain* 1987; **31**: 53–64.
35. Carroll L, Mercado AC, Cassidy JD et al. A population-based study of factors associated with combinations of active and passive coping with neck and low back pain. *J Rehabil Med* 2002; **34**: 67–72.
36. Buitenhuis J, Spanjer J, Fidler V. Recovery from acute whiplash: the role of coping styles. *Spine* 2003; **28**: 896–901.
37. Sobel JB, Sollenberger P, Robinson R et al. Cervical nonorganic signs: a new clinical tool to assess abnormal illness behavior in neck pain patients: a pilot study. *Arch Phys Med Rehabil* 2000; **81**: 170–175.
38. Polatin PB, Cox B, Gatchel RJ et al. A prospective study of Waddell signs in patients with chronic low back pain. When they may not be predictive. *Spine* 1997; **22**: 1618–1621.
39. Ferrari R. Waddell signs in patients with chronic low back pain. *Spine*1999; **24**: 306–307.

40. Hoffman JR, Mower WR, Wolfson AB et al. Validity of a set of clinical criteria to rule out injury to the cervical spine in patients with blunt trauma, for the National Emergency X-Radiography Utilization Study Group. *N Engl J Med* 2000; **343**: 94–99.

41. Stiell IG, Clement CM, McKnight RD et al. The Canadian c-spine rule versus the NEXUS low-risk criteria in patients with trauma. *N Engl J Med* 2003; **349**: 2510–2518.

42. Ferrari R. *The Whiplash Encyclopedia. The Facts and Myths of Whiplash*, 2nd edn. Aspen, Gaithersburg, MD, 2005.

43. Özdemir F, Birtane M, Kokino S. The clinical efficacy of low-power laser therapy on pain and function in cervical osteoarthritis. *Clin Rheumatol* 2001; **20**: 181–184.

44. Johnson MJ, Lucas GL. Value of cervical spine radiographs as a screening tool. *Clin Orthop Res* 1997; **340**: 102–108.

45. Ferrari R, Russell AS. Pain in the neck for a rheumatologist. *Scand J Rheum* 2000; **29**: 1–7.

46. Suissa S Harder S, Veilleux M. The relation between initial symptoms and signs and the prognosis of whiplash. *Euro Spine J* 2001; **10**: 44–49.

47. Spitzer WO, Skovron ML, Salmi LR et al. Scientific monograph of the Quebec Task Force on Whiplash-Associated Disorders: redefining 'whiplash' and its management. *Spine* 1995; **20**(8 Suppl): 1S-73S.

48. Kjellman GV, Skargren EI, Öberg BE. A critical analysis of randomised clinical trials on neck pain and treatment efficacy. A review of the literature. *Scand J Rehab Med* 1999; **31**: 139–152.

49. Peeters GG, Verhagen AP, de Bie RA et al. The efficacy of conservative treatment in patients with whiplash injury: a systematic review of clinical trials. *Spine* 2001; **26**: E64–E73.

50. Seferiadis A, Rosenfeld M, Gunnarsson R. A review of treatment interventions in whiplash-associated disorders. *Eur Spine J* 2004; **13**: 387–397.

51. Borchgrevink GE, Kaasa A, McDonagh D et al. Acute treatment of whiplash neck sprain injuries. A randomized trial of treatment during the first 14 days after a car accident. *Spine* 1998; **23**: 25–31.

52. Burton AK, Waddell G, Tillotson KM et al. Information and advice to patients with back pain can have a positive effect. A randomized controlled trial of a novel educational booklet in primary care. *Spine* 1999; **24**: 2484–2491.

53. McClune T, Burton AK, Waddell G. Evaluation of an evidence based patient educational booklet for management of whiplash associated disorders. *Emerg Med J* 2003; **20**: 514–517.

54. Ferrari R, Rowe BH, Majumdar S et al. Simple educational intervention to improve the recovery from acute whiplash: results of a randomized, controlled trial. *Acad Emerg Med* 2005; **12**: 699–706.

55. Vendrig AA, van Akkerveeken PF, McWhorter KR. Results of a multimodal treatment program for patients with chronic symptoms after a whiplash injury of the neck. *Spine* 2000; **25**: 238–244.

56. Bronfort G, Evans R, Nelson B et al. A randomized clinical trial of exercise and spinal manipulation for patients with chronic neck pain. *Spine* 2001; **26**: 788–799.

57. Gross AR, Hoving JL, Haines TA et al. A Cochrane Review of manipulation and mobilization for mechanical neck disorders. *Spine* 2004; **29**: 1541–1548.

58. Taimela S, Takala EP, Asklöf T et al. Active treatment of chronic neck pain. *Spine* 2000; **25**: 1021–1027.

59. Chiu TT, Lam TH, Hedley AJ. A randomized controlled trial on the efficacy of exercise for patients with chronic neck pain. *Spine* 2005; **30**: E1–E7.

60. Waling K, Sundelin G, Ahlgren C et al. Perceived pain before and after three exercise programs – a controlled clinical trial of women with work-related trapezius myalgia. *Pain* 2000; **85**: 201–207.

61. Lord SM, Barnsley L, Wallis B et al. Percutaneous radio-frequency neurotomy for chronic cervical zygapophyseal-joint pain. *N Engl J Med* 1996; **335**: 1721–1726.

62. Sapir DA, Gorup JM. Radiofrequency medial branch block neurotomy in litigant and nonlitigant patients with cervical whiplash. *Spine* 2001; **26**: E268–E273.

63. Ferrari R. The many facets of whiplash. *Spine* 2001; **26**: 2063–2064.

64. Wheeler AH, Goolkasian P, Gretz SS. Botulinum toxin A for the treatment of chronic neck pain. *Pain* 2001; **94**: 255–260.

65. van Wieringen S, Jansen T, Smits MG et al. Melatonin for chronic whiplash syndrome with delayed melatonin onset. *Clin Drug Invest* 2001; **21**: 813–820.

66. Buchbinder R, Jolley D, Wyatt M. Population based intervention to change back pain beliefs and disability: three part evaluation. *BMJ* 2001; **322**: 1516–1520.

67. van der Windt D, Croft P, Pennix B. Neck and upper limb pain: more pain is associated with psychological distress and consultation rate in primary care. *J Rheumatol* 2002; **29**: 564–569.

Chapter 8

Low back pain

Maurits van Tulder, Bart Koes and Claire Bombardier

DESCRIPTIVE EPIDEMIOLOGY

Low back pain is a major health and socio-economic problem in western countries.[1] Many people will experience one or more episodes of low back pain in their life. Low back pain is also associated with high costs of healthcare utilization, work absenteeism and disability.[2] Low back pain has important consequences for patients, but also for their families, employers and society in general.[3]

A description of the epidemiology of low back pain should start with a clear definition of relevant concepts and include classification criteria, possible causes and risk factors. The epidemiological information available in the literature usually comes from a variety of selected populations. Epidemiological figures from the general population are usually not directly comparable with those from occupational, general practice or hospital settings. Also, occupational data from a blue collar workers' population are not directly comparable with data from white collar workers. Consequently, incidence and prevalence figures should always be presented for a specific population.

This chapter summarizes the epidemiology of low back pain. Epidemiology is defined as the study of the occurrence of illness.[4] Some important epidemiological concepts that are used to express the occurrence of low back pain are:

- *Incidence*: the proportion of the population at issue that experiences low back pain for the first time in a particular time period.
- *Point prevalence*: the proportion of the population at issue that experiences low back pain at a particular point in time.
- *Period prevalence*: the proportion of the population at issue that experiences low back pain during a specific period.
- *'Lifetime' prevalence*: the proportion of the population at issue that ever experienced an episode of low back pain during their life.

Epidemiological studies can use experimental or observational study designs. Epidemiological studies in the field of low back pain typically evaluate factors or interventions that may influence or change the occurrence of low back pain or the occurrence of chronicity in those who already have back pain. The results of these studies on risk factors, prevention and treatment are summarized in this chapter.

Definitions

Low back pain is usually defined as pain, muscle tension, or stiffness localized below the costal margin and above the inferior gluteal folds, with or without leg pain (sciatica). Low back pain is typically classified as being 'specific' or 'non-specific'. Specific low back pain is defined as symptoms caused by a specific pathophysiological mechanism, such as herniated disc, infection, inflammation, osteoporosis, rheumatoid arthritis, fracture or tumour. A study in the USA showed that of all back pain patients in primary care 4% had a compression fracture, 3% spondylolisthesis, 0.7% a tumour or metastasis, 0.3% spondylitis ankylopoetica and 0.01% an infection.[5] Non-specific low back pain is defined as symptoms without clear specific cause (i.e. low back pain of unknown origin). Approximately 90% of all low back pain patients will have non-specific low back pain. Although many healthcare professionals use a variety of diagnostic labels, at present no reliable and valid classification system exists for the large majority of non-specific low back pain cases.

The most important symptoms of non-specific low back pain are pain and disability. Physical measures such as stiffness, strength and poor mobility correlate poorly with back pain.[6] There is an increasing body of evidence showing that psychosocial problems play an important role in chronic non-specific low back pain.[7] There seems to be no strong association between abnormalities on x-rays and magnetic resonance imaging (MRI) and non-specific low back pain.[8, 9]

Non-specific low back pain is usually classified according to the duration of the complaints in the patients at issue.[10] Low back pain is defined as acute when it persists for less than 6 weeks, subacute when it lasts between 6 weeks and 3 months, and chronic when it lasts for longer than 3 months.

In general, the clinical course of an episode of low back pain seems to be favourable and most pain will resolve within a couple of weeks. Approximately 90% of patients with low back pain in primary care will have stopped consulting their physician within 3 months.[11] However, von Kor and Saunders[12] stated that this traditional view of low back pain consisting of single episodes of acute and chronic low back pain is inadequate. Back pain among primary care patients typically has a recurrent course characterized by variation and change, rather than an acute, self-limiting course.[12] Croft et al.[13] suggested that low back pain symptoms fluctuate (Figure 8.1). The majority of back pain patients will have experienced a previous episode, and acute attacks often occur as exacerbations of chronic low back pain. Recurrences are frequent, with the percentage of subsequent low back pain episodes ranging from 20% to 44% within 1 year in occupational populations to lifetime recurrences of up to 85%.[14] In general, recurrences will occur more frequently and be more severe if patients have had frequent or long-lasting low back pain complaints in the past.

The course of sick leave due to low back pain has similarly been reported to be favourable. Waddell[15] reported that 67% of patients on sick leave due to low back pain will have returned to work within 1 week and 90% will have done so within 2 months. However, the longer the period of sick leave the less likely return to work becomes. Less than half of the low back pain patients who have been off work for 6 months will return to work. After 2 years of work absenteeism, the chance of returning to work is virtually zero (Figure 8.2). Recently, it has been suggested that a substantial proportion of patients with chronic back pain actually have chronic widespread pain.[16, 17] There is also some evidence that widespread pain is associated with more severe, long-lasting disabling low back pain.[18] Thus,

the large proportion of subjects with widespread pain may be responsible for the major burden that chronic low back pain has on individuals and society.

Summarizing the epidemiological literature regarding low back pain in terms of incidence and prevalence is hampered by the lack of agreement on classification.[1] A variety of classification systems is used in epidemiological studies, e.g. the International Classification of Primary Care (ICPC), the International Classification of Diseases (ICD), the International Classification of Human Functioning (formerly the International Classification of Impairments, Disabilities and Handicaps (ICIDH)), the International Classification of Health Problems in Primary Care (ICHPPC-2-Defined) and the Reason for Encounter Classification (RFEC). The confusion is increased by the numerous terms for low back pain that are used for the same concept, e.g. non-specific low back pain, lumbago, idiopathic low back pain and mechanical low back pain.

Another related problem in this respect is 'recall bias', the limited ability of people to remember their pain experience or healthcare utilization. Longer periods covered by a retrospective survey will lead to more unreliable answers than will shorter periods.

Furthermore, in epidemiological studies the answer to the question of whether someone has low back pain might depend upon the way this question was asked. 'Have you ever had low back pain?' 'Do you have low back pain now?' 'Do you sometimes have low back pain?' 'Did you have low back pain during the last week?' 'Have you not been able to work due to low back pain?' 'Have you visited your family doctor because of

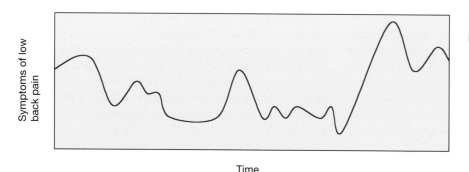

Figure 8.1. The actual course of low back pain as suggested by Croft et al.[13]

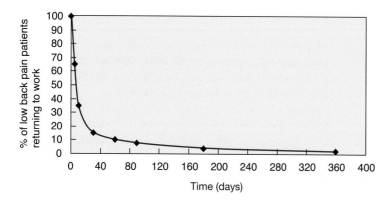

Figure 8.2. Return to work after an acute attack of back pain. Redrawn from Waddell (1998).[15]

low back pain during the last week?', are some examples of the various ways the incidence and prevalence of low back pain have been measured in epidemiological studies.

Validity and reliability of epidemiological data should always be reviewed critically and carefully. A description of the epidemiology of low back pain should take into account the definitions, classification systems and terminology used in the original studies.

Incidence

Epidemiological data reported in the literature have usually been collected in different populations. Lumping together data from open populations (e.g. the general population) and closed populations (e.g. general practice patients) is not very useful, and incidence and prevalence data need to be reported for specific populations. Only a few studies have reported incidence data.

General practice

A large epidemiological study in The Netherlands included data from a random sample of 161 general practitioners (GPs) in 103 practices with a total population of 335,000 patients.[19] The registration period was from April 1987 to April 1988 using the ICPC classification. The incidence of low back pain was 28.0 episodes/1000 persons per year. The reported incidence of low back pain with sciatica was 11.6/1000 per year. The incidence of low back pain was higher for men (32.0) than for women (23.2). The incidence was highest for people between 25 and 64 years of age.[19]

Another epidemiological study from The Netherlands reported data collected by 59 GPs in 21 practices with a population of 41,000 patients.[20] The ICPC criteria were used for classification. The incidence of low back pain (ICPC code L03) was 30 episodes/1000 persons per year. The incidence of low back pain with sciatica (ICPC code L86; including herniated disc and discopathy) was 6 episodes/1000 persons per year. The incidences of both low back pain and low back pain with sciatica were highest for patients between 45 and 64 years of age.[20]

The South Manchester Back Pain Study in the UK included 2715 adults who were free of low back pain during the month prior to the baseline survey. Subsequently, all primary care consultations were prospectively monitored.[21] The 12-month cumulative incidence of new consulting episodes was 3% in males and 5% in females. Those with a history of previous low back pain had twice the rate of new episodes compared with those with no low back pain in the past.

General population

The South Manchester Back Pain Study also included a follow-up survey after 1 year to determine new episodes that had not led to consultation (non-consulting episodes) during that 1-year period. The 12-month cumulative incidence of new non-consulting episodes was 31% in males and 32% in females. Those with a history of previous low back pain and those with widespread pain had a much higher incidence than those with no low back pain in the past.[21]

Prevalence

A summary of prevalence data from epidemiological studies in various countries is presented in Table 8.1.[1]

Reported lifetime prevalence ranges widely (49–70%), as do point prevalence (12–30%) and period prevalence (25–42%). A large epidemiological study on low back pain among the general population in The Netherlands was conducted from 1993 to 1995.[22] The study population consisted of a sample of 13,927 men and women aged 20–59 years. Almost half of the respondents (49.2%, of whom 45.5% were men and 52.4% women) reported low back pain in the previous year. More than 40% of the respondents reported that the episode lasted for more than 12 weeks (7.1%) or that the low back pain was continuously present (34.7%). Chronic low back pain was more common among women (22.6%) than men (18.3%) and increased with age from 12% at 20–29 years of age to 27.1% at 50–59 years of age.

In general, the conclusion from these prevalence estimates is quite clear: low back pain is a common disorder in western countries. The estimates of prevalence may vary because of national variations, age or gender of the population and the sampling method used.

Costs

The total costs of back pain in The Netherlands in 1991 were estimated to be more than US $3.7 billion, equalling 1.7% of the gross national product. The total direct costs of healthcare for back pain were approximately US $290 million, while the total indirect costs of back pain were approximately US $3.4 billion ($2.4 billion due to work absenteeism and $1.0 billion due to disability).[2]

The economic consequences of back pain have also been estimated in other countries such as the USA, the UK, Sweden, Canada and Australia. A comparison of cost estimates between countries is difficult because of the differences in methods, diagnoses and classification, study populations, healthcare and social security systems, medico-legal aspects and socio-economic variables. Furthermore, the perspective of the cost evaluation will have implications for the cost categories that will be included, and consequently for the final cost estimates. For example, cost estimates can be conducted from a societal perspective including all relevant costs, or from a perspective of employers in which only the costs of production losses are included. The latter perspective has often been used in the USA where the total cost of back pain between 1972 and 1978 was estimated to be US $16 billion per year[23] and in 1986 it was estimated at US $11.1 billion.[24] Table 8.2 presents the costs of back pain in three European countries, The Netherlands (1991), the UK (1991/1992) and Sweden (1995), in which costs were estimated from the societal perspective.[25]

Table 8.2 shows two important characteristics of total costs for back pain. Firstly, approximately 90% of the total costs for back pain are indirect costs due to work absenteeism and disability, reflecting the fact that back pain typically affects the working population. Secondly, costs are not normally distributed. The small subgroup of patients with chronic back pain is responsible for most of the costs; 15% of the employees with back pain for more than 1 month are responsible for half of the work absenteeism.[26] Others have reported that approximately 10–25% of back pain patients account for 75% of the costs.[23]

Although the data on costs for back pain are far from complete, they clearly show that low back pain is a major burden to society.

RISK FACTORS

Many epidemiological studies have been conducted to evaluate the association between risk factors and the occurrence of non-specific low back pain. Relatively little is known about risk factors for the transition from acute to chronic low back pain. Usually variables associated with non-specific low back pain are

classified as individual, psychosocial or occupational factors. Risk factors are summarized in Table 8.3.

Risk factors for occurrence
Individual risk factors

Although the results from epidemiological studies are not necessarily consistent, factors that have been reported to be associated with low back pain are age, physical fitness and strength of back and abdominal muscles. There seems to be no association between low back pain and other individual factors such as gender, height, weight, body mass index, flexibility/mobility and structural deformities of the spine.

Recent systematic reviews found that smoking and body weight should be considered to be weak risk indicators and not causes of low back pain,[27, 28] and that alcohol consumption,[29]

Table 8.1. Prevalence of low back pain in cross-sectional studies

Study	Prevalence (%)			Study population		
	Lifetime	Point	Period	Number	Age (years)	Sex (M/F)
Biering-Sørensen	62.6	12.0	–	449	30–60	M
Biering-Sørensen	61.4	15.2	–	479	30–60	F
Frymoyer	69.9	–	–	1221	28–55	M
Gyntelberg	–	–	25	–	40–59	M
Hirsch	48.8	–	–	692	15–72	F
Hult	60.0	–	–	1193	25–59	M
Magora	–	12.9	–	3316	–	M, F
Nagi	–	18.0	–	1135	18–64	M, F
Papageorgiou	59.0	–	35	1884	>18	M
Papageorgiou	59.0	–	42	2617	>18	F
Svensson	61	–	31	716	40–47	M
Svensson	67	–	35	1640	38–64	F
Valkenburg	51.4	22.2	–	3091	>20	M
Valkenburg	57.8	30.2	–	3493	>20	F
Walsh	58.3	–	36	2667	20–59	M, F

Reprinted, with permission from Andersson (1997)[1] where full details of the studies included can be found.

Table 8.2. Costs of back pain in the UK, Sweden and The Netherlands

Cost type	UK		Sweden		The Netherlands	
	Costs in US $ million (% of total)	Costs/capita	Costs in US $ million (% of total)	Costs/capita	Costs in US $ million (% of total)	Costs/capita
Direct costs	385 (11.5)	7	213 (8)	24	368 (7.4)	24
Indirect costs	2948 (88.5)	113	2262 (92)	266	4600 (92.6)	299
Total costs	3333 (100)	120	2475 (100)	290	4968 (100)	323

Source: Moffeh et al. (1995).[26]

Table 8.3. Risk factors for occurrence and chronicity of low back pain

Factor type	Occurrence	Chronicity
Individual factors	Age	Obesity
	Physical fitness	Low educational level
	Strength of back and abdominal muscles	High levels of pain and disability
	Smoking	
Psychosocial factors	Stress	Distress
	Anxiety	Depressive mood
	Mood/emotions	Somatization
	Cognitive functioning	
	Pain behaviour	
Occupational factors	Manual handling of materials	Job dissatisfaction
	Bending and twisting	Unavailability of light duty on return to work
	Whole-body vibration	Job requirement of lifting for 75% of the day
	Job dissatisfaction	
	Monotonous tasks	
	Work relations/social support	
	Control	

standing or walking, sitting, sports and total leisure-time physical activity[30] do not seem to be associated with low-back pain.

Psychosocial risk factors

Psychosocial factors that traditionally have been reported to be associated with low back pain are anxiety, depression, emotional instability and alcohol or drug abuse.[1]

A recent systematic review of observational studies of psychosocial factors for the occurrence of back pain found insufficient evidence for an effect of psychosocial factors in private life, such as family support, presence of a close friend or neighbour, social contact, social participation, instrumental support and emotional support.[31]

A recent prospective cohort study provided evidence that psychological distress at 23 years of age more than doubled the risk of low back pain onset 10 years later, while other factors (e.g. social class, childhood emotional status, body mass index, job satisfaction) did not increase the risk.[32] Another systematic review found a clear link between psychological variables and low back pain.[33] Psychological variables that are associated with low back pain are stress, distress, or anxiety as well as mood and emotions, cognitive functioning and pain behaviour.

Occupational risk factors

Occupational factors, such as physically heavy work, lifting, bending, twisting, pulling and pushing (or a combination of these last three with lifting), and vibrations, have often been associated with low back pain.[34]

A recent systematic review of aspects of physical load found strong evidence that manual handling of materials, bending and twisting, and whole-body vibration are risk factors for back pain.[31] Two systematic reviews of psychological workplace variables in back pain found strong evidence that job dissatisfaction, monotonous tasks, work relations, social support in the workplace, demands, stress and perceived ability to work were associated with the occurrence of low back pain.[31, 35] Moderate evidence was found for work pace, control, emotional effort at work and the belief that work is dangerous, while insufficient evidence was found for an association with high work pace, high qualitative demands,[35] low job content and low job control.[31]

Studies on the association between occupational risk factors and low back pain are hampered by the difficulties of measuring exposure to specific factors. Exposure to specific risk factors may vary among employees with the same job, but also the tasks they perform may vary. In addition, the 'healthy worker effect' may considerably affect results of epidemiological studies in occupational settings. That is, healthy workers may stay on the same job or perform the same task for years, while workers with low back pain may have moved to another job or function or their tasks may have been adjusted.

Risk factors for chronicity

It is important to identify as early as possible those low back pain patients who are at risk for long-term disability and sick leave, because early and specific interventions may be developed and used in this subgroup of patients. As stated previously, most patients are likely to recover within a couple of days or weeks, but recovery for those who develop chronic low back pain and disability becomes increasingly less likely the longer the problems continue. The small group of patients with long-term, severe, low back pain also account for substantial health-care utilization and sick leave, with the associated costs.

Evidence suggests that psychosocial factors are important in the transition from acute to chronic low back pain and disability.[33] A recently published systematic review of prospective cohort studies found that some psychological factors (distress, depressive mood and somatization) are associated with an increased risk of chronic low back pain.[36]

Individual and workplace factors, such as job dissatisfaction, low educational level and high levels of pain and disability, have also been reported to be associated with the transition to chronic low back pain.[37, 38] A prospective cohort study recently found that severe leg pain, obesity, functional disability, poor general health status, unavailability of light duties on return to work and a job requirement of lifting for three-quarters of the day or more were associated with the transition from acute to chronic occupational back pain.[39] Job dissatisfaction or poor workplace relations were not associated with chronic low back pain.[39] Another prospective cohort study of 328 employees identified prognostic factors for return to work of employees with 3–4 months' sick leave due to low back pain.[40] Risk factors included poor general health status, low job satisfaction, not being a breadwinner, lower age and higher pain intensity. The authors concluded that psychosocial aspects of health and work in combination with economic aspects have a significantly larger impact on return to work when compared to the relatively more physical aspects of disability and physical requirements of the job.[40]

The transition from acute to chronic low back pain seems complicated, and many individual, psychosocial and workplace factors may play a role. Since the identification of patients who are at risk for chronicity will depend on the identification of these risk factors, the implication for clinical management is unclear. Although psychosocial yellow flags are, at present, expected to play an important role in screening high-risk patients with acute and subacute low back pain,[41] and a screening instrument has been suggested for this purpose in clinical practice,[42] future research is definitely needed to test the predictive value of these factors and instruments in clinical practice.

PREVENTION

Since low back pain is a frequently occurring problem associated with high healthcare utilization and work absenteeism, prevention seems to be important to reduce the enormous suffering and related high costs. Several approaches to the prevention of back pain have been reported in the literature, but it is still unclear which types of interventions are most commonly employed, and little is known about the effectiveness of these interventions.[43–45] An important distinction is often made between primary and secondary prevention. Primary prevention usually refers to preventing the onset of a given disease in healthy people, while secondary prevention refers to preventing further development of a disease (recurrences or chronicity).[46] However, since most people suffer from low back pain at some point in their life, the difference between primary and secondary prevention of low back pain is not always clear.

Usually there is some underlying mechanism that suggests a preventive effect for a specific intervention, e.g. based on biomechanical or pathophysiological research. However, the evidence for the rationale of preventive interventions is usually not strong.[44, 46, 47] Lumbar supports may prevent low back pain because they provide support of the trunk, preventing pain-producing events caused by overflexion. Also, they remind the wearer to lift properly and they increase intra-abdominal pressure and decrease intradiscal pressure.[47] Back schools are based on the assumption that people have an increased risk of back pain because they lack knowledge about a variety of relevant topics such as anatomy, body mechanics and stress. These programmes aim to reduce the risk for problems by increasing the participant's knowledge, which in turn should alter that person's behaviour.[44] Exercises may prevent low back pain because they strengthen the back muscles and increase trunk flexibility, increase blood supply to the spine muscles, joints and intervertebral discs and, consequently, minimize injury and enhance repair. Furthermore, exercise may improve mood and have a positive effect on the perception of pain.[44] Ergonomic interventions are directed towards occupational risk factors, such as lifting, physically heavy work, a static work posture, frequent bending and twisting, repetitive work and exposure to vibration. Ergonomic interventions can be divided into job-related and worker-related types, and can include a variety of interventions.[46] Minimizing the impact of risk factors is obviously expected to result in a lower frequency or lower intensity of low back pain. Risk-factor modification is usually directed towards factors other than occupational risk factors, e.g. individual risk factors (weight, strength, smoking) and psychosocial risk factors (job control, job dissatisfaction).

A review of controlled trials on prevention included 27 studies on educational efforts, lumbar supports, exercises, ergonomics and risk-factor modification.[46] The results showed strong evidence that back schools and lumbar supports were not effective in the prevention of low back pain.[46] There was strong evidence that exercises were an effective preventive intervention. No controlled trials were found for ergonomic interventions or risk-factor modification, despite the fact that these are often promoted as preventive interventions for low back pain.[46] The authors suggested a number of factors that might account for the relatively disappointing results of these prevention studies: (1) many studies on prevention had small sample sizes and consequently lacked power to detect positive effects; (2) most studies had relatively short follow-up periods; (3) there was considerable heterogeneity in the study populations, the content of the interventions, the control interventions and the outcome measures; (4) most studies evaluated single-modal rather than multimodal interventions, which does not seem to fit with the idea that multiple risk factors usually play a role; and (5) compliance was either not high or not measured in the studies.

TREATMENT

At present, the results from more than 600 randomized controlled trials evaluating all types of conservative or complementary treatments for low back pain that are commonly used in primary care have been published. The establishment of the Cochrane Back Review Group in 1997 was an important step forward in promoting the systematic collection, review and synthesis of the low back pain literature.[48] Within the framework of the Cochrane Back Review Group, method guidelines have been developed and published to improve the quality of reviews in this field, and to facilitate comparison across reviews and enhance consistency among reviewers.[49] The evidence on treatment for acute and chronic low back pain from Cochrane and other systematic reviews has recently been updated with the results of additional trials.[50, 51] The results are summarized below.

Acute low back pain[50]

There is strong evidence that non-steroidal anti-inflammatory drugs (NSAIDs) relieve pain more than placebo. Advice to stay active speeds up symptomatic recovery and reduces chronic disability. There is strong evidence that muscle relaxants relieve pain more than placebo, but potential side-effects, including drowsiness, have been reported. There is also strong evidence that bed rest and specific back exercises (strengthening, flexibility, stretching, flexion and extension exercises) are not effective, i.e. these interventions were not more effective than no treatment, some type of placebo or sham treatment. There is moderate evidence that analgesics and spinal manipulation are effective for pain relief. There is no evidence that other interventions (e.g. lumbar supports, traction, massage or acupuncture) are effective for acute low back pain.

Various clinical guidelines on the management of low back pain in primary care have been issued. At present, guidelines exist in at least 11 different countries: Australia, Denmark, Finland, Germany, Israel, The Netherlands, New Zealand, Sweden, Switzerland, the UK and the USA. In general, the recommendations in these guidelines are quite consistent:[52]

- reassure patients (favourable prognosis)
- advise patients to stay active
- prescribe medication if necessary (preferably time-contingent): (1) paracetamol (acetaminophen), (2) NSAIDs
- discourage bed rest
- consider spinal manipulation for pain relief
- do not advise back-specific exercises.

Routine use of passive treatment modalities (e.g. bed rest, ultrasound, electrotherapy and massage) as monotherapy is not recommended, because they increase the risk of illness behaviour and chronicity. Most guidelines state that referral to secondary healthcare and x-ray examination are not indicated in the great majority of acute low back pain patients.

Chronic low back pain[51]

The evidence is summarized in Table 8.4. There is strong evidence that exercise therapy, behavioural therapy and multidisciplinary pain treatment programmes are effective for chronic low back pain, and moderate evidence for the effectiveness of analgesics, NSAIDs and back schools in occupational settings. Recent evidence also suggests that

massage may have some effect. There is no evidence that other interventions (e.g. antidepressants, steroid injections and acupuncture) are effective. However, effects are usually only small and for a short term. Sufficient evidence on long-term effects is still lacking for many commonly used interventions.

Although national guidelines do not exist, recommendations for the management of chronic low back pain have been published recently.[15, 53] The most important objectives of treatment of chronic low back pain in primary care are: (1) to prevent or reduce disability, both physically and mentally; and (2) to limit sick leave. In cases of long-lasting chronic low back pain it is important to identify an increase in disability early, to avoid long-term medical treatment and to help the patient to live with chronic low back pain. Management of chronic low back pain should focus on the problems that patients have with activities of daily living, but emotional problems, depression and other psychosocial factors may play a role. Referral for exercise therapy may be considered if patients need help to improve daily functioning. If exercise therapy has failed, if there is serious disability, or if medical consumption is high, patients should be referred for multidisciplinary biopsychosocial rehabilitation.

SUMMARY

Low back pain is a tremendous medical and socio-economic problem. Low back pain has a high incidence and prevalence, can lead to severe, long-lasting disability and is associated with high costs to society. Recent epidemiological data suggest that there is a need to revise our views regarding the course of low back pain. Low back pain is not simply either acute or chronic, but fluctuates over time with frequent recurrences or exacerbations. Also, low back pain may frequently be part of a widespread pain problem instead of being isolated, regional pain.

Epidemiological studies have identified many individual, psychosocial and occupational risk factors for the onset of low back pain, but their independent prognostic value is usually low.

PRACTICE POINTS

- Episodes of low back pain may be regarded as a natural part of human life due to its high prevalence and worldwide distribution.

- No treatment has been shown to beat the natural history of episodes of low back pain.

- Physically demanding tasks for the back, such as bending, twisting and lifting, may give increased back pain, but have little or no impact on the development of structural changes.

- There is no treatment shown to have any effect other than rather modest pain reduction.

- High intensity of pain is usually no indication of any serious structural derangement.

Table 8.4. Effectiveness of treatments for acute and chronic low back pain

Effectiveness	Acute low back pain	Chronic low back pain
Beneficial	Advice to stay active	Exercise therapy
	NSAIDs	Behavioural therapy
	Muscle relaxants	Multidisciplinary treatment programmes
Likely to be beneficial	Analgesics	Analgesics
	Spinal manipulation	Back schools in occupational settings
		Massage
		NSAIDs
Unknown effectiveness	Acupuncture	Acupuncture
	Back schools	Antidepressants
	Epidural steroid injections	Epidural steroid injections
	Lumbar supports	Lumbar supports
	Massage	Muscle relaxants
	TENS	Spinal manipulation
	Traction	TENS
	Trigger-point injections	Trigger-point injections
	Thermal therapy	Thermal therapy
	Ultrasound	Ultrasound
Unlikely to be beneficial	Specific exercises	Bed rest
		EMG biofeedback
Ineffective or harmful	Bed rest	Facet joint injections
		Traction

EMG, electromyography; NSAIDs, non-steroidal anti-inflammatory drugs; TENS, transcutaneous electrical nerve stimulation.

Similarly, a number of factors have now been identified that may increase the risk of chronic disability, but no single factor seems to have a strong impact.

Exercises seem to be the only intervention that has proven to be effective for the prevention of low back pain. There is strong evidence that advice to stay active, NSAIDs and muscle relaxants are effective treatments for acute low back pain, and moderate evidence for the effectiveness of analgesics and spinal manipulation. There is also strong evidence that exercise therapy, behavioural therapy and multidisciplinary pain treatment programmes are effective for chronic low back pain, and moderate evidence for the effectiveness of analgesics, NSAIDs and back schools in occupational settings.

RESEARCH AGENDA

- Prospective studies on the prognostic value of symptoms, signs and diagnostic labels for identifying low back pain are needed.

- The development of valid and reliable instruments identifying patients at high risk for chronicity and disability is needed.

- There is a need for future high-quality trials on prevention of chronic low back pain with sufficiently long follow-up periods and large study populations.

- Full economic evaluations should be carried out to assess the cost-effectiveness of preventive and therapeutic interventions.

REFERENCES

1. Andersson GBJ. The epidemiology of spinal disorders. In: Frymoyer JW (ed.), *The Adult Spine: Principles and Practice.* Lippincott-Raven, Philadelphia, PA, 1997, pp. 93–141.
2. Van Tulder MW, Koes BW, Bouter LM. A cost-of-illness study of back pain in The Netherlands. *Pain* 1995; **62**: 233–240.
3. Waddell G. The epidemiology of low back pain. In: *The Back Pain Revolution.* Churchill Livingstone, Edinburgh, 1998, pp. 69–84.
4. Rothman KJ, Greenland S. *Modern Epidemiology.* Lippincott-Raven, Philadelphia, PA, 1998.
5. Deyo RA, Rainville J, Kent DL. What can the history and physical examination tell us about low back pain? *JAMA* 1992; **268**: 760–765.

6. Deyo RA. Measuring the functional status of patients with low back pain. *Arch Phys Med Rehab* 1988; **69**: 1044–1053.

7. Waddell G. 1987 Volvo award in clinical sciences. A new clinical model for the treatment of low-back pain. *Spine* 1987; **12**: 632–644.

8. Van Tulder MW, Assendelft WJ, Koes BW et al. Spinal radiographic findings and nonspecific low back pain. A systematic review of observational studies. *Spine* 1997; **22**: 427–434.

9. Jensen MC, Brant-Zawadzki MN, Obuchowski N et al. Magnetic resonance imaging of the lumbar spine in people without back pain. *N Engl J Med* 1994; **331**: 69–73.

10. Frymoyer JW. Back pain and sciatica. *N Engl J Med* 1988; **318**: 291–300.

11. Croft PR, Macfarlane GJ, Papageorgiou AC et al. Outcome of low back pain in general practice: a prospective study. *BMJ* 1998; **316**: 1356–1359.

12. Von Kor M, Saunders K. The course of back pain in primary care. *Spine* 1996; **21**: 2833–2837.

13. Croft PR, Papageorgiou AC, McNally R. Low back pain. In: Stevens A, Raffery J (eds), *Health Care Needs Assessment.* Radcliffe Medical, Oxford, 1997, pp. 129–182.

14. Andersson GB. Epidemiological features of chronic low-back pain. *Lancet* 1999; **354**: 581–585.

15. Waddell G. The clinical course of low back pain. In: *The Back Pain Revolution.* Churchill Livingstone, Edinburgh, 1998, pp. 103–107.

16. Bergman S, Herrstrom P, Hogstrom K et al. Chronic musculoskeletal pain, prevalence rates, and sociodemographic associations in a Swedish population study. *J Rheumatol* 2001; **28**: 1369–1377.

17. Natvig B, Bruusgaard D, Eriksen W. Localized low back pain and low back pain as part of widespread musculoskeletal pain: two different disorders? A cross-sectional population study. *J Rehab Med* 2001; **33**: 21–25.

18. Thomas E, Silman AJ, Croft PR et al. Predicting who develops chronic low back pain in primary care: a prospective study. *BMJ* 1999; **318**: 1662–1667.

19. Van den Velden J, De Bakker DH, Claessens AAMC et al. *Een Nationale Studie Naar Ziekten en Verrichtingen in de Huisartspraktijk.* Morbiditeit in de huisartspraktijk, Basisrapport/NIVEL, Utrecht, 1991.

20. Lamberts H. *In Het Huis Van de Huisarts. Verslag van het Transitieprojekt.* Meditekst, Lelystad, 1991.

21. Papageorgiou AC, Croft PR, Thomas E et al. Influence of previous pain experience on the episode incidence of low back pain: results from the South Manchester Back Pain Study. *Pain* 1996; **66**: 181–185.

22. Picavet HSJ, Schouten JSAG, Smit HA. *Prevalences and Consequences of Low Back Pain in the MORGEN-Project 1993–1995.* Reference No. 263200004. Rijksinstituut voor volksgezondheid en milieu, Bilthoven, 1996.

23. Frymoyer JW, Cats-Baril W. An overview of the incidences and costs of low back pain. *Orthop Clin North Am* 1991; **22**: 263–271.

24. Webster BS, Snook SH. The cost of compensable low back pain. *J Occup Med* 1990; **32**: 13–15.

25. Moffett JK, Richardson G, Sheldon TA et al. *Back Pain: Its Management and Costs to Society.* Discussion Paper 129. Centre for Health Economics, University of York, York, 1995.

26. Watson PJ, Main CJ, Waddell G et al. Medically certified work loss, recurrence and costs of wage compensation for back pain: a follow-up study of the working population of Jersey. *Br J Rheumatol* 1998; **37**: 82–86.

27. Leboeuf-Yde C. Smoking and low back pain. A systematic literature review of 41 journal articles reporting 47 epidemiologic studies. *Spine* 1999; **24**: 1463–1470.

28. Leboeuf-Yde C. Body weight and low back pain. A systematic literature review of 56 journal articles reporting on 65 epidemiologic studies. *Spine* 2000; **25**: 226–237.

29. Leboeuf-Yde C. Alcohol and low-back pain: a systematic literature review. *J Manip Physiol Ther* 2000; **23**: 343–346.

30. Hoogendoorn WE, van Poppel MNM, Bongers PM et al. Physical load during work and leisure time as risk factors for back pain. *Scand J Work Environ Health* 1999; **25**: 387–403.

31. Hoogendoorn WE, van Poppel MNM, Bongers PM et al. Systematic review of psychosocial factors at work and private life as risk factors for back pain. *Spine* 2000; **25**: 2114–2125.

32. Power C, Frank J, Hertzman C et al. Predictors of low back pain onset in a prospective British study. *Am J Pub Health* 2001; **91**: 1671–1678.

33. Linton SJ. A review of psychological risk factors in back and neck pain. *Spine* 2000; **25**: 1148–1156.

34. Bongers PM, de Winter CR, Kompier MAJ et al. Psychosocial factors at work and musculoskeletal disease: a review of the literature. *Scand J Work Environ Health* 1993; **19**: 297–312.

35. Linton SJ. Occupational psychological factors increase the risk for back pain: a systematic review. *J Occup Rehab* 2001; **11**: 53–66.

36. Pincus T, Burton AK, Vogel S et al. A systematic review of psychological factors as predictors of chronicity/disability in prospective cohorts of low back pain. *Spine* 2002; **27**: E109–E120.

37. Cats-Baril WL, Frymoyer JW. Identifying patients at risk of becoming disabled because of low back pain: the Vermont Rehabilitation Engineering Center predictive model. *Spine* 1991; **16**: 605–607.

38. Gatchel RJ. The dominant role of psychosocial risk factors in the development of chronic low back pain disability. *Spine* 1995; **20**: 2702–2709.

39. Fransen M, Woodward M, Norton R et al. Risk factors associated with the transition from acute to chronic occupational back pain. *Spine* 2002; **27**: 92–98.

40. van der Giezen AM, Bouter LM, Nijhuis FJ. Prediction of return-to-work of low back pain patients sicklisted for 3–4 months. *Pain* 2000; **87**: 285–294.

41. Kendall N, Linton S, Main C. *Guide to Assessing Psychosocial Yellow Flags in Acute Low Back Pain: Risk Factors for Long-Term Disability and Work Loss.* National Advisory Committee on Health and Disability and ACC (Accident Rehabilitation and Compensation Insurance Corporation), Wellington, 1997.

42. Linton SJ, Hallden K. Can we screen for problematic back pain? A screening questionnaire for predicting outcome in acute and subacute back pain. *Clin J Pain* 1998; **14**: 209–215.

43. Frank JW, Kerr MS, Brooker AS et al. Disability resulting from occupational low back pain. Part I. What do we know about primary prevention? *Spine* 1996; **21**: 2908–2917.

44. Lahad A, Malter AD, Berg AO et al. The effectiveness of four interventions for the prevention of low back pain. *JAMA* 1994; **272**: 1286–1291.

45. van Poppel MNM, Koes BW, Smid T et al. A systematic review of controlled clinical trials on the prevention of back pain in industry. *Occup Environ Med* 1997; **54**: 841–847.

46. Linton SJ, Van Tulder MW. Preventive interventions for back and neck pain problems: what is the evidence? *Spine* 2001; **26**: 778–787.

47. van Poppel MN, de Looze MP, Koes BW et al. Mechanisms of action of lumbar supports: a systematic review. *Spine* 2000; **25**: 2103–2113.

48. Bombardier C, Esmail R, Nachemson AL. Back Review Group Editorial Board. The Cochrane Collaboration Back Review Group for spinal disorders. *Spine* 1997; **22**: 837–840.

49. Van Tulder MW, Assendelft WJJ, Koes BW et al. Method guidelines for systematic reviews in the Cochrane Collaboration Back Review Group for Spinal Disorders. *Spine* 1997; **22**: 2323–2330.

50. Van Tulder MW, Koes BW. Acute low back pain and sciatica. *Clin Evidence* 2002; **7**: 1018–1031.

51. van Tulder MW, Koes BW. Chronic low back pain and sciatica. *Clin Evidence* 2002; **7**: 1032–1048.

52. Koes BW, Van Tulder MW, Ostelo R et al. Clinical guidelines for the management of low back pain in primary care: an international comparison. *Spine* 2001; **26**: 2504–2513.

53. Nachemson A, Jonsson E. *Neck and Back Pain: the Scientific Evidence of Causes, Diagnosis, and Treatment.* Lippincott Williams & Wilkins, Philadelphia, PA, 2000.

Low back pain from a clinical point of view

Aage Indahl

New research on low back pain is published almost daily. For a clinician it is hard to stay up to date at all times. In this context, writing a book chapter is challenging from many perspectives, not least for the fear that it is already out of date at the time of publication. To meet this need, a variety of systematic reviews is published at an increasing rate, and these seem to be popular with both researchers and clinicians. For clinicians there is also a need for an overview of such different aspects of low back pain as prevention and treatment in order to stay in line with best practice. For this reason publications such as this book serve a good cause and are very useful. The introduction of evidence-based medicine seems to be gradually changing our way of thinking. We are becoming increasingly aware of what we really know and what we think we know. For many of us, as clinicians, this has brought a sense of unrest into our practice. Increasingly, we are faced with patients challenging our handling, procedures and diagnoses based on information they have obtained on the Internet.

The question now is whether there is any new evidence available that alters the recommendations and conclusions of the preceding chapter. The short answer is 'No', but if you need more details they can be found in the new European guidelines on low back pain.[1] Here you will also find the background data and the discussion behind the recommendations and conclusions.

From a clinical point of view one wonders what is the bottom line so far and what it is we need to know in order to stay in line with best practice. Let us take a look at the different areas of low back pain. The epidemiology tells us that the majority of mankind is afflicted with this condition at one time or another. It does not seem that it is a result of living and working in an industrialized part of the world. Acute low back pain may in the future prove to be like the common flu, a real nuisance but unavoidable, and maybe have some kind of constructive effect.

PREVENTION OF THE CONSEQUENCES OF LOW BACK PAIN

There is no indication that primary prevention is feasible. There is also little evidence that secondary prevention (prevention of recurrences) is effective or highly successful. What seems possible is the prevention of the consequences of low back pain. The pain itself may be treated in different ways, but what is feared is the development of an acute episode into a chronic pain condition. The consequences of developing chronic pain are important from the perspectives of both the individual and society. They include broad issues such as recurrence (including severity and disability), work loss, care seeking, health-related quality of life and compensation.

The traditional thinking along the lines of an 'injury model' seems to be losing support and recommendations based on a biomechanical approach are no longer recommended.[2] This means that we do not have to give our patients any restrictions on activities or how to carry out their activities. There seems to be no need to learn 'proper' lifting techniques or 'correct' ways of using your back. Lifetime exposure to high physical loading of the back does not seem to cause any clinically important increase in 'degeneration' of the spine (spondylosis), including disc herniations. Heavy work seems only to be a factor for aggravating low back pain and does not seem to predict chronic back pain.[3, 4] Thus optimal progress in prevention in low back pain will likely require a cultural shift in how low back pain is viewed, its relationship with activity and work, how it might best be tackled, and just what is reasonable to expect from preventive strategies. However, there is evidence to suggest that prevention of various consequences of low back pain is feasible.

The most promising approaches seem to involve physical activity and exercise, and appropriate education for all target groups, at least for adults (Box 8.1). In other words, preventing the consequences of low back pain is in line with the treatment recommendations for low back pain, namely to encourage the patient to stay active and keep fit, regardless of how this is done. Overall, there is limited robust evidence for many aspects of prevention of low back pain. For those interventions where there is acceptable evidence, the effect sizes are rather modest.

TREATMENTS

It is difficult to treat something when the cause is unknown. The vast majority of patients are labelled as having non-specific low back pain, in other words pain of unknown origin. Even if the origin of the pain is unknown the sufferer is in no way unknown to us. It is our patient who is seeking help and expecting us to perform best practice in so doing. Before focusing on how to resolve this issue, we need to look at the evidence.

For the treatment of low back pain there is no proof that any treatment has a curative effect on the condition or alters the natural course. All treatments should therefore be regarded as pain management and applied with this in mind. The effect of those modalities that seem to be successful is not impressive. There is no proven treatment that seems to have a superior benefit over other treatments. The effect size is at best rather modest. In other words a combination of non-steroidal anti-inflammatory drugs (NSAIDs) and paracetamol (acetaminophen) seems to have largely the same effect as manipulations. It has been argued that there are subgroups that respond to different treatments in a much more favourable way than the results seem to indicate. That may be the case, but to date there have been no reports of a practical method of how to divide patients adequately into such subgroups. So for now we have to live with the challenge of finding the best treatment for our patient without the benefit of a good selection tool.

Acute and subacute low back pain

It is very seldom that acute low back pain is a sign of serious pathology, but still we must rule out this possibility. In low back pain that means, for all practical purposes, the occurrence of fractures, tumours or infections in the spine. There is no simple diagnostic procedure that will resolve the matter, but three questions will most likely suffice. As primary tumours of the spine are rare, but metastasis to the spine is common, the first question to ask is: 'Have you had a malignant or cancerous condition before?' The next thing to ask is about infection, and a simple question such as 'Do you feel unwell?' will most likely be sufficient. Finally, it is important to ask about any recent major fall

or injury. A negative answer to all three questions will allow you to go on treating the pain as a common low back pain condition.

In taking the patient's history, focus on the patient's situation rather than on finding any connection with some activity that may have coincided with the onset of the pain. There is no evidence that any of the procedures done in a physical examination will bring us any closer to finding out where the pain is coming from. Taking the patient's history and listening to his or her symptoms gives you the diagnosis.[5] In treating acute low back pain there is still no magic bullet. The most recent research confirms the trend we have seen over recent years: a more positive approach to keeping patients active and with no specific restrictions on activity. This seems to be the uniform message from all recent guidelines on treating low back pain (see the preceding chapter).

In addition, there is a trend towards emphasizing the need for reassurance of the favourable prognosis of the condition and removing unwarranted fear in order to keep the patient active. In this respect the physical examination may be our best tool in undertaking a cognitive intervention designed to remove fear and uncertainties and reassure the patient that there is no serious spinal pathology. The examination procedure will take on the character of a guided tour for the patient, where what we are looking for and what we find is explained. When the tour is finished the patient will hopefully be reassured and determined to stay active and thankful for your suggestions for pain management.

As stated before, there is no evidence that any of the treatment modalities offered to patients have any other effect than pain relief. So the bottom line for treatments is: if it works, it has some effect on pain and the effect size seems to be roughly the same, regardless of the treatment. The best effect of treatment seems to be when both the provider and the patient believe in the treatment, so choose whichever treatment you prefer (Box 8.2).

Long-lasting (chronic) low back pain

The best treatment of chronic pain is probably good handling of acute low back pain. Even if best practice is applied we will in some cases inevitably end up with patients having a more chronic pain condition. The term 'chronic pain' is problematic in itself because it conveys a message both to the health provider and patient that this may be more or less permanent. I think it is important to regard it as long-lasting pain, and that it eventually will get better.

What do we do then? At this stage many patients have tried different treatments or are on the lookout for treatments that will resolve their pain problem. There is still no evidence that any of the treatments offered have a curative effect on chronic low back pain. There are no new treatments, either invasive or non-invasive, that have been proven to be effective, even if they initially looked promising. As for acute low back pain, the treatment modalities shown to have some effect also seem to have at most a modest effect on long-lasting back pain. The only treatment for which this is not true is exercise. For acute low back pain exercise does not seem to have any effect and is not recommended, while in long-lasting low back pain it seems to be one of the best approaches. There is still no evidence for recommending a specific type of exercise, so the patient can choose whatever he or she prefers. While high-impact exercise, such as jogging on hard surfaces, is beneficial and is not harmful, it may be too painful to be a realistic option.

The evidence suggests that combining exercise with a cognitive approach designed to reduce pain-related fear seems to be effective, but it is still unknown what type of patient is most likely to benefit from what kind of behavioural treatment.[6] Hindrance towards resuming activity and work seems to be complex. 'Fear-avoidance behaviour' has been proposed as an important factor in not resuming activity.[7–12] In this model the patient's disability is not only a function of their pain, but also of their response to pain. This model also maintains that there are two extreme responses to pain, either a confronting response or an avoidance response. Since the relationship between pain and disability has been shown to be low,[12, 13] it is proposed that the fear is more linked to fear of injury or re-injury than to pain.[8] Fear-avoidance behaviour has been shown to be an important factor in the development and maintenance of chronic low back pain.[9, 14]

The focus on fear as a factor in developing persistent low back pain may not lead us far enough to solving the puzzle of chronicity. Our behaviour is based on experience, cognition, memory, beliefs and anticipation. A certain behaviour that can be described as fear avoidance may in reality be a logical reaction based on the cognition the patient has of the situation without any aspect of fear. If the patient believes that he has sustained an injury, avoidance of certain activities would be logical and founded on judgement rather than on fear. In other words, fear-avoidance behaviour may be the normal response of normal people to conflicting and confusing explanations from care providers. Clinical examination coupled with education designed to remove uncertainty and give the patient an understanding that the spine is strong and will not suffer any injury through activity, has proved to be beneficial.[15–18] In a recent study comparing spinal fusion surgery with a cognitive intervention and exercise treatment, emphasis was put on giving the patient a new understanding of his or her pain, which

was designed to remove misunderstanding and uncertainty. This approach proved to be equal in effect when compared with surgical fusion.[19] The inability to show for specific targeted interventions a substantial effect in treating specific entities strongly suggests that the modalities applied in the cure for non-specific low back pain have non-specific pain-modulating effects. This may be important for patients during the time when the condition heals itself and may have an effect on return to work. The trend in the treatment of low back pain seems to be focused on giving the patient support through physical examination and education to resume activity, in other words to focus on treating the disability rather than the pain itself.[20] Treating the pain will, in this context, be part of the effort to get patients back to participating in social and work life as soon as possible (Box 8.3).

FURTHER RESEARCH

Where should we go from here? There seems to be less and less evidence in support of an injury model for the changes found in painful conditions of the spine. Popular terms such as 'stability' and 'instability' seem to form the basis of many treatments, both invasive (e.g. fusion surgery) and non-invasive (e.g. different exercises). None of these have been proven to be successful. There is a great need for the development of new models that may result in novel research. We need to ask questions like: 'Why does lifelong heavy physical loading on the spine not result in disc degeneration and disc herniation?' and 'What are the real mechanisms behind disc herniations?' Our injury model may prevent us from asking the crucial questions.

In the task of having the patient keep on with normal activity despite pain, we must find out how this can be done most efficiently. We must find out how and by whom reassurance is

---

Box 8.3. Treatment of long-standing (chronic) low back pain

- Take a history, focusing on the patient's situation and identifying any complicating factors
- To rule out serious conditions ask 'Have you had a malignant disease before?', 'Do you feel unwell?' and 'Have you had a recent major fall or injury?'
- Do a physical examination as a guided tour, where the findings are explained and designed to rule out misconceptions and uncertainties in order for the patient to stay active
- Provide adequate pain management
- Urge the patient to keep on with light normal activity as best as they can
- Assure the patient that such activity will do no harm
- Advise the patient to do some exercise of their own choosing
- Use imaging to rule out pathology and as a cognitive tool, not for finding the cause of pain
- Reassess if progress is not as expected

delivered most effectively and how it can be targeted to the patient's specific need. Overall there is a great need for the development of highly effective treatment modalities, even if the chances of finding the magic bullet seem rather bleak at present.

RESEARCH AGENDA

- There is a need for new models to replace the injury model.

- Mechanisms underlying disc herniations need to be elucidated.

- Pain mechanisms in the spine need to be determined.

- We need to find out what patients need in order to stay active.

- We need to determine how our message of reassurance is best delivered and by whom.

- There is a need for novel treatments that can be proven to be highly effective.

- We need to find the magic bullet!

REFERENCES

1. European Commission Research Directorate General. *Low Back Pain: Guidelines for its Management.* Available at: http://www.backpaineurope. org/web/files/WG4_Guidelines.pdf (accessed 28 August 2006).
2. Burton AK, Balague F, Cardon G et al. How to prevent low back pain. *Best Pract Res Clin Rheumatol* 2005; **19**: 541–555.
3. Nachemson AL, Jonsson E. *Neck and Back Pain. The Scientific Evidence of Causes, Diagnosis, and Treatment.* Lippincott Williams & Wilkins, Philadelphia, PA, 2000.
4. Hansson T, Westerholm P. *Arbete och besvär i rörelseorganen. En vetenskaplig värdering av frågor om samband.* Arbetslivsinstitutet, Stockholm, 2001.
5. Indahl A. Low back pain: diagnosis, treatment, and prognosis. *Scand J Rheumatol* 2004; **33**: 199–209.
6. Tulder van MW, Ostelo RWJG, Vlaeyen JWS et al. *Behavioural Treatment for Chronic Low Back Pain.* Cochrane Review, Issue 4. Cochrane Library/Wiley, Chichester, 2003.
7. Lethem J, Slade PD, Troup JDG et al. Outline of a fear-avoidance model of exaggerated pain perception. *Behav Res Ther* 1983; **21**: 401–408.
8. Vlaeyen JW, Kole-Snijders AM, Boeren RG et al. Fear of movement/(re)injury in chronic low back pain and its relation to behavioral performance. *Pain* 1995; **62**: 363–372.
9. Vlaeyen JW, Linton SJ. Fear-avoidance and its consequences in chronic musculoskeletal pain: a state of the art. *Pain* 2000; **85**: 317–332.
10. Vlaeyen JWS, Haazen IW, Schuerman JA et al. Behavioural rehabilitation of chronic low back pain: comparison of an operant treatment, an operant–cognitive treatment and an operant–respondent treatment. *Br J Clin Psychol* 1995; **34**: 95–118.
11. Waddell G, Main CJ, Morris EW et al. Chronic low back pain, psychologic distress, and illness behavior. *Spine* 1984; **9**: 209–213.
12. Waddell G, Newton G, Henderson WI et al. A fear-avoidance beliefs questionnaire (FABQ) and the role of fear-avoidance beliefs in chronic low back pain and disability. *Pain* 1993; **52**: 157–168.
13. Linton SJ, Buer N. Working despite pain: factors associated with work attendance versus dysfunction. *Int J Behav Med* 1995; **2**: 252–262.
14. Burton AK, Tillotson KM, Main CJ et al. Psychosocial predictors of outcome in acute and subchronic low back trouble. *Spine* 1995; **20**: 722–728.
15. Indahl A, Haldorsen EH, Holm S et al. Five-year follow-up study of a controlled clinical trial using light mobilization and an informative approach to low back pain. *Spine* 1998; **23**: 2625–2630.
16. Indahl A, Velund L, Reikeraas O. Good prognosis for low back pain when left untampered. A randomized clinical trial. *Spine* 1995; **20**: 473–477.
17. Karjalainen K, Malmivaara A, Pohjolainen T et al. Mini-intervention for subacute low back pain: a randomized controlled trial. *Spine* 2003; **28**: 533–541.
18. McGuirk B, King W, Govind J et al. Safety, efficacy, and cost-effectiveness of evidence-based guidelines for the management of acute low back pain in primary care. *Spine* 2001; **26**: 2615–2622.
19. Brox JI, Sørensen R, Friis A et al. Randomized clinical trial of lumbar instrumented fusion and cognitive intervention and exercises in patients with chronic low back pain and disc degeneration. *Spine* 2003; **28**: 1919–1921.
20. Loisel P, Durand M-J, Berthelette D et al. Disability prevention. New paradigm for the management of occupational back pain. *Dis Manage Health Outcome* 2001; **9**: 351–360.

Chapter 9
Self-care techniques for acute episodes of low back pain

Sherri Weiser, Marco A. Campello, Margareta Nordin and Markus Pietrek

INTRODUCTION

Up to 80% of adults have had at least one episode of low back pain during their lifetime. Clinicians and researchers have dichotomized low back pain as specific or non-specific. Specific back pain indicates spinal pathology such as fracture, tumour, infection, cauda equina syndrome or systemic diseases, which are often called 'red flags'.[1] Specific diagnoses also include non-spinal conditions such as vascular, abdominal, urinary or pelvic pathology causing referred back pain. Non-specific low back pain (NSLBP) is pain that occurs in the absence of red flags and any other referred conditions. NSLBP usually resolves spontaneously within 1 month.[1, 2] However, it is unclear how often and how disabling recurrences are in the population at large.

Despite efforts to reduce its impact, NSLBP remains a growing problem in western cultures. In the past decade evidence-based guidelines for the management and treatment of low back pain have suggested that minimal medical intervention is necessary in the majority of cases of acute (duration up to 1 month) NSLBP.[1, 3, 4] For example, guidelines advise that the resumption of normal activities should be encouraged and non-prescribed or over-the-counter medications should be used as needed in the acute phase of a NSLBP episode.[1, 3, 5] However, many NSLBP patients continue to seek treatment from healthcare practitioners that may be unnecessary or even harmful. Overtreatment can result in a 'validation' of the back problem as a serious disorder that becomes increasingly hard to challenge. It is contended that the recommendation of self-care for early low back pain can prevent these problems and teach the patient life-long habits that may control future episodes of pain.

SHIFTING PERSPECTIVE

Experts in the field of back pain have supported the concept of self-care since the introduction of the first evidence-based guidelines.[6] However, minimizing medical intervention involves important philosophical shifts on the part of the individual with NSLBP as well as on the part of the healthcare practitioner. Patients must change their perception of NSLBP as a serious disorder requiring the attention of a healthcare professional to a common disorder that is self-limiting. Such a change in perception would put the emphasis on alleviating symptoms and preventing future episodes instead of the often fruitless search for aetiology. The healthcare provider must also view the problem in a new way. A professional who is trained to heal may have difficulty relying on the patient's own ability to self-heal. Yet this shift must occur if the concept of self-care is to be conveyed to the patient in a convincing manner. Understanding the advantages of self-care is necessary to facilitate a change in philosophy.

Advantages of self-care techniques

Teaching patients to manage their own back pain is desirable for several reasons. Reducing healthcare visits can diminish the risk of iatrogenic complications, alter the individual's beliefs about NSLBP and significantly reduce the costs associated with low back pain.

Iatrogenic complications

The risk of complications from medical treatment can vary from mild to severe. For example, pain medications may cause unpleasant side-effects and injections can lead to infection. In a qualitative study, Schers et al.[7] found that physicians were willing to order unnecessary tests or treatment to appease a patient who is expecting a certain type of care. Some of these problems can be avoided by encouraging the patient to engage in self-care.

In addition to the risks posed from unnecessary or inappropriate treatment, inaccurate or incomplete information given to the patient by the healthcare provider may have equally damaging results. Such information forms the basis of the patient's beliefs about their medical status. Failure to describe the natural history of low back pain and to minimize the severity of the disorder can cause anxiety, depression and fear of movement.[8, 9] This is often the prelude to chronicity.

Studies have found that most healthcare providers address only medical issues at the first encounter and do not adequately address the patient's concerns.[9, 10] The potential impact is dissatisfaction with the provider. The patient may thus seek care elsewhere or become a 'treatment shopper' until a satisfactory relationship is obtained.

Another potential outcome of miscommunication between the patient and the provider is that the patient does not fully understand or adhere to treatment. Suggestions for improving communication between healthcare providers and patients are given at the end of this chapter.

BACK PAIN BELIEFS

Beliefs about health are important in the course and outcome of low back pain. Self-care promotes the view that individuals have control over their back pain. Research has found that active approaches are superior to passive modalities for NSLBP. This may be moderated, in part, by feelings of control. It has been shown that individuals who perceive that they have control over their low back pain and the ability to affect the necessary behaviours have better outcomes than those who do not.[11]

A belief in one's ability to control health has been related to active coping strategies and to lower levels of psychological distress in a correlational study of chronic patients.[11] It has also been associated with greater benefits from treatment in a prospective study of individuals with chronic or recurrent low back pain.[12] A lack of perceived control over health was found to predict prolonged sick leave when combined with other variables in a prospective study of subacute patients.[13] However, prospective studies of asymptomatic individuals found no predictive value for belief in control over one's health.[14, 15]

General health beliefs about control may be less helpful in acute low back pain than specific beliefs, such as self-efficacy, in one's ability to control pain and function. This is an area that requires further research. However, in prospective studies of chronic low back pain patients, self-efficacy beliefs about function predicted actual behaviour[16, 17] and, therefore, may be an important determinant of disability. Some studies of chronic patients indicated that self-efficacy beliefs about pain had no relationship to functional performance.[16–18] However, others have found this variable to be predictive.[19–21]

In a study by Damush et al.,[22] inner-city patients with acute low back pain maintained gains in physical and mental functioning and reported greater self-efficacy to manage recurrences after self-care education at 1 year follow-up than did a control group receiving usual care. Despite a low participation rate, this study indicates that the advantages of self-care may be moderated by cognitive factors.

It may be concluded that increasing perceptions of control and self-efficacy can have beneficial effects. Providing patients with self-care techniques and the encouragement they need to use them can increase psychological well-being, improve adherence and result in good outcomes.

MEDICAL COSTS

Different estimates of the cost of NSLBP have been reported. However, the range is estimated to be between US $25 million to US $25 billion per year in direct costs and US $50 billion to more than US $100 billion for the total cost in the USA.[23] Medical costs comprise a large percentage of these costs.[9, 23, 24] Guidelines are intended to reduce costs. However, little empirical evidence is available to support this claim. One randomized controlled study compared a guideline-based intervention with usual care in a group of subacute low back pain patients. The intervention group returned to work faster than the control group and had statistically lower costs in the first year at follow-up. However, at a 3-year follow-up there were no differences in costs between the two groups.[25]

Medical costs, such as medical visits, hospitalization, rehabilitation and/or diagnostics for NSLBP, may be reduced by promoting self-care that is consistent with guidelines, since self-care implies fewer visits to healthcare professionals. Whether or not this is true is a matter for future research. However, given the considerable costs associated with low back pain, teaching patients to use self-care techniques seems prudent.

SELF-CARE TECHNIQUES

Self-care techniques are techniques that individuals can use independently, without the help of a healthcare professional. Self-care techniques include oral medication, physical activity and modalities, and mind–body techniques. Guideline recommendations are aimed at healthcare providers who treat low back pain and are not often read by patients. The following is information that may be given to patients to encourage self-care. The techniques here are limited to methods that can be easily described by the healthcare provider and implemented by the individual.

Medication

According to the guidelines for the management of acute low back pain,[1, 2] paracetamol (acetaminophen) as an over-the-counter pharmaceutical is recommended as the first choice for treatment. Besides being prescription-free and inexpensive, paracetamol has a low potential for side-effects at usual doses.[1–3] In comparison, non-steroidal anti-inflammatory drugs (NSAIDs), such as the prescription-free acetylsalicylic acid (Aspirin), or the prescription-bound diclofenac or ibuprofen, have a number of potential side-effects, particularly gastro-intestinal complications, which also occur but at a lower incidence rate in the new cyclooxygenase-2 inhibitors such as celecoxib.[26] The other commonly used drugs for low back pain, muscle relaxants (which are generally prescription-bound) and opioid analgesics (prescription-bound), may cause drowsiness, physical dependence (only opioids), decreased reaction time and clouded judgement.[1, 2]

Patients should be advised to use paracetamol at regular intervals and usual doses for acute NSLBP. It is a safe and inexpensive drug and with its over-the-counter availability it is least likely to encourage 'medicalization' of the low back problem, since it does not necessitate visits to the treating physician to obtain a prescription. If paracetamol does not provide adequate pain control, NSAIDs may be used as a replacement, but side-effects, patients' age and comorbidities as well as the costs must be taken into consideration. Due to their side-effects and potential complications, muscle relaxants and, in particular, opioids should be used only as a short-course treatment (less than 1–2 weeks) if the other two possibilities do not achieve adequate pain relief. An extensive review of the use of medication for low back pain has been published elsewhere.[27]

Empirical support   Literature reviews[2, 28, 29] have shown that paracetamol is comparable to NSAIDs, which are effective in reducing back pain. Different types of NSAIDs are equally effective.[30] Muscle relaxants and opioids are an additional option, but have not been shown to be more effective than the other, safer drugs.[31] The use of other oral medication such as antidepressants and corticosteroids is not recommended for the treatment of acute low back pain.

Physical activities and modalities
Activity
Bed rest and inactivity have been shown to be detrimental for patients. They promote muscle atrophy, cardiorespiratory de-conditioning, bone mineral loss and a sense of being seriously ill.[32] The Paris Task Force recommendation for patients with acute NSLBP is: 'Patients must be strongly encouraged to maintain or resume their normal activities as far as the pain allows'.[3] This statement is strongly supported by experts in the primary care, rheumatology, surgical and physical therapy fields.[3, 27, 30, 33] It is also recommended that specific exercises be avoided in the acute stage of low back pain as they have been shown to have no benefit or to be less effective than the recommendation to resume normal activities.

Activity limitations   Commonly the healthcare practitioner will recommend against certain activities. These recommendations are usually based on the patient's symptoms, activity requirements, such as work tasks, and the practitioner's beliefs. Biomechanical and epidemiological studies have underlined the fact that lifting, awkward positions and exposure to whole-body vibration increase reporting of low back pain, and therefore should be avoided during an episode of acute low back pain. However, gradually returning to normal activities seems to have better long-term outcome for the patient than 'avoidance' recommendations.[34]

Fear of movement   Fear of movement is common among patients with acute NSLBP.[9] It is natural for patients to associate hurt with harm. Explaining the difference between these concepts in NSLBP is crucial for a good outcome.

One simple way to detect fear of movement is to ask the patient directly. For example, you may ask 'Do you think movement will harm you?' Another way is to use standardized scales such as The Fear Avoidance Beliefs Questionnaire or The Tampa Scale for Kinesiophobia (TSK).[35] If fear of movement is suspected, the patient should be given accurate and current information that indicates that avoiding normal activities can have a detrimental effect on low back pain. A referral to a pain specialist or psychologist is not necessary unless the patient's resistance to movement persists.[3, 4]

Empirical support   Hagen et al.[36] reviewed 11 trials that included 1962 participants and concluded that for acute low back pain patients advice to stay in bed is less effective than the advice to stay active. Likewise, the Paris Task Force[3] scrutinized six randomized controlled trials[34, 37–41] of acceptable to excellent quality. They found that exercise prescription during the first week of acute NSLBP is also not indicated. In fact, they stated: 'The prescription of active physical exercises or re-education is contraindicated in the first week of acute low back pain and sciatica. Dynamic, active exercises, in particular are contra-indicated'.[3] This recommendation is consistent with the concept of resuming normal activities gradually. However, there are some caveats to this recommendation. The six randomized controlled trials appraised acute NSLBP of no more than 7 days duration. Three of the studies of high quality[38–40] clearly demonstrated the ineffectiveness of prescribed exercise in the treatment of acute NSLBP. In the three other studies[34, 37, 41] exercise was somewhat effective but only under certain conditions and in certain patient groups. In general, the evidence was stronger for maintaining activity than for prescribing specific exercises during the acute phase of NSLBP.

Molde Hagen et al.[25] conducted a randomized, controlled trial in subacute patients with low back pain to assess the benefits of the recommendation to stay active. One group received this recommendation by the physician and the other did not. The study showed that the group exposed to the 'stay active' message showed greater health gains 3 years after injury than the group that was not exposed.

Exercises
After 4 weeks of NSLBP, exercises have been shown to be effective when used in conjunction with a behavioural approach.[42, 43] The same holds true for the patient with intermittent or recurrent low back pain. A behavioural approach to exercise suggests a goal-oriented or graded-exercise programme, where exercises are gradually increased to achieve the desired level of physical ability (Box 9.1). No one type of exercise has been shown to be more effective than any other. However, the

patient's preference for a certain type of exercise may increase compliance and improve outcome.

Most specific exercise techniques require some instruction and training from a specialist such as a physical therapist. A general exercise programme that combines aerobic training, stretching and strengthening exercises can be easily taught as part of self-care. However, little is known about establishing the exact parameters for intensity, duration and frequency of exercises for the patient with non-acute NSLBP. The type of exercise prescribed is often dependent on the training and preferences of the provider and may vary considerably. For example, some therapists advocate the use of weights and aerobic training, while others endorse movement therapies. Since the clinical examination of a patient with NSLBP rarely indicates specific findings, a general fitness programme of any type is usually safe.

Empirical support   A variety of exercises have been studied in a small number of randomized controlled trials for patients with NSLBP. They include flexion/extension exercises for the trunk, various dynamic exercises, aerobics, stretching, the Williams method, McKenzie-style exercises, isometric exercises and walking and jogging.[3] There is no evidence that one type of exercise achieves a better outcome than another type of exercise in the treatment of subacute NSLBP. There is some evidence, however, that graded-exercise is effective in decreasing sick leave in patients with subacute low back pain (Table 9.1).[44, 45]

Exercise recommendations   Individuals who maintain a regular exercise regimen should be encouraged to resume their programme as soon as possible. The following guidelines are recommended for a disease-free, sedentary population and can be used for a patient interested in self-care who is in the subacute stage of NSLBP.

A walking programme   Aerobic training (cardiorespiratory endurance) can be achieved through a walking programme that includes brisk walking, jogging or stair climbing. Such a programme is easy to do and does not require special equipment. The guidelines for cardiorespiratory training for a population with no underlying disease are the following: engaging in activities that will require moderate intensity (40–60% of functional capacity) within 20–30 minutes' duration. The recommended frequency is at least three times per week.[46]

Self-care monitoring   One way of controlling the intensity of the exercises is to monitor the heart rate. Wristwatch heart monitors may be used. Teaching patients how to monitor their heart rate through pulse can be difficult. An alternative way to monitor the amount of effort is by instructing patients in the use of a perceived exertion scale. One such scale is the Borg Scale,[47] which will be used for illustrative purposes. Maintaining effort at a level of 12 on the Borg Scale (indicating a heart rate of approximately 120 beats/minute in a normal healthy population of active age (30–40 years old)) is safe and provides the aerobic benefit desired. Patients should be instructed to increase their pace or distance to maintain the same effort as the exercise progresses.

Flexibility   Flexibility is the ability to move a joint through a range of motion and may be achieved by a stretching programme. Flexibility exercises usually require 3–5 repetitions of dynamic movement with a static stretch to be held for 10–30 seconds. Stretches should be done two to three times per week (see Box 9.1).[46]

Strengthening exercises   Strength may be thought of as the ability of a muscle or a muscle group to overcome resistance. Strengthening exercises are a major component in the rehabilitation of patients with low back pain. The exercises

---

Box 9.1. Exercise and modalities for self-care

Modalities
- Hot packs: 10 ± 20 minutes
- Cold packs: As often as needed

Flexibility exercises
- Lower extremity (hamstring, hip flexors, hip extensors): 3 ± 5 repetitions; holding time 15–30 seconds; done 2 ± 3 times weekly
  1. Supine
  2. Sitting
  3. Standing
- Back muscles (back extensors)
  1. Kneeling quadruped position
  2. Standing
- Knee to chest
  1. Supine

Strengthening exercises
- Active back extension: 1 ± 3 sets of 8 ± 12 repetitions done 2 ± 3 times weekly
  1. Prone
  2. Prone leaning on gym ball
- Abdominal strengthening
  1. Supine
- Pelvic tilt
  1. Supine
  2. Sitting
  3. Standing

Aerobic conditioning
- Walking programme: 20 ± 30 minutes, 3 times weekly
  1. Outdoor/indoor track
  2. Treadmill
- Stationary bike
  1. Recumbent
  2. Upright

This protocol can be safely recommended to patients.

Table 9.1. Graded scale of mobility-related activities based on selected functional and quality-of-life indices from the literature

Activity	Quantitative description	Qualitative description
Walking	More than 10, 20 or 30 min, several consecutive hours	Ability to walk for a short/long time
	Several metres, several hundred metres, several kilometres	Ability to walk for a short/long time
Sitting	Needing to remain seated for most of the day	Need support for oneself to get up, have difficulty to get up
	Remain seated for more than 10, 30 or 60 min or for more than several consecutive answers	Sitting in a favourite chair, ability to sit in any chair
Standing	10, 20–30 or more than 30 min, more than 1 hour	For prolonged periods, for as long as one desires
Lying down and getting up	Not applicable	Have difficulty getting into bed, turning over in bed, getting out of bed
Staying in bed	Number of hours	Lying down most of the time or more than normal
	Number of days	Not lying down to rest
Climbing stairs	Five steps, one storey, several storeys	Using a banister, climbing more slowly
Transportation	Travelling less than 30 min, less than 1 hour, more than 2 hours	Travelling in cars, travelling anywhere

Source: Abenhaim et al.[3]

usually consist of body-weight resistance against gravity, machines or free weights and elastic band resistance.

Physical modalities

The most common physical modalities that patients can use on their own to treat low back pain include electrotherapy (transcutaneous electrical nerve stimulation (TENS)), therapeutic heat (superficial heat), therapeutic cold (cold packs, sprays), massage and magnetic therapy.[48] There is no proof that these physical modalities improve the outcome of low back pain.[3] However, as a source of short-term relief and as an aid for activity resumption some of them, such as the use of moist heat and ice, can be easily taught to the patient. It is important that patients understand that these physical modalities are for controlling symptoms only and that an active approach will provide the best outcome.[49]

Physical modalities that can be safely recommended for self-care to patients include: hot packs or cold packs for 20–30 minutes as needed for pain relief. Alternatively, patients should be advised to follow the heating or cooling directions of the manufacturer. Vapocoolant sprays (e.g. ethyl chloride) require local application and can be used in combination with stretching exercises.[49]

In summary, if the benefits and limitations of the physical modalities are explained to the patient they can be used easily and safely. Patients should be encouraged to use these physical modalities as part of an active approach to NSLBP.

Empirical support   There are no empirical studies that support the use of physical modalities for the treatment of low

back pain. However, since they pose no threat of harm and there are no studies to warn against their use, they may be used for symptom relief. They should not be used as a substitute for self-care approaches that have been shown to be successful, such as activity resumption.

Mind–body techniques

The introduction of the gate control theory and biopsychosocial model to the problem of low back pain and disability has resulted in an understanding of pain as a multidimensional experience. Pain may be modulated by stress, beliefs, mood and attention.[5] A number of simple self-help techniques exist that address the mind–body connection in low back pain. They usually fall under the heading of cognitive–behavioural interventions. The easiest techniques to learn independently are relaxation and creative visualization or imagery.

Relaxation and visualization for self-care

Stress has been implicated as a cause of low back pain, for several reasons. Perceived tension results in the activation of the sympathetic nervous system that causes muscles to tighten. This can result in painful spasms, ischaemia and vulnerability to injury during movement due to muscle contraction. Stress is associated with negative mood states that enhance pain perception, such as depression and anxiety.[50] Stress can also affect work habits by causing workers to assume repetitive and constrained postures without sufficient rest breaks. This can result in cumulative trauma injuries.

The most common mind–body technique for alleviating low back pain is relaxation. All relaxation exercises involve relaxed breathing and focused attention on a neutral or pleasant stimulus (Boxes 9.2 and 9.3). Relaxation exercises evoke the 'relaxation response' in the parasympathetic nervous system and counteract the effects of the stress response.[51] Visualization, or imagery, is often used in conjunction with a relaxation technique. It involves creating and focusing on a peaceful or healing image to maintain a deep level of relaxation and promote positive beliefs about recovery.

Many relaxation techniques exist. Meditation, self-hypnosis, forms of yoga and other movement therapies and progressive muscle relaxation (Box 9.4) are all good examples. Patients may be encouraged to practise the one they feel most comfortable with. Deep breathing with progressive muscle relaxation and imagery is one of the simplest forms of relaxation and can be instructed as shown in Box 9.4.

Empirical support In a review of randomized controlled studies, van Tulder et al.[52] found strong evidence that behavioural treatment has a small to moderate effect on outcome in chronic low back pain when compared with no treatment, but virtually no effect when added to other treatments. However, few high-quality studies exist and it is suggested that patients at risk may benefit from cognitive–behavioural treatment earlier in a low back pain episode.

In a prospective randomized study, Hasenbring et al.[53] compared psychological intervention including relaxation techniques with usual medical care in acute back pain patients. They found a positive effect of these techniques, especially in the group of patients deemed to be at high risk for chronicity based on psychological risk factors that were assessed at baseline. In fact, patients in the intervention groups did as well as the low-risk patients at follow-up.

Linton and Andersson[54] conducted a randomized controlled study that compared cognitive–behavioural intervention with the provision of information to patients. Patients in the treatment group received six sessions of cognitive–behavioural intervention, including relaxation training. The comparison groups received either a pamphlet or an extensive information packet. While all groups improved, the cognitive–behavioural group had significantly lower levels of perceived risk of chronicity and healthcare use, and was much less likely to be out of work long-term.

More recently, Linton et al.[55] found that adding cognitive–behavioural treatment or cognitive–behavioural treatment and physical therapy to information from a physician about how to manage low back pain was more effective in reducing sick leave and healthcare utilization than information alone. Chapman and Turner[56] reported that results from randomized controlled trials show that cognitive–behavioural treatment is an effective treatment for pain, particularly when it is given early.

There are several limitations of current research. Few randomized controlled studies on acute low back pain exist. This makes it difficult to assess the effectiveness of mind–body techniques in the early stages of low back pain. A related problem is the fact that there are few studies that have compared relaxation or creative visualization alone with other treatments. Cognitive–behavioural interventions that include relaxation and imagery are typically compared with other treatments by themselves or as part of a multidisciplinary intervention. Therefore, the effective component of the treatment is not known. Finally, existing studies have examined interventions that require several

---

Box 9.2. Deep breathing

Deep breathing is the common thread in all relaxation techniques. It reflects the absence of tension.

Initiating deep breathing provokes the parasympathetic reaction consonant with relaxation.

- Breathe deeply from your diaphragm. Avoid shallow chest breathing
- Inhale through your nose and exhale through your mouth
- As you inhale, let your stomach expand. As you exhale, let it contract
- Practise controlling the speed at which you breathe. Breathe slowly but naturally
- Allow your mind to focus on your breathing instead of negative thoughts or feelings

Deep breathing may be practised alone or as an introduction to other relaxation techniques

---

Box 9.3. Creative visualization

Relaxation exercises work well with creative visualization or imagery. These exercises tap into the mind–body connection by purposely creating pleasant mental images that promote salubrious physical responses. Visualizations can have a motivational effect as well. Imagining an achieved goal can motivate the individual to adopt the behaviours necessary to meet that challenge. Creative visualization can be taught as follows: The success of creative visualization is based on your ability to make the images as real as possible, so that your body behaves as if they are true. Think about the last time you had a very vivid dream. When you awoke, your body probably felt like the dream really happened. Applying this approach while you are awake requires the use of all five senses and some practice. One popular image among pain sufferers is a golden healing light. Here is a creative visualization exercise using healing light.

1. Imagine the beautiful golden colour and the warmth of the light.
2. As you inhale, allow the light to enter the body, healing and soothing any area in pain or discomfort.
3. As you exhale, let the light leave your body through the skin, removing pain and tension. You may use any other image that you find relaxing.

It can also be helpful to imagine yourself exactly the way you want to look and feel. See yourself doing all the things you want to do in perfect health. This image of yourself can move you closer to achieving your goals

sessions with a healthcare provider. Repeated cognitive–behavioural interventions may increase perceptions of control and motivate self-care behaviours. However, the focus of this chapter is self-care techniques that patients can use without the help of a healthcare provider. These have not been studied.

Despite the lack of research to support mind–body techniques in the self-care of acute low back pain, they are highly recommended for the following reasons: the cost of these exercises is low, they are easy to learn and can be done anywhere with no special equipment. In addition, the evidence from the chronic low back pain literature suggests that the benefits are potentially high for low back pain outcomes. These techniques may have generalized health benefits as well.

IMPROVING THE ODDS OF SUCCESS

Patients want information about the likely course of their low back pain, the associated activity limitations, how to manage their back pain, how to return to normal activities as soon as possible, and how to avoid or deal with recurrences.[9, 57] Appropriate information and advice can reduce anxiety and improve patient satisfaction with care.[1, 2, 58]

Waddell[9] suggested that the same advice should be given by all members of the healthcare team, and should reflect clinical guidelines and any other written information provided to the patient to avoid ambiguity. Waddell and Burton's recommendations[5] are listed in Box 9.5.

Certain ways of interacting may promote the concept of self-care better than others and may avoid iatrogenic complications. The first encounter with a healthcare professional is most important, since it is an opportunity to build trust in the patient–healthcare provider 'team'. If trust is established, the patient is more likely to accept the prognosis and the recommended course of treatment.

Information should be evidence based as often as possible, communicated in several ways (verbally, handouts, brochures, video tape, internet site, referral to back education, other means) and repeated by the healthcare-providing team. The same message must be provided by the physician, chiropractor, physical therapist, nurse and others involved.

In a randomized controlled study with geographic stratification, Coudeyre et al.[59] provided an advice book on back pain and consistent oral information to the treatment group. The control group received only oral information. After 3 months the treatment group reported less persistent pain. Damush et al.[22] also found positive effects of self-care strategies consisting of education, fear reduction and advice to stay active in a randomized sample of inner-city patients with acute low back pain.

Patients should be encouraged to form a partnership with the healthcare provider.[60] The patient and the provider have equal responsibility for the outcome of treatment. Today, patients have access to more information from non-traditional sources, such as the Internet or alternative care practitioners, than in years past. The healthcare provider must be willing to

---

Box 9.4. Progressive muscle relaxation

Progressive muscle relaxation (PMR) is a systematic method of tightening and releasing muscles to reduce muscle tension. PMR helps you to relax by focusing your attention on different muscle groups.

1. Get in a comfortable position, either sitting or lying down.
2. Find a quiet place where you know you will not be interrupted for about 20 minutes.
3. Wear comfortable clothing.
4. Close your eyes.
5. Take three deep, slow relaxing breaths. Maintain this slow, deep breathing throughout your PMR.
6. When you exhale, tell yourself to 'relax' or 'let go'.
7. Tense each muscle group and hold for about 5 seconds.
8. Go slowly, muscle group by muscle group.
9. Start with your forehead, then your face, your neck, your shoulders, etc.
10. Move slowly down your body until you reach your toes.
11. After you are completely relaxed, scan your body mentally. If you come across any tension spots, repeat the tensing and releasing in that area.
12. Keep going until you feel fully relaxed.
13. Keep your eyes closed and just enjoy feeling totally relaxed.
14. Before you open your eyes, picture your surroundings. Wiggle your fingers and toes. When you feel comfortable, open your eyes.

Practise this technique at least once a day.

Box 9.5. Communication to patients

- Reassure the patient that there is no serious damage or disease
- Explain that back pain is a symptom that the back 'is not working properly'
- Avoid labelling as injury, disc trouble, degeneration, or wear and tear
- Reassure the patient that the natural history is good providing he or she stays active, but also give accurate information about recurrent symptoms and how to deal with them
- Advise the patient to use simple, safe treatments to control symptoms
- Encourage staying active, continuing daily activities as normally as possible and staying at work. This gives the most rapid and complete recovery and less risk of recurrent problems
- Avoid the 'let pain be your guide' idea
- Encourage patients to take responsibility for their own continued management

Adapted from Waddell.[9]

discuss the patient's questions and concerns.[9, 61] Patients' beliefs about their condition and the proposed course of treatment must be taken very seriously, as it can affect compliance and satisfaction with care and, ultimately, the outcome.[58]

Empirical support   Moore et al.[10] conducted a large randomized controlled trial to evaluate a brief intervention for primary care back pain patients. The intervention consisted of accurate information about back pain, suggestions for self-care, reduction of fears and worries, and the development of personalized action plans for pain management. They found that the intervention group showed significantly greater reductions in back-related worry and fear-avoidance beliefs as well as in pain ratings and interference with activities compared with the control group that received usual care.

LIMITATIONS OF SELF-CARE TECHNIQUES

Adherence to healthcare practitioner recommendations is a challenge in many treatment protocols. This is especially true for self-care treatment. Passive medical interventions have the advantage of ensuring a certain level of intervention if the patient merely attends the sessions. It is much more difficult to monitor adherence in self-care. In addition, some studies suggest that patients tend to adhere more to prescribed exercises when they are supervised.[12, 62, 63] Patients may have difficulty with self-care for a variety of reasons. One is that the healthcare provider has failed to convince the patient that self-care is as, or more, effective than traditional treatment in acute NSLBP episodes. In some cases, it may be impossible to convince patients that they have NSLBP. Despite reassurance and education, some patients remain convinced that there is a structural problem in their back that needs to be 'fixed' for them to feel better. The idea that back pain is not serious and requires no special treatment is a new concept for many individuals. The initial

healthcare provider–patient interaction is critical in determining the extent to which the patient will be able to accept responsibility for their low back pain.

Some patients may have difficulty with self-care because of deeply entrenched beliefs in the power of modern medicine to cure them. Attempts to shift the control to the patient may backfire and result in feelings of rejection, confusion and anger on the patient's part. For these patients, evidence-based treatment by the healthcare provider may be the best approach to a positive outcome.

Finally, even patients who believe that their back pain is self-limiting and not serious may still desire immediate pain relief by means of passive modalities such as manipulation, massage, injections, electrotherapy, hot or cold packs, magnetic therapy or acupuncture. As long as these methods are not contraindicated, they should not be discouraged. However, it can be emphasized that self-care is an important adjunct to any passive treatment.

In many ways the promotion of self-care for low back pain relies on the attitudes that are communicated by society. Attempts are underway to educate the general public about self-care for low back pain. Buchbinder et al.[64] found that citizens who were exposed to a television media campaign regarding evidence-based early care for low back pain fared better than those who did not in terms of health beliefs and medical management. The intervention population received strong messages about the importance of self-management and information about how to cope with acute episodes of low back pain. These types of public service messages may be important in improving low back pain outcomes.

It is important to remember that no intervention works for everybody. Even evidence-based treatment recommendations are not a substitute for common sense and individualized assessment. Self-care should be encouraged. However, responding to the patient's needs should always be paramount.

PRACTICE POINTS

- Deep breathing is the common thread in all relaxation techniques.
- Relaxation exercises work well with creative visualization or imagery.
- Progressive muscle relaxation can be used to help the patient to relax.
- Communication with the patient is vitally important.
- There is strong evidence against recommending bed rest for acute NSLBP.
- There is strong evidence for recommending the maintenance or resumption of gradual activity in an episode of acute NSLBP for long-term well-being.

RESEARCH AGENDA

- The type, amount and frequency of exercises and their relationship to outcome of NSLBP is not well established.
- Research is needed on how to educate patients about the mind–body connection.
- A comparison of the effectiveness of different types of mind–body approaches to low back pain is needed.
- How to communicate more effectively to the patient with acute NSLBP that the best treatment is staying active needs to be carefully assessed.
- How to better convince primary healthcare providers to communicate that the best treatment for the patient with acute NSLBP is to stay active needs to be investigated.
- More community-based studies of the exposure to self-care messages for low back pain through the media are needed.

SUMMARY

Guidelines recommend minimal intervention in the early stages of low back pain. Yet patients often seek medical care in cases of NSLBP that do not resolve quickly. In response to this request, healthcare providers may overtreat patients at the expense of their well-being. It is suggested that healthcare providers shift their emphasis to educating patients to care for back pain on their own. This can be accomplished by improving communication with patients, engaging them as partners in healthcare and encouraging simple self-care techniques. This may be an important step in curtailing the exorbitant costs and the pain and suffering that result from NSLBP.

REFERENCES

1. Bigos SJ, Bowyer O, Braen G. *Acute Low Back Problems in Adults, Clinical Practice Guideline, No. 14.* Vol. AHCPR Pub 95–0642. US Department of Health and Human Services, Public Health Service, Agency for Health Care Policy and Research, Rockville, MD, 1994.
2. Waddell G, McIntosh A, Hutchinson A et al. *Low Back Pain Evidence Review.* Royal College of General Practitioners, London, 1999.
3. Abenhaim L, Rossignol M, Valat JP et al. The role of activity in the therapeutic management of back pain. Report of the International Paris Task Force on Back Pain. *Spine* 2000; 25(4 Suppl): 1S–33S.
4. Kendall N, Linton S, Main C. *Guide to Assessing Psychosocial Yellow Flags in Acute Low Back Pain: Risk Factors for Long Term Disabilities and Work Loss.* New Zealand Guidelines and National Health Committee, Wellington, 1997.
5. Waddell G, Burton AK. Occupational health guidelines for the management of low back pain at work evidence review. *Occup Med London* 2001; 51: 124–135.
6. Snook SH. Self-care guidelines for the management of nonspecific low back pain. *J Occup Rehab* 2004; 14: 243–253.
7. Schers H, Wensing M, Huijsmans Z et al. Implementation barriers for general practice guidelines on low back pain a qualitative study. *Spine* 2001; 26: E348–E353.
8. Linton S. Psychological risk factors for neck and back pain. In: Nachemson A, Jonsson E (eds), *Neck and Back Pain. The Scientific Evidence of Causes, Diagnosis, and Treatment.* Lippincott Williams & Wilkins, Philadelphia, PA, 2000, pp. 57–78.
9. Waddell G. *The Back Pain Revolution.* Churchill Livingston, Edinburgh, 1998.
10. Moore JE, Von Korff M, Cherkin D et al. A randomized trial of a cognitive–behavioral program for enhancing back pain self care in a primary care setting. *Pain* 2000; 88: 145–153.
11. Harkapaa K. Relationships of psychological distress and health locus of control beliefs with the use of cognitive and behavioral coping strategies in low back pain patients. *Clin J Pain* 1991; 7: 275–282.
12. Harkapaa K, Jarvikoski A, Mellin G et al. A controlled study on the outcome of inpatient and outpatient treatment of low back pain. Part I. Pain, disability, compliance, and reported treatment benefits three months after treatment. *Scand J Rehab Med* 1989; 21: 81–89.
13. Haldorsen EM, Indahl A, Ursin H. Patients with low back pain not returning to work. A 12-month follow-up study. *Spine* 1998; 23: 1202–1207; discussion 1208.
14. Adams MA, Mannion AF, Dolan P. Personal risk factors for first-time low back pain. *Spine* 1999; 24: 2497–2505.
15. Mannion AF, Dolan P, Adams MA. Psychological questionnaires: do 'abnormal' scores precede or follow first-time low back pain? *Spine* 1996; 21: 2603–2611.
16. Lacker JM, Carosella AM, Feuerstein M. Pain expectancies, pain, and functional self-efficacy expectancies as determinants of disability in patients with chronic low back disorders. *J Consult Clin Psychol* 1996; 64: 212–220.
17. Lackner JM, Carosella AM. The relative influence of perceived pain control, anxiety, and functional self efficacy on spinal function among patients with chronic low back pain. *Spine* 1999; 24: 2254–2260; discussion 2260–2251.
18. Keller A, Johansen JG, Hellesnes J et al. Predictors of isokinetic back muscle strength in patients with low back pain. *Spine* 1999; 24: 275–280.
19. Al-Obaidi SM, Nelson RM, Al-Awadhi S et al. The role of anticipation and fear of pain in the persistence of avoidance behavior in patients with chronic low back pain. *Spine* 2000; 25: 1126–1131.
20. Council JR, Ahern DK, Follick MJ et al. Expectancies and functional impairment in chronic low back pain. *Pain* 1988; 33: 323–331.
21. Estlander AM, Takala EP, Viikari-Juntura E. Do psychological factors predict changes in musculoskeletal pain? A prospective, two-year follow-up study of a working population. *J Occup Environ Med* 1998; 40: 445–453.
22. Damush TM, Weinberger M, Perkins SM et al. The long-term effects of a self-management program for inner-city primary care patients with acute low back pain. *Arch Intern Med* 2003; 163: 2632–2638.
23. Leigh JP, Markowitz SB, Fahs M et al. Occupational injury and illness in the United States. Estimates of costs, morbidity, and mortality. *Arch Intern Med* 1997; 157: 1557–1568.
24. Liu AC, Byrne E. Cost of care for ambulatory patients with low back pain. *J Fam Prac* 1995; 40: 449–455.
25. Molde Hagen E, Grasdal A, Eriksen HR. Does early intervention with a light mobilisation program reduce long-term sick leave for low back pain: a 3-year follow-up study. *Spine* 2003; 28: 2309–2315.
26. Silverstein FE, Faich G, Goldstein JL et al. Gastrointestinal toxicity with celecoxib vs nonsteroidal anti-inflammatory drugs for osteoarthritis and rheumatoid arthritis: the CLASS study: a randomized controlled trial. Celecoxib Long-term Arthritis Safety Study. *JAMA* 2000; 284: 1247–1255.
27. van Tulder M, Waddell G. Conservative treatment of acute and subacute low back pain. In: Nachemson A, Jonsson E (eds), *Neck and Back Pain. The Scientific Evidence of Causes, Diagnosis, and Treatment.* Lippincott Williams & Wilkins, Philadelphia, PA, 2000, pp 241–265.
28. Deyo RA, Phillips WR. Low back pain. A primary care challenge. *Spine* 1996; 21: 2826–2832.
29. van Tulder MW, Scholten RJ, Koes BW et al. Nonsteroidal anti-inflammatory drugs for low back pain: a systematic review within the framework of the Cochrane Collaboration Back Review Group. *Spine* 2000; 25: 2501–2513.
30. Deyo RA, Weinstein JN. Low back pain. *N Engl J Med* 2001; 344: 363–370.
31. Bernstein E, Carey TS, Garrett JM. The use of muscle relaxant medications in acute low back pain. *Spine* 2004; 29: 1346–1351.
32. Deyo RA. Non-operative treatment of low back disorders. Differentiating useful from useless therapy. In: Frymoyer J (ed.), *The Adult Spine: Principles and Practice.* Raven, New York, 1991, pp. 1567–1580.
33. Rozenberg S, Delval C, Rezvani Y et al. Bed rest or normal activity for patients with acute low back pain: a randomized controlled trial. *Spine* 2002; 27: 1487–1493.
34. Malmivaara A, Hakkinen U, Aro T et al. The treatment of acute low back pain – bed rest, exercises, or ordinary activity? *N Engl J Med* 1995; 332: 351–355.
35. Kori SH, Miller RP, Todd DD. Kinesiophobia: a new view of chronic pain behavior. *Pain Manage* 1990; Jan/Feb: 35–43.
36. Hagen KB, Hilde G, Jamtvedt G et al. Bed rest for acute low-back pain and sciatica. *Cochrane Database Syst Rev* 2004; 4: CD001254.
37. Dettori JR, Bullock SH, Sutlive TG et al. The effects of spinal flexion and extension exercises and their associated postures in patients with acute low back pain. *Spine* 1995; 20: 2303–2312.
38. Evans C, Gilbert J, Taylor W et al. A randomized controlled trial of flexion exercises, education, and bed rest for patients with acute low back pain. *Physiother Can* 1987; 39: 96–101.
39. Faas A, Chavannes AW, van Eijk JT et al. A randomized, placebo-controlled trial of exercise therapy in patients with acute low back pain. *Spine* 1993; 18: 1388–1395.
40. Fordyce WE, Brockway JA, Bergman JA et al. Acute back pain: a control-group comparison of behavioral vs traditional management methods. *J Behav Med* 1986; 9: 127–140.
41. Stankovic R, Johnell O. Conservative treatment of acute low back pain. A 5-year follow-up study of two methods of treatment. *Spine* 1995; 20: 469–472.
42. Hayden JA, van Tulder MW, Malmivaara AV et al. Meta-analysis: exercise therapy for nonspecific low back pain. *Ann Intern Med* 2005; 142: 765–775.
43. Kellett KM, Kellett DA, Nordholm LA. Effects of an exercise program on sick leave due to back pain. *Phys Ther* 1991; 71: 283–291; discussion 291–283.
44. Lindström I, Ohlund C, Eek C et al. The effect of graded activity on patients with subacute low back pain: a randomized prospective clinical study with an operant-conditioning behavioral approach. *Phys Ther* 1992; 72: 279–290.
45. Staal JB, Hlobil H, Twisk JW et al. Graded activity for low back pain in occupational health care: a randomized, controlled trial. *Ann Intern Med* 2004; 140: 77–84.
46. American College of Sports Medicine. *American College of Sport Medicine's Guidelines for Exercise Testing and Prescription*, 4th edn. Lea & Febiger, Philadelphia, PA, 1991.
47. Borg G. Perceived exertion: a note on 'history' and methods. *Med Sci Sport* 1973; 5: 90–93.
48. Tan J. *Practical Manual of Physical Medicine and Rehabilitation: Diagnostics, Therapeutics, and Basic Problems.* Mosby Year Book, St. Louis, MO, 1998.

49. Nordin M, Campello M. Physical therapy: exercises and the modalities: when, what, and why? *Neurol Clin* 1999; **17**: 75–89.

50. Fishbain DA, Cutler RB, Rosomoff HL et al. Impact of chronic pain patients' job perception variables on actual return to work. *Clin J Pain* 1997; **13**: 197–206.

51. Syrjala K. Relaxation and imagery techniques. In: Bonica JJ (ed.), *The Management of Pain*, Vol. 1, 2nd edn. Lea & Febiger, Philadelphia, PA, 1990.

52. van Tulder MW, Ostelo R, Vlaeyen JW et al. Behavioral treatment for chronic low back pain: a systematic review within the framework of the Cochrane Back Review Group. *Spine* 2001; **26**: 270–281.

53. Hasenbring M, Ulrich HW, Hartmann M et al. The efficacy of a risk factor-based cognitive behavioral intervention and electromyographic biofeedback in patients with acute sciatic pain. An attempt to prevent chronicity. *Spine* 1999; **24**: 2525–2535.

54. Linton SJ, Andersson T. Can chronic disability be prevented? A randomized trial of a cognitive–behavior intervention and two forms of information for patients with spinal pain. *Spin* 2000; **25**: 2825–2831; discussion 2824.

55. Linton SJ, Boersma K, Jansson M et al. The effects of cognitive–behavioral and physical therapy preventive interventions on pain-related sick leave: a randomised controlled trial. *Clin J Pain* 2005; **21**: 109–119.

56. Chapman RC, Turner J. Psychological aspects of pain. In: Loeser JD (ed.), *Bonica's Management of Pain*, 3rd ed. Lippincott Williams & Wilkins, Philadelphia, PA, 2001, pp. 180–190.

57. Von Korff M, Saunders K. The course of back pain in primary care. *Spine* 1996; **21**: 2833–2837; discussion 2838–2839.

58. Deyo RA, Diehl AK. Patient satisfaction with medical care for low-back pain. *Spine* 1986; **11**: 28–30.

59. Coudeyre E, Rannou F, Coriat F et al. Impact of the back book on acute low back pain outcome. *32nd Annual Meeting of the International Society for the Study of the Lumbar Spine*, New York, 10–14 May 2005.

60. Nordin M, Cedraschi C, Skovron ML. Patient–health care provider relationship in patients with non-specific low back pain: a review of some problem situations. *Baillières Clin Rheumatol* 1998; **12**: 75–92.

61. Cedraschi C, Reust P, Lorenzi-Cioldi F et al. The gap between back pain patients' prior knowledge and scientific knowledge and its evolution after a back school teaching programme: a quantitative evaluation. *Patient Educ Counsel* 1996; **27**: 235–246.

62. Friedrich M, Gittler G, Halberstadt Y et al. Combined exercise and motivation program: effect on the compliance and level of disability of patients with chronic low back pain: a randomized controlled trial. *Arch Phys Med Rehab* 1998; **79**: 475–487.

63. Reilly K, Lovejoy B, Williams R et al. Differences between a supervised and independent strength and conditioning program with chronic low back syndromes. *J Occup Med* 1989; **31**: 547–550.

64. Buchbinder R, Jolley D. Effects of a media campaign on back beliefs is sustained 3 years after its cessation. *Spine* 2005; **30**: 1323–1330.

Chapter 10

Advances in analgesics and NSAIDs for the treatment of spinal disorders

Jules A. Desmeules, Victoria Rollason, Christine Cedraschi, Valérie Piguet, Anne-Françoise Allaz and Pierre Dayer

INTRODUCTION

Non-malignant back pain encompasses a heterogeneous group of syndromes that are treated in a variety of ways. In contrast to acute pain, chronic back pain very often defies satisfactory treatment. One of the major developments with regard to chronic non-malignant pain in recent years has been a better understanding of the mechanisms that act to maintain pain, while inferences about the pathophysiology have clarified therapeutic decision-making.

Pain syndromes fall into two main categories: the term 'nociceptive pain' is applied to pain presumed to be maintained by continuous tissue injury such as bone, joint, or muscle inflammation. The term 'neuropathic' pain is used when pain is believed to be sustained by aberrant somatosensory processing in the peripheral or central nervous systems. Although neuropathic pain can respond well to conventional analgesics, these syndromes are disproportionately represented among patients whose pain responds poorly to opioid drugs.[1, 2] As a result, the diagnosis of a neuropathic pain syndrome often implies the need to turn to other therapies, including the use of specific non-traditional analgesic drugs such as anticonvulsants and antidepressants.[3]

Nociceptive and neuropathic pain can be acute or chronic. The latter is commonly defined as pain that persists for longer than the expected time frame for healing or pain associated with a progressive disease of malignant or non-malignant origin. Chronic or persistent pain may be due to the persistent stimulation of nociceptors in areas of ongoing tissue damage (e.g. chronic pain due to osteoarthritis).

Chronic nociceptive or neuropathic pain needs to be distinguished from particular chronic pain syndromes that persist long after the tissue damage that initially triggered their onset has resolved, or pain syndromes without any identified ongoing tissue damage or antecedent injury. These syndromes, such as myofascial pain syndrome, fibromyalgia and somatoform pain disorders, are currently diagnosed on the basis of clinical criteria alone. Knowledge of the underlying pathophysiology of these disorders has excluded most of the possible peripheral origins and has pointed out possible central dysfunction of the nervous system.[4, 5] The pharmacological approaches remain unsatisfactory but partially effective. The trend over the past decade has been to emphasize the biopsychosocial model and the advantages of a multidisciplinary approach provided by pain centres that carry out comprehensive somatic and psychosocial assessments, in addition to providing pharmacological, physical and psychological treatments.[6] Back pain may refer to various or even mixed components of chronic pain, and it is thus not surprising that in most multidisciplinary pain centres back pain is one of the main reasons for consultation.

There is extensive experimental and clinical evidence documenting the major prevalence of persistent pain and the deleterious biological and psychological consequences of undertreated pain. Experimental studies have confirmed long-standing clinical impressions about the dynamic nature of pain and have shown that inadequately managed acute pain sometimes becomes more difficult to suppress. In fact, if tissue damage is unavoidable, a set of excitability changes in the peripheral and central nervous systems takes place and sometimes builds in a slowly reversible or irreversible pain hypersensitivity in the inflamed and surrounding tissues.[7, 8] Biological and pharmacological evidence has shown that the induction and maintenance of central hyperexcitability and secondary hyperalgesia is mainly mediated by N-methyl-D-aspartate (NMDA) receptor activation, which offers a new target for pain modulation in chronic pain patients. Persistent pain syndromes offer no biological advantage and lead to profound biological changes in both the peripheral and central nervous systems with potential 'central sensitization' and suffering.[2, 9] Furthermore, persistent pain profoundly affects patients' social relationships, mood and physical functioning. Concomitant depression and sleep disturbance further decrease overall physical functioning, and working disability is typically experienced by chronic pain patients.[10] Thus, in order to reduce the neurobiological and psychosocial consequences of pain, prompt, vigorous and tailored management of severe pain is mandatory in acute situations and should run concurrently with the aetiological treatment.

The comprehensive management of quality of life in rheumatology encompasses control of inflammation, the prevention of joint destruction, the maintenance of optimal function and the management of pain. Non-pharmacological interventions, including patient education, psychological support and physical and occupational therapy, play a crucial role in the management of chronic pain.

Chronic pain often remains a complex syndrome where analgesic prescription is only one part of the treatment. However, when analgesics are tailored by taking into account their pharmacological properties and the patient's pain syndrome and comorbidities, they may contribute to a favourable risk–benefit ratio.

PHARMACOLOGICAL APPROACHES TO NOCICEPTIVE PAIN

Various chemicals (bradykinin, histamine, serotonin (5-hydroxytryptamine (5-HT)), prostaglandins, potassium, protons) released after tissue damage induce nociceptive reactions and modify the activity of nociceptors, either by direct activation or by modulation.[8, 11]

Several peptides are present within primary afferent fibres and their profile can be altered by sustained stimulation or by damage to the nerve. Apart from these substances, which are liberated soon after tissue damage, other factors such as the cytokines (interleukins, interferon, tumour necrosis factor (TNF) and nerve growth factor) are released by phagocytic cells and cells of the immune system and have an important role in the inflammatory process.[8, 11]

To treat acute or persistent nociceptive pain in rheumatological conditions, pharmacological approaches, which encompass anti-inflammatory and immunomodulatory agents, such as glucocorticoids, methotrexate, ciclosporin, anti-TNF, leflunomide, mycophenolate mofetil and disease-modifying antirheumatic drugs (DMARDs), are targeted at the originating factors.

However, many patients remain insufficiently relieved and symptomatic analgesic therapy is needed. The World Health Organization (WHO) recommends a three-step ladder approach to the use of analgesic drugs, with an initial treatment choice of a non-opioid analgesic, either non-steroidal anti-inflammatory drugs (NSAIDs) or paracetamol (acetaminophen). If one of these agents fails to relieve pain, a 'weak' opioid for mild to moderate pain is used, either alone or in combination with a non-opioid analgesic. If pain persists or increases, a 'strong' opioid for moderate to severe pain should be substituted. Current non-opioid and opioid analgesics have their limitations, and physicians' and patients' fear of adverse effects associated with opioids and NSAIDs contribute to the undertreatment of pain. The 'analgesic ladder' approach of the WHO is widely accepted as the basis for treatment guidelines for cancer-related nociceptive syndromes,[12] and this approach is nowadays extended to non-cancer pain, although scientific evidence is still lacking.

BENEFITS AND LIMITS OF NSAIDS AND PARACETAMOL

Finding the best available clinical evidence for making decisions about the selection of an analgesic in painful spinal disorders remains a necessary goal. Systematic reviews of randomized controlled trials provide the best level of evidence for selecting a treatment, despite some pitfalls such as the inclusion of low-quality trials, unpublished trials and the numerous different options available among drugs, doses, routes of administration and pain conditions, which make meaningful comparisons difficult.[13, 14]

Single-dose analgesic trials using reproducible clinical procedures (dental extraction, postsurgical or post-partum models) are not sufficient to assess their value in clinical practice, although such trials may be helpful in determining the relative efficacy of NSAIDs. Effective relief can be achieved in these models with oral non-opioids and NSAIDs. The results of a meta-analysis including 42 randomized controlled trials using these models allowed the comparison of the dose–response curves for diclofenac and ibuprofen, for example. Although diclofenac has long been regarded by clinicians as a more effective NSAID than ibuprofen, they both showed the same level of efficacy when the dose was adjusted, diclofenac 50 mg orally not being more efficient than ibuprofen 600 mg.[15] With regard to back pain, a systematic review that included 51 randomized controlled trials (6057 patients) that assessed the benefit of NSAIDs suggested that there was a significant clinical benefit over placebo and a strong level of evidence that various types of NSAIDs were, somehow, equally effective for the short-term relief of acute back pain.[16] For chronic inflammatory back pain, one study has suggested that a 1-year trial might be of optimum value compared with a 6-week assessment in order better to define the efficacy and tolerability of NSAIDs in ankylosing spondylitis. Evidence of long-term (exceeding 6 months of treatment) efficacy from randomized controlled trials is still lacking, and safety issues remain the most important problem.[17]

Gastrointestinal effects

The most commonly prescribed NSAIDs reduce the synthesis of prostaglandins and thromboxane by the inhibition of the enzyme cyclo-oxygenase 1 (COX-1), a constitutive form of the enzyme. Inhibition of COX-1 is responsible for the gastrointestinal irritation and ulceration and for the blockade of platelet aggregation. The COX-2 inducible form of the enzyme is selectively inhibited by various new COX-2 NSAIDs that reduce the risk of these adverse effects and are effective in relieving the chronic pain conditions associated with rheumatoid arthritis or osteoarthritis.[18, 19] The rate of confirmed gastrointestinal events in 8076 randomized rheumatoid arthritis patients who received rofecoxib 50 mg/day was 50% lower than the rate observed with naproxen 500 mg twice daily (2.1 events/100 patient-years with rofecoxib versus 4.5 events/100 patient-years with naproxen). A number of studies in patients with osteoarthritis, rheumatoid arthritis and acute pain have confirmed that the clinical efficacy of COX-2 selective inhibitors is similar to that of conventional NSAIDs.[20] Before its withdrawal from the worldwide market, rofecoxib was licensed in Europe only for the treatment of osteoarthritis, but some other selective COX-2 NSAIDs, such as nimesulide, have been investigated in back pain. A randomized, prospective, double-blind trial evaluated the efficacy of nimesulide 100 mg twice daily for 10 days, which is claimed to be a COX-2 selective agent, versus ibuprofen 600 mg three times daily in 104 patients (age 18–65 years) suffering from acute common back pain. There was a clear improvement in all parameters of pain and back function from the third day of treatment onwards with both treatments versus placebo.[21] A 6-week, randomized controlled study in 246 patients with ankylosing spondylitis showed an improvement in pain and functional impairment that was greater in the celecoxib 200 mg/day or ketoprofen 200 mg/day treatment groups than in the placebo group.[22]

Since the available COX-2 selective inhibitors are still not 'pure' COX-2 drugs, especially if considering nimesulide, they may not display as dramatic an improvement on the gastrointestinal adverse effects profile as was previously hoped. Although rare, well-documented cases of acute hepatic injury have been reported with nimesulide and with a number of NSAIDs such as diclofenac.[23] Age was the main risk factor identified in a cohort study that included 400,000 users of NSAIDs.[24] Furthermore, COX-2 selective agents are not expected to differ in terms of cardiovascular and renal adverse events, particularly when one takes into account the long half-life of rofecoxib or celecoxib, compared with the short-acting non-selective NSAIDs, and, indeed, this cardiovascular toxicity has lately been pointed out.

Cardiovascular effects

A case–control study showed that the use of NSAIDs other than low-dose aspirin in the preceding week was associated with a doubling of the odds of a hospital first admission with cardiac failure (adjusted odds ratio (OR) = 2.1) with a greater increase when patients had a history of heart disease (OR = 10.5) compared to those without such a history (OR = 1.6). The odds of a first admission to hospital with cardiac failure was positively related to the NSAID intake dose in the previous week and was increased to a greater extent with long half-life NSAIDs. Assuming these relationships are causal, it was estimated that NSAIDs were responsible for approximately 19% of hospital admissions for cardiac heart failure.[25] Therefore, long half-life NSAIDs in particular should be used with caution in patients with a history of cardiovascular disease.

As demonstrated recently, the cardiovascular safety profile of the COX-2 selective inhibitors is also a concern. As early as 1999 the rate of serious thrombotic adverse events (e.g. myocardial infarction) was significantly higher in patients receiving rofecoxib in the VIGOR study.[19] Analysis of the data showed a relative risk of 2.38 (95% confidence interval (CI) 1.39–4.00, $p = 0.002$).[26] At that time the most likely explanation for the difference in cardiovascular events was a protective effect of naproxen, possibly related to an antiplatelet activity. However, rofecoxib was withdrawn from the market on 30 September 2004 following an interim analysis of a prospective, randomized, placebo-controlled, double-blind trial, the APPROVE (Adenomatous Polyp Prevention on Vioxx) trial. This study was designed to determine the effect of a 3-year treatment with rofecoxib 25 mg/day on the risk of recurrent neoplastic polyps of the large bowel in patients with a history of colorectal adenomas. The data of this trial showed that after 18 months of treatment the relative risk (RR) for a confirmed thrombotic event in the rofecoxib group was twice that in the placebo group (RR = 1.92, 95% CI 1.19–3.11, $p = 0.008$).[27] Use of aspirin was not allowed in this study. A recent meta-analysis that included a total of 21,432 patients evaluated 18 controlled randomized clinical studies of patients suffering from osteoarthritis or rheumatoid arthritis and 11 observational studies where the indication for the NSAID was often not described.[29] The relative risk from the randomized trials was 2.24 (95% CI 1.24–4.02, $p = 0.007$). This relative risk did not seem to depend on the control group or the duration of the trial. In the observational studies, the cardioprotective effect of naproxen was small (RR = 0.86, 95% CI 0.75–0.99) and cannot explain the findings of the VIGOR trial. A few months later, the Adenoma Prevention with Celebrex (APC) trial was suspended due to an intermediate analysis that also revealed an increased risk of cardiovascular events. This study had already included 2035 patients with a history of colorectal neoplasia who received 400 or 800 mg/day of celecoxib for 2.8–3.1 years. Analysis of deaths due to cardiovascular causes revealed seven cases in the placebo group, 16 in the low-dose group (hazard ratio 2.3, 95% CI 0.9–5.5) and 23 in the high-dose group (hazard ratio 3.4, 95% CI 1.4–7.8).[29] However, two other studies, the PreSAP (Prevention of Spontaneous Adenomatous Polyps) trial and the ADAPT trial (Alzheimer's Disease Anti-Inflammatory Prevention Trial), evaluating the efficacy of celecoxib 400 mg/day, did not show an increased risk for cardiovascular events compared with placebo. The PreSAP trial is still ongoing, but the ADAPT trial was suspended due to an increased risk for cardiovascular events in the naproxen group (50% increased risk compared to placebo). Valdecoxib and its prodrug parecoxib also showed an increased risk for cardiovascular adverse events in two studies that evaluated their efficacy on postoperative pain after cardiac surgery.[30, 31] Both drugs have been suspended for treatment of chronic pain, primarily due to serious adverse skin reactions.

Therefore, a large number of the elderly should remain on aspirin if they receive a COX-2 inhibitor and, in this case, the advantage in terms of gastrointestinal tract security remains an open question. In 2000, 1120 safety issues were reported to the Committee on Safety of Medicines in the UK for rofecoxib on 557,000 estimated prescriptions. Half of these issues concerned the gastrointestinal tract, while 12% concerned bleeding, ulcers and perforations. Five patients had a fatal outcome. Over two-thirds of the patients were over 65 years old and a quarter were taking aspirin.[32] The Committee on Safety of Medicines in the UK also reminded practitioners that COX-2 selective inhibitors were contraindicated in the presence of active peptic ulceration or gastrointestinal bleeding. Celecoxib, in the CLASS study, at doses greater than those indicated clinically, was associated with a lower incidence of symptomatic ulcers and ulcer complications, as compared with NSAIDs at standard doses; however, this benefit was reduced in patients taking aspirin concomitantly[18] and disappeared when one looks at the 1-year outcomes of the study.[33]

Renal effects

Regarding renal toxicity, the available data demonstrate that the same frequency and type of renal toxicity should be expected with selective COX-2 inhibitors as with the NSAIDs. When used in high-risk patients or with other drugs that influence renal haemodynamics, their prescription should be restricted as with the other NSAIDs. This assertion is borne out by clinical studies showing that the COX-2 inhibitors rofecoxib and celecoxib produce qualitative changes in urinary prostaglandin excretion, glomerular filtration rate and sodium retention.[34] It is therefore unlikely that these COX-2 selective inhibitors will have greater renal safety benefits over non-selective NSAID therapies, and it is reasonable to assume that all NSAIDs, including COX-2 selective inhibitors, share a similar risk of adverse renal effects.[35] These adverse effects include functional acute renal failure, sodium and water retention, hyperkalaemia and immunoallergic nephritis. Moreover, it is possible that the improved gastrointestinal safety will increase the use of the selective COX-2 inhibitors in older and high-risk patients, which may lead to more renal adverse effects. The overall incidence of adverse renal events after celecoxib was similar to that observed after NSAID use in a post hoc analysis of the renal toxicity of celecoxib, using the safety database generated during its clinical development programme, which included data from more than 5000 subjects.

Therapeutic strategies for the use of NSAIDs

In the light of the above discussion, in terms of safety and cost short half-life NSAIDs should be used in acute painful conditions. This is particularly the case when chronic persistent nociceptive pain is affected by short-lasting acute exacerbation. When moderate pain persists and when digestive risk factors have been identified, the combination of classical NSAIDs with a proton pump inhibitor can be used. A COX-2 selective agent such as celecoxib is also an option for patients without cardiovascular disease. For all NSAIDs (including COX-2 inhibitors)

the lowest dose should be used for the shortest possible time. The patient should be informed of the potential risks.

Several non-NSAID, non-narcotic therapies are available when inflammation is not the foremost issue in pain management. Since its introduction in 1893, paracetamol has been widely used for the treatment of pain. Despite many attempts to elucidate its mechanism of action, it remains unclear. It has been shown that paracetamol selectively inhibits central nervous tissue COX but has little effect on enzyme preparations from peripheral tissues.[36–38] Although this is not unequivocally accepted,[39] many experiments in animals[40–42] and humans[43] have suggested that descending spinal serotonergic pathways are essential for maintaining its efficacy.[44] This centrally acting analgesic is devoid of the gastric or renal adverse-event profile usually seen with NSAIDs. Paracetamol is as effective as NSAIDs for the management of mild-to-moderate osteoarthritic pain. The reported advantages of NSAIDs over paracetamol in spinal painful conditions remain, at best, conflicting, and paracetamol is still the first-line therapy recommended by the European and American societies of rheumatology[45] for treating pain associated with osteoarthritis, and is safer in the elderly population.[46]

OPIOIDS IN LOW BACK PAIN

Primary care physicians frequently face the challenge of treating chronic debilitating pain. Whether or not treatment with opioids is effective and justified in the treatment of pain that is unrelated to cancer is a matter of great controversy. Growing experience with opioid administration in cancer patients and the publication of some controlled studies have promoted a more liberal attitude. Some carefully selected patients could benefit from short-term opioid treatment within the context of a more permanent pain-treatment regimen. However, potential pitfalls, such as prescribing opioids for myofascial pain syndrome, fibromyalgia, or somatoform pain disorders, should be taken into account, as should the psychosocial dimensions surrounding the prescription of opioids.

In chronic nociceptive pain conditions, regular use of low-dose, long-acting opioids, although controversial, can effectively control chronic pain in selected patients.[47–49] Opioids can improve the quality of life of patients in pain, but their use requires particular precautions, both in the choice of the specific opioid and in singling out patients with a high risk of drug abuse. Several randomized controlled studies have been performed in rheumatological chronic pain conditions evaluating the efficacy of opioids in back pain.

An open randomized 4-month comparison of naproxen and two opioid regimens of oxycodone and sustained-release morphine sulphate in 36 patients with chronic back pain has been performed. The opioid groups were significantly better than the naproxen-alone group, with less pain and emotional distress, but opioids had little impact on daily activity and sleep, and one of the participants showed signs of abuse.[50]

Another study evaluated 380 chronic back pain outpatients (age 21–79 years) enrolled in an enriched 1-month randomized, placebo-controlled trial.[51] During the preceding 4-week open-label phase patients were treated with tramadol in doses up to 400 mg/day. Because of adverse events 20% withdrew, but 254 patients entered the double-blind phase, during which daily doses were maintained (tramadol 200–400 mg) and compared to placebo. The Kaplan–Meier estimate of the cumulative discontinuation rate due to therapeutic failure was 20% in the opioid group as compared with 51% in the placebo group.

A randomized, double-blind, placebo-controlled trial evaluated the efficacy and the safety of the tramadol + paracetamol combination in chronic low back pain.[52] The study assessed 336 patients over a 3-month period. Intention-to-treat analysis showed a better mean final pain score and mean final pain relief score with the combination compared to placebo. The cumulative estimate for treatment discontinuation due to insufficient pain relief was 22.9% in the treatment group versus 54.7% in the placebo group. Adverse events in the tramadol + paracetamol group were those commonly encountered with tramadol and other opioids: nausea (12%), dizziness (11%), constipation (10%) and somnolence (9%).

Another study based on the same design yielded the same results.[53] A recent randomized, double-blind study evaluated the efficacy and safety of an extended-release form of oxymorphone versus oxycodone and placebo in chronic low back pain.[54] During 7–14 days, the patients ($n = 330$) were randomized to receive either oxymorphone or oxycodone in a dose-titration phase. The patients that achieved effective analgesia ($n = 235$) were then randomized to receive either an opioid or a placebo for 18 days. Of these patients, 139 completed the study. The two opioid groups were significantly superior to placebo for the mean change from baseline in pain intensity. Lack of efficacy was the reason for discontinuation of the study in 57% of the patients included in the placebo group, compared to 20% in the oxymorphone group and 16% in the oxycodone group.

Finally, a 3-year retrospective analysis of opioid use in an orthopaedic spine clinic was performed.[55] Opioids were prescribed for 152 of the 230 patients evaluated, treatment being for less than 3 months in 94 patients and more than 3 months in 58. The control group received NSAIDs or nothing. The different medications prescribed were codeine, oxycodone, propoxyphene, tramadol, morphine, meperidine, fentanyl and hydroxycodone, alone or in combination. Opioid treatment reduced spinal pain from 8.3 to 4.5 on a 0 to 10 point scale, results that were statistically and clinically significant and equal for long- and short-term therapy. Adverse effects appeared in all treatment groups: 59% in the short-term group, 73% in the long-term group and 37% in the NSAID group, with the most common toxicities in the opioid groups being sedation and constipation. The authors concluded that opioids were effective and safe for the treatment of spinal disorders. One must, however, bear in mind that retrospective analyses have limitations; in this case, especially, there was recall bias regarding pain relief and side-effects. Long-term, randomized, prospective, double-blind controlled studies are the only way to demonstrate a benefit of opioids in these clinical conditions.

In osteoarthritis, a randomized controlled study on 236 patients (mean age 60 years) in an 8-week, double-blind phase showed that the addition of an opioid allows for a reduction in NSAIDs without compromising pain relief.[56] This can be of benefit in the mainstay of chronic pain management, since NSAIDs are known to be associated with cardiac and renal toxicities, which is a particular problem for the elderly population.

Although some open-label studies have suggested a possible benefit of long-term opioid analgesic therapy for some well-selected patients with refractory back pain,[57] factors responsible for chronification, such as the patient's psychosocial situation, should systematically be taken into account and an multidisciplinary approach to the treatment of pain should be proposed. Such is the case in common back pain, fibromyalgia[58] or failed back surgery, where nociceptive and neuropathic pain syndromes may, moreover, coexist. One should therefore be extremely cautious as far as opioid prescription is concerned. Choosing the optimal analgesic treatment is not easy considering the multitude of currently available opioid derivatives, the commercialization of new preparations (e.g. slow-release or transdermal formulations) and the difficulty of evaluating their risk/benefit ratio. Basic principles for selecting an opioid treatment on an individual basis rely on various selection criteria such as the pharmacodynamic and pharmacokinetic properties of available opioids, the presence of comorbidities and concomitant medications, and pharmacokinetic situations that are prone to increase the risk of substance abuse.

Addiction is a concern among patients and healthcare providers, and drug-seeking behaviour is seen among patients with chronic pain. When opioids are used appropriately, addiction is rare, but patients should be monitored to ensure that they are using the opioid correctly. The risk can be minimized by prescribing opioids to patients with a history of drug abuse only with great caution and under strict medical supervision. To reduce the risk even further, the drug chosen should be given at the lowest effective dose, with regular monitoring, have the least addictive potential and not be prescribed indefinitely. The risk of addiction can be reduced by avoiding their prescription in pain syndromes that are poorly responsive to opioids, such as psychogenic or neuropathic pain, and by selecting an opioid with an appropriate pharmacokinetic and pharmacodynamic profile. Some pharmacokinetic characteristics of drugs lower the addiction potential. The rate of central nervous system drug delivery, for example, influences positive reinforcement. Giving an oral formulation, a slow-release formulation, or even a drug the opiate component of which necessitates bioactivation, such as codeine or tramadol, reduces the risk of addiction. An optimal pharmacokinetic profile would also avoid negative reinforcement, such as physical dependence, and this can be accomplished with slow-release formulations or long half-life opioids. Physical dependence should be clearly differentiated from addiction. Physical dependence can occur in the clinical setting, but does not involve inappropriate drug-seeking behaviour. Withdrawal symptoms and signs can be prevented by gradually decreasing the dose of the opioid. An optimal pharmacodynamic profile would favour selectivity on μ opioid receptors, and avoid a high intrinsic activity.

Pain is often inadequately treated due in part to reluctance to use opioid analgesics and fear of abuse behaviour. Every day throughout the world, patients, caregivers and their governments face difficulties obtaining opioid analgesics for the relief of severe pain. The WHO has promoted guidelines to avoid national narcotic laws that interfere with making these drugs available for medical use. These guidelines, recognizing that physicians should have the flexibility to decide the dose and duration of opioid treatment based on individual patients' needs, recommend that a country's narcotic legislation should not restrict the amount of opioids prescribed at one time, and a survey conducted by the International Narcotics Control Board shows that 52% of governments do not have this provision in their legislation.[59]

A retrospective survey of medical records from 1990 to 1996 stored in the databases of the Drug Abuse Warning Network and the Automation of Reports and Consolidated Orders System in the USA from 1990 to 1996 showed an increased medical use of opioid analgesics to treat pain, but this did not seem to contribute to an increase in opioid abuse.[60] Among opioids, tramadol is not scheduled in the USA and Europe. A proactive postmarketing surveillance programme was carried out; monthly population exposure to tramadol had grown to just under 1 million patients over a 3-year period. Reports of abuse over the same period, however, grew no higher than 2/100,000 patients, recorded during a brief period of experimentation in the first 18 months. Since then the reported rate of abuse has significantly declined, to levels of less than 1/100,000 patients by the year 2000.[61] Despite new branded and generic formulations of tramadol, the average rate of abuse at June 2003 was approximately 0.5/100,000 patients. The abuse rate for the tramadol + paracetamol combination in the first 2 years after its commercialization was of 0.25/100,000 patients.[62] Moreover, 97% of abuse cases occurred in patients with a history of drug abuse. Because of its dual mode of action, tramadol may have a better safety profile compared with other opioids. On the down side, however, the monoaminergic profile may increase central nervous system susceptibility. Convulsions, for instance, have been described with tramadol, although this occurred mainly after overdoses. In addition, due to the monoaminergic action of tramadol, concomitant antidepressants should be used with caution to avoid a serotonergic syndrome.

In cases of insufficient control of pain symptoms the use of a 'stronger' opioid, such as a slow-release morphine formulation, can be recommended when one keeps in mind the prescribing guidelines in non-cancer pain (Box 10.1).[63]

Box 10.1. Recommendations for the prolonged administration of opioids in chronic pain patients*

- A history of drug abuse or other substances (alcohol), of severe personality disorders, and of a disturbed social environment should be considered as relative contraindications
- Only one physician should be responsible for prescribing opioids. At each visit (at least once a month), the physician should evaluate the analgesia, the adverse effects and possible behavioural signs of psychological dependence. The preset goal is a partial analgesia as well as an improvement of physical activity and quality of life
- The physician should know the pharmacology of the opioid and the kinetic consequences of renal or hepatic insufficiency
- Start the treatment progressively, with low doses of opioids having pharmacological characteristics adapted to the clinical situation
- Adjust the route of administration to the patient's needs, while favouring the new forms (e.g. slow-release or transdermal formulations), which offer stable plasma concentrations
- Repeated administration at fixed intervals is needed in order to maintain efficient plasma levels and prevent anticipation anxiety
- Anticipate a 'rescue' dose for the predictable or unpredictable breakthrough pain
- The optimal dose should be determined after reaching the steady state (four half-lives to reach stable plasma concentrations)
- Avoid interactions between opioids and sedative non-analgesic drugs (benzodiazepines and neuroleptics used as tranquillizers) or the association of opioids such as tramadol with other serotoninergic psychotropic drugs (antidepressants)
- Anticipate and treat adverse effects (constipation, nausea, vomiting, sedation) or neurological complications (myoclonia, confusion, hallucinations)
- Discuss with the patient his or her representations about the use of morphine or of any other opioid. The patient should give informed consent before being prescribed opioids, and after having received information about the low risk of dependence and the possible cognitive problems due to opioids
- Assess the appearance of tolerance (increase doses, change of analgesic)
- Anticipate a withdrawal syndrome by stopping opioid treatment progressively

*Adapted from the recommendations of the American Pain Society, the consensus of the Canadian Pain Society and Limoges recommendations.

ANTIDEPRESSANTS IN THE MANAGEMENT OF PAINFUL SPINAL DISORDERS

There is evidence that antidepressants have pain-relief effects that are either acute, as observed in experimental pain studies, or chronic, as demonstrated in patients.[64–66] Therefore, they have been commonly used to treat chronic pain for years. There are many assumptions about the mechanisms involved in the analgesic effects of antidepressants. Tricyclic antidepressants are known to inhibit noradrenaline (NA) and 5-HT presynaptic reuptake but also to block α_1 adrenergic, muscarinic and H_1 histaminergic receptors. Some of the tricyclics present a balanced inhibition of NA and 5-HT reuptake, such as amitriptyline or imipramine, or a relatively selective inhibition of NA reuptake, such as desipramine or the tetracyclic antidepressant maprotiline. The selective serotonergic reuptake inhibitors (SSRIs) act mainly on 5-HT. A new agent, venlafaxine, chemically distinct from tricyclics and SSRIs, has shown an inhibition in reuptake of NA and 5-HT, with a relatively selective action on 5-HT, particularly at low doses.[67]

Some authors have argued that antidepressants might decrease pain through the improvement of masked or manifest depression. Although an improvement in mood may contribute to reports of decreased pain in some patients, there is clear evidence for pain relief in patients without pre-existing mood disorders and with smaller doses than the usual doses recommended for depression.[68, 69] The relationship between depression and pain could be even more complex, since an antagonist for substance P, which is a peptide involved in pain endings in the spinal cord, has shown antidepressant properties that are equivalent to paroxetine.[70] As well as their inhibitory mechanisms on 5-HT and/or NA reuptake, their analgesic effects could also be mediated through an involvement in the opioidergic system. Antidepressants have additional effects on various ion channels, such as inhibition of cardiac or neuronal sodium channels. This latter blockade could be involved in analgesic effects of antidepressants. Some authors have claimed that the analgesic effect of antidepressants could be an epiphenomenon of their sedative effects.

Meta-analyses have shown that non-sedative antidepressants are as effective as sedative ones. Furthermore, lorazepam, a benzodiazepine, did not relieve neuropathic pain, in contrast to amitriptyline.[71] The majority of clinical trials that have assessed the analgesic effects of antidepressants have done so using subjective scales, usually rating pain intensity, fatigue, sleep, physical or social activities, and quality of life. Numerous clinical trials have been performed with antidepressants in various chronic pain syndromes. Evidence of their efficacy is conclusive for diabetic neuropathy, postherpetic neuralgia, atypical facial pain, tension and migraine headache, fibromyalgia, rheumatic pain and chronic pain of mixed aetiologies.[66]

Evidence is less clear for chronic back pain, given the methodological biases in many of the studies (e.g. small sample sizes that lack statistical power, inadequate specification of inclusion and exclusion criteria, failure to use standardized outcomes measures, absence of a rigorous assessment for major depressive disorder and failure to maintain study blinding).[72] Furthermore, the differences among the chronic back pain studies in terms of patients' characteristics, medications, doses and outcome measures limit the use of a meta-analysis for a synthesis of this literature. In two recent placebo-controlled studies, which included patients suffering from chronic back pain referred to primary practice, nortriptyline and maprotiline showed an analgesic effect in non-depressed individuals and were also associated with a lreduction of disability in daily functioning, predominantly in the psychosocial domain.[68] These gains seemed more important for patients with radicular pain. Further studies are needed to investigate the effect of antidepressants on chronic back pain with a neuropathic pain component. As in the experimental assays, the numerous clinical studies used the whole range of antidepressants from the first tricyclics to the newest antidepressants, such as the SSRIs, which cause fewer severe adverse effects. A large majority of these studies used a tricyclic, particularly amitriptyline, which was superior to placebo or to an SSRI. More specifically, in neuropathic pain, most of the studies showed a higher efficacy of tricyclics compared to SSRIs.[64, 73] These conclusions were confirmed in meta-analyses, and non-selective tricyclics remain the most effective.[74]

Several dose–response studies in patients did not produce consistent findings regarding the relationship between dose, serum levels and analgesic effect. There is no established therapeutic concentration of antidepressants, and as a consequence no dosing recommendations for antidepressant use in any chronic pain disorder, reflecting the importance of first considering individual metabolism capacity. Thus, the monitoring of plasma drug concentrations should be restricted to compliance or toxicity problems or inefficiency after an adequate period of treatment. Antidepressants are associated with a relatively high incidence of adverse effects in therapeutic usage. Many of the commonly observed adverse effects, such as dryness of mouth, blurred vision and drowsiness, can be troublesome, particularly at the start of tricyclic treatment. Studies have shown higher adverse effect scores at the start of treatment than 4–6 weeks later. The most common cardiovascular adverse effects appear to be orthostatic hypotension, although more severe cardiac complications could arise in patients with pre-existing cardiovascular disease. There appears to be a dose-dependent relationship, such as has been found for venlafaxine, and increased frequency of hypertension. In a meta-analysis, the risk of central toxicity (e.g. tremor, ataxia) was positively correlated with plasma drug concentration.

ANALGESICS AND COMPLIANCE

Compliance has been defined as 'the extent to which a person's behaviour (in terms of taking medication or executing lifestyle changes) coincides with medical or health advice'.[75] Non-compliance may refer to many behaviours, such as: not having a prescription filled; taking an incorrect dose; taking the medication at the wrong times; forgetting one or more doses of the medication; increasing the frequency of doses; and stopping the treatment too soon, either by ceasing to take the medication sooner than the physician recommended or by failing to obtain a refill prescription. The most common forms of non-compliance, except with narcotic analgesics and benzodiazepines, are delaying or omitting doses.[76]

Although consistently found to occur in about one-half of all patients, non-compliance has been found to vary according to the type and state of disease. Chronicity is associated with decreased compliance, as has been shown in some chronic pain problems such as headache,[77] rheumatoid arthritis[78] and ankylosing spondylitis.[79]

During the last decade many methods have been devised to assess compliance, but the complexity of the problem has prevented the development of a 'gold standard' method of measurement. The most frequently used methods are drug levels in blood or urine as direct measures, and interviews, diaries and tablet counts (e.g. medication event monitoring system (MEMS)) as indirect measures.

For patients, compliance is not an issue: they do not perceive taking drugs entirely in terms of obeying the doctor's orders. Instead, they weigh up the costs and benefits of taking a particular medication, as they perceive them within the context and the constraint of their everyday lives and needs. This perspective implies the patient's active participation in the therapeutic relationship, leading to a shared decision-making process. It also implies that non-compliance may not be due to disregard for doctor's orders, but may result from reasoned behaviour based on the patient's beliefs and previous experiences. Compliance appears to be high when practitioners and patients have common representations, agree on treatment procedures and share criteria for outcome appraisals.[80]

Studies have shown that adverse effects and beliefs about adverse effects are major determinants of non-compliance in patient populations suffering from a variety of diseases or problems. The occurrence and severity of adverse effects have been reported to decrease compliance to cholesterol-altering drugs, antiepileptic drug regimens and migraine medication.[81] Non-compliance due to fear of becoming dependent on the medication has been pointed out in populations as divergent as asthmatic patients, general practice patients taking long-term medication and patients suffering from ankylosing spondylitis.[79] Such findings in rheumatoid arthritis and ankylosing spondylitis patients may lead one to consider compliance with medication intake as being a last resort, when the symptoms are more unacceptable than the fears of adverse effects and possible dependence.[82]

For antidepressants, a fear of adverse effects has been evidenced in depressive patients as well as in the general population.[83] The results of a large opinion survey in Germany showed that, even for the treatment of severe mental disease, psychotropic drugs are not well accepted in comparison to cardiac drugs: they are believed to cause significantly more severe adverse effects and raise a greater fear of losing control.[83] However, a patient's attention to adverse effects does not only lead to compliance problems. Wynne and Long's study[84] showed that this attention might help the patient to cope adequately with his or her medication intake, and thus avoid detrimental adverse effects. Adverse effects are thus of major interest when dealing with medication intake.

Since information on the beliefs of chronic pain patients about antidepressants is scarce, we conducted a pilot study to investigate these beliefs.[85] Seventy-six chronic pain patients (CPPs) and 54 pain-free non-patient controls were included. The CPPs were representative of the population referred to the Geneva Multidisciplinary Pain Centre. The sample included 30 chronic back pain patients (CBPs) and 46 patients suffering from other chronic pain problems. Controls were matched for age, gender, socio-economic status and nationality. Semistructured interviews were conducted, explicitly referring to individuals' definitions of medication and antidepressants. We chose to ask the individuals to give their own definitions instead of using multiple-choice questionnaires, as the latter mainly call up recognition memory. Moreover, the items in a questionnaire might inhibit a further search for alternative answers. The data analysis procedure was a content analysis. All responses were transcribed and categorized. Bivariate statistical procedures were used to evaluate within-group and between-group differences.

Aside from depression, the CBPs' description of the indications for antidepressants included mood improvement, soothing effects, but also loss of desire. Pain was more often mentioned in this group (Table 10.1). However, this response was much less frequent than expected on the basis of the CBPs' reported antidepressant intake and their medical records.

One-third of CBPs considered antidepressants were used to address severe psychological problems, including madness, and 19% of them expected antidepressants to induce personality changes. Accordingly, 24% of CBPs considered antidepressants to be a dangerous medication, having many adverse effects, including addiction (37%). Up to 19% would refuse to take antidepressants, 41% would accept but with great reluctance, and 33% would accept only if they were convinced that it would affect their pain problem. The effect of antidepressants on pain is barely known among chronic pain patients. Patients' beliefs may hinder their understanding of the physician's prescription and their compliance with it. Non-congruence between patients' beliefs and physicians' prescriptions may account for part of the difficulties when prescribing such medication.

We have also been investigating the way individuals get information about medication.[86] Patient information leaflets (PILs) were the main reported source of information about medication in the patients and the controls. Expected 'ideal' information included the possibility of discussing PILs and adverse effects with the physician. Content analysis of PILs showed that leaflets on antidepressants point to indications that have a clear psychological, if not psychiatric, connotation. This is in line with patients' and controls' representations of antidepressants, so that they may consider such medication inappropriate for the treatment of pain. In the context of chronic pain, where the causes of pain persistence often remain elusive, prescription of antidepressants may be seen as a 'delegitimation', i.e. a denial of the patient's experience of pain and suffering.[87] Even when antidepressants are prescribed because of their

Table 10.1. Intake of antidepressants and beliefs about antidepressant medication

	Chronic back pain patients	Chronic pain patients	Controls	Significance
Intake of antidepressants				
Present intake of antidepressants (%)	37	33	7	$p < 0.001$
Ever taken antidepressants (%)	63	69	33	$p < 0.001$
Beliefs about antidepressants				
Against pain (%)	33	20	8	$p = 0.001$
Mood improvement (%)	30	41	63	$p = 0.008$
Severe psychological problems (%)	33	27	24	NS
Dangerous medication (%)	24	20	17	NS
Somatic adverse effects (%)	63	53	41	NS
Psychological adverse effects (%)	45	35	30	NS

NS, not significant.

analgesic effect, indications as described in the PILs may lead the patient to think that the physician does not truly believe he or she is in pain. Thus, non-congruence between the motive for prescribing antidepressants and the PILs may also account for part of the difficulties when prescribing such medication.

A study conducted with a sample of the Geneva population aged 18–75 years showed that a vast majority of the interviewees did not differentiate between the various classes of psychotropic drugs and between the various psychiatric illnesses.[88] Similarly, for psychotropic drugs, more than 80% of the subjects referred to real or presumed somatic and/or psychological harmful effects (e.g. lethargy or drowsiness, loss of contact with reality, changes of personality). They criticized, in the same proportion, the addiction and the dependency created by psychotropic drugs, and society, which promoted their use. Subjects' attitudes regarding psychotropic drugs, as well as medication in general, and compliance were strongly associated. Thus, both aspects seemed to be related to the subjects' degree of adherence to medication and to its therapeutic approaches.

SUMMARY

Experimental studies have confirmed long-standing clinical impressions about the dynamic nature of pain and have shown that inadequately managed acute pain may become more difficult to suppress. Persistent pain syndromes offer no biological advantage; they could be the result of profound neurobiological alterations and be complicated by major psychosocial consequences. In order to reduce the neurobiological peripheral or central sensitization and the psychosocial consequences of severe pain, one should uncompromisingly handle acute pain in parallel to the aetiological treatment.

Chronic pain syndromes fall into main categories that imply different therapeutic strategies. As a result, nociceptive pain can be adequately reduced using NSAIDs, paracetamol or opioids, whereas neuropathic pain often implies the need for other ther-

apeutic approaches, including the use of specific non-traditional analgesic drugs such as antidepressants or anticonvulsants.

For nociceptive pain, the selective COX-2 inhibitors were thought to be a real therapeutic advance with a better gastrointestinal safety profile, but their renal and particularly their cardiovascular safety have been shown to be a major concerns.

Indeed, in terms of efficacy, safety and cost, short half-life NSAIDs should be suggested for use in acute painful conditions. This is especially the case when chronic persistent nociceptive pain is affected by short-lasting acute exacerbations. When moderate pain persists and digestive risk factors are identified, the combination of classical NSAIDs with a proton pump inhibitor can be used. COX-2 selective agents, such as celecoxib, are also an option, but only for patients without a cardiovascular disease. For all NSAIDs (including COX-2 inhibitors) the lowest dose should be prescribed for the shortest time. The patients should be informed of the potential risks. Several non-NSAID, non-narcotic therapies, such as paracetamol, are available when inflammation is not the foremost issue in pain management, and they remain the first choice analgesic for mild to moderate nociceptive non-malignant pain. In chronic nociceptive pain conditions, regular use of low-dose long-acting opioids, although controversial, can effectively control chronic pain in selected patients. Opioids can improve the quality of life of patients in pain, but their use requires particular precautions, both when choosing the opioid and when singling out patients at risk of drug abuse. There is evidence that antidepressants offer benefits in chronic pain: meta-analyses have confirmed that non-selective tricyclic antidepressants remain the most effective, especially when a neuropathic component is present. Like any pharmacological treatment, antidepressants raise the issue of patients' compliance. Various factors, such as beliefs and previous experiences, may affect this. The analgesic effect of antidepressants is barely known, whereas the adverse effects are highly emphasized. Regarding beliefs, the case of opioids has not yet been settled by either patients or therapists.

Chronic pain remains a complex syndrome where analgesic treatment is only one part of the treatment. However, when analgesics are tailored to the individual, taking into account the drug's pharmacological properties and the patient's comorbidities, they may contribute to a favourable risk–benefit ratio in these complex clinical conditions.

PRACTICE POINTS

- Distinguishing nociceptive from neuropathic and somatoform pain disorders (or components) will help in selecting the best therapeutic approach.

- In terms of efficacy, safety and cost, short half-life NSAIDs can be proposed in acute painful conditions. This is especially the case when chronic persistent nociceptive pain is affected by short-lasting acute exacerbations.

- When moderate pain persists and digestive risk factors are identified, the combination of classical NSAIDs with a proton pump inhibitor can be used. COX-2 selective agents, such as celecoxib, are also an option, but only for patients without a cardiovascular disease.

- For all NSAIDs (including COX-2 inhibitors) the lowest dose should be prescribed for the shortest time.

- Paracetamol is available when inflammation is not the foremost issue in pain management, and remains the first-choice analgesic for mild to moderate nociceptive non-malignant pain.

- Opioids can improve the quality of life of patients in pain, but their use requires particular precautions, both when choosing the specific opioid and when singling out patients at risk of drug abuse.

- There is evidence that antidepressants have analgesic properties in chronic pain conditions, with non-selective tricyclic antidepressants being the most effective.

RESEARCH AGENDA

- Epidemiological studies are needed to evaluate the prevalence and incidence of the different pain components in common chronic back pain, and experimental studies should evaluate the importance of central sensitization in chronic back pain.

- Prospective longitudinal studies must be undertaken to evaluate the efficacy and the incidence of renal and cardiovascular incidents related to NSAIDs versus paracetamol or opioids in chronic back pain.

- Prospective longitudinal studies are needed to evaluate the efficacy and the safety of different opioids in chronic back pain.

- Further studies are needed to investigate the dose–response effect of antidepressants on chronic back pain and to determine the influence of the neuropathic pain component when present.

REFERENCES

1. Ossipov MH, Lai J, Malan TP Jr et al. Spinal and supraspinal mechanisms of neuropathic pain. *Ann NY Acad Sci* 2000; **909**: 12–24.
2. Woolf CJ, Mannion RJ. Neuropathic pain: aetiology, symptoms, mechanisms, and management. *Lancet* 1999; **353**: 1959–1964.
3. Anon. Drug treatment of neuropathic pain. *Drug Ther Bull* 2000; **38**: 89–93.
4. Desmeules JA, Cedraschi C, Rapiti E et al. Neurophysiologic evidence for a central sensitization in patients with fibromyalgia. *Arthritis Rheum* 2003; **48**: 1420–1429.
5. Goldenberg DL, Burckhardt C, Crofford L. Management of fibromyalgia syndrome. *JAMA* 2004; **292**: 2388–2395.
6. Allaz AF, Vannotti M, Desmeules J et al. Use of the label 'litigation neurosis' in patients with somatoform pain disorder. *Gen Hosp Psychiatry* 1998; **20**: 91–97.
7. Woolf CJ, Salter MW. Neuronal plasticity: increasing the gain in pain. *Science* 2000; **288**: 1765–1769.
8. Woolf CJ. Pain: moving from symptom control toward mechanism-specific pharmacologic management. *Ann Intern Med* 2004; **140**: 441–451.
9. Perrot S, Guilbaud G. Pathophysiology of joint pain. *Rev Rhumatol (English Edn)* 1996; **63**: 485–492.
10. Ashburn MA, Staats PS. Management of chronic pain. *Lancet* 1999; **353**: 1865–1869.
11. Besson J-M. The neurobiology of pain. *Lancet* 1999; **353**: 1610–1615.
12. Anon. *Cancer Pain Relief and Palliative Care*. WHO, Geneva, 1996.
13. Furlan AD, Clarke J, Esmail R et al. Critical review of reviews on the treatment of chronic low back pain. *Spine* 2001; **26**: E155–E162.
14. McQuay HJ, Moore RA (eds). *An Evidence-Based Resource for Pain Relief.* Oxford University Press, Oxford, 1998.
15. McQuay HJ, Moore RA. Oral ibuprofen and diclofenac in postoperative pain. In: McQuay HJ, Moore RA (eds), *An Evidence-Based Resource for Pain Relief.* Oxford University Press, Oxford, 1998, pp. 78–83.
16. Van Tulder MW, Scholten RJ, Koes BW et al. Nonsteroidal anti-inflammatory drugs for low back pain: a systematic review within the framework of the Cochrane Collaboration Back Review Group. *Spine* 2000; **25**: 2501–2513.
17. Dougados M, Gueguen A, Nakache JP et al. Ankylosing spondylitis: what is the optimum duration of a clinical study? A one year versus a 6 weeks non-steroidal anti-inflammatory drug trial. *Rheumatology* 1999; **38**: 235–244.
18. Silverstein FE, Faich G, Goldstein JL et al. Gastrointestinal toxicity with celecoxib vs nonsteroidal anti-inflammatory drugs for osteoarthritis and rheumatoid arthritis. The CLASS study: a randomized controlled trial. Celecoxib Long-term Arthritis Safety Study. *JAMA* 2000; **284**: 1247–1255.
19. Bombardier C, Laine L, Reicin A et al. Comparison of upper gastrointestinal toxicity of rofecoxib and naproxen in patients with rheumatoid arthritis. *N Engl J Med* 2000; **343**: 1520–1528.
20. Cannon GW, Breedveld FC. Efficacy of cyclooxygenase-2-specific inhibitors. *Am J Med* 2001; **110**(Suppl 1): 6–12.
21. Pohjolainen T, Jekunen A, Autio L et al. Treatment of acute low back pain with the COX-2-selective anti-inflammatory drug nimesulide: results of a randomized, double-blind comparative trial versus ibuprofen. *Spine* 2000; **25**: 1579–1585.
22. Dougados M, Behier JM, Jolchine I et al. Efficacy of celecoxib, a cyclooxygenase 2-specific inhibitor, in the treatment of ankylosing spondylitis: a six-week controlled study with comparison against placebo and against a conventional nonsteroidal antiinflammatory drug. *Arthritis Rheum* 2001; **44**: 180–185.
23. Van Steenbergen W, Peeters P, De Bondt J et al. Nimesulide-induced acute hepatitis: evidence from six cases. *J Hepatol* 1998; **29**: 135–141.
24. Traversa G, Bianchi C, Da Cas R et al. Cohort study of hepatotoxicity associated with nimesulide and other non-steroidal anti-inflammatory drugs. *BMJ* 2003; **327**: 18–22.
25. Page J, Henry D. Consumption of NSAIDs and the development of congestive heart failure in elderly patients: an underrecognized public health problem. *Arch Intern Med* 2000; **160**: 777–784.
26. Mukherjee D, Nissen SE, Topol EJ. Risk of cardiovascular events associated with selective COX-2 inhibitors. *JAMA* 2001; **286**: 954–959.
27. Bresalier RS, Sandler RS, Quan H et al. Cardiovascular events associated with rofecoxib in a colorectal adenoma chemoprevention trial. *N Engl J Med* 2005; **352**: 1092–1102.
28. Juni P, Nartey L, Reichenbach S et al. Risk of cardiovascular events and rofecoxib: cumulative meta-analysis. *Lancet* 2004; **364**: 2021–2029.
29. Solomon SD, McMurray JJ, Pfeffer MA et al. Cardiovascular risk associated with celecoxib in a clinical trial for colorectal adenoma prevention. *N Engl J Med* 2005; **352**: 1071–1080.

30. Ott E, Nussmeier NA, Duke PC et al. Efficacy and safety of the cyclooxygenase 2 inhibitors parecoxib and valdecoxib in patients undergoing coronary artery bypass surgery. *J Thorac Cardiovasc Surg* 2003; **125**: 1481–1492.

31. Nussmeier NA, Whelton AA, BrownMT et al. Complications of the COX-2 inhibitors parecoxib and valdecoxib after cardiac surgery. *N Engl J Med* 2005; **352**: 1081–1091.

32. Committee on Safety of Medicines. *Current Problems Pharmacovigilance* 2000; **26**: 13.

33. Juni P, Rutjes AW, Dieppe PA. Are selective COX 2 inhibitors superior to traditional non steroidal anti-inflammatory drugs? *BMJ* 2002; **324**: 1287–1288.

34. Whelton A, Maurath CJ, Verburg KM et al. Renal safety and tolerability of celecoxib, a novel cyclooxygenase-2 inhibitor. *Am J Ther* 2000; **7**: 159–175.

35. Brater DC, Harris C, Redfern JS et al. Renal effects of cox-2-selective inhibitors. *Am J Nephrol* 2001 **21**: 1–15.

36. Flower RJ, Vane JR. Inhibition of prostaglandin synthetase in brain explains the antipyretic activity of acetaminophen. *Nature* 1972; **240**: 410–411.

37. Tolman EL, Fuller BL, Marignan BA et al. Tissue selectivity and variability of effect of acetaminophen on arachidonic acid metabolism. *Prostaglandin Leukotriene Med* 1983; **12**: 347–356.

38. Ferrari RA, Ward SJ, Zobre CM. Estimation of the in vivo cyclooxygenase inhibitors on prostaglandin E2 levels in mouse brain. *Eur J Pharmacol* 1990; **179**: 25–34.

39. Lanz R, Polster P, Brune K. Antipyretic analgesics inhibit prostaglandin release from astrocytes and macrophages similarly. *Eur J Pharmacol* 1986; **130**: 105–109.

40. Carlsson KH, Jurna I. Central analgesic effect of paracetamol manifested by depression of nociceptive activity in thalamic neurones of the rat. *Neurosci Lett* 1987; **77**: 339–343.

41. Ferreira SH, Lorenzetti BB, Correa FMA. Central and peripheral antialgesic action of aspirin-like drugs. *Eur J Pharmacol* 1978; **53**: 39–48.

42. Tjolsen A, Lund A, Hole K. Antinociceptive effect of paracetamol in rats is partly dependant on spinal serotoninergic systems. *Eur J Pharmacol* 1991; **193**: 193–201.

43. Piletta P, Porchet H, Dayer P. Central analgesic effect of acetaminophen but not of aspirin. *Clin Pharmacol Ther* 1991; **41**: 350–354.

44. Pelissier T, Alloui A, Paeile C et al. Evidence of central antinociceptive effect of paracetamol involving spinal 5HT$_3$ receptors. *Neuroreport (England)* 1995; **6**: 1546–1548.

45. Schnitzer TJ Non-NSAID pharmacologic treatment options for the management of chronic pain. *Am J Med* 1998; **105**: 45S–52S.

46. Ray WA, Stein MC, Byrd V et al. Educational program for physicians to reduce use of non-steroidal anti-inflammatory drugs among community-dwelling elderly persons: a randomized controlled trial. *Med Care* 2001; **39**: 425–435.

47. Bannwarth B. Risk–benefit assessment of opioids in chronic noncancer pain. *Drug Safety* 1999; **21**: 283–296.

48. Federation of State Medical Boards of the US. *Model Guidelines for the Use of Controlled Substances for the Treatment of Pain.* Federation of State Medical Boards of the United States, Dallas, TX, 1998.

49. Dellimijn P, van Duijn H, Vanneste J. Prolonged treatment with transdermal fentanyl in neuropathic pain. *J Pain Symp Manage* 1998; **16**: 220–229.

50. Jamison RN, Raymond SA, Slawsby EA et al. Opioid therapy for chronic non-cancer back pain. A randomized prospective study. *Spine* 1998; **23**: 2591–2600.

51. Schnitzer TJ, Gray WL, Paster RZ et al. Efficacy of tramadol in treatment of chronic low back pain. *J Rheumatol* 2000; **27**: 772–778.

52. Peloso PM, Fortin L, Beaulieu A et al. Analgesic efficacy and safety of tramadol/acetaminophen combination tablets (Ultracet®) in treatment of chronic low back pain: a multicenter, outpatient, randomized, double blind, placebo controlled trial. *J Rheumatol* 2004; **31**: 2454–3463.

53. Ruoff GE, Rosenthal N, Jordan D et al. Tramadol/acetaminophen combination tablets for the treatment of chronic lower back pain: a multicenter, randomised, double-blind, placebo-controlled outpatients trial. *Clin Ther* 2003; **325**: 1123–1141.

54. Hale ME, Dvergsten C, Gimbel J. Efficacy and safety of oxymorphone extended release in chronic low back pain: results of a randomised, double-blind, placebo- and active-controlled phase III study. *J Pain* 2005; **1**: 21–28.

55. Mahowald ML, Singh JA, Majeski P. Opioid use by patients in an orthopedic spine clinic. *Arthritis Rheum* 2005; **52**: 312–321.

56. Schnitzer TJ, Kamin M, Olson WH. Tramadol allows reduction of naproxen dose among patients with naproxen-responsive osteoarthritis pain: a randomized, double-blind, placebo-controlled study. *Arthritis Rheum* 1999; **42**: 1370–1377.

57. Schofferman J. Long-term opioid analgesic therapy for severe refractory lumbar spine pain. *Clin J Pain* 1999; **15**: 136–140.

58. Buskila D. Drug therapy. *Baillière's Best Practice Res Clin Rheumatol* 1999; **13**: 479–485.

59. WHO. New Guidelines to Evaluate National Opioid Policy 2001; **14**: 1.

60. Joranson DE, Ryan KM, Gilson AM et al. Trends in medical use and abuse of opioid analgesics. *JAMA* 2000; **283**: 1710–1714.

61. Cicero TJ, Adams EH, Geller A et al. A postmarketing surveillance program to monitor Ultram (tramadol hydrochloride) abuse in the United States. *Drug Alcohol Depend* 1999; **57**: 7–22.

62. Cicero TJ, Inciardi JA, Adams EH et al. Rates of abuse of tramadol remain unchanged with the introduction of new branded and generic products: results of an abuse monitoring system, 1994–2004. *Pharmacoepidemiol Drug Safety* 2005; **14**: 851–859.

63. Perrot S, Bannwarth B, Bertin P et al. Use of morphine in nonmalignant joint pain: the Limoges recommendations. The French Society for Rheumatology. *Rev Rhumatol (English Edn)* 1999; **66**: 571–576.

64. McQuay HJ, Tramer M, Nye BA et al. A systematic review of antidepressants in neuropathic pain. *Pain* 1996; **68**: 217–227.

65. Fishbain D. Evidenced-based data on pain relief with antidepressants. *Ann Med* 2000; **32**: 305–316.

66. Ansari A. The efficacy of newer antidepressants in the treatment of chronic pain: a review of current literature. *Harvard Rev Psychiatry* 2000; **7**: 257–277.

67. Tatsumi M, Groshan K, Blakely RD et al. Pharmacological profile of antidepressants and related compounds at human monoamine transporters. *Eur J Pharmacol* 1997; **340**: 249–258.

68. Atkinson JH, Slater MA, Williams RA et al. A placebo-controlled randomized clinical trial of nortriptyline for chronic low back pain. *Pain* 1998; **76**: 287–296.

69. Max MB. Antidepressant drugs as treatments for chronic pain: efficacy and mechanisms. *Adv Pain Res Ther* 1995; **22**: 501–515.

70. Nutt D. Substance-P antagonists: a new treatment for depression? *Lancet* 1998; **352**: 1644–1645.

71. Max MB, Schafer SC, Culnane M et al. Amitriptyline, but not lorazepam, relieves postherpetic neuralgia. *Neurology* 1988; **38**: 1427–1432.

72. Turner JA, Denny C. Do antidepressant medications relieve chronic low back pain? *J Fam Prac* 1993; **37**: 545–553.

73. Sindrup SH, Gram LF, Brosen K et al. The selective reuptake serotonin inhibitor paroxetine is effective in the treatment of diabetic neuropathy symptoms. *Pain* 1990; **42**: 135–144.

74. Hempenstall K, Nurmikko TJ, Johnson RW et al. Analgesic therapy in post-herpetic neuralgia: a quantitative systematic review. *PLoS Med* 2005; **2**: e164.

75. Haynes RB, Taylors DW, Sackett DL. *Compliance in Health Care.* Hopkins, London, 1979.

76. Kouyanou K, Pither CE, Wessely S. Medication misuse, abuse and dependence in chronic pain patients. *J Psychosom Res* 1997; **43**: 497–504.

77. Ferrari A, Stefani M, Sternieri S et al. Analgesic drug taking: beliefs and behavior among headache patients. *Headache* 1997; **37**: 88–94.

78. Brus H, van de Laar M, Taal E et al. Compliance in rheumatoid arthritis and the role of formal patient education. *Semin Arthritis Rheum* 1997; **26**: 702–710.

79. De Klerk E, van der Linden SJ. Compliance monitoring of NSAID drug therapy in ankylosing spondylitis experiences with an electronic monitoring device. *Br J Rheumatol* 1996; **35**: 60–65.

80. Nordin M, Cedraschi C, Skovron ML. Patient–health care provider relationship in patients with non-specific low back pain: a review of some problem situations. *Baillière's Clinic Rheumatol* 1998; **12**: 75–92.

81. McGregor EA. The doctor and the migraine patient: improving compliance. *Neurology* 1997; **48**: S16–S20.

82. Donovan JL, Blake DR. Patient non-compliance. Deviance or reasoned decision-making? *Soc Sci Med* 1992; **34**: 507–513.

83. Benkert O, Graf-Morgenstern M, Hillert A et al. Public opinion on psychotropic drugs: an analysis of the factors influencing acceptance or rejection. *J Nerve Mental Dis* 1997; **185**: 51–58.

84. Wynne HA, Long A. Patient awareness for the adverse effects of non-steroidal anti-inflammatory drugs (NSAIDs). *Br J Clin Pharmacol* 1996; **42**: 253–256.

85. Cedraschi C, Piguet V, Fischer W et al. Beliefs about antidepressants in back pain patients: a clue to non-compliance? The Annual Meeting of the International Society for the Study of the Lumbar Spine, Adelaide, 2000.

86. Cedraschi C, Piguet V, Fischer W et al. Patient information leaflets and antidepressant prescription in chronic pain patients. *Prog Pain Res Manage* 2000; **16**: 887–895.

87. Piguet V, Cedraschi C, Fischer W et al. Antidepressants representations in chronic pain patients [abstract]. The 9th World Congress on Pain, Vienna, 1999, p. 471.

88. Fischer W, Goerg D, Zbinden E et al. Determining factors and the effects of attitudes towards psychotropic medication. In: Guimón J, Fischer W, Sartorius N (eds), *The Image of Madness. The Public Facing Mental Illness and Psychiatric Treatment.* Karger, Basel, 1999, pp. 162–186.

Chapter 11
The contribution of psychosocial factors to long-term disability and work loss

Amanda C. de C. Williams and Nicholas A. S. Kendall

INTRODUCTION

Different factors contribute to the onset of a low back pain problem, the decision to seek care and support, and early treatment.[1-4] The onset of pain, usually followed closely by the onset of disability or loss of the ability to perform certain activities, may be produced by a wide range of factors. These include occupational variables (e.g. heavy physical work, static work postures, frequent bending and twisting, repetitive work, vibration and psychosocial conditions) and individual factors (e.g. age and sex, posture and physical fitness).[5, 6] For a given individual, factors combine in complex ways to produce the onset of low back symptoms.

Next comes the decision to seek healthcare and/or financial support (e.g. social security benefit or compensation). Where pain affects work, and particularly when the onset of pain is perceived to be work related, job satisfaction and support in the workplace, and management policies and practices concerning sickness absence, affect progress of the problem.[5, 6]

The third phase involves the initial treatment and management of the pain problem. Most people with a new episode of low back pain recover without intervention, but a minority fail to do so, and pain and disability increasingly disrupt their lives.[7] This small group has been repeatedly identified as seriously disabled and the most expensive in terms of health and welfare costs and work days lost.[8] This is a significant waste, as prevention seems a real possibility. Musculoskeletal pain problems, back pain prominent among them, are now a very common cause of long-term disability in most developed countries. This is not due to an increased incidence, but to how the pain and disability are managed or mismanaged within the healthcare system and at work.[8, 9] These behaviours and practices can be changed.

CONVENTIONAL CLINICAL MANAGEMENT

Recent decades have witnessed a proliferation of physical interventions based on theoretical assumptions about the cause of the symptoms. Many of these interventions have become common practice without proper evaluation and continue largely unexamined, while the majority of patients recover within weeks without intervention. The lack of evidence for the efficacy of some interventions, and the possible harm done by others, is evident from the European guidelines,[10] but concerns about inappropriate or ineffective treatments are not new.[11-13] Such treatments also have worrying non-specific effects: they confirm to the patient the appropriateness of the biomechanical model of low back pain; the patient delays return to normal activity until the pain has resolved; and patients who do not recover acquire pejorative labels (e.g. 'non-compliant' or 'heartsink') that compromise their future healthcare.[14] The issue is therefore to provide appropriate treatment at an early stage, with the aim of speeding recovery or of delaying progression to persistent pain and disability. The recovery of individuals from persistent pain is expensive and difficult, and is complicated by associated problems such as the adverse health effects of long-term unemployment.[15] Agencies that fund and purchase healthcare are under increasing pressure to ensure that treatments purchased represent good value. One response has been the production of several major task force reports and guideline documents around the world: those published in the last decade are listed in Box 11.1.

PSYCHOSOCIAL FACTORS IN ACUTE LOW BACK PAIN

What predicts longer term pain and disability varies with the population, the context, and which of the stages (onset,

Box 11.1. Recent back pain guidelines

1996: Accident Rehabilitation & Compensation Insurance Corporation and National Health Committee, New Zealand[15]
- Reprint of Agency for Health Care policy and research (AHCPR) guidelines released at 'Spine in Action' Conference, Christchurch, 1996
- Post-conference seminars emphasized the prevention of chronicity

1996: Royal College of General Practitioners, UK[16]
- Revised edition of Clinical Standards Advisory Group (CSAG) guidelines
- Recognition at highest level of evidence that psychosocial factors are important in chronic low back pain and disability
- Recognition that psychosocial factors are more important at early stages than previously considered
- Stronger recommendations about return to usual activities

1997: Accident Rehabilitation & Compensation Insurance Corporation and National Health Committee, New Zealand[17]
- Publication of the *New Zealand Acute Low Back Pain Guide*
- Publication of the *Guide to Assessing Psychosocial Yellow Flags: Risk Factors for Long-Term Disability and Work Loss*

1999: Royal College of General Practitioners, UK[18]
- Updated version of UK guide, little changed
- Adopted the concept of psychosocial yellow flags developed in New Zealand[19]

1999: Accident Rehabilitation & Compensation Insurance Corporation and National Health Committee, New Zealand[20]
- Updated 1999 version of the *New Zealand Acute Low Back Pain Guide*, based on a systematic review of the back pain literature since January 1997

2000: Faculty of Occupational Medicine, UK. Occupational health guidelines for the management of low back pain at work[21–23]
- Evidence-based and graded by evidence level
- Advises caution in attributing pain in worker to work conditions
- States that there is no current satisfactory screening for suitability of physical work demands: low back pain is widespread among non-workers as well as workers
- Management as Royal College of General Practitioners guidelines; encourages return to work, as caution risks perpetuating the problem

2003: Australian Acute Musculoskeletal Pain Guidelines Group. Evidence-based management of acute musculoskeletal pain[24, 25]
- Summaries marked by evidence levels
- Emphasizes weak level of confidence in diagnostic tests, findings on such tests, and rarity of serious conditions as the cause of acute low back pain
- Highlights advice to stay active
- Excellent two-sided information sheet of explanation and advice for patients (Australian Government National Health and Medical Research Council 2004)

2004: European Union. European guidelines for the management of chronic non-specific low back pain[10]
- Some reference to acute and recurrent low back pain, although mainly about chronic low back pain
- Strict adherence to evidence levels in recommending treatments or not

2005: Royal College of General Practitioners, UK[26]
- Updated in line with the 2004 European guidelines
- More integrated psychosocial with biomedical treatment
- Says little about decision to investigate and/or refer
- Less stringent on evidence for some treatments than are the European guidelines

healthcare seeking or work loss, or persistence of symptoms beyond 6 months) is at issue. What is clear is that psychosocial factors are fundamental and can no longer be considered as secondary reactions;[1–3, 27–29] they may also contribute significantly to the outcome of surgical interventions.[30, 31] In a prospective study,[32] one-third of individuals with high pain scores, many fearful beliefs about pain and activity, and low function at baseline, had significantly poorer work status and sickness records than those with fewer or less strongly held fearful beliefs. Of those who were also distressed at baseline, two-thirds had taken more than 2 weeks' sick leave or had not returned to work. Disability consists in part of behaviours learned and shaped within the healthcare and welfare systems, and of others that arise from mistaken and negative beliefs about the meaning and implications of pain. The picture is far from complete,[32] and studies of the process of developing persistent pain are needed to interpret existing epidemiological information.

Fear of pain and of its longer term implications for activity are particularly important,[32–34] but cannot be dealt with adequately here. Those who encounter the patient early in his or her pain episode, particularly primary care physicians and physical therapists, are in a good position to examine, explain, reassure and advise, but may be handicapped by their own erroneous beliefs and anxieties about the meaning of the pain and about best treatment.[35]

PSYCHOSOCIAL RISK FACTORS (YELLOW FLAGS)

A significant conceptual advance to integrating cognitive and behavioural approaches into the early management of acute low back pain is that of psychosocial yellow flags[19] (analogous to the widely used red flags). Yellow flags are best conceptualized as barriers to recovery. Ideally, every primary care practitioner should recognize particular barriers to recovery in each patient, and deal with them appropriately, using cognitive and behavioural methods. Several screening questionnaires have been developed covering similar ground,[19, 36, 37] but all have been found to have limited predictive accuracy.[38] This presents problems in that a significant proportion of patients are categorized as at risk of persistent pain at a point where they still have a reasonable chance of spontaneous recovery.

However, screening measures are unlikely to improve substantially in their discriminative power until we understand better the development of persistent low back pain. At present, there is a risk that variables drawn from a broad spectrum (demographic, medical, psychological, occupational), rather than from a clear developmental model, may be spuriously identified as risk factors. In addition, some of the factors bearing on patients' successful return to work consist of employment practices, discrimination (institutional or informal) against those with disabilities, and the broader context of the job market.[38]

Factors that consistently predict poor outcomes include the belief that back pain is harmful or potentially severely disabling, the avoidance of normal activities because of the inaccurate belief that they will result in greater pain or in physical harm, a tendency to low mood and withdrawal from social interaction, and an expectation that effective treatment can only be delivered by an expert healthcare practitioner, rather than achieved by activities under the patient's own control (although using expert advice). Suggested questions for eliciting these risk factors, low expectations, and barriers to recovery are listed in Box 11.2.

EARLY INTERVENTION AND PREVENTING PERSISTENT PAIN

Given that cognitive and behavioural aspects of persistent musculoskeletal pain are amenable to change[39] and are often the aspects that are most treatable, it is reasonable to expect 'better' early management to produce clear benefits, including

---

Box 11.2. Useful questions for identifying psychosocial risk factors

These questions should be phrased in treatment provider's own words.

- Have you had time off work in the past with back pain?
- What do you understand is the cause of your back pain?
- What do you expect will help you?
- What are you doing to cope with your back pain?
- How is your employer responding to your back pain? Your coworkers? Your family?
- When do you think that you will return to work? What will help you to do that?

---

prevention, in at least some cases, of persistent low back pain. Several high-quality, randomized controlled trials show reduction in disability, pain experience, days of work lost, healthcare usage and distress.[10, 40, 41] However, the size of the effect is often rather small, and some trials show no detectable benefit.[42]

Some of the assumptions about early intervention to prevent low back pain are now being re-examined.[38, 43] The recurrent nature of acute low back pain makes the notion of 'early' intervention difficult to apply. Apparent risk factors identified in epidemiological studies may be associated indirectly, rather than causally, with functional outcomes. Both the risk factor and the outcome may be functions of an overarching factor that is so far unrecognized (perhaps social class). The effect of a risk factor may be limited to a very brief period, shorter than is represented in study design. Recruiting patients to treatment early in an episode of pain relies on early presentation, and on the referrer's recognition of the problem. Screening tools to identify those at high risk are blunt, and treatment of false-positives represents a waste of resources. Even with early identification, the organization of early intervention can be practically difficult, particularly where populations are geographically widely distributed, and treatment may only be cost-effective above certain group sizes. Furthermore, to maximize cost-effectiveness the intervention needs to be lightweight in comparison with cognitively and behaviourally based management for persistent pain.[39] This has meant delivering psychological components via minimally trained physiotherapists[40] or primary care physicians,[42] which, in practice, may further underpower the intervention.

Ideally, secondary prevention should become an integral and usual part of primary care for low back pain.[19, 44] Reviews of guidelines for acute back pain management (see Box 11.1) agree that these are generally consistent where they use strong evidence, mainly systematic reviews, but their recommendations become more subjective when the evidence is weaker.[45, 46] Implementation appears to be cost-effective,[47] but remains very partial.[48, 49] Even an evidence-based intervention[50] failed to reduce referral to secondary care, which UK guidelines advise against. It appears that primary care physicians still value a specialist opinion on acute musculoskeletal pain. Suggestions are provided in Box 11.3 on how the primary or secondary care

Box 11.3. Helping a patient at risk of persistent disability or work loss

These points are intended to assist in the prevention of long-term disability and work loss. They are not intended to be prescriptive or to suggest ignoring individual needs.

- Provide a positive expectation that the individual will return to normal activities, including work
- Explain the causes of pain in terms accessible to the patient; avoid using words that imply irreparable damage or inevitable deterioration. Listen to the patient's account for indications that he or she holds such beliefs; they can be unambiguously and authoritatively corrected at this stage
- Plan short-term activity goals; review progress towards goals regularly rather than discuss pain: what is the patient doing despite pain, and how can they do it in a way that minimizes or controls pain? Acknowledge difficulties with activities, without implying that these must be avoided until pain is resolved. Demonstrate interest in improvements, however small
- Try to keep the individual at work if at all possible, even for a short part of the day, to help maintain work habits and relationships. If in touch with the employer, encourage regular supportive contact with the worker. Consider reasonable requests for selected duties and modifications to the workplace, but avoid putting too much faith in the many expensive adaptations and equipment supported only by manufacturers' claims: these may be ineffective and perpetuate disability
- At 4–6 weeks, if there is little improvement, review barriers to return to work, including psychosocial problems at work and residual fears about pain and damage. Outline the psychosocial and career risks of taking further time off work and the increasing difficulties of returning to work. If complex barriers to return to work are identified, referral to a multidisciplinary team may be required
- Promote self-management and confidence in self-management: positive feedback from healthcare professionals can be effective, but the experience of successful self-management is most persuasive
- Distressed people seek more help, and have been shown to be more likely to receive medical intervention, but overinvestigation and overtreatment can be physically and psychologically harmful. Involvement of a healthcare professional with psychological expertise may be necessary

health provider can minimize work loss in the patient with musculoskeletal pain.

SUMMARY

Together, the problems with guideline implementation and the somewhat disappointing results of early interventions based on risk-reduction strongly suggest that we do not fully understand the process by which acute low back pain becomes persistent pain and disability.[43] There are complexities of timing and interaction of risk factors that remain to be elucidated.

Furthermore, we have underestimated the strength of lay and medical beliefs and anxieties that underpin the search for diagnosis and technical fixes, and which undermine brief and minimal interventions and maintenance of the gains that they

PRACTICE POINTS

- Impairment, pain and disability are conceptually related, but are also distinct.
- The discovery of an impairment (e.g. disc prolapse) does not imply that psychosocial factors are unimportant.
- Negative findings on investigation for impairment do not imply that psychosocial factors are primary.
- Interventions based on cognitive and behavioural principles aim primarily to reduce disability, with or without pain reduction.
- Disability, including work loss and activity reduction, is influenced by many psychosocial factors, from those particular to the patient and his or her circumstances, to those common across the host culture (or culture of origin).

RESEARCH AGENDA

- A prospective study is needed of the development of persistent pain from an acute episode, investigating to what extent individual predictors are those identified at a population level.
- Key events (e.g. interactions with healthcare providers and/or employer) in changing the course of progression from acute to persistent pain need to be identified (this progression may be discontinuous and event-related rather than steady and time related).
- Further exploration is needed of the barriers to implementation of guidelines, particularly those that render primary care physicians unwilling to start reactivation without further investigation and treatment.
- Employment practices that establish a cooperative rather than an adversarial relationship with the worker on sick leave need to be identified.
- Effectiveness of physical therapists in using cognitive and behavioural techniques to change the beliefs and behaviour of people with acute musculoskeletal pain and substantial fears and avoidance of activity needs to be evaluated, as does the patient's experience of psychological messages delivered by trained physical therapists.

produce. Consequently, the difficulty of changing these beliefs and practices has also been underestimated. Perhaps their persistence is because they inevitably relate to broader technological tendencies in medicine and to the concerns of practitioners to exclude rare but serious pathologies in each individual patient. Employers, occupational health physicians, and union advisers will also share concerns about whether pain indicates a serious and treatable medical problem, and will be under pressure to be cautious in their decisions about return to work. These concerns are embedded in societal values and may prove hard to change in the case of acute musculoskeletal pain.

REFERENCES

1. Pengel LHM, Herbert RD, Maher CG et al. Acute low back pain: systematic review of its prognosis. *BMJ* 2003; **327**: 323–327.

2. Pincus T, Burton AK, Vogel S et al. A systematic review of psychological factors as predictors of chronicity/disability in prospective cohort of low back pain. *Spine* 2002; **27**: 109–120.

3. Linton SJ. A review of psychological risk factors in back and neck pain. *Spine* 2000; **25**: 1148–1156.

4. Gureje O, Simon GE, Von Korff M. A cross-national study of the course of persistent pain in primary care. *Pain* 2001; **92**: 195–200.

5. Crook J, Milner R, Schultz IZ et al. Determinants of occupational disability following a low back injury: a critical review of the literature. *J Occup Rehab* 2002; **12**: 277–295.

6. Waddell G, Aylward M, Sawney P. *Back Pain, Incapacity for Work and Social Security Benefit: An International Literature Review and Analysis.* Royal Society of Medicine, London, 2002.

7. Turk DC. The role of demographic and psychosocial factors in transition from acute to chronic pain. In: Jensen TS, Turner JA, Wiesenfeld-Hallin Z (eds), *Proceedings of the 8th World Congress on Pain, Progress in Pain Research and Management*, vol. 8. IASP, Seattle, WA, 1997, pp. 185–213.

8. Waddell G. *The Back Pain Revolution*, 2nd edn. Churchill Livingstone, Edinburgh, 2004.

9. Kendall NAS. Manual therapy round – low back pain: treatment and prevention. *J Manual Manip Ther* 1997; **5**: 134–139.

10. European Union (EU) COST B13 Working Group on Guidelines for Chronic Low Back Pain. *European Guidelines for the Management of Chronic Nonspecific Low Back Pain.* 2004. Available at: http://www.backpaineurope.org/web/files/WG2_Guidelines.pdf (accessed 27 August 2006).

11. Deyo RA. Conservative therapy for low back pain: distinguishing useful from useless therapy. *JAMA* 1983; **250**: 1057–1062.

12. Deyo RA. Practice variations, treatment fads, rising disability: do we need a new clinical research paradigm? *Spine* 1993; **18**: 2153–2162.

13. Loeser JD. Mitigating the dangers of pursuing cure. In: Cohen MJM, Campbell JN (eds), *Pain Treatment Centers at a Crossroads: A Practical and Conceptual Reappraisal. Progress in Pain Management*, Vol. 7. IASP, Seattle, WA, 1996, pp 101–108.

14. Daykin AR, Richardson B. Physiotherapists' pain beliefs and their influence on the management of patients with chronic low back pain. *Spine* 2004; **29**: 783–95

15. Kendall NAS, Thompson BF. A pilot programme for dealing with the comorbidity of chronic pain and long-term unemployment. *J Occup Rehab* 1998; **8**: 5–26.

16. Waddell G, Feder G, McIntosh A et al. *Low Back Pain Evidence Review.* Royal College of General Practitioners, London, 1996.

17. ACC and National Health Committee. *New Zealand Acute Low Back Pain Guide.* Accident Rehabilitation & Compensation Insurance Corporation of New Zealand/National Health Committee, Ministry of Health, Wellington, New Zealand, 1997.

18. Royal College of General Practitioners. *Clinical Guidelines for the Management of Acute Low Back Pain.* Royal College of General Practitioners, London, 1999.

19. Kendall NAS, Linton SJ, Main CJ. *Guide to Assessing Psychosocial Yellow Flags in Acute Low Back Pain: Risk Factors for Long-Term Disability and Work Loss.* Accident Rehabilitation & Compensation Insurance Corporation of New Zealand/National Health Committee, Ministry of Health, Wellington, New Zealand, 1997.

20. ACC and the National Health Committee. *New Zealand Acute Low Back Pain Guide*, 1999 edn. Accident Rehabilitation & Compensation Insurance Corporation of New Zealand/National Health Committee, Ministry of Health, Wellington, New Zealand, 1999.

21. Waddell G, Burton K (eds). *Occupational Health Guidelines for the Management of Low Back Pain at Work.* Faculty of Occupational Medicine, London, 2000. Available at: http://www.facoccmed.ac.uk (accessed 27 August 2006).

22. Carter JT, Birrell LN (eds). *Occupational Health Guidelines for the Management of Low Back Pain At Work – Principal Recommendations.* Faculty of Occupational Medicine, London, 2000. Available at: http://www.facoccmed. ac.uk (accessed 27 August 2006).

23. Waddell G, Burton AK. Occupational health guidelines for the management of low back pain at work: evidence review. *Occup Med* 2001; **51**: 124–135.

24. Australian Acute Musculoskeletal Pain Guidelines Group. *Evidence-based Management of Acute Musculoskeletal Pain.* Australian Academic Press, Brisbane, 2003. Available at: http://www.nhmrc.gov.au/publications/synopses/cp94syn.htm (accessed 27 August 2006).

25. Spearing N, March L, Bellamy N et al. Review: management of acute musculoskeletal pain. *Asia Pacific League Assoc Rheumatol J Rheumatol* 2005; **8**: 5–15.

26. Royal College of General Practitioners. *Clinical Guidelines on Acute Low Back Pain.* Royal College of General Practitioners, London, 2005. Available at: http://www.prodigy.nhs.uk/back_pain_lower (accessed 27 August 2006).

27. Boersma K, Linton S. How does persistent pain develop? An analysis of the relationships between psychological variables, pain and function across stages of chronicity. *Behav Res Ther* 2005; **43**: 1495–1507.

28. Manninen P, Helivaara M, Riihimiki H et al. Does psychological distress predict disability? *Int J Epidemiol* 1997; **26**: 1063–1070.

29. Symonds TL, Burton AK, Tillotson KM et al. Do attitudes and beliefs influence work loss due to low back trouble? *Occup Med* 1996; **46**: 25–32.

30. Hasenbring M, Marienfeld G, Kuhlendahl D et al. Risk factors of chronicity in lumbar disc patients. A prospective investigation of biologic, psychologic, and social predictors of therapy outcome. *Spine* 1994; **19**: 2759–2765.

31. Junge A, Fröhlich M, Ahrens S et al. Predictors of bad and good outcome of lumbar spine surgery. A prospective clinical study with 2 years' follow up. *Spine* 1996; **21**: 1056–1064.

32. Boersma K, Linton S. Screening to identify patients at risk. Profiles of psychological risk factors for early intervention. *Clin J Pain* 2005; **21**: 38–43.

33. Vlaeyen JWS, Linton SJ. Fear-avoidance and its consequences in chronic musculoskeletal pain: a state of the art. *Pain* 1999; **85**: 317–332.

34. Asmundson GJG, Vlaeyen JWS, Crombez G (eds). *Understanding and Treating Fear of Pain.* Oxford University Press, Oxford, 2004.

35. Balderson BHK, Lin EHB, Von Korff M. The management of pain-related fear in primary care. In: Asmundson GJG, Vlaeyen JWS, Crombez G (eds), *Understanding and Treating Fear of Pain.* Oxford University Press, Oxford, 2004, pp. 267–291.

36. Main CJ, Wood PLR, Hollis S et al. The distress and risk assessment method: a simple patient classification to identify distress and evaluate the risk of poor outcome. *Spine* 1992; **17**: 42–52.

37. Linton SJ, Boersma K. Early identification of patients at risk of developing a persistent back problem: the predictive validity of the Örebro Musculoskeletal Pain Questionnaire. *Clin J Pain* 2003; **19**: 80–86.

38. Linton SJ, Gross D, Schulz IZ et al. Prognosis and the identification of workers risking disability: research issues and directions for future research. *J Occup Rehab* 2005; **15**: 459–474.

39. Morley S, Eccleston C, Williams A. Systematic review and meta-analysis of randomized controlled trials of cognitive behaviour therapy and behaviour therapy for chronic pain in adults, excluding headache. *Pain* 1999; **80**: 1–13.

40. Hay E, Mullis R, Lewis M et al. Comparison of physical treatments versus a brief pain-management programme for back pain in primary care: a randomised clinical trial in physiotherapy practice. *Lancet* 2005; **365**: 2024–2030.

41. Damush TM, Weinberger M, Perkins SM et al. The long-term effects of a self-management program for inner-city primary care patients with acute low back pain. *Arch Intern Med* 2003; **163**: 2632–2638.

42. Jellema P, van der Windt D, van der Horst H et al. Should treatment of (sub)acute low back pain be aimed at psychosocial prognostic factors? Cluster randomised clinical trial in general practice. *BMJ* 2005; **331**: 84.

43. Sullivan MJL. Introduction: emerging trends in secondary prevention of back pain disability. *Clin J Pain* 2003; **19**: 77–79.

44. Von Korff M. Pain management in primary care: an individualized stepped-care approach. In: Gatchel RJ, Turk DC (eds), *Psychosocial Factors in Pain: Critical Perspectives.* Guilford Press, New York, 1999, pp. 360–373.

45. Koes BW, van Tulder MW, Ostelo R et al. Clinical guidelines for the management of low back pain in primary care: an international comparison. *Spine* 2001; **26**: 2504–2513.

46. van Tulder MW, Tuut M, Pennick V et al. Quality of primary care guidelines for acute low back pain. *Spine* 2004; **29**: E357–E362.

47. McGuirk B, King W, Govind J et al. Safety, efficacy, and cost effectiveness of evidence-based guidelines for the management of acute low back pain in primary care. *Spine* 2001; **26**: 2615–2622.

48. Barnett AG, Underwood MR, Vickers MR. Effect of UK national guidelines on services to treat patients with acute low back pain: follow-up questionnaire survey. *BMJ* 1999; **318**: 919–920.

49. Schers H, Wensing M, Huijsmans Z et al. Implementation barriers for general practice guidelines on low back pain a qualitative study. *Spine* 2001; **26**: E348–353.

50. Dey P, Simpson CWR, Collins SI et al. Implementation of RCGP guidelines for acute low back pain: a cluster randomised controlled trial. *Br J Gen Pract* 2004; **54**: 33–37.

Chapter 12

Steroid injections: effect on pain of spinal origin

Les Barnsley, Mary McLoone and Andrew Baranowski

INTRODUCTION

Injections of steroids for the relief of spinal pain syndromes have achieved both popularity and notoriety. The proponents of the various procedures point to the convenience and ease of administration of steroid injections, particularly where they are administered without radiological guidance (probably not to be recommended), and a low rate of adverse effects. Belief in the efficacy of a procedure has often been based on anecdotal evidence, personal experience or extrapolation from other interventions, such as the use of intra-articular steroid injections for peripheral joint arthropathy. On the other hand, detractors argue that the procedures have uncertain efficacy, are poorly targeted and are used to treat patients with poorly defined anatomical diagnoses.

This chapter adopts an unashamedly evidence-based approach to the question of the efficacy and effectiveness of various steroid injections for the relief of spinal pain syndromes. It is explicitly not a technical manual for the performance of these procedures, although the broad principles and examples are presented where appropriate. This chapter has been updated by Dr Mary McLoone and Dr Andrew Baranowski to take on board publications since the original paper was published. The basic text remains the same as published by Dr Les Barnsley. Additions and changes have been made where there is new evidence or the views of the review authors differ.

SEARCH STRATEGY

Although not a formal systematic review, this chapter follows the protocol of explicit searching strategies for papers of interest. Unless otherwise stated, all searches for the papers retrieved in this review were performed on the following databases to April 2006:

- Cochrane Collaboration Database of Systematic Reviews
- Cochrane Database of Abstracts of Reviews of Effectiveness
- Cochrane Controlled Trials Register (CENTRAL/CCTR)
- EMBASE
- MEDLINE.

The MESH headings used for all searches were Adrenal Cortex Hormones/ad, ae, tu, to [Administration & Dosage, Adverse Effects, Therapeutic Use, Toxicity]. This group of terms was then combined with appropriate descriptors of the target conditions. Retrieved articles were hand-searched for pertinent references.

Retrieved papers were classified according to the level of evidence provided (Table 12.1). The summaries comprise the author's (L.B.) opinions, based on the retrieved evidence on efficacy and adverse effects.

Table 12.1. Level of evidence in the retrieved papers

Evidence level	Description
I	Systematic review of all randomized controlled trials
II	At least one randomized controlled trial
III-1	Well-designed, pseudo-randomized trial
III-2	Comparative study with a concurrent control group
III-3	Comparative study with a non-concurrent control group or two single-arm studies
IV	Case series

RATIONALE

Corticosteroids have a wide range of biological effects but their putative therapeutic utility in pain of spinal origin is afforded by their anti-inflammatory effects. There is some evidence that they may have long-acting local anaesthetic-like actions on peripheral nerves by actions on sodium channels. Corticosteroids are potent suppressors of inflammation. This action is achieved primarily through the modification of protein synthesis at a nuclear level. At therapeutic doses corticosteroids upregulate the production of lipocortin, a protein that inhibits phospholipase A_2. This enzyme converts membrane-bound phospholipids into arachidonic acid derivatives, including leukotrienes and prostaglandins that are potent inflammatory mediators. Other effects of corticosteroids include the suppression of production of other proinflammatory cytokines such as interleukin-1 (IL-1) and tumour necrosis factor (TNF). Corticosteroids also directly suppress production of proinflammatory enzymes, including collagenase, elastase and plasminogen activator, by downregulating the nuclear transcription of their RNA.

PREPARATIONS

The most commonly available oral corticosteroids have half-lives that vary from 8 to 72 hours. To prolong these effects for local, depot injection therapy, various slowly dissolving salts of corticosteroids have been developed. Several commonly used preparations are summarized in Table 12.2.

RADICULAR PAIN

Radicular pain is defined as pain arising from irritation of a nerve root. It is typically lancinating or electrical in character and follows the course of the nerve root. As such it is differentiated from somatic pain, which is deep and aching. This differentiation is occasionally difficult, and the recognition of radicular pain is made more complex by the observation that irritation of cervical nerve roots can produce pain in a non-dermatomal distribution.[1] At a clinical level, it would seem reasonable to diagnose radicular pain when clinical features are matched by appropriate abnormalities on cross-sectional imaging, such as magnetic resonance imaging (MRI) or computed tomography (CT) scanning.

It is suspected that radicular pain stems from irritation or inflammation of the nerve root. Experimental studies have shown that simply compressing a nerve root in the inter-vertebral foramen produces 'negative' symptoms, i.e. absence of sensation or weakness. Prolonged compression, presumably accompanied by pathological change in the nerve root or structures such as the dorsal root ganglion, causes radicular pain to develop. It is suspected that these changes are related to inflammation in the nerve roots or surrounding tissues. This inflammation is then thought to lead to swelling that further compromises the exiting nerve root. In the lumbar spine, the principal cause of radicular pain is compression by a herniated intervertebral disc. Numerous experiments attest to the potential of nucleus pulposus components to incite local inflammation. It would therefore seem a reasonable construct to treat such problems with anti-inflammatory measures. However, in the cervical spine, it is bony stenoses of the exit foramen that are thought to be the leading cause of radicular pain, so the cause of inflammation, if any, is less clear.

Little research attention has been given to the demonstration of nerve root inflammation in vivo. It might be reasonable to study cerebrospinal fluid in patients with radiculopathy, but the limited information available shows little evidence of pleocytosis, which might be expected if there were significant inflammation. Notwithstanding the lack of definitive evidence for nerve root inflammation, corticosteroid injections have been used widely on the basis that they decrease inflammation of and around the nerve root.

Injections of corticosteroid can be placed on or around the nerve roots, either through a translaminar approach or a 'selective' or root sleeve injection. The former involves placing a reasonable volume of fluid in the epidural space with the intention that it flows around the epidural space to bathe the affected nerve root. The latter approach is more targeted, seeking to place the injectate into the sleeve around the exiting nerve root. These approaches are quite different and are considered separately below.

Cervical injections
Techniques

Cervical translaminar epidural steroid injections are performed by placing a needle into the epidural space from a posterior approach. The principal concern is inadvertent puncture of the thecal sac or even contusion of the spinal cord. The cervical canal is narrow in comparison to the lumbar canal, and there is little margin for error. There is no consensus as to the correct volume to be injected or whether the corticosteroid should be mixed with other agents or injected alone.

Table 12.2. Some commonly used oral corticosteroid preparations

Preparation	Dose to provide equivalent therapeutic effect (mg)	Propensity for systemic effects
6-Methylprednisolone acetate*	40	++
Triamcinolone acetonide*	20	+
Betamethasone acetate/sodium phosphate 6	+++	

*Opinions differ as to the equivalent dose range between these two drugs; they may differ with mode and site of application.

Clinical data

There have been randomized controlled trials of cervical epidural corticosteroids for radicular pain. For example, in the study by Stav et al.[2] 68% of the epidural steroid group had good or very good pain relief after 1 year, versus only 12% in the placebo group. There is also evidence from case series,[3, 4] with no controls, constituting level IV evidence. There is a systematic review of mechanical neck disorder therapies, which cites limited effectiveness of epidural injection of methylprednisolone for patients with radicular findings compared with intramuscular steroid and lidocaine.[5] Before evaluating these data further it is important to consider the issue of the natural history of the condition. In his monograph on acute cervical radicular pain, Bogduk[6] concluded that the clinical natural history was quite favourable, with as many as 90% of patients normal or only mildly incapacitated at follow-up. Against this background, the two available studies of cervical epidural steroids for cervical radicular pain report that around two-thirds of patients achieved greater than 75% relief to the end of follow-up. Consequently, the true efficacy of cervical epidural steroid injections is not known, but would have to be most impressive to impact positively upon what appears to be a favourable natural history.

Adverse effects

The available literature on cervical epidural injections does not systematically evaluate adverse effects. It is therefore difficult to state with any confidence what the rate and nature of any adverse effects are. An attempt to gather the evidence concerning complications of epidural steroids revealed few data on which to base conclusions, with retrieved articles primarily concerning lumbar epidural injections.[7] However, several complications of cervical epidurals have been reported, including epidural abscess,[8] dural puncture, transient upper limb weakness, facial flushing, and nausea and vomiting.[9] There is also one documented case of cardiac arrest and irreversible quadriparesis following a fluoroscopically guided C6–7 epidural steroid injection. The subsequent MRI at 6 hours and 6 months after the procedure did not demonstrate any abnormality, and it is thought that the patient may have suffered a vascular event.[10]

Lumbar injections

Techniques

There are three techniques for entering the lumbar epidural space: translaminar or lumbar epidural; caudal epidural, where the injection is made into the sacral hiatus and root sleeve; or periradicular (which is considered in a later section). The two former techniques aim to place the injectate into the epidural space within the spinal canal. This can be performed either 'blind' (i.e. without imaging guidance) or by using imaging, typically CT or fluoroscopy.

Translaminar or lumbar procedures are performed by introducing a needle perpendicular to the skin over the midline of the interspinous space at a level below L2. The needle is advanced until the ligamentum flavum is pierced. The arrival of the needle into the epidural space is typically detected by the loss of resistance to injection.

Caudal epidurals are performed by palpating the sacral hiatus at the posterior inferior part of the sacrum and then introducing a needle-directed cephalad through this space.

Formal study of the accuracy of placement of these injections under different circumstances reveals that translaminar lumbar epidural injections performed blindly (i.e. without imaging guidance) miss the epidural space in up to 30% of attempts.[11] Similarly, about 25% of blind caudal injections are not correctly placed, particularly (and predictably) where landmarks are not readily palpable.[12] There is again no agreement as to what constitutes a standard epidural. Typically, the equivalent of methylprednisolone 80 mg is mixed with an equal volume of local anaesthetic, and then sterile saline is added to constitute a volume of 5–10 mL.

Clinical data

The efficacy or otherwise of epidural corticosteroid injections for lumbar radiculopathy has been a controversial topic for some time. A systematic review published in 2005 showed short-term improvement from lumbar/caudal epidural injection, but at 6 weeks the evidence was limited for long-term benefit.[13]

An important contribution to the evidence in this area was the publication of a high-quality, carefully designed, randomized controlled trial of corticosteroid epidural injections for sciatica. It measured a number of outcomes and found that in the first few weeks after injection there was some improvement favouring the steroid group in leg pain and finger–floor distance, whereas other measures of pain and disability were not significantly improved.[14] No significant differences were found between active and control groups after 3 months.

This was backed up by a randomized controlled trial that compared translaminar epidural steroid injection with intramuscular steroid and local anaesthetic. In the short term there was an improvement in the epidural group, but there was no difference in the long term and subsequent operation rates were similar in both groups.[15] A prospective trial of 100 patients with large symptomatic herniated discs who were randomized to surgery or epidural steroid injection, however, demonstrated that 42–56% of the epidural group derived benefit for up to 3 years.[16]

A prospective, randomized controlled trial published in 2005 showed a transient benefit in Oswestry Disability Questionnaire (ODQ) score compared with placebo up to 3 weeks after epidural steroid injection, but at 6–52 weeks there was no difference.[17] There was also no difference in other indices, including function, return to work or need for surgery. This study also investigated the cost of carrying out treatment using quality-adjusted life-years (QALYs), and epidural steroid injection failed to meet the threshold recommended by the National Institute for Health and Clinical Excellence (NICE). Therefore, epidural steroid injections do not seem to provide good value for money.[17] Further work may need to be carried out to target this treatment to appropriate subgroups.

A further randomized controlled trial done in 2003 showed no benefit of using an epidural steroid over saline alone.[18] The contemporary, higher quality literature therefore offers little positive news for proponents of this procedure, but there may be a role in patients awaiting surgery for a significant herniated lumbar disc. The best available evidence suggests a small and temporary effect for lumbosacral radicular pain.

Adverse effects

Untoward effects of lumbar and caudal epidural corticosteroid injections can be divided into systemic and local. It is clear that there is significant systemic absorption of corticosteroid from the epidural space. This can cause symptoms such as insomnia, flushing and mood changes, as well as metabolic and endocrine effects, notably exacerbation of hyperglycaemia and pituitary suppression.[19] For the most part, these symptoms are rarely of clinical significance, but it is prudent to advise patients that they may occur. Diabetic patients should be carefully observed for any severe sequelae of hyperglycaemia.

Local adverse effects occurring in 1% or more of procedures include exacerbation of pain, headache and hypotension. Rare events include spinal anaesthesia, bloody tap and nerve root injury. Inadvertent dural puncture occurs relatively frequently. The consequences of subarachnoid infiltration of corticosteroids are not fully known, but in their careful and exhaustive review for the Australian National Health and Medical Research Council, Bogduk et al.[20] concluded that there were no grounds for concern in the absence of excessive and repeated injections. Rare but significant adverse effects include the development of epidural lipomatosis[21] and central serous chorioretinopathy.[22] There has been one documented case of paraplegia after an intracord injection of steroid in an awake patient.[23]

Thoracic injections

The search strategy failed to recover any articles addressing the treatment of thoracic radicular pain with corticosteroids. No comment as to their utility can be made.

Conclusions

There is level IV evidence supporting some benefit of cervical translaminar epidural injections for cervical radiculopathy but the available evidence does not allow the true efficacy to be known. Consequently, where the procedure is being considered for a patient, this uncertainty of benefit should be revealed to the patient and there should be a frank discussion regarding the potential risks.

There are no extant data on thoracic epidural steroid injections that allow any conclusion to be reached.

For lumbar translaminar corticosteroid injections in the treatment of lumbar radiculopathy, there is level I evidence that suggests some short-term benefit. More contemporary level II studies indicate similar findings, but there is no evidence of any long-term benefit; the best available study shows no decrease in the eventual need for surgery. If such procedures are to be performed, the operator should be aware of the potential for inaccurate placement when 'blind' (i.e. non-imaging-guided) techniques are used. Patients should again be consulted about the risks and benefits of the procedure. There is no available evidence to support the use of multiple injections where the first one fails to achieve any benefit, and such practice is not cost-effective.

ROOT SLEEVE (SELECTIVE) EPIDURAL INJECTIONS

Cervical injections

In an attempt to improve the accuracy of placement of epidural injections, selective epidurals (also referred to as periradicular, transforaminal, selective nerve root blocks or root sleeve injections) have been advocated as a more reliable technique for the placement of steroid onto symptomatic nerve roots. Smaller volumes are used, typically 1–2 mL of a mixture of steroid preparation and a local anaesthetic.

Techniques

Cervical selective epidurals are performed under direct imaging control, either fluoroscopy or CT guidance, and involve the placement of the needle immediately adjacent to the exiting nerve root outside the spinal canal. The approach is typically posterior oblique or lateral.

Clinical data

An initial study in 1996 considered the effects of selective cervical epidural injections. This was an uncontrolled, observational study involving 42 patients with cervical radicular pain who had not responded to 'paravertebral' injections of steroid.[4] Of these, 31 were described as responders, as they did not go on to receive translaminar epidural injections. This is level IV evidence, and must again be considered in the context of a condition with a favourable natural history, as discussed above.

A further retrospective study in 2001 of 20 patients with atraumatic cervical radicular pain demonstrated a significant reduction in pain at 21 months, with an excellent result in 60% of patients.[24] This was not the case when the study was repeated by the same group in traumatically induced pain.[25] A prospective outcome study in 2001 involving 32 patients also demonstrated 50–75% pain relief in 56% of patients, with return to their full lifestyle.[26] A group of 21 patients awaiting cervical disc surgery were treated with two transforaminal steroid injections. Five of the 21 patients decided to cancel surgery and reported a statistically significant reduction in radicular pain score at 4 months.[27] A more recent case series of 30 patients with periradicular foraminal steroid infiltration under CT control reported good–excellent pain relief in 60% of patients. There was no rebound of pain at 6 months' follow-up, and duration of symptoms before treatment and cause of radiculalgia were not predictive of the pain relief derived.[28] All this evidence is level IV and has to be interpreted as such, but there seems to be encouragement for more randomized controlled studies in this area.

Adverse effects

There is significant literature describing serious adverse effects as a consequence of cervical transforaminal injections. A prospective study observing fluoroscopy in 504 injections demonstrated intravascular injection in 19.4% of cases. The absence of observed blood in the needle hub despite aspiration is not a completely reliable method of detecting intravascular injection, and contrast should always be used to confirm needle placement.[29] A retrospective survey also demonstrated two cases of radicular artery injection out of 354 by digital subtraction angiography.[30] An anatomical study of ten cadavers showed that there are variable anastomoses between the vertebral and cervical arteries. These arteries are located in the posterior aspect of the intervertebral foramen and may be vulnerable to injection or injury during transforaminal epidural steroid injection.[31]

Case reports published in the literature include a spinal cord infarction after a fluoroscopically guided C6 nerve root injection despite using contrast. There was no associated hypotension and no large volume of injectate was used to account for the infarction.[32] There is also a report of a patient who died following a C7 nerve root block. Dissection of the left vertebral artery resulted in thrombosis and massive cerebral oedema.[33]

Although cervical transforaminal injections seem to have a useful role in the management of radicular pain, the serious nature of the adverse effects would argue against the pursuit of this technique. As in all clinical decisions, the decision to use a particular intervention rests on a careful consideration of the benefits and risks inherent in the intervention in a particular patient. In this case, periradicular injections should probably be reserved for those with contained disc herniations and radicular pain, where other conservative means have failed and the patient remains highly symptomatic but desirous to avoid surgery. Then, patients should be informed of the possibility of these severe and permanent adverse reactions and informed consent obtained.

Lumbar injections
Techniques
Selective lumbar epidural injections also require real-time imaging, either CT or fluoroscopy, to ensure accurate placement of the injectate around the exiting nerve root. A posterior oblique approach is used and the needle tip is placed at the posterior margin of the intervertebral foramen. Correct placement is confirmed by injecting a small amount of contrast medium, which should outline the nerve root (Figure 12.1).

Clinical data
Initial reports of the use of transforaminal corticosteroid injections for lumbar radicular pain were encouraging. Two studies of case series (level IV evidence) considered the effect of the procedure on patients destined for surgery for refractory pain who had failed conservative measures. In the first of these studies, 30 patients with demonstrated lumbar radicular pain, all of whom had failed to respond adequately to traditional epidural injections, underwent a transforaminal injection of corticosteroids. Only three went on to surgery, with 14 having complete relief of pain that lasted from 1 to 10 years.[34] The second study considered 69 patients with MRI-proven disc herniation and lumbar radiculopathy. Three-quarters of these patients achieved greater than 50% relief of pain. These results encouraged some commentators to suggest transforaminal epidural steroid injections for patients with refractory lumbar

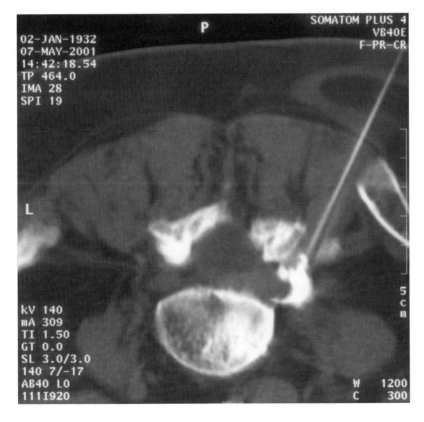

Figure 12.1. Axial CT scan view of a lumbar periradicular injection. Contrast has been injected from a needle inserted via a posterior oblique approach and is seen to outline the exiting nerve root.

radicular pain.[35] Further uncontrolled series followed, also with positive results.[36–38] There is also a retrospective study demonstrating that 27% of patients with radiculopathy secondary to degenerative lumbar scoliosis had good relief at 2 years post-injection,[39] and a prospective case series reporting successful long-term outcome in 75% of the same population.[40] A pseudo-randomized controlled trial (level III evidence) compared transforaminal epidural injections with saline trigger-point injections and found a greater number of positive outcomes, using a composite score of pain and disability ratings, in the transforaminal group.[41]

There have been two randomized controlled trials of the technique. In the first, patients were randomized to an injection of either saline or steroid and local anaesthetic.[42] At 2 weeks there were benefits from the steroids in terms of leg pain, straight leg raising and lumbar flexion, but back pain was lower in the saline group at 3 and 6 months. The authors concluded that the steroid and local anaesthetic group experienced a short-term effect, but there seemed to be a 'rebound' later. A subsequent subgroup analysis of this study, which included a positive cost-effectiveness analysis favouring periradicular injection, suggested that better results were seen in patients with contained herniations than in those with disc extrusions.[43] Another randomized controlled trial, using patient preference for surgery as an outcome, compared the effects of up to four selective nerve root sleeve injections of bupivacaine versus bupivacaine and betamethasone.[44] Sixty-seven per cent of the control group and 28% of the betamethasone group went on to have surgery – a highly significant outcome.

Adverse effects

In contrast to many other spinal injection procedures, there have been systematic attempts to document adverse effects of lumbar transformational steroid injections. An independent reviewer assessed adverse effects in over 200 patients, using both chart review and telephone interview.[45] The commonest adverse effect was a transient headache, occurring in 3.1%; back pain was temporarily increased in 2.4%, and leg pain in 0.6%. Systemic effects were infrequent, with one patient having a vasovagal episode and one having increased blood glucose. Two formal studies attest to a significant rate of intravascular injection, with approximately 10% of injections being into vascular structures.[46, 47] One case of intradiscal needle placement has also been described; if not recognized, such placement could result in a discitis.[48] This underscores the need for the injection of contrast medium to confirm the correct positioning of the needle before steroid is injected. However, in spite of contrast injection under fluoroscopic control, spinal cord infarction and permanent paraplegia have occurred.[49] More cases of spinal cord infarction have been reported following transforaminal injections.[50]

Conclusions

Cervical transforaminal epidural injections may help some patients with cervical radicular pain, but this conclusion is based on weak studies. Potentially disabling and lethal adverse events make the use of this technique difficult to justify, especially in the setting of a favourable natural history. It is essential that, if this technique is employed, practitioners are able to recognize intra-arterial injection of contrast before particulate steroid is injected.

Lumbar transforaminal epidural steroid injections have been found in level II studies to have a short-term effect on pain and to decrease the need for surgery in patients with lumbar radicular pain, particularly in the setting of disc herniations rather than extrusions. It is recommended that these procedures be performed under direct imaging guidance and using contrast medium injections to confirm correct placement. More work needs to be done in this area in the form of randomized controlled trials.

There are no data on thoracic transforaminal selective epidural injections.

DISCOGENIC PAIN

There is an increasing awareness that lumbar discs can hurt in their own right, without protruding into the spinal canal or compressing nerve roots. The pathology is thought to be internal disruption of the annulus fibrosus, eventually resulting in circumferential tears of the innervated, outer third of the annulus and, consequently, pain. It is suspected, but not proven, that inflammation has an important role in this process.[51] Far less is understood about the mechanisms of pain production from cervical discs, although it is clear that their structure and function are quite different to those of the lumbar discs.[52] It is not therefore legitimate simply to extrapolate from the lumbar spine to the cervical spine.

Intradiscal injections
Techniques

Techniques for intradiscal injection are essentially those approaches used for discography. A needle is placed into the centre of the nucleus pulposus, under direct imaging, from a posterior approach in the lumbar spine, and an anterior approach in the cervical spine. A high degree of technical skill is required in the performance of these injections. In the light of the poor clinical results described below, further details are not furnished in this chapter, and the interested reader is referred to radiology texts for specific technical details.

Clinical data

The literature on intradiscal corticosteroid injections for any part of the spine is very limited: no articles were retrieved in the Cochrane Collaboration's systematic review of injection therapy for low back pain.[13] A single, small case series (level IV evidence) involving both lumbar and cervical procedures has been reported.[53] In the lumbar group over half the patients with 'lumbar disc disease' achieved short-lived pain relief, with only one in five having longer term relief. In the cervical group 14 patients with 'cervical disc disease' fared less well, with only 15% of patients experiencing relief for more than 3 months. A subsequent case series of 85 patients demonstrated long-term benefit (2 years) in 21% of patients.[54] No further data are available on cervical intradiscal steroid injections, but two randomized controlled trials studying patients with proven painful lumbar discs found no benefit of intradiscal methylprednisolone over intradiscal bupivacaine[55] or saline.[56] A randomized controlled trial has also been carried out with patients randomized to steroid or not at discography. The patients with inflammatory end-plate changes showed greater improvement in their Oswestry Disability Index.[57]

No information is available concerning thoracic disc injections.

Adverse effects

No studies specifically addressing intradiscal injections of corticosteroids are available, but the adverse effects of any intradiscal injection include allergy to the injected agents, introduction of infection and systemic effects from the corticosteroids. In the cervical spine reported adverse effects after discography include discitis, subdural empyema, spinal cord injury, vascular injury and prevertebral abscess. A formal assessment of the frequency of such events revealed an incidence of significant complications of 0.16%.[58] Similar adverse effects have been noted in the lumbar spine, but their frequency is not known.

Conclusions

There is no evidence of a significant beneficial effect from intradiscal corticosteroid injection for cervical or lumbar pain. Given the high degree of technical skill required and the potential for adverse events, these procedures cannot be recommended.

ZYGAPOPHYSEAL JOINT PAIN: INTRA-ARTICULAR INJECTIONS

Cervical injections
Techniques

Intra-articular injections of the cervical zygapophyseal joints are performed under fluoroscopic control, using either a posterior or a lateral approach. A narrow-gauge spinal needle is directed towards the centre of the target joint. Once the needle is felt to have pierced the joint capsule, a minimal volume of contrast medium must be injected to confirm intra-articular placement. Thereafter, 0.7–1.0 mL of local anaesthetic can be injected to anaesthetize the joint.

The total injected volume should not exceed the joint capacity (generally accepted to be 1.0 mL) because distension beyond this volume may cause capsular rupture. Nevertheless, even when smaller volumes have been employed, extra-articular leakage has been observed in up to 17% of cases. Epidural spread has been reported, but it is believed to be rare and has been reported only when more than 1.0 mL of injectate was used.

Clinical data

When a definitive diagnosis of cervical zygapophyseal joint pain has been made (typically through cervical medial branch

blocks[59]), therapy can be targeted at the specific joint. Injection of these joints with corticosteroids has been advocated on the basis of open studies, which demonstrated some benefits in pain relief. However, a randomized, controlled trial of corticosteroid injected into painful cervical zygapophyseal joints after whiplash injury (level II evidence) has shown no benefit over injections of local anaesthetic, with neither group obtaining useful relief.[60] It is not known whether patients whose pain arises spontaneously also fail to respond to intra-articular corticosteroids. A systematic review done in 2005 showed negative evidence for cervical facet joint injection.[61]

Adverse effects

The adverse effects of intra-articular injections of corticosteroids into cervical zygapophyseal joints have not been formally studied. Reported series do not systematically report adverse effects, and the overall numbers are small. Theoretically, the potential problems include allergy to one of the injected agents, inadvertent intravascular injection, infection and epidural spread of the injectate. Appropriate technique with a sound knowledge of the radiographic anatomy should eliminate the likelihood of damage to other nearby structures.

Lumbar injections

The lumbar zygapophyseal joints have been demonstrated to be a source of pain in about 10–15% of patients with chronic low back pain.[62] The diagnosis should be established by either intra-articular or medial branch, local anaesthetic blocks.

Techniques

The lumbar zygapophyseal joints are injected under direct imaging, either with CT or fluoroscopy. The plane of the posterior joint space of these curved joints lies in a posterior oblique plane, at approximately 20° to the sagittal plane. Once the joint space has been identified on fluoroscopy, a narrow-gauge spinal needle is directed into the middle of the joint space, with the correct position being confirmed by injecting a small amount of contrast medium. The capacity of these joints is taken to be about 1 mL.

Clinical data

As is becoming a clear pattern, earlier enthusiasm for the use of corticosteroid injections into lumbar zygapophyseal joints was reflected in case series that reported an improvement in significant proportions of patients.[63] However, a subsequent, carefully designed, randomized controlled trial again failed to provide support for these observations. One hundred and one patients who had experienced pain reduction following intra-articular injections of local anaesthetic were randomized to receive an intra-articular injection of either methylprednisolone or isotonic saline into a painful zygapophyseal joint.[64] No benefit was observed on overall self-rating or pain at rest or on lumbar flexion and extension. The previously mentioned systematic review of facet joint injections in spinal pain demonstrated moderate evidence for short-term benefit and limited evidence for long-term benefit,[61] the main outcome measures being pain relief, functional improvement, improvement of psychological status and return to work.

Adverse effects

The adverse effects of intra-articular injections in the lumbar spine are similar to those in the cervical spine, as discussed above.

Thoracic injections

The thoracic zygapophyseal joints are suspected of being a source of pain in the chest and over the thoracic spine,[65] and denervation procedures have been advocated for pain control. However, the author (L.B.) was unable to find any studies pertaining to the use of corticosteroid injections into thoracic zygapophyseal joints.

Conclusions

There is limited level II evidence that corticosteroid injections into the cervical and lumbar zygapophyseal joints are not efficacious for chronic neck and back pain, respectively. The use of injections into cervical and spinal zygapophyseal joints may be of use in localizing painful joints.

OTHER SPINAL JOINTS

Sacroiliac joints

The sacroiliac joints are a recognized cause of pain in patients with spondyloarthropathies, such as ankylosing spondylitis and psoriatic arthritis. In these patients, with documented sacroiliitis, there is level II evidence from a small, randomized controlled trial that injection of corticosteroid provides a high likelihood of prolonged relief of pain, typically in the order of several months.[66] These injections can be performed under CT or MRI guidance. The lower, synovial component of the joint is targeted. The joint is complex in shape and orientation, so that care must be taken during injection using non-axial imaging that the appropriate part of the joint is being targeted.[67] Details of injection techniques for the sacroiliac joints are available elsewhere.[68] It is important to emphasize that it is virtually impossible to inject these joints without imaging guidance. Practitioners who describe being able to do so are justifiably viewed with scepticism.

It is also known that the sacroiliac joints can be a source of pain in the lower back without underlying inflammatory arthropathy.[69] However, there are no data on the effectiveness of corticosteroid injections in this latter group. The author's (L.B.) anecdotal experience in patients with demonstrated sacroiliac pain, but not sacroiliitis, has been that few patients have experienced any significant or prolonged relief of pain.

A systematic review of all the evidence cites moderate evidence for short-term benefit and limited evidence for long-term relief of pain with sacroiliac joint injections.[70]

Conclusions

Intra-articular injections of corticosteroids into the sacroiliac joint for patients with inflammatory sacroiliitis are supported by level II evidence of efficacy. No data exist for patients with mechanical sacroiliac pain, but anecdotal evidence does not support a significant effect.

Atlantoaxial joint

Provocation studies in normal volunteers have demonstrated that the atlantoaxial joint can be a source of pain.[71] Injections of the lateral atlantoaxial (C1–2) joint require needles to be placed adjacent to vital structures such as vertebral and carotid arteries and the upper spinal cord. All injections aiming for these joints must be performed under direct imaging, typically fluoroscopy. Both posterior and lateral approaches have been described, and these are considered in detail elsewhere.[72, 73] Whereas in other parts of the spine it might be considered reasonable to inject local anaesthetic as a diagnostic procedure, the potential hazards involved in performing injections of these upper joints have led to the common practice of injecting corticosteroids into these joints as presumptive treatment when they are suspected of being a source of pain. Evidence for the efficacy of these injections is limited to a retrospective case series of 26 patients, ten with inflammatory disorders (principally rheumatoid arthritis) and 16 with 'mechanical' pain.[74] The study reported superior results in the inflammatory group, with 100% responding compared with 50% in the mechanical group. In the mechanical group, the decrease in pain score was 34% and the duration of relief varied from a few weeks to over 2 years. This is in keeping with anecdotal suggestions reported in other papers.[75] No randomized controlled trials of the technique have been published, and these injections have not been considered in any systematic reviews.

Atlanto-occipital joint

The atlanto-occipital joints have been shown to be a potential source of pain through intra-articular injections.[76] This study reported relief of pain following injection of the atlanto-occipital joint in three cases, and constitutes the extent of the literature recovered on the topic. The risks and benefits of this procedure, and its role in the management of neck pain and headaches, remain unknown.

Conclusions

Corticosteroid injection into the upper cervical synovial joints is a potentially hazardous procedure of possible but uncertain benefit in patients with non-inflammatory joint pain.

SPINAL PAIN – SOURCE UNSPECIFIED

Comprehensive evaluation of patients with spinal pain using provocation procedures, such as discography, or anaesthetic procedures, such as zygapophyseal joint blocks or sacroiliac joint blocks, permits an anatomical source of pain to be identified in the majority of cases. However, where such procedures are not available or prove negative, treatment is pragmatic rather than targeted. Included in the many non-specific interventions for chronic spinal pain are local injections into tender areas typically identified by palpation. Rarely are these injections administered under direct imaging. The targets of these injections are typically tender areas, sometimes defined as trigger points, or anatomical structures purported to be painful (i.e. muscle attachments, iliolumbar ligament and paravertebral muscles).

Local steroid infiltration

Most studies of local injection therapy have involved local anaesthetic alone, or in combination with sclerosants or corticosteroids. These studies were grouped together in the Cochrane Collaboration review of injections for back pain.[77] The conclusion for all types of local injections was that there was insufficient evidence to determine the effectiveness of local therapy. However, this was based principally on the finding of a non-significant pooled odds ratio when three of the available five studies were combined. These studies were of different agents, administered into different parts of the back with different outcomes. The legitimacy of pooling such data is open to question.

Two studies have specifically included local steroid injections. Sonne et al.[78] injected either saline or a mixture of lignocaine and methylprednisolone acetate into the iliolumbar ligament in 30 patients with low back pain. Significant improvement in the patients' pain score was found in the steroid group. Garvey et al.[79] studied the outcomes of 63 patients with low back sprain. The patients were given one of four regimens: lignocaine, lignocaine combined with triamcinolone, acupuncture, or vapocoolant spray with acupressure. Non-injection treatment achieved no significantly higher rate of improvement (63%) than drug injections (42%). The authors argue that the injected substance is not the critical factor because direct mechanical stimulus to the trigger point seems to give symptomatic relief equal to that of treatment with various injections. No studies specifically addressing the efficacy of local steroid injections for cervical or thoracic pain were found.

Adverse effects

Although there are no extant data on the adverse effects of local injections into the superficial back musculature and muscle attachments, the risks of needle injury to important structures would be low. Any adverse effects are those common to all steroid injections, principally local infection and the metabolic consequences of systemic absorption.

Conclusions

There is conflicting, level II evidence for the effects of local steroid injections into the iliolumbar ligament for patients with low back pain. From first principles, these would appear to have a low likelihood of serious adverse effects. The clear superiority of corticosteroids over local anaesthetic injections has not been demonstrated. If local injection therapy is to be used, it would seem reasonable to try local anaesthetic alone before corticosteroids.

EPIDURAL INJECTIONS FOR NON-RADICULAR PAIN

As well as being used as treatment for radicular pain, epidural (but not transforaminal) injections of corticosteroid have been advocated for non-specific spinal pain. The rationale is that pain may be originating from inflammation of structures that might be accessible to injections placed into the epidural space, such as the intervertebral discs, and dura. However, any positive response to steroid injections near these structures could be attributed to the effects of systemic absorption and cannot be taken to imply a particular source of pain.

Cervical injections

Only case series (level IV evidence) are available on the efficacy of cervical epidurals for neck pain without radiculopathy. Cicala et al.[80] reported good or excellent results (equating to 75% improvement and 50% improvement) in 70% of patients. This must be viewed against a variable and generally benign natural history.

Lumbar injections

There is little evidence to support the use of lumbar epidural injections for back pain alone. In a small study of patients with chronic back pain or postsurgical spinal pain but negative radiculography, Andersen and Mosdal[81] found such poor results that a planned double-blind, randomized controlled trial was abandoned. Other studies are difficult to interpret as it is unclear whether they concern radicular symptoms or simple low back pain. The review by Bogduk et al.[20] in 1994 concluded that there were no worthwhile data vindicating the use of lumbar epidurals for lumbar pain problems other than sciatica. The present author has been unable to find any controlled studies since then that would lead to any change in this conclusion.

Conclusions

The value of cervical or lumbar epidural corticosteroids for non-radicular neck or back pain remains unproven and cannot be recommended at this time.

SUMMARY

Although their use is widespread, corticosteroid injections for spinal pain are poorly supported by the available literature. The best studied techniques are those directed at radicular pain where neural or perineural inflammation is thought to contribute to pain production. Translaminar lumbar epidural injections for lumbar radicular pain (sciatica) appear to have a small and short-lived effect. The efficacy of translaminar injections in the cervical spine for cervical radicular pain is uncertain from the available evidence. The available evidence does not support a role for epidural corticosteroids in non-radicular pain.

Lumbar transforaminal injections result in significant improvement of lumbar radicular pain, delaying or obviating the need for surgery in some patients. Cervical transforaminal injections are of uncertain efficacy and have the potential to cause rare but disabling or lethal complications.

Corticosteroid injections into painful cervical and lumbar intervertebral discs have not been shown to be clinically useful. Similarly, there is evidence from controlled clinical trials against a beneficial effect of intra-articular corticosteroids for painful cervical or lumbar zygapophyseal joints.

Although the atlantoaxial and atlanto-occipital joints are known to be sources of upper neck pain and headaches, there is little evidence to enable a judgement to be made about the value of intra-articular corticosteroid. Painful, inflammatory sacroiliitis has been shown to respond well to intra-articular corticosteroids, whereas mechanical sacroiliac joint pain seems to be far less responsive. Injections of corticosteroid and/or local anaesthetic into tender areas or the iliolumbar ligament may have some benefit in helping to resolve non-specific low back pain.

PRACTICE POINTS

- There is insufficient supportive evidence for the use of translaminar epidural steroid injection in cervical and lumbar radicular pain.

- There is supportive evidence for the use of lumbar and cervical transforaminal epidural steroid injection, but the significant risks, particularly in the latter procedure, need to be taken into account.

- Steroid injections into intervertebral discs have not been shown to be useful.

- There is evidence against the use of intra-articular steroids in painful cervical and lumbar zygapophyseal joints.

- Inflammatory sacroiliitis has been shown to respond well to intra-articular steroids, but mechanical joint pain seems less responsive.

- There is insufficient evidence to support intra-articular steroid injection in atlantoaxial and atlanto-occipital joint pain.

RESEARCH AGENDA

- Carefully designed and conducted, randomized, controlled clinical trials are needed to determine the efficacy of corticosteroid injections into painful atlantoaxial and atlanto-occipital joints, thoracic joints and sacroiliac joints where sacroiliitis is not present.

- Clinical trials should attempt to identify those patients whose conditions are more likely to respond to corticosteroids, through demonstrating the presence of inflammation at the target structure.

REFERENCES

1. Slipman CW, Plastaras CT, Palmitier RA et al. Symptom provocation of fluoroscopically guided cervical nerve root stimulation. Are dynatomal maps identical to dermatomal maps? *Spine* 1998; **23**: 2235–2242.

2. Stav A, Ovadia L, Sternberg A et al. Cervical epidural steroid injection for cervicobrachialgia. *Acta Anaesth Scand* 1995; **37**: 562–566.

3. Rowlingson JC, Kirschenbaum LP. Epidural analgesic techniques in the management of cervical pain. *Anesthes Analges* 1986; **65**: 938–942.

4. Peloso P, Gross A, Haines T et al. *Medicinal and Injection Therapies for Mechanical Neck Disorders*. Cochrane Database of Systematic Reviews 2004, Issue 2.

5. Bush K, Hillier S. Outcome of cervical radiculopathy treated with periradicular/epidural corticosteroid injections: a prospective study with independent clinical review. *Eur Spine J* 1996; **5**: 319–325.

6. Bogduk N. *Medical Management of Acute Cervical Radicular Pain: An Evidence-Based Approach*. Newcastle Bone and Joint Institute, Newcastle, Australia, 1999.

7. Abram SE, O'Connor TC. Complications associated with epidural steroid injections. *Regional Anesthes* 1996; **21**: 149–162.

8. Cicala RS, Westbrook L, Angel JJ. Side effects and complications of cervical epidural steroid injections. *J Pain Symptom Manage* 1989; **4**: 64–66.

9. Waldman SD. Cervical epidural abscess after cervical epidural nerve block with steroids. *Anesthes Analges* 1991; **72**: 717–718.

10. Bose B. Quadraparesisi following cervical epidural steroid injections. *Spine J* 2005; **5**: 1529–9430.

11. White AH, Derby R, Wynne G. Epidural injections for the diagnosis and treatment of low-back pain. *Spine* 1980; **5**: 78–86.

12. Stitz MY, Sommer HM. Accuracy of blind versus fluoroscopically guided caudal epidural injection. *Spine* 1999; **24**: 1371–1376.

13. Abdi S, Datta S, Lucas LF. Role of epidurals in the management of chronic spinal pain: a systematic review of effectiveness and complications. *Pain Physician* 2005; **8**: 1533–3159.

14. Carette S, Leclaire R, Marcoux S et al. Epidural corticosteroid injections for sciatica due to herniated nucleus pulposus. *N Engl J Med* 1997; **336**: 1634–1640.

15. Wilson-MacDonald J, Burt G, Griffin D et al. Epidural steroid injection for nerve root compression. *J Bone Joint Surg* 2005; **87**: 352–355.

16. Buttermann GR. Treatment of lumbar disc herniation: epidural steroid injection compared with discectomy. A prospective, randomized study. *J Bone Joint Surg* 2004; **86**: 670.

17. Price C, Arden N, Coglan L et al. Cost effectiveness and safety of epidural steroids in the management of sciatica. *Health Technol Assess* 2005; **9**: 1–58.

18. Valat JP, Giraudeau B, Rozenberg S et al. Epidural corticosteroid injections for sciatica: a randomised, double blind, controlled clinical trial. *Ann Rheum Dis* 2003; **62**: 639–643.

19. Ward A, Watson J, Wood P et al. Glucocorticoid epidural for sciatica: metabolic and endocrine sequelae. *Rheumatology* 2002; **41**: 68–71.

20. Bogduk N, Christophidis N, Cherry D et al. *Epidural use of Steroids in the Management of Back Pain and Sciatica of Spinal Origin. Report of the Working Party on Epidural Steroid Use of Steroids in the Management of Low Back Pain*. National Health and Medical Research Council, Canberra, 1994.

21. McCullen GM, Spurling GR et al. Epidural lipomatosis complicating lumbar steroid injections. *J Spinal Disord Tech* 1999; **12**: 526–529.

22. Iida T, Spaide RF, Negrao SG et al. Central serous chorioretinopathy after epidural corticosteroid injection. *Am J Ophthalmol* 2001; **132**: 423–425.

23. Tripath M, Nath SG, Gupta RK. Paraplegia after intracord injection during attempted epidural steroid injection in an awake patient. *Anesthes Analges* 2005; **101**: 1209–1211.

24. Slipman CW, Lipetz JS, DePalma MJ et al. Theraputic selective nerve root block in the non surgical treatment of traumatically induced cervical spondylitic radicular pain. *Am J Phys Med Rehab* 2004; **83**: 446–454.

25. Slipman CW, Lipetz JS, Jackson HB et al. Therapeutic selective nerve root block in the nonsurgical treatment of atraumatic cervical spondylitic radicular pain: a retrospective analysis with independent clinical review. *Am J Phys Med Rehab* 2000; **81**: 741–746.

26. Vallee JN, Feydy J, Carlier RY et al. Chronic cervical radiculopathy: lateral approach periradicular corticosteroid injection. *Radiology* 2001; **218**: 886–892.

27. Kolstad F, Leivseth G, Nygaard OP. Transforaminal steroid injections in the treatment of cervical radiculopathy. A prospective outcome study. *Acta Neurochir* 2005; **147**: 1065–1070.

28. Cyteval C, Thomas E, Decoux E et al. Cervical radiculopathy: open study on percutaneous periradicular foraminal steroid infiltration performed under CT control in 30 patients. *Am J Neuroradiol* 2004; **25**: 441–445.

29. Furman MB, Giovanniello MT, O'Brien EM. Incidence of intravascular penetration in transforaminal cervical epidural steroid injections. *Spine* 2003; **28**: 1528–1159.

30. Derby R, Lee SH, Kim BJ et al. Complications following cervical epidural steroid injections by expert interventionalists in 2003. *Pain Physician* 2004; **7**: 1533–3159.

31. Huntoon MA. Anatomy of the cervical intervertebral foramina: vulnerable arteries and ischaemic neurologic injuries after transforaminal epidural injections. *Pain* 2005; **117**: 104–111.

32. Ludwig MA, Burns SP. Spinal cord infarction following cervical transforaminal epidural injection: a case report. *Spine* 2005; **30**: 1528–1159.

33. Rozin L, Rozin R, Koehler SA et al. Death during transforaminal epidural steroid nerve root block (C7) due to perforation of the left vertebral artery. *Am J Forensic Med Pathol* 2003; **24**: 351–355.

34. Weiner BK, Fraser RD. Foraminal injection for lateral lumbar disc herniation. *J Bone Joint Surg (Britain)* 1997; **79**: 804–807.

35. Bogduk N, Govind J. *Medical Management of Acute Lumbar Radicular Pain: An Evidence-based Approach*, 1st edn. Newcastle Bone and Joint Institute, Newcastle, Australia, 1999.

36. Lutze M, Stendel R, Vesper J et al. Periradicular therapy in lumbar radicular syndromes: methodology and results. *Acta Neurochir* 1997; **139**: 719–724.

37. Viton JM, Rubino T, Peretti-Viton P et al. Short-term evaluation of periradicular corticosteroid injections in the treatment of lumbar radiculopathy associated with disc disease. *Rev Rhumatis (English Edn)* 1998; **65**: 195–200.

38. Narozny M, Zanetti M, Boos N. Therapeutic efficacy of selective nerve root blocks in the treatment of lumbar radicular leg pain. *Swiss Med Week* 2001; **131**: 75–80.

39. Cooper G, Lutz GE, Boachie AO et al. Effectiveness of transforaminal epidural steroid injections in patients with degenerative lumbar scoliotic stenosis and radiculopathy. *Pain Physician* 2004; **7**: 311–317.

40. Botwin KP, Gruber RD, Bouchlas CG et al. Fluoroscopically guided lumbar transforaminal epidural steroid injections in degenerative lumbar stenosis: an outcome study. *Am J Phys Med Rehab* 2002; **81**: 898–905.

41. Vad VB, Bhat AL, Lutz GE et al. Transforaminal epidural steroid injections in lumbosacral radiculopathy: a prospective randomized study. *Spine* 2002; **27**: 11–16.

42. Karppinen J, Malmivaara A, Kurunlahti M et al. Periradicular infiltration for sciatica: a randomized controlled trial. *Spine* 2001; **26**: 1059–1067.

43. Karppinen J, Ohinmaa A, Malmivaara A et al. Cost effectiveness of periradicular infiltration for sciatica: subgroup analysis of a randomized controlled trial. *Spine* 2001; **26**: 2587–2595.

44. Riew KD, Yin Y, Gilula L et al. The effect of nerve-root injections on the need for operative treatment of lumbar radicular pain. A prospective, randomized, controlled, double-blind study. *J Bone Joint Surg (Am)* 2000; **82A**: 1589–1593.

45. Botwin KP, Gruber RD, Bouchlas CG et al. Complications of fluoroscopically guided transforaminal lumbar epidural injections. *Arch Phys Med Rehab* 2000; **81**: 1045–1050.

46. Furman MB, O'Brien EM, Zgleszewski TM. Incidence of intravascular penetration in transforaminal lumbosacral epidural steroid injections. *Spine* 2000; **25**: 2628–2632.

47. Sullivan WJ, Willick SE, Chira-Adisai W et al. Incidence of intravascular uptake in lumbar spinal injection procedures. *Spine* 2000; **25**: 481–486.

48. Finn KP, Case JL. Disk entry: A complication of transforaminal epidural injection – a case report. *Arch Phys Med Rehab* 2005; **86**: 1489–1491.

49. Glaser SE, Falco F. Paraplegia following thoracolumbar transforaminal epidural steroid injection. *Pain Physician* 2005; **8**: 309–314.

50. Rathmell JP, Benzon HT. Transforaminal epidural injection of steroids: should we continue? *Reg Anesth Pain Med* 2004; **29**: 397–399.

51. Saifuddin A, Mitchell R, Taylor BA. Extradural inflammation associated with annular tears: demonstration with gadolinium-enhanced lumbar spine MRI. *Eur Spine J* 1999; **8**: 34–39.

52. Mercer S, Bogduk N. The ligaments and annulus fibrosus of human adult cervical intervertebral discs. *Spine* 1999; **24**: 619–626.

53. Wilkinson HA, Schuman N. Intradiscal corticosteroids in the treatment of lumbar and cervical disc problems. *Spine* 1980; **5**: 385–389.

54. Koning HM, Koning AJ, Bruinen TCM et al. Long term efficacy of intradiscal steroids for low back syndromes. *Pain Clin* 2001; **13**: 133–143.

55. Simmons JW, McMillin JN, Emery SF et al. Intradiscal steroids. A prospective double-blind clinical trial. *Spine* 1992; **17**(6 Suppl): S172–S175.

56. Khot A, Bowditch M, Powell M et al. The use of intradiscal steroid therapy for lumbar spinal discogenic pain: a randomized controlled trial. *Spine* 2004; **29**: 833–836.

57. Buttermann GR. The effect of spinal steroid injections for degenerative disc disease. *Spine J* 2004; **4**: 495–505.

58. Zeidman SM, Thompson K, Ducker TB. Complications of cervical discography: analysis of 4400 diagnostic disc injections. *Neurosurgery* 1995; **37**: 414–417.

59. Barnsley L, Lord SM, Bogduk N. Comparative local anaesthetic blocks in the diagnosis of cervical zygapophyseal joint pain. *Pain* 1993; **55**: 99–106.

60. Barnsley L, Lord SM, Wallis BJ et al. Lack of effect of intra-articular corticosteroids for chronic cervical zygapophyseal joint pain. *New Engl J Med* 1994; **330**: 1047–1050.

61. Boswell MV, Colson JD, Spillane WF. Theraputic facet joint interventions in chronic spinal pain: a systematic review of effectiveness and complications. *Pain Physician* 2005; **8**: 101–114.

62. Schwarzer AC, Wang S, Laurent R et al. The role of the zygapophyseal joint in chronic low back pain [Abstract]. *Austr NZ J Med* 1992; **22**: 185.

63. Murtagh FR. Computed tomography and fluoroscopy guided anesthesia and steroid injection in facet syndrome. *Spine* 1988; **13**: 686–689.

64. Carette S, Marcoux S, Truchon R et al. A controlled trial of corticosteroid injections into facet joints for the treatment of chronic low back pain. *N Engl J Med* 1991; **325**: 1002–1007.

65. Dreyfuss P, Tibiletti C, Dreyer SJ. Thoracic zygapophyseal joint pain patterns. A study in normal volunteers. *Spine* 1994; **19**: 807–811.

66. Maugars Y, Mathis C, Berthelot JM et al. Assessment of the efficacy of sacroiliac corticosteroid injections in spondylarthropathies: a double-blind study. *Br J Rheumatol* 1996; **35**: 767–770.

67. Ebraheim NA, Mekhail AO, Wiley WF et al. Radiology of the sacroiliac joint. *Spine* 1997; **22**: 869–876.

68. Braun J, Bollow M, Seyrekbasan F et al. Computed tomography guided corticosteroid injection of the sacroiliac joint in patients with spondyloarthropathy with sacroiliitis: clinical outcome and followup by dynamic magnetic resonance imaging. *J Rheumatol* 1996; **23**: 659–664.

69. Schwarzer AC, Aprill C, Bogduk N. The sacroiliac joint in chronic low back pain. *Spine* 1995; **20**: 31–37.

70. McKenzie-Brown AM, Shah RV, Sehgal N et al. A systematic review of sacroiliac joint interventions. *Pain Physician* 2005; **8**: 115–125.

71. Dreyfuss P, Michaelsen M, Fletcher D. Atlanto-occipital and atlantoaxial joint pain patterns. *Spine* 1994; **19**: 1125–1131.

72. Dreyfuss P. Atlanto-occipital and lateral atlantoaxial joint injections. In: Lennard TA (ed.), *Physiatric Procedures*. Hanley and Belfus, Philadelphia, PA, 1995, pp. 227–237.

73. McCormick C. Arthrography of the atlanto-axial (C1–C2) joints: techniques and results. *J Intervent Radiol* 1987; **2**: 9–13.

74. Glemarec J, Guillot P, Laborie Y et al. Intraarticular glucocorticosteroid injection into the lateral atlantoaxial joint under fluoroscopic control. A retrospective comparative study in patients with mechanical and inflammatory disorders. *Joint Bone Spine* 2000; **67**: 54–61.

75. Dreyfuss P. Atlanto-occipital and lateral atlantoaxial joint injections. In: Lennard TA (ed.), *Physiatric Procedures*. Hanley and Belfus, Philadelphia, PA, 1995, pp. 227–237.

76. Dreyfuss P, Rogers J, Dreyer S et al. Atlanto-occipital joint pain. A report of three cases and description of an intraarticular joint block technique. *Region Anesthes* 1994; **19**: 344–351.

77. Nelemans PJ, De Bie RA, de Vet HC et al. *Injection Therapy for Subacute and Chronic Benign Low Back Pain*. Cochrane Database of Systematic Reviews 2000; Issue 2: CD001824.

78. Sonne M, Christensen K, Hansen SE et al. Injection of steroids and local anaesthetics as therapy for low-back pain. *Scand J Rheumatol* 1985; **14**: 343–345.

79. Garvey TA, Marks MR, Wiesel SW. A prospective, randomized, double-blind evaluation of trigger-point injection therapy for low-back pain. *Spine* 1989; **76**: 962–964.

80. Cicala RS, Thoni K, Angel JJ. Long-term results of cervical epidural steroid injections. *Clin J Pain* 1989; **5**: 143–145.

81. Andersen KH, Mosdal C. Epidural application of cortico-steroids in low-back pain and sciatica. *Acta Neurochir* 1987; **87**: 52–53.

Chapter 13
Radiofrequency procedures in chronic pain

Nikolai Bogduk and Susan M. Lord

INTRODUCTION

The adjective 'radiofrequency' (RF) is used to qualify several procedures used to treat chronic pain. They all have in common the delivery of an alternating current to an electrode; the current having the same frequency as radio waves (100,000–500,000 Hz). Certain procedures differ, however, with respect to the purpose to which the current is put and the target structure.

Originally, the current was used to produce a heat lesion at the electrode. In historical order, target structures have included the trigeminal ganglion, the spinothalamic tract in the spinal cord, and various peripheral nerves. In order to distinguish them from other applications, such procedures are known as *thermal RF* or *RF thermocoagulation* procedures. They are qualified further by specifying the target structure (e.g. ganglionotomy, tractotomy, cordotomy or neurotomy).

Subsequently, an application was developed in which the target is the dorsal root ganglion (DRG), and heating is minimized. This procedure became known as *RF-DRG*. In another development, the current is delivered in a pulsed fashion without heating the target; this procedure is known as *pulsed RF*.

RADIOFREQUENCY THERMOCOAGULATION

Mechanism

Conventional thermal RF lesion generation requires a ground plate with a large surface area, and a needle electrode that is insulated along its length, save for the tip for a distance of 2–10 mm. The needle is directed into, or onto, the target structure, while the ground plate is applied onto a convenient region of the surface of the body. The generator delivers the alternating current between the ground plate and the electrode.

At the ground plate the electric field is diffuse, because of the large surface area of the plate, but as it passes through the body the electric field concentrates onto the uninsulated tip of the

needle electrode (Figure 13.1). The alternating electrical field oscillates charged molecules in the intervening body tissues,[1] and this molecular oscillation generates heat. The oscillation is of greatest amplitude where the electric field density is greatest, namely near the electrode (Figure 13.2). Consequently, heating is maximal close to the electrode. When so heated, tissues near the electrode will secondarily transfer heat to the electrode, and if a thermocouple is inserted into or incorporated in the electrode that temperature can be monitored. At distances progressively further from the electrode the temperature achieved will be progressively less, in proportion to the decreasing density of the electric field. In effect, isotherms can be identified in a concentric pattern extending from the electrode (see Figure 13.2).

The size of the lesion produced by the electrode is a function of the magnitude of the current applied, the temperature achieved at the electrode, the size of the electrode and the duration of heating. Soft tissues will coagulate if they are heated above 60–65°C.[2, 3] If sufficient current is applied to establish a temperature of 80–85°C at the surface of the electrode, tissues

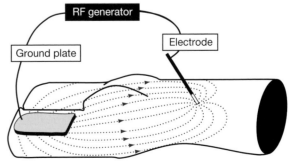

Figure 13.1. A sketch of the circuitry and electric field of thermal RF neurotomy. From the ground plate the electric field is concentrated onto the exposed tip of the electrode.

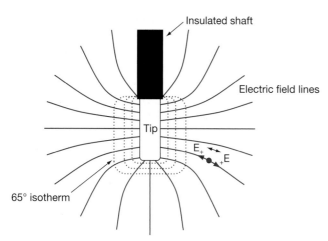

Figure 13.2. Effects near the tip of the electrode subjected to a RF current. Electric-field lines converge onto the tip of the electrode. Charged molecules oscillate with the electric field (E). Temperatures are higher where the electric field is denser. Isotherms radiate concentrically from the surface of the electrode.

within a short distance from the surface will be heated to 60–65°C or more. Those tissues are coagulated in the form of a prolate spheroid, the long axis of which is formed by the uninsulated tip of the electrode (Figure 13.3). The electrode coagulates principally in a transverse direction; little tissue distal to the tip is coagulated. The actual size of the lesion is proportional to the diameter (width) of the electrode, and can be normalized in terms of electrode-widths. On average, tissues within about two electrode-widths from the surface of the electrode will be coagulated, but sometimes the lesion will be smaller than this. The lower two standard deviation limit of

lesion size (see Figure 13.3) dictates that often the electrode will coagulate tissues only to within about one electrode-width from its surface. This becomes the critical distance within which operators can expect to coagulate a target nerve consistently. Furthermore, because the electrode coagulates transversely, not distally, the electrode must be placed into, across or parallel to the target nerve in order for the lesion to be optimally effective.[2] If the electrode is placed perpendicular to the target, the lesion made may fail to incorporate the target (Figure 13.4).

Once a temperature of 80°C has been achieved at the electrode, lesion size increases with time as the temperature is maintained. The effect of time is logarithmic. Most of the increase in size occurs within 60 seconds, but an appreciable growth continues between 60 and 90 seconds.[3] Thereafter, further growth is clinically insignificant. Growth is impeded, and eventually arrested, because the coagulated tissue has a high impedance and resists flow of current sufficient to heat additional tissue.

Pathology

If the electrode is placed sufficiently close to a target nerve, that nerve will be incorporated into the lesion formed around the electrode. If an electrode is inserted into a DRG, heating it to 67°C produces a haemorrhagic lesion with total loss of myelinated fibres.[4] If a large electrode (14G) is placed beside a DRG, thermal lesions of 45°C, 55°C, 65°C, 75°C and 85°C produce total loss of unmyelinated nerve fibres and near total loss of myelinated fibres.[5] In the sciatic nerve, an 80°C thermal lesion produces extensive Wallerian degeneration of the axons, and disruption of their myelin sheaths and epineurium.[6] In the saphenous nerve, lesions made at 70°C destroy both myelinated and unmyelinated fibres.[7]

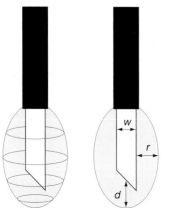

	Electrode	
	SMK	RRE
w	0.7 mm	1.6 mm
r	2.3w	1.6w
SD	0.4w	0.3w
d	1.4w	0.4w
SD	0.4w	0.2w

Figure 13.3. The geometry of the lesion generated by a thermal RF current. The volume of tissue coagulated assumes the shape of a prolate spheroid (i.e. elliptical in longitudinal section and circular in transverse section). The radial extent (r) of the lesion beyond the surface of the electrode, and its distal extent (d) beyond the tip of the electrode are functions of the width (w) of the electrode. The inset shows the actual dimensions of lesions generated by two types of electrode:[3] the SMK electrode and the RRE electrode (Radionics, Burlington, MA).

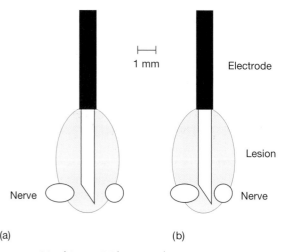

Figure 13.4. Matching an RF lesion to the target nerve. (a) Because of the shape and limited size of the lesion an electrode placed close to the nerve may fail to incorporate it completely. The larger the nerve the less it will be encompassed by the lesion. (b) Even if the electrode is placed in contact with the nerve, parts of it escape coagulation, more so if the nerve is large.

Physiology

An early study claimed that RF coagulation selectively destroyed only A-δ and C fibres, and hence could be selective for preventing nociception,[8] but this contention is incompatible with the results of pathology studies, which show that RF coagulation affects all nerves, both myelinated and unmyelinated.[4–7] Electromyography (EMG) studies have shown that even alpha motor neurons are coagulated.[9] RF neurotomy, therefore, is a nonselective method of coagulating nerves.

Applications

Thermal RF procedures have been used to target: the trigeminal ganglion, for the treatment of trigeminal neuralgia; the dorsal root entry zone, for deafferentation pain; and the medial branches of the dorsal rami, for the treatment of certain types of spinal pain; as well as other cranial and peripheral nerves. The nature and extent of evidence differs for these procedures.

Trigeminal RF thermocoagulation

In the treatment of trigeminal neuralgia, the target for RF thermocoagulation has been the region between the trigeminal ganglion and its sensory root. Accordingly, the procedure has variously been referred to as RF thermocoagulation of the Gasserian ganglion, retrogasserian thermorhizotomy, RF rhizotomy, RF trigeminal neurolysis and RF ganglionolysis. The electrode is introduced through the foramen ovale, until its tip reaches the posterior end of Meckel's cave. Its position is adjusted until electrical stimulation evokes sensation in the territory of that division of the nerve in which the patient perceives their pain. Lesions are generated according to various protocols, which involve applying the current in cycles of 45–90 seconds[10] or continuously for up to 300 seconds,[11] at temperatures increasing from 60°C to 90°C,[10] or at 55–70°C[12] or 70–80°C.[11]

Trigeminal thermal RF has a strongly established reputation of efficacy.[13] This reputation is based on numerous observational studies, some encompassing over 1000 patients. Nevertheless, despite a large literature, dating back to the original report by Sweet and Wepsic,[14] a systematic review[15] found much of the literature to have methodological shortcomings. It found only four studies upon which sound conclusions could be based.[11, 12, 16, 17] Those studies, however, corroborate the impression engendered by the literature at large. Some 90% of patients achieve complete relief of pain immediately after treatment. This success deteriorates, albeit slowly, over ensuing years, such that just over 50% remain completely pain free at 5 years. In one series, 41% of patients sustained relief for 20 years.[12] The cardinal side-effects are: sensory loss, sufficient to affect quality of life, in more than 30% of patients; keratitis in some 10%; and dysaesthesia in 4–10%. Complications are rare.

Dorsal root entry zone

Dorsal root entry zone (DREZ) lesioning was developed as a treatment for central pain caused by peripheral nerve injuries or diseases.[18, 19] The rationale is that deafferentation results in spontaneous activity in apical dorsal horn neurons, and that ablation of these neurons should relieve the pain that they

cause. Ablation is achieved by introducing a small RF electrode posterolaterally into the DREZs of the spinal cord at segments affected by the peripheral nerve injury. Electrical stimulation is used to confirm the relevant segments.[20, 21]

Controlled trials have not been performed, but the reputation of effectiveness of DREZ lesioning relies on multiple observational studies that describe remarkable relief in sizeable proportions of patients with otherwise intractable pain. DREZ lesioning has been particularly effective for the pain of brachial plexus avulsion (more than 70% relief in 54–83% of cases),[22–27] the pain of spinal cord injuries ('good' outcomes in 50–60% of cases)[28–33] and phantom limb pain.[34] It has not been particularly effective for postherpetic neuralgia.[26, 27] For intractable facial pain, the DREZ of the nucleus caudalis can be targeted. Success rates of 60–70% have been reported.[35–38]

The proximity of the site of the DREZ lesion to the lateral corticospinal tract and the dorsal column is an inherent problem with the procedure that can lead to unwanted neurological deficits.[19] Motor weakness, bladder or sexual dysfunction, and paraesthesia occur in various proportions of patients, depending on the nature of the index pathology, the skill and experience of the operator, and the technique used.

The effect of DREZ lesioning is not enduring in all cases. Recurrences occur; but although follow-up periods of 50 months, 84 months, 1–7 years and 1–20 years have been reported there is no clear picture of the expected rate of enduring success, as there is for trigeminal thermocoagulation.[12, 15] The study with the longest follow-up reported that good long-term results were obtained in 68% of the patients who had a segmental pain distribution, compared with 0% in patients with predominant infralesional pain; and in 88% of patients with predominantly paroxysmal pain, compared with 26% with continuous pain.[31]

Lumbar medial branch neurotomy

The lumbar zygapophysial joints are innervated by the medial branches of the lumbar dorsal rami. Back pain stemming from these joints can be diagnosed by performing controlled diagnostic blocks of the nerves that supply them. If these blocks completely relieve the patient's pain, it can be treated by RF thermocoagulation of the nerves responsible for mediating the pain.

RF denervation of the lumbar zygapophysial joints was initiated by Shealy,[39–42] who called the procedure 'facet denervation'. He claimed excellent results, and others adopted his technique, also claiming excellent outcomes. However, anatomical studies showed that the surgical anatomy of Shealy's technique was fatally flawed: there were no nerves where he recommended putting electrodes.[43, 44] Thus, despite the large literature that had developed, there was no anatomical and physiological basis for the successes claimed for facet denervation.

The anatomical studies prescribed accurate target points, and recommended renaming the procedure as RF lumbar medial branch neurotomy.[44] Those studies, however, overlooked the manner in which thermal RF lesions are produced. A later study showed that RF electrodes coagulate principally transversely, not distally.[45] Therefore, for optimal efficacy electrodes should be placed parallel to the target nerve, not perpendicular to it, as had been previously recommended. A recent study illustrated, in cadavers, the potential flaws in the technique and how accurate placement of electrodes was critical.[46]

Few practitioners have heeded these recommendations, and many have persisted with older versions of the procedure, even the flawed 'facet denervation'. Consequently, because accurate techniques have not been used, there is virtually no literature on the effectiveness of lumbar medial branch neurotomy. Systematic reviews[47, 48] have looked for evidence of efficacy but they did not recognize the flaws in technique in the available studies.[49, 50] Nevertheless, two studies have provided data.

A randomized, placebo-controlled trial showed that active lumbar thermocoagulation was, indeed, more effective than sham therapy.[51] However, optimal technique was not used. Consequently, few patients had satisfying degrees of relief. Also, the study had a short follow-up period, which was sufficient to test for placebo response but not to determine the duration of effect, the latter being provided by a descriptive study.[52] In patients carefully selected using controlled diagnostic blocks, and using accurate electrode placement (Figure 13.5), RF lumbar medial branch neurotomy provided greater than 60% relief of pain in 80% of patients at 12 months, and greater than 80% relief in 60% of patients. This study sets the benchmark for the magnitude and duration of relief achievable by lumbar medial branch neurotomy.

Since lumbar medial branch neurotomy targets the peripheral axons, and not the cell bodies, of the medial branches, the nerves are not permanently destroyed. The nerves regenerate, typically within 12 months. However, relief can be reinstated by repeating the procedure. A descriptive study reported that relief can be successfully reinstated, after one, two or more repeat treatments.[53]

A second placebo-controlled trial[54] tested an inaccurate technique, but nevertheless one that is commonly practised in The Netherlands. Furthermore, patients were not selected on the basis of controlled diagnostic blocks, which is another feature of practice in The Netherlands. The trial showed no difference between active treatment and placebo. This result underscores the significance of correct technique and correct patient selection. If both are neglected, the intervention is no more than a sham.

Cervical medial branch neurotomy

The typical cervical zygapophysial joints are innervated by each of the medial branches that bear the same segmental number as the joint. The C2–3 joint is innervated by the third occipital nerve. Pain stemming from these joints can be diagnosed using cervical medial branch blocks under controlled conditions.

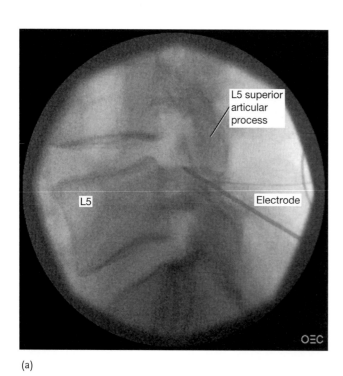

(a)

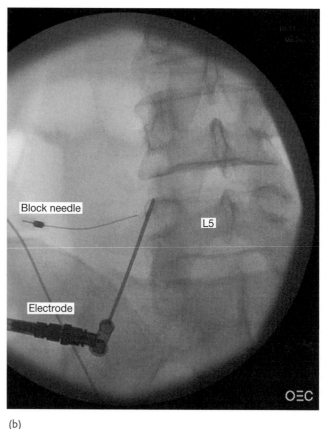

(b)

Figure 13.5. Radiographs of an electrode in place for L4 medial branch neurotomy. The electrode crosses the neck of the L5 superior articular process, dorsal to the L5 transverse process. (a) Lateral view; (b) anteroposterior view.

The early literature on cervical medial branch thermocoagulation was confounded by poor selection criteria and questionable operative techniques.[55] On the basis of accurate anatomy, a revised technique was piloted.[55] That study achieved poor results from third occipital neurotomy, to treat C2–3 zygapophysial joint pain, and recommended that a better technique be developed. For medial branch neurotomy at typical cervical levels, however, the pilot study produced sufficiently encouraging results that a randomized, placebo-controlled trial was conducted. The technique requires placing multiple lesions across and along the course of each target nerve, across both the lateral and the anterolateral aspect of the articular pillar (Figure 13.6).

For the placebo-controlled trial, power calculations indicated that 24 patients were sufficient, and the sample was restricted to that size by ethical considerations.[56] It transpired that the treatment was so effective that a sample of 24 had 100% power for the results obtained. The procedure involved between 2–3 hours operating time, in order to thoroughly coagulate each of the two target nerves. Randomization required only that half the patients received lesions generated at 80°C for 90 seconds, while the other half endured the same procedure, save that no electricity was supplied to the generator. Patients, operator and assessor were blind to treatment allocation. Success was defined as complete relief of pain, corroborated by the following: a visual–analogue pain scale score of 0–5/100; a total word count on the McGill Pain Questionnaire of 0–3/20, accompanied by restoration of four activities of daily living nominated preoperatively by the patient; and denial by the patient of any need for further treatment. The median duration of relief of pain following active treatment was 263 days, while in the placebo group it was 8 days.[56] Systematic reviews[47, 48] have misrepresented this study as having only a 3-month follow-up, while in fact the follow-up was for 12 months. The only relevance of the 3-month figure is that patients who obtained no relief were classified as 'failed' at 3 months in order that they could have escape treatment.

Subsequent follow-up studies have shown that cervical medial branch neurotomy is effective in providing complete relief of pain in some 70% of patients whose pain is completely relieved by controlled blocks of the cervical medial branches.[57, 58] In those patients in whom cervical medial branch neurotomy achieves complete relief of pain, the median duration of effect is 422 days.[58] Those studies also showed that, if pain recurs, relief can be reinstated by repeating the procedure. The duration of response to the first treatment dictates the likelihood of response in the event of recurrence. If patients initially obtain relief for longer than 90 days, they have an 82% chance of relief being reinstated by a repeat procedure. If the initial relief lasts less than 90 days the chance of successful repeat treatment drops to 33%.[58]

A revised technique for third occipital neurotomy has been developed.[59] This requires a larger diameter electrode than was used in the pilot study, careful and accurate placement of electrodes so as to cover all possible locations of the third occipital nerve, and holding the electrode in place so that it does not displace during coagulation. Using these modifications success rates of 85% can be achieved for the relief of headache stemming from the C2–3 zygapophysial joint.[59] The duration of complete relief is similar to that achieved by medial branch neurotomy at typical cervical levels. Relief can be reinstated in the event of recurrence of pain. Multiple annual repetitions

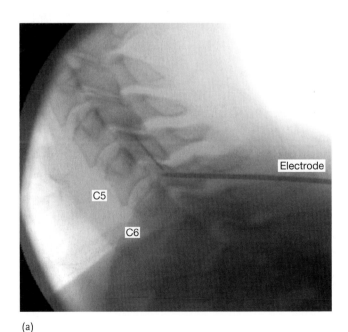

(a)

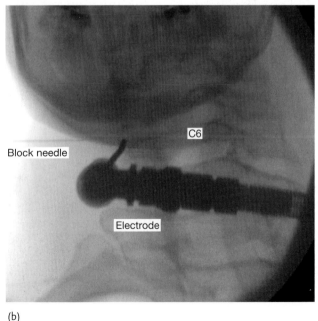

(b)

Figure 13.6. Radiographs of an electrode in place for a C6 medial branch neurotomy. The electrode lies against the lateral aspect of the C6 articular pillar. (a) Lateral view; (b) anteroposterior view.

have kept some patients recurrently free of pain for in excess of 7 years.[59]

A study, conducted in a conventional practice, has corroborated the outcomes described from research centres.[60] The success rate and the duration of effect are the same as those in formal research studies. Provided that the same operative technique is used, this observation allows the results from highly specialized, research centres to be generalized.[60] Cervical medial branch neurotomy is the only procedure that has been validated for cervical zygapophysial joint pain, and is the only procedure shown to be able to achieve complete relief of chronic neck pain. An independent inquiry concluded that cervical medial branch neurotomy establishes a benchmark for the treatment of chronic neck pain.[61]

It is critical that patients selected for this procedure obtain complete relief of pain following controlled diagnostic blocks of the target nerves. Response to cervical medial branch neurotomy is not affected whether placebo-controlled or comparative local anaesthetic blocks are used,[58] and the response is not affected by litigation status.[49, 56, 58, 60, 62] Although cervical medial branch neurotomy is slightly less effective in patients with litigation pending, the differences are not statistically significant.

Other applications

A variety of nerves and structures have been targets for RF thermocoagulation. For each application the literature is scant and of limited quality, in the form of case reports or case series, with few outcome measures having been used.

Neurosurgeons have applied RF techniques to perform cordotomy and myelotomy for the treatment of cancer pain.[63] These procedures have an established reputation, and are not considered controversial, for they are used sparingly. Improvements in palliative care have reduced the need for neuro-destructive procedures.

Some practitioners have reported performing RF neurotomy of the medial branches of the thoracic dorsal rami.[64] A dissection study, however, revealed that the target points used in that study were remote from the medial branches and, therefore, that those nerves could not have been coagulated.[65] A technique for thoracic medial branch neurotomy based on accurate anatomy has not been developed.

RF neurotomy of the upper cervical sympathetic trunk has been championed by one authority,[66] but the literature is sparse. An attempted review[67] found only one publication, which provided inadequate data.[68] That review offered its own outcome data, claiming that one-third of patients achieved more than 50% reduction of pain. Follow-up, however, was limited, with a dropout rate of 69%. Otherwise, the literature has concentrated on relief of sympathetic features in vascular disorders; relief of pain has been described in only a limited fashion.[66]

Some practitioners have coagulated the sphenopalatine ganglion for the treatment of cluster headache.[69, 70] They and others have coagulated cranial nerves other than the trigeminal nerve to treat oral and facial pain.[71, 72]

In various ways, RF technology has been applied to treat low back pain stemming from the lumbar intervertebral discs.

Placing lesions in the nucleus pulposus[73] was based on a false premise,[74, 75] and has been refuted as no more than a sham treatment.[76] More vexatious is placing lesions in or near the annulus fibrosus. Two devices have been used to this end: a radiant heating electrode[77, 78] and an RF electrode.[79] Each has been evaluated in comparison studies. Both interventions appear more effective than conservative therapy.[77–79] In those patients who benefit, active treatment with the radiant-heat electrode is more effective than placebo.[80] However, for both procedures only a minority of patients benefit. Technical problems, in matching the placement of the electrode, and the size of lesion that it makes, with the location and size of the pathology, seem to be the cardinal reason for limited benefit from these procedures.[81] Newer technologies may overcome these limitations.

RADIOFREQUENCY-DORSAL ROOT GANGLION

RF-DRG was developed in response to patients failing to obtain relief of pain following medial branch neurotomy. The development involved two changes. First, the target became the DRG of a spinal nerve (cervical, thoracic, lumbar or sacral). Secondly, the intention was not to destroy the nerve completely. Instead, a heat lesion was placed sufficiently near the DRG to produce what was described as a partial lesion, but not so close as to destroy the ganglion completely. The intention was to produce a lesion that might relieve pain, but would not interrupt other sensations in the dermatome of the target nerve. A further measure, to this end, was to reduce the temperature attained at the electrode to 67°C.

The procedure was first called 'partial RF rhizotomy'.[82,83] Later it became known as 'RF lesion adjacent to the DRG'.[84] This name was contracted to 'RF dorsal root ganglion', and abbreviated to RF-DRG.[84,85]

Rationale

Proponents of RF-DRG believe that a therapeutic effect is achieved by the partial lesion produced in the DRG. Explicitly, they have stated that it is not the intention of this procedure to coagulate the ganglion. Rather, 'the procedure is intended to expose the DRG to temperatures that prevail in the peripheral part of an RF lesion to preserve the large myelinated fibers and to deactivate the small myelinated fibers'.[86]

Critics are perplexed by the inherent paradox in the rationale: the DRG is referred to as the target but the lesion must not be so close as to actually damage the ganglion.[87] The literature[8] cited by the proponents[86] as evidence of a differential effect on small-diameter and large-diameter afferents has been refuted.[5–7] A pathology study showed that an electrode placed next to the DRG produced a lesion in the neighbouring tissues but not in the ganglion itself.[4] An anatomical study showed that, although placed according to the prescribed protocol, electrodes are often too remote from the target ganglion for a lesion to have a thermal effect.[88] This paradox invites the interpretation that perhaps the lesion does nothing to the nerve, and the outcomes are due to no more than a placebo effect. This paradox is reflected in the empirical, clinical data.

Efficacy

Descriptive studies promoted the use of RF-DRG for cervical,[82] thoracic[83,84] and, eventually, lumbar[89] pain syndromes. Outcomes were reported in terms of whether the patients were 'pain-free' or had 'good' (50–100%) relief of their pain. Other outcome measures were not provided.

The first of the cervical studies[82] reported that 2/20 patients (10%) were pain-free at 3 months; 4/20 were so at 6 months and 2/17 (11%) at 12 months. Eight patients had good relief at 3 months, but this number dropped to two at 6 months and two at 12 months. The authors did not conclude that their treatment was successful. They portrayed it as a 'reversible procedure' that can be useful to provide a relatively pain-free period that can be used to obtain the maximum benefit from conservative forms of treatment. No studies have documented such ancillary benefit.

The first of the thoracic studies[83] announced astounding results. At 2 months 30/45 (67%) patients were pain-free, and a further 11 (24%) had a greater than 50% reduction in pain. At long-term follow-up, ranging from 13 to 46 months, 20 patients were pain-free, and 15 had greater than 50% relief of pain. The second thoracic study[84] did not reproduce these outcomes. At 8 weeks only 8/43 (18%) patients had complete relief of pain, and 9/43 (21%) had greater than 50% relief. At follow-up beyond 36 weeks only five patients (12%) were pain-free and eight (18%) had greater than 50% relief.

There is no obvious explanation for the discrepancy between these studies. Differences in technique are unlikely because the authors are known to one another, and have collaborated with one another on other studies of RF-DRG. Patient selection may have been the source of difference. The first study had a large proportion (38%) of patients with postsurgical pain (thoracotomy, mastectomy, abdominal scar), in whom good outcomes were achieved. Such patients were absent from the second study. Conversely, the second study had a large proportion (47%) of patients with neuralgia. In the first study, patients with neuralgias had less than average outcomes. (The second study did not stratify its results according to diagnosis.)

The first of the lumbar studies[89] was a retrospective review of 361 patients, but results were available for only 279. At 2 months 61 patients were pain-free. This number became 23 at a mean follow-up of 22.9 months, but the range of that period was 2–70 months. A further 103 patients reported incomplete but greater than 50% relief at 2 months. This number dropped to 73 at longer term follow-up.

Despite the less than modest outcomes of the first cervical study, investigators from the same institution undertook a placebo-controlled trial.[90] Success was defined as a reduction by 2 points or more on a 10-point visual–analogue scale. A significantly greater proportion of patients (8/9) had a successful outcome following active treatment than those (2/11) who underwent sham treatment. Follow-up, however, was limited to only 8 weeks. At this time the actively treated patients

had reduced their mean pain scores from 6.4 to 3.3, whereas the sham-treated patients maintained the same scores (5.9 and 6.0).

Although this study provided data to the effect that the initial effects of cervical RF-DRG were not due to placebo, they do not attest to a successful, lasting effect. Unlike the preceding study, this controlled study did not report on the number of patients completely relieved. Success was defined only as a 2-point decrease in pain scores. The duration of effect beyond 8 weeks was not measured. These data attest only to a modest and short-lived therapeutic effect. The data of the preceding observational study would predict that outcomes would attenuate substantially beyond 8 weeks.

The reported effects of lumbar RF-DRG[89] have also been tested in a placebo-controlled trial.[91] In all patients, the DRG was anaesthetized and a RF electrode was placed in position. The active treatment was RF-DRG at 67°C. The control treatment was no generation of current. At 3 months 16% of the 44 patients treated with RF-DRG had greater than 50% reduction in pain, and 25% of the 36 patients who had sham treatment experienced the same outcome. These proportions are not significantly different statistically. Patients whose DRG was anaesthetized, without a lesion being produced, had the same outcomes as actively treated patients.

Comment

The outcomes of RF-DRG are not consistent across the cervical, thoracic and lumbar levels. The outcomes of cervical RF-DRG have been less than modest, even in a controlled trial. For lumbar RF-DRG, a rigorous controlled trial has shown that sham therapy achieves at least equivalent outcomes to those of active therapy. Since this study was conducted by the same workers as the foregoing observational study, that trial surely refutes lumbar RF-DRG as a valid treatment, and by extrapolation casts doubt on the validity of RF-DRG in general.

Thoracic RF-DRG has not been subjected to a controlled trial, but it might be effective for certain types of thoracic pain for which there is no analogue at cervical and lumbar levels. The available data hint at the possibility that thoracic RF-DRG could be useful for postsurgical pain, although not for neuralgias.

PULSED RADIOFREQUENCY

A pivotal study precipitated what was to become the most recent evolution of RF treatment. Slappendel et al.[92] compared the outcomes of cervical RF-DRG in patients treated with lesions made at 40°C or 67°C. They found no significant difference (Table 13.1) between the outcomes in the two groups. The investigators interpreted this result as indicating that 40°C lesions and 67°C lesions were equally effective, and inferred that the efficacy was due to an effect other than a thermal lesion. A competing interpretation – that neither intervention was effective and that all responses were due to a placebo effect – was declined.

The interpretation of equal 'effectiveness' prompted a search for an explanation of a mechanism other than a heat lesion. The

Table 13.1. The results of RF-DRG at two different temperatures[92]

	Temperature	
	67°C	**40°C**
No. of patients	32	29
VAS pain scale (0–10) score (mean ± SD)		
Baseline	6.7 ± 1.6	6.3 ± 2.1
6 weeks	4.8 ± 3.5	4.9 ± 2.7
3 months	5.0 ± 2.9	4.4 ± 2.9
No. with a VAS score of 0–1 at 3 months	4	3

following hypothesis emerged: irrespective of the heat produced, a RF current is therapeutic because of electrical effects it had on the target nerve, which gave rise to another mode of applying RF current. That procedure became pulsed RF.[93]

Theory

The theory of pulsed RF is that the tip of the electrode delivers a large current density, estimated as 2×10^4 A/m²[.93] This current can be applied to a nerve, without heating it, and without creating a histological lesion, by delivering the current in very brief pulses. The recommended protocol involves delivering a current of 500,000 Hz in 20-ms pulses, at a frequency of 2/second. By limiting the delivery of current in this manner, the relatively long pause between pulses allows any heat generated to dissipate and thereby prevents the development of any thermal lesion. Heat is further minimized by limiting the electrode-tip temperature to less than 42°C. Meanwhile, the electric current, and its purported therapeutic effect, is delivered to the nerve. As the greatest density of the electric field is near the tip of the electrode, the applied current is densest distal to the tip of the electrode. This rationale allows the electrode to be applied perpendicular to the target nerve.

Physiology

The pulsed RF theory explicitly maintains that no lesion is created in the nerve.[93] The fact that no histological lesion is created has been borne out by laboratory studies.

A study that predated the concept of pulsed RF showed that applying a continuous RF current to a peripheral nerve, with a tip temperature of 40–45°C, resulted in reversible conduction block in the nerve.[94] Upon cessation of the current, conduction promptly reverted to normal. The same effect was achieved by heating the nerve using water circulated through a coil around the nerve.[94]

Thus, heating a nerve to low temperatures (40–45°C) temporarily blocks conduction along the nerve, but the rapid recovery of function indicates that no physiological lesion is produced. These experiments do not exclude a possible induced electrical effect of the RF current, but the fact that heated water

achieved the same effect strongly suggests that it is the low level of heat produced, not the current itself, which is responsible for the temporary conduction block.

In a study using slices of hippocampus as the target tissue,[95] two protocols of pulsed RF (one at 38°C and one at 42°C) and a 42°C continuous ('thermal') RF current were applied for 120 seconds. The continuous current reduced the excitatory postsynaptic potentials (EPSPs) to less than 50% of normal amplitude, for the duration of the experiment (25 minutes). The 38°C pulsed RF reduced the EPSPs to 75% of normal amplitude for 5 minutes after application; thereafter, normal amplitudes recovered. The 42°C pulsed RF reduced the EPSPs to 50% of normal amplitude for 5 minutes; thereafter normal amplitudes recovered.

Beyond 2000 µm from the electrode (which had a diameter of 1mm), neither of the pulsed RF protocols produced any lesions in the tissue; neither did the continuous thermal protocol. Between 500 and 1000 µm tissue damage occurred with the thermal protocol but not with either pulsed protocols. Within 500 µm all of the protocols tested produced tissue damage.

These results show the expected effect of even a low-temperature, continuous RF thermal RF lesion. Tissues were coagulated to a distance slightly greater than one electrode-width from the surface of the electrode. This coagulation was consistent with marked reduction in function of the affected tissues (EPSP > 50% reduced for at least 25 minutes).

In contrast, both pulsed RF protocols produced only a minimal lesion immediately around the surface of the electrode (< 0.5 mm). Although neural function was suppressed, the effect was only transient (5 minutes), which is consistent with no significant permanent lesion having been made.

A third study examined the effects on cells in the dorsal horn of the rat spinal cord following pulsed RF application to the C6 DRG.[96] The C6 DRG was exposed to continuous RF or pulsed RF at 38°C. The animals were sacrificed 3 hours after exposure, and immunohistochemical assays for c-fos reactivity performed. Animals treated with pulsed RF at 38°C exhibited increased expression of c-fos in lamina I and lamina II. These effects were not seen in animals treated with continuous RF at 38°C.

Somewhat contrary results were obtained in another study,[97] which examined the effects on dorsal horn cells of both continuous and pulsed RF applied to the C6 DRG. Sham treatment was used for comparison. Both forms of RF application induced increased c-fos expression in the dorsal horn. This contradicts a specific effect attributable to delivering the current in pulses.

Collectively the results of these studies provide extremely limited insight into the potential physiological effects of pulsed RF. The study by Brodkey et al.[94] did not address the effects of pulsed RF; but it established a reference point. Heating a nerve temporarily blocks the conduction along it. This is compatible with the effects, observed by Cahana et al.,[95] caused by a continuous 42°C RF lesion, but not pulsed RF at 38°C or 42°C.

In contrast to continuous RF lesions, pulsed RF seems to have limited effects. It transiently suppresses, but does not abolish, EPSPs in tissue slices,[94] and also seems to activate a subset of central spinal cord neurons.[95] Specifically, however, pulsed RF does not produce a tissue lesion. Any therapeutic effect, therefore, would seem to be akin to a brief and mild electrical stimulation, perhaps not unlike the effects of a brief application of transcutaneous nerve stimulator or an implanted nerve stimulator.

Finding that pulsed RF, and continuous RF for that matter, increase expression of *c-fos* does not provide an explanation for the effects of RF. Expression of *c-fos* is no more than a marker of increased cellular metabolic activity; it is not even specific for nociceptive pathways. It indicates only that cells are activated by RF. It does not distinguish between inhibitory and excitatory activity. It is not evidence that patients will be relieved of their pain. For such reasons, an editorial[98] concluded that basic scientific studies in the neurobiology of pain models and analgesic techniques are not a substitute for randomized controlled clinical trials, and studies such as that by van Zundert et al.[97] do not justify using the technique clinically.

Pathology

Studies have explicitly examined the pathological effects of pulsed RF in laboratory animals. In one study, neither continuous RF nor pulsed RF, at 42°C, produced any lasting effects on a DRG.[6] Both types of treatment produced oedema at 2 days, which was resolved by 21 days; but the DRG cells remained structurally normal. Similar effects were observed when the same lesions were applied to a sciatic nerve.[6]

In another study no structural lesions were found on light microscopy following application to a DRG of either a continuous RF current at 67°C or a pulsed RF current at 42°C.[99] Electron microscopy, however, did show some changes. In the ganglia treated with continuous RF at 67°C, DRG neurons exhibited numerous, giant cytoplasmic vacuoles fused with each other, and enlarged endoplasmic reticulum cisterns; in some cells there was loss of integrity of nuclear and neurolemma membranes. In the ganglia treated with pulsed RF at 42°C enlargements of endoplasmic reticulum cisterns were observed, along with some vacuole groups, in DRG cells, but membranes were intact. Following either treatment, myelinated and unmyelinated nerve fibres remained morphologically normal. These morphology studies corroborated the inference from the physiology studies, i.e. that pulsed RF does not produce a lesion in the nerves treated.

Efficacy

Clinical data on the efficacy of pulsed RF are extremely limited. The worldwide popularity of pulsed RF treatment is severely disproportionate to the volume and quality of the available peer-reviewed literature.

One publication[93] has reported two briefly described studies. In the first, patients were said to be treated either with pulsed RF or with continuous RF applied to a DRG. The anatomical location of the target nerve (cervical, lumbar) was not given. Both forms of RF were delivered at 42°C. Table 13.2 shows the results at 6 weeks. No other outcome measures were provided.

The effects of continuous RF were dismal. Indeed, the authors commented that they abandoned this intervention

Table 13.2. The reported results of pulsed RF treatment[93]

Treatment	No. of patients	Global perceived effect		
		> 75%	50–75%	< 50%
Continuous RF	24	1 (4%)	2 (8%)	21 (88%)
Pulsed RF	36	20 (56%)	11 (30%)	5 (14%)

because of the high failure rate.[1] Intriguingly, this outcome and appraisal of continuous RF is at direct odds with how Slappendel et al.[92] portrayed their outcomes with the same procedure. Slappendel et al.[92] considered their meagre outcomes with 40°C RF-DRG to be sufficient to warrant exploration of the mechanism by which it was 'therapeutic'; which in turn was the step that gave rise to pulsed RF. It is clearly ironic, therefore, that Sluijter et al.[93] found and considered the results of the identical procedure to be so dismal as to warrant abandonment.

Meanwhile, the results of pulsed RF in this study were obviously better, at least at 6 weeks. Unfortunately, the report of outcomes was severely limited. Global perceived effect is not the same as relief of pain; and no other outcome measures were provided. Nor was there any longer term follow-up. At best, it can only be deduced from this study that pulsed RF appears to offer a short-term benefit to some patients with radicular pain.

The second study[93] involved 15 patients with persistent leg pain after surgery, who responded to diagnostic spinal nerve blocks. Eight were said to have obtained a 'satisfactory' result, defined as a greater than 2-point improvement in pain scores (range 2–4) at 6 months after treatment. Two of these patients had a recurrence of pain between 6 and 12 months. The fate of the others was not reported.

This definition of success is somewhat generous, and the sample size is quite small. Although these data suggest some degree of benefit, the results cannot be attributed to pulsed RF, as no controls were used.

Much of the remaining literature on pulsed RF is limited to case reports, in which authors have claimed success in treating post-traumatic headache,[100] post-tonsillectomy pain,[101] inguinal pain and orchialgia[102] or trigeminal neuralgia.[103] Without controls, these case reports do not provide evidence of efficacy. In some instances, patients received cointerventions at the target site, in the form of injection of local anaesthetic and corticosteroids.[100, 101]

In one study,[104] the target for pulsed RF was the medial branches of the cervical and lumbar dorsal rami. The authors reported that 68/114 (60%) patients obtained at least 50% relief of pain for a minimum of 1.5 months. On average, the relief lasted for 3.9 ± 1.9 months. These results paint, at best, a very modest picture of the efficacy of pulsed RF delivered to the medial branches. No patients were rendered pain-free, and relief persisted for only a very short period. Meanwhile, the benchmark set by cervical medial branch neurotomy is complete relief of pain in 70% of patients for up to a year or more. Furthermore, there was no control group. For relief that is moderate in

PRACTICE POINTS

Basic science

- RF lesions are small.
- Accurate placement requires knowledge of the size, course and radiographic landmarks of target nerves, and extreme surgical precision.
- RF lesions do not selectively destroy only nociceptive afferents.

Trigeminal neuralgia

- RF thermocoagulation is indicated when conservative treatment fails or is not tolerated.
- It offers advantages over open surgery for the aged, medically unfit or younger patients who elect not to accept the risks of posterior fossa surgery.
- Its role in pain management has been established on the basis of a large, but uncontrolled, documented clinical experience.

DREZ procedures

- The indication for this procedure is intractable deafferentation pain, particularly after brachial plexus avulsion or spinal cord injury.
- Evidence of effectiveness is limited to uncontrolled case series.
- The potential for neurological side-effects is considerable.

Lumbar medial branch neurotomy

- Much effort has been squandered promulgating and perpetuating versions of this procedure that lack a correct anatomical basis.
- Controlled trials have refuted those techniques with a flawed anatomical basis.
- For anatomically valid versions of this procedure, the literature is almost non-existent.
- Nevertheless, in carefully selected patients, good outcomes can be achieved, provided correct technique is used.

Cervical medial branch neurotomy

- Provided that a correct technique is used, this procedure has proven efficacy.
- It is applicable only to patients whose neck pain can be relieved by controlled medial branch blocks.
- There is no evidence to support less rigorous techniques.

Radiofrequency-DRG

- A controlled trial has refuted any efficacy for this procedure in the lumbar spine.
- The same study also cast doubt on the efficacy of this procedure at the cervical or thoracic level.

Pulsed RF

- This procedure is based on an untested theory.
- Laboratory studies have provided no biological basis for efficacy.
- Due to lack of controls, case studies do not provide evidence of efficacy.
- Case series indicate marginal effectiveness that may not be greater than placebo.

magnitude and limited in duration, such as that reported for pulsed RF of the medial branches, controls are essential in order to exclude non-specific treatment effects. For reference, Marks et al.[105] found that 21% of their patients reported good relief continuing at 1 month, and 14% at 3 months, simply after undergoing anaesthetic medial branch blocks.

An audit of selected patients, by advocates of pulsed RF[106] introduced an additional indication. The authors described 18 patients with chronic neck and arm pain, who were selected for treatment if they obtained at least 50% relief of their pain following diagnostic segmental nerve blocks. They underwent pulsed RF of the DRG of the previously anaesthetized nerve. Of these patients, 13 reported a greater than 50% improvement at 6–8 weeks, this number diminishing to 10 by 3–11 months and to 6 at 1 year. The authors were guarded in their discussion. They wrote that: 'this clinical audit ... does not allow us to draw definitive conclusions'. Nevertheless, they offered that the results justify 'the start of a randomized controlled trial'. That trial has been concluded, but the results have not yet been published.

DISCUSSION

Only two RF procedures used for pain are based on solid evidence. Trigeminal thermocoagulation has a long history of success, audited over many years, by many practitioners. So established is its reputation that there is no justification for a controlled trial. Cervical medial branch neurotomy has a shorter history, but the results of a placebo-controlled trial have been resoundingly positive, and supported by several, long-term follow-up studies.

Lumbar medial branch neurotomy has a chequered past, characterized by enthusiasm based on contentious outcome data, and in the absence of a controlled trial. Much clinical and

RESEARCH AGENDA

Basic science

- Repeat experiments to determine the physiological effects of RF thermocoagulation on peripheral nerves are overdue.
- Such experiments should assess the effects on conduction in A-α, A-β, A-δ and C fibres of heat lesions generated at different temperatures and at different displacements from the target nerve.
- The duration of effect should be compared with the reported duration of effect in clinical studies.

Radiofrequency procedures

- A controlled trial of the effect of pulsed RF is needed to determine its efficacy.
- Controlled trials are required to determine the efficacy of lumbar RF neurotomy when performed using accurate techniques.
- Replication studies of cervical RF neurotomy are required to allay persisting resistance to this intervention.

intellectual effort was wasted generating publications that did not recognize the anatomical errors of the technique, and which did not advance the cause of evidence. This social phenomenon set the scene for subsequent developments.

RF-DRG was rapidly adopted once it was conceived. Enthusiasm rose despite the absence of compelling evidence of efficacy, and despite a specious rationale. It took 10 years for a controlled trial to be conducted. That trial vindicated the scepticism that the procedure had attracted. The trial showed an effect no greater than that of placebo, and perhaps even less.

The history, to date, of pulsed RF has followed the same pattern. The procedure has been widely adopted, despite a lack of evidence, and despite a particularly questionable rationale. The scene is set for a controlled trial to refute this procedure as well.

REFERENCES

1. Organ LW. Electrophysiologic principles of radiofrequency making. *Appl Neurophysiol* 1976; **39**: 69–76.
2. Bogduk N, Macintosh J, Marsland A. A technical limitation to efficacy of radiofrequency neurotomy for spinal pain. *Neurosurgery* 1987; **20**: 529–535.
3. Lord SM, McDonald GJ, Bogduk N. Percutaneous radiofrequency neurotomy of the cervical medial branches: a validated treatment for cervical zygapophyseal joint pain. *Neurosurg Quart* 1998; **8**: 288–308.
4. de Louw AJA, Vles HSH, Freling G et al. The morphological effects of a radiofrequency lesion adjacent to the dorsal root ganglion (RF-DRG) – an experimental study in the goat. *Eur J Pain* 2001; **5**: 169–174.
5. Smith HP, McWhorter JM, Challa VR. Radiofrequency neurolysis in a clinical model: neuropathological correlation. *J Neurosurg* 1981; **55**: 246–253.
6. Podhajsky RJ, Sekiguchi Y, Kikuchi S et al. The histological effects of pulsed and continuous radiofrequency lesions at 42°C to rat dorsal root ganglion and sciatic nerve. *Spine* 2005; **30**: 1008–1013.
7. Hamann W, Hall S. Acute effect and recovery of primary afferent nerve fibres after graded radiofrequency lesions in anaesthetized rats. *Br J Anaesth* 1992; **68**: 443P.
8. Letcher FS, Goldring S. The effect of radiofrequency current and heat on peripheral nerve action potential in the cat. *J Neurosurg Sci* 1968; **29**: 42–47.
9. Dreyfuss P, Halbrook B, Pauza K et al. Efficacy and validity of radiofrequency neurotomy for chronic lumbar zygapophyseal joint pain. *Spine* 2000; **25**: 1270–1277.
10. Peters G, Nurmikko TJ. Peripheral and Gasserian ganglion-level procedures for the treatment of trigeminal neuralgia. *Clin J Pain* 2002; **18**: 28–34.
11. Zakrzewska JM, Jassim S, Bulman JS. A prospective, longitudinal study on patients with trigeminal neuralgia who underwent radiofrequency thermo-coagulation of the Gasserian ganglion. *Pain* 1999; **79**: 51–58.
12. Kanpolat Y, Savas A, Bekar A et al. Percutaneous controlled radiofrequency trigeminal rhizotomy for the treatment of idiopathic trigeminal neuralgia: 25-year experience with 1600 patients. *Neurosurgery* 2001; **48**: 524–534.
13. Wilkins RH. Trigeminal neuralgia: historical overview, with emphasis on surgical treatment. In: Burchiel K (ed.), *Surgical Management of Pain*. Thieme, New York, 2002, pp. 288–303.
14. Sweet WH, Wepsic JG. Controlled thermocoagulation of trigeminal ganglion and rootlets for differential destruction of pain fibres: 1st trigeminal neuralgia. *J Neurosurg* 1974; **39**: 143–157.
15. Lopez BC, Hamlyn PJ, Zakrzewska JM. Systematic review of ablative neurosurgical techniques for the treatment of trigeminal neuralgia. *Neurosurgery* 2004; **54**: 973–983.
16. Latchaw JP, Hardy RW, Forsythe SB et al. Trigeminal neuralgia treated by radiofrequency coagulation. *J Neurosurg* 1983; **59**: 479–484.
17. Oturai AB, Jensen K, Eriksen J et al. Neurosurgery for trigeminal neuralgia: comparison of alcohol block, neurectomy, and radiofrequency coagulation. *Clin J Pain* 1996; **12**: 311–315.
18. Nashold BS, Urban B, Zorub DS. Phantom pain relief by focal destruction of the substantia gelatinosa of Rolando. *Adv Pain Res Ther* 1976; **1**: 959–963.
19. Nashold BS, Ostdahl RH. Dorsal root entry zone lesions for pain relief. *J Neurosurg* 1979; **51**: 59–69.
20. Nashold BS, Ovelmen-Levitt JM, Sharp R et al. Intraoperative evoked potentials recorded in man directly from dorsal roots and spinal cord. *J Neurosurg* 1985; **62**: 680–693.
21. Tomas R, Haninec P. Dorsal root entry zone (DREZ) localization using direct spinal cord stimulation can improve results of the DREZ thermocoagulation procedure for intractable pain relief. *Pain* 2005; **116**: 159–163.
22. Friedman AH, Bullitt E. Dorsal root entry zone lesions in the treatment of pain following brachial plexus avulsion, spinal cord injury and herpes zoster. *Appl Neurophysiol* 1988; **51**: 164–169.
23. Campbell JN, Solomon CT, James CS. The Hopkins experience with lesions of the dorsal horn (Nashold's operation) for pain from avulsion of the brachial plexus. *Appl Neurophysiol* 1988; **51**: 170–174.
24. Friedman AH, Nashold BS Jr, Bronec PR. Dorsal root entry zone lesions for the treatment of brachial plexus avulsion injuries: a follow-up study. *Neurosurgery* 1988; **22**: 369–373.
25. Thomas DG, Kitchen ND. Long-term follow up of dorsal root entry zone lesions in brachial plexus avulsion. *J Neurol Neurosurg Psychiatry* 1994; **57**: 737–738.
26. Rath SA, Seitz K, Soliman N et al. DREZ coagulations for deafferentation pain related to spinal and peripheral nerve lesions: indication and results of 79 consecutive procedures. *Stereotact Funct Neurosurg* 1997; **68**: 161–167.
27. Prestor B. Microsurgical junctional DREZ coagulation for treatment of deafferentation pain syndromes. *Surg Neurol* 2001; **56**: 259–265.
28. Nashold BS, Bullitt E. Dorsal root entry zone lesions to control central pain in paraplegics. *J Neurosurg* 1981; **55**: 414–419.
29. Friedman AH, Nashold BS. DREZ lesions for relief of pain related to spinal cord injury. *J Neurosurg* 1986; **65**: 465–9.
30. Sampson JH, Cashman RE, Nashold BS Jr et al. Dorsal root entry zone lesions for intractable pain after trauma to the conus medullaris and cauda equina. *J Neurosurg* 1995; **82**: 28–34.
31. Sindou M, Mertens P, Wael M. Microsurgical DREZotomy for pain due to spinal cord and/or cauda equina injuries: long-term results in a series of 44 patients. *Pain* 2001; **92**: 159–171.
32. Spaic M, Markovic N, Tadic R. Microsurgical DREZotomy for pain of spinal cord and Cauda equina injury origin: clinical characteristics of pain and implications for surgery in a series of 26 patients. *Acta Neurochir* 2002; **144**: 453–462.
33. Falci S, Best L, Bayles R et al. Dorsal root entry zone microcoagulation for spinal cord injury-related central pain: operative intramedullary electrophysiological guidance and clinical outcome. *J Neurosurg* 2002; **97**(Suppl 2): 193–200.
34. Saris SC, Iacono RP, Nashold BS Jr. Successful treatment of phantom pain with dorsal root entry zone coagulation. *Appl Neurophysiol* 1988; **51**: 188–197.
35. Bullard DE, Nashold BS Jr. The caudalis DREZ for facial pain. *Stereotact Funct Neurosurg* 1997; **68**: 168–174.
36. Gorecki JP, Nashold BS. The Duke experience with the nucleus caudalis DREZ operation. *Acta Neurochir* 1995; **64**(Suppl): 128–131.
37. Rossitch E Jr, Zeidman SM, Nashold BS Jr. Nucleus caudalis DREZ for facial pain due to cancer. *Br J Neurosurg* 1989; **3**: 45–49.
38. Bernard EJ Jr, Nashold BS Jr, Caputi F et al. Nucleus caudalis DREZ lesions for facial pain. *Br J Neurosurg* 1987; **1**: 81–91.
39. Shealy CN. Facets in back and sciatic pain. A new approach to a major pain syndrome. *Minn Med* 1974; **57**: 199–203.
40. Shealy CN. The role of the spinal facets in back and sciatic pain. *Headache* 1974; **14**: 101–104.
41. Shealy CN. Percutaneous radiofrequency denervation of spinal facets. *J Neurosurg* 1975; **43**: 448–451.
42. Shealy CN. Facet denervation in the management of back sciatic pain. *Clin Orthop* 1976; **115**: 157–164.
43. Bogduk N, Long DM. The anatomy of the so-called 'articular nerves' and their relationship to facet denervation in the treatment of low back pain. *J Neurosurg* 1979; **51**: 172–177.
44. Bogduk N, Long DM. Percutaneous lumbar medial branch neurotomy. A modification of facet denervation. *Spine* 1980; **5**: 193–200.
45. Bogduk N, Macintosh J, Marsland A. Technical limitations to the efficacy of radiofrequency neurotomy for spinal pain. *Neurosurgery* 1987; **20**: 529–535.
46. Lau P, Mercer S, Govind J et al. The surgical anatomy of lumbar medial branch neurotomy (facet denervation). *Pain Med* 2004; **5**: 289–298.
47. Geurts JW, van Wijk RM, Stolker RJ et al. Efficacy of radiofrequency procedures for the treatment of spinal pain: a systematic review of randomized clinical trials. *Region Anesth Pain Med* 2001; **26**: 394–400.
48. Niemisto L, Kalso E, Malmivaara A et al. Radiofrequency denervation for neck and back pain: a systematic review within the framework of the Cochrane Collaboration Back Review Group. *Spine* 2003; **28**: 1877–1888.
49. Bogduk N. In defense of radiofrequency neurotomy [Letter to the Editor]. *Reg Anesth Pain Med* 2002; **27**: 439–440.
50. Hooten WM, Martin DP, Huntoon MA. Radiofrequency neurotomy for low back pain: evidence-based procedural guidelines. *Pain Med* 2005; **6**: 129–138.

51. van Kleef M, Barendse GAM, Kessels A et al. Randomized trial of radiofrequency lumbar facet denervation for chronic low back pain. *Spine* 1999; **24**: 1937–1942.

52. Dreyfuss P, Halbrook B, Pauza K et al. Efficacy and validity of radiofrequency neurotomy for chronic lumbar zygapophysial joint pain. *Spine* 2000; **25**: 1270–1277.

53. Schofferman J, Kine G. Effectiveness of repeated radiofrequency neurotomy for lumbar facet pain. *Spine* 2004; **29**: 2471–2473.

54. Van Wijk RMA, Geurts JWM, Wynne HJ et al. Radiofrequency denervation of lumbar facet joints in the treatment of chronic low back pain. A randomized, double-blind sham lesion-controlled trial. *Clin J Pain* 2004; **21**: 335–344.

55. Lord SM, Barnsley L, Bogduk N. Percutaneous radiofrequency neurotomy in the treatment of cervical zygapophysial joint pain: a caution. *Neurosurgery* 1995; **36**: 732–739.

56. Lord SM, Barnsley L, Wallis B et al. Percutaneous radio-frequency neurotomy for chronic cervical zygapophyseal joint pain. *N Engl J Med* 1996; **335**: 1721–1726.

57. Lord SM, McDonald GJ, Bogduk N. Percutaneous radiofrequency neurotomy of the cervical medial branches: a validated treatment for cervical zygapophyseal joint pain. *Neurosurg Quart* 1998; **8**: 288–308.

58. McDonald GJ, Lord SM, Bogduk N. Long term follow-up of patients treated with cervical radiofrequency neurotomy for chronic neck pain. *Neurosurgery* 1999; **45**: 61–68.

59. Govind J, King W, Bailey B et al. Radiofrequency neurotomy for the treatment of third occipital headache. *J Neurol Neurosurg Psychiatry* 2003; **74**: 88–93.

60. Barnsley L. Percutaneous radiofrequency neurotomy for chronic neck pain: outcomes in a series of consecutive patients. *Pain Med* 2005; **6**: 282–286.

61. Centre for Health Services and Policy Branch. *Percutaneous Radio-Frequency Neurotomy Treatment of Chronic Cervical Pain following Whiplash Injury.* Report No. 01: 5T. University of British Columbia, British Columbia Office of Health Technology Assessment, Vancouver, 2001.

62. Sapir DA, Gorup JM. Radiofrequency medial branch neurotomy in litigant and nonlitigant patients with cervical whiplash. *Spine* 2001; **26**: E268–E273.

63. Kanpolat Y. Percutaneous sterotactic pain procedures: percutaneous cordotomy, extralemniscal myelotomy, trigeminal tractotomy–nucleotomy. In: Burchiel K (ed.), *Surgical Management of Pain.* Thieme, New York, 2002, pp. 745–761.

64. Stolker RJ, Vervest ACM, Groen GJ. Percutaneous facet denervation in chronic thoracic spinal pain. *Acta Neurochir* 1993; **122**: 82–90.

65. Chua WH, Bogduk N. The surgical anatomy of thoracic facet denervation. *Acta Neurochir* 1995; **136**: 140–144.

66. Wilkinson HA. Percutaneous radiofrequency upper thoracic sympathectomy. *Neurosurgery* 1996; **38**: 715–725.

67. Forouzanfar T, van Kleef M, Weber WEJ. Radiofrequency lesions of the stellate ganglion in chronic pain syndromes: retrospective analysis of clinical efficacy in 86 patients. *Clin J Pain* 2000; **16**: 164–168.

68. Geurts JWR, Stolker RJ. Percutaneous radiofrequency lesion of the stellate ganglion in the treatment of pain in the upper extremity reflex sympathetic dystrophy. *Pain Clin* 1993; **6**: 17–25.

69. Sanders M, Zuurmond WW. Efficacy of sphenopalatine ganglion blockade in 66 patients suffering from cluster headache: a 12- to 70-month follow-up evaluation. *J Neurosurg* 1997; **87**: 876–880.

70. Salar G, Ori C, Iob I et al. Percutaneous thermocoagulation for sphenopalatine ganglion neuralgia. *Acta Neurochir* 1987; **84**: 24–28.

71. Salar G, Iob I, Ori C. Combined thermocoagulation of the 5th and 9th cranial nerves for oral pain of neoplastic aetiology. *J Maxillofac Surg* 1986; **14**: 1–4.

72. Salar G, Ori C, Baratto V et al. Selective percutaneous thermolesions of the ninth cranial nerve by lateral cervical approach: report of eight cases. *Surg Neurol* 1983; **20**: 276–279.

73. Van Kleef, Barendse GAM, Wilmink JT. Percutaneous intradiscal radiofrequency thermocoagulation in chronic non-specific low back pain. *Pain Clin* 1996; **9**: 259–268.

74. Troussier B, Lebas JF, Cirosel JP et al. Percutaneous intradiscal radio-frequency thermocoagulation: a cadaveric study. *Spine* 1995; **20**: 1713–1718.

75. Houpt JC, Conner ES, McFarland EW. Experimental study of temperature distributions and thermal transport during radiofrequency current therapy of the intervertebral disc. *Spine* 1996; **21**: 1808–1813.

76. Barendse GAM, van den Berg SGM, Kessels AHF et al. Randomized controlled trial of percutaneous intradiscal radiofrequency thermocoagulation for chronic discogenic back pain. *Spine* 1996; **26**: 287–292.

77. Karasek M, Bogduk N. Twelve-month follow-up of a controlled trail of intradiscal thermal anuloplasty for back pain due to internal disc disruption. *Spine* 2000; **25**: 2601–2607.

78. Bogduk N, Karasek M. Two-year follow-up of a controlled trial of intradiscal electrothermal anuloplasty for chronic low back pain resulting from internal disc disruption. *Spine J* 2002; **2**: 343–350.

79. Finch PM, Price LM, Drummond PD. Radiofrequency heating of painful annular disruptions. One-year outcomes. *J Spinal Disord Tech* 2005; **18**: 6–13.

80. Pauza KJ, Howell S, Dreyfuss P et al. A randomised, placebo-controlled trial of intradiscal electrothermal therapy for the treatment of discogenic low back pain. *Spine J* 2004; **4**: 27–35.

81. Bogduk N, Lau P, Govind J et al. Intradiscal electrothermal therapy. *Techniques Region Anesthes Pain Manage* 2005; **9**: 25–34.

82. van Kleef M, Spaans F, Dingemans W et al. Effects and side effects of a percutaneous thermal lesion of the dorsal root ganglion in patients with cervical pain syndrome. *Pain* 1993; **52**: 49–53.

83. Stolker RJ, Vervest ACM, Groen GJ. The treatment of chronic thoracic segmental pain by radiofrequency percutaneous partial rhizotomy. *J Neurosurg* 1994; **80**: 986–992.

84. van Kleef M, Barendse GAM, Dingemans WAAM et al. Effects of producing a radiofrequency lesion adjacent to the dorsal root ganglion in patients with thoracic segmental pain. *Clin J Pain* 1995; **11**: 325–332.

85. van Kleef M, Liem L, Lousberg R et al. Radiofrequency lesion adjacent to the dorsal root ganglion for cervicobrachial pain. a prospective double-blind study. *Neurosurgery* 1996; **38**: 1127–1132.

86. van Kleef M, Barendse G, Sluijter M. Assessing a new procedure: thoracic radiofrequency dorsal root ganglion lesions [Response to Invited Commentary]. *Clin J Pain* 1996; **12**: 76–78.

87. Bogduk N. Assessing a new procedure: thoracic radiofrequency dorsal root ganglion lesions [Invited Commentary]. *Clin J Pain* 1996; **12**: 76–78.

88. Stolker RJ, Vervest ACM, Ramos LMP et al. Electrode positioning in thoracic percutaneous partial rhizotomy: an anatomical study. *Pain* 1994; **57**: 241–251.

89. van Wijk RMAW, Geurts J, Wynne HJ. Long-lasting analgesic effect of radiofrequency treatment of the lumbosacral dorsal root ganglion. *J Neurosurg (Spine 2)* 2001; **94**: 227–231.

90. van Kleef M, Liem L, Lousberg R et al. Radiofrequency lesion adjacent to the dorsal root ganglion for cervicobrachial pain. a prospective double-blind study. *Neurosurgery* 1996; **38**: 1127–1132.

91. Geurts JWM, can Wijk MAW, Wunne H et al. Radiofrequency lesioning of dorsal root ganglia for chronic lumbosacral radicular pain: a randomized, double-blind, controlled trial. *Lancet* 2003; **361**: 21–26.

92. Slappendel R, Crui BJP, Braak GJJ et al. The efficacy of radiofrequency lesioning of the cervical spinal dorsal root ganglion in a double blinded randomized study: no difference between 40°C and 67°C treatments. *Pain* 1997; **73**: 159–163.

93. Sluijter ME, Vosman ER, Rittman WB et al. The effects of pulsed radiofrequency fields applied to the dorsal root ganglion – a preliminary report. *Pain Clin* 1998; **11**: 109–117.

94. Brodkey JS, Miyazaki Y, Ervin FR et al. Reversible heat lesions with radiofrequency current. A method of stereotactic localization. *J Neurosurg* 1964; **21**: 49–53.

95. Cahana A, Vutskits L, Muller D. Acute differential modulation of synaptic transmission and cell survival during exposure to pulsed and continuous radiofrequency energy. *J Pain* 2003; **4**: 197–202.

96. Higuchi Y, Nashold B, Sluijter M et al. Exposure of the dorsal root ganglion in rats to pulsed radiofrequency currents activates dorsal horn lamina I and II neurons. *Neurosurgery* 2002; **50**: 850–856.

97. van Zundert J, de Louw AJA, Joosten EAJ et al. Pulsed and continuous radiofrequency current adjacent to the cervical dorsal root ganglion of the rat induces late cellular activity in the dorsal horn. *Anesthesiology* 2005; **102**: 125–131.

98. Richebe P, Rathmell JP, Brennan T. Immediate early genes after pulsed radiofrequency treatment: neurobiology in need of clinical trials. *Anesthesiology* 2005; **102**: 1–3.

99. Erdine S, Yucel A, Cunen A et al. Effects of pulsed versus conventional radiofrequency current on rabbit dorsal root ganglion morphology. *Eur J Pain* 2005; **9**: 251–256.

100. Shah RV, Racz G. Long-term relief of posttraumatic headache by spheno-palatine ganglion pulsed radiofrequency lesioning: a case report. *Arch Phys Med Rehab* 2004; **85**: 1013–1016.

101. Shah RV, Racz BG. Pulsed mode radiofrequency lesioning to treat chronic post-tonsillectomy pain (secondary glossopharyngeal neuralgia). *Pain Pract* 2003; **3**: 232–237.

102. Cohen SP, Foster A. Pulsed radiofrequency as a treatment for groin pain and orchialgia. *Urology* 2003; **61**: 645xxi–645xxiii.

103. van Zundert J, Brabant S, van de Kelft E, Vercruyssen A et al. Pulsed radiofrequency treatment of the Gasserian ganglion in patients with idiopathic trigeminal neuralgia. *Pain* 2003; **104**: 449–452.

104. Mikeladze G, Espinal R, Finnegan R et al. Pulsed radiofrequency application in treatment of chronic zygapophyseal joint pain. *Spine J* 2003; **3**: 360–362.

105. Marks RC, Houston T, Thulbourne T. Facet joint injection and facet nerve block: a randomised comparison in 86 patients with chronic low back pain. *Pain* 1992; **49**: 325–328.

106. Van Zundert A, Lamé IE, de Louw A et al. Percutaneous pulsed radiofrequency treatment of the cervical dorsal root ganglion in the treatment of chronic cervical pain syndromes: a clinical audit. *Neuromodulation* 2003; **6**: 6–14.

SECTION 5
Regional pain

Chapter 14

Clinical examination as a tool to identify the origin of regional musculoskeletal pain

Bernard Fouquet

INTRODUCTION

Pain is the most prominent symptom and the commonest reason for seeking medical help for people with musculoskeletal disorders. The clinical assessment of pain must be both qualitative and quantitative. The physical examination may localize the anatomical origin of the pain and sometimes indicate the mechanical or inflammatory mechanisms underlying it.

The usual definition of pain is 'an unpleasant sensory and emotional experience, associated with actual or potential tissue damage or described in terms of such damage'.[1] Nociception refers to the reception of signals by the central nervous system evoked by the activation of specialized receptors, called nociceptors, by a noxious stimulus. Such a noxious stimulus is potentially or actually damaging to body tissue. Pain is always an individual and subjective experience.

Pain can be caused by nociceptive mechanisms and, in the absence of nerve tissue injury, is called nociceptive pain. Pain caused by nerve tissue injury is called neuropathic pain. Psychological mechanisms are often involved in the subjective experience of pain. Pain syndromes are nociceptive, neuropathic or psychogenic in nature, or combinations of two or three of these.[2] Because not all pain experience is the result of a noxious stimulus or an injury, and not all noxious stimuli lead to the experience of pain through neurological processes,[3, 4] it is the duty of the practitioner to understand that each painful condition is a complex individual state that can be influenced by several physiological and psychological factors. Some painful conditions may be 'just a window on the predicament of life'.[5]

Musculoskeletal pain is one of the commonest causes of primary care office visits and regional musculoskeletal pain (RMP) from the back, shoulder, neck, knee, hip, foot or hand is a major cause of morbidity, both in the community and in the workplace.[6] RMP may be analysed in two ways: as an actual or potential lesion of the musculoskeletal system causing nociceptive pain, or as aberrant somatosensory processing in the peripheral or central nervous system causing neuropathic pain. These two features of pain may coexist. There are many causes of RMP (Table 14.1). Taking an appropriate history and a clinical examination assists in differentiating these causes.

RMP should not be considered separately from the cognitive and behavioural components of pain. For example, in the work place organizational and economic factors (i.e. downsizing) affect sick leave in individuals who complain of musculoskeletal pain.[7–9] The observed increase in musculoskeletal disorders, particularly localized to the back, neck and shoulders, in association with these economic factors may be explained by an associated increase in physical demands placed on the workers, a reduction in their skill discretion and increased job insecurity.[10] In workplaces with a high proportion of older employees, major down-sizing may lead to a ten-fold increase in the risk of an individual developing musculoskeletal disorders when compared with a more minor downsizing.[7] Women are more prone to musculoskeletal problems than are men. Women seem to be vulnerable to the development and maintenance of musculoskeletal pain conditions due to a state of increased pain sensitivity from peripheral or central origin; biological and psychosocial factors may account for these differences.[11] Compared with men, women with mental distress have more primary care consultations in the workplace.[12]

Genetic factors, race and ethnicity may influence the experience of acute pain.[13] These genetic factors may underlie differences in the molecular biology of pain, but may also affect pain coping styles – the meaning of pain to the individual. Disparities in socio-economic status may also be important. Pain can have a major influence on pain-related emotional responses, such as depression, guilt and anxiety. Age is associated with impairment of the early warning functions of pain, mainly an increase in the pain perception threshold. This may place the older person at a greater risk of injury. A reduced efficacy of the endogenous analgesic systems may decrease tolerance to pain and slow the resolution of postinjury hyperalgesia.[14]

The clinical evaluation of RMP should be, as far as possible, completed at the initial interview.

In the following, the pathophysiology of the two main types of pain (nociceptive and neuropathic) is analysed and the main clinical characteristics associated with the two types of pain described.

THE PHYSIOLOGY OF PAIN

Understanding the pathogenesis of nociceptive and neuropathic pain is fundamental to understanding the objectives of the physical examination. The main elements and functions involved are: the nociceptors and their fibres; the locoregional reflexes associated with pain and leading to peripheral and central sensitization to pain-provoking stimuli; and the ascending and descending pathways of pain impulses and their modulations. All these factors are related to cerebral and spinal sensitization to pain.[15-20] Some of these elements associated with the transmission and modulation of a nociceptive stimulus may be detected during the clinical examination.

Table 14.1. Localizations and causes of RMP

	Joint or soft-tissue pain	Neuropathic pain
Localization	Capsule	Peripheral nerve
	Ligaments	Nerve root
	Muscle	Central nervous system
	Vascular components	
	Tendon	
	Peritendon	
	Bursa	
	Enthesis	
	Synovium	
Aetiology	*Soft-tissue diseases*	*Nerve*
	Tendinitis	Nerve Entrapment
	Tendinosis	Mononeuritis
	Enthesopathy	Polyneuritis
	Paratendon inflammation	
	Tendon rupture	*Radiculopathy*
	Tendon sheath diseases	Disc herniation
	Bursal inflammation	Spinal osteoarthritis or spondylosis
	Capsulitis	Radiculitis
	Muscle strain	Polyneuritis
	Delayed muscle soreness	
	Muscle cramps	*Central nervous system*
	Myopathies	Degenerative diseases
	Fatigue?	Vascular diseases
		Syringomyelia
	Joint diseases	Myelitis
	Osteoarthritis	Spinal cord compression
	Infectious monoarthritis	Metabolic diseases of the spinal cord
	Non-infectious inflammatory arthritis	

Joint and soft tissue pain

Sensory receptors are diffusely distributed not only in the joint in the capsule, ligaments and synovium, but also around the joint, in tendons, muscles, fascia, skin and perhaps in bone, and around the blood vessels.[20, 21] Two main types of receptor are identified: encapsulated receptors; and free nerve endings, which are predominantly near blood vessels.

Nociceptive pain

Pain impulses arise from nociceptors. A noxious stimulus activates a receptor responding to stimuli that cause tissue damage. Some receptors respond to mechanical stimuli (uni-modal receptors), others to mechanical and thermal stimuli, and others to chemical, thermal and mechanical (polymodal receptors).[20] Many data have established a dynamic competence of the sensory receptors which, as a function of the quality of the stimulus, send a noxious signal or not. Some receptors do not react to any mechanical stimulus (silent nociceptors). Many of these are C-fibres that are normally inactive and unresponsive to acute nociceptive stimuli. These C-fibres undergo gradual activation if the nociceptive stimuli persist, contributing to hyperalgesia.[21]

Three main types of fibres convey sensory input: heavily myelinated A-β fibres, which have a high conduction velocity and are associated with proprioception; thinly myelinated A-δ fibres, which have an intermediate conduction velocity; and unmyelinated C-fibres, which have a slow conduction velocity. Two main types of fibre conduct the inputs of the nociceptors: the A-δ fibres and the C-fibres.

Different anatomical structures in and around the joint are able to signal nociception. The cartilage is not normally innervated. The human synovium contains free nerve endings – sympathetic efferent fibres and unmyelinated C nociceptive afferents. The ligaments contain A-δ receptors and the capsule has unmyelinated C afferent fibres. In the tendons and muscles, a very wide distribution of receptors is observed from high to low threshold, including A-β, A-δ and free-nerve-ending receptors. The cell bodies of all somatic afferent fibres are located in the dorsal root ganglia. All the afferent sensory fibres converge to the dorsal horn, where they synapse with spinal neurons in the dorsal grey matter. Afferents from the noci-ceptors have synaptic connections with efferent neurons to skeletal ipsilateral or contralateral muscles, from the same spinal segment, but also from adjacent levels,[22] and with sympa-thetic efferents that cause localized vasoconstriction.

After a tissue injury, the nociceptors, both polymodal and silent, are sensitized by a decrease in their response threshold. This *primary sensitization* may be provoked or enhanced by prostaglandins, leucotrienes, a decrease in the pH, adenosine triphosphate (ATP) release from the muscle, bradykinin, different neurotransmitters (e.g. substance P (SP)), calcitonin gene-related peptide (CGRP), neurokinin, catecholamines, dynorphine, excitatory amino acids (e.g. glutamate) and nitric oxide. Prostaglandin, serotonin (protein kinase A) and bradykinin or histamine (protein kinase C) act on the C fibre membrane sodium channels, potentiating the hyperalgesia-inducing mechanisms.[23] These neurotransmitters may act directly on the free-nerve-ending nociceptors or indirectly through a sequential process initiated at spinal level. Some of them, such as SP and CGRP, promote hyperexcitability of the dorsal horn neurons and an expansion of the receptive fields. This sensitization explains alterations of sensitivity to light touch,[24] extension of the painful area (*secondary sensitization – secondary hyperalgesia*) and, to some degree, also explains the referred pain that is a zone of radiation of the perceived pain. This area of radiation is almost never in a clear neurological distribution, i.e. it does not follow the distribution of a peripheral nerve.

In the inflammatory rheumatic disorders, proinflammatory cytokines, such as tumour necrosis factors and other cytokines, including interleukin-1β (IL-1β), IL-6 and IL-8, augment activity in nociceptive pathways. They may cause sensitization directly or indirectly by triggering other cytokines or classical mediators of hyperalgesia such as prostanoids. Other cytokines, such as IL-4, IL-10 and IL-13, may inhibit the release of proinflammatory cytokines or inhibit cyclo-oxygenase activity and expression.

The liberation of SP and CGRP by the non-myelinated fibres, which are closely associated with blood vessels, may induce modifications of vascular tone, with resultant oedema, redness, heat and pain (*neurogenic inflammation*). In osteoarthritis, neurogenic inflammation, without any biological changes, may be associated with vascular changes in the synovial membranes.[25]

Subsequently, the nociceptive input through the nerve cells of the dorsal horn follows two principal routes of transmission: via the spinothalamic tract to the midbrain; and via a more diff-use polysynaptic tract that projects bilaterally to the brainstem reticular formation, which is called the spinoreticular tract and connects to the lateral thalamic nuclei (Figure 14.1). Different cortical areas that are involved in motor processes also seem to be active in acute and, particularly, in chronic pain states, probably through modifications of the motor memory process and of the motor anticipation process. It is only at this stage that the noxious input or stimulus is integrated as pain and associated with all the cortical and subcortical areas implicated in the cognitive and behavioural processing of pain. The subcortical and cortical areas are differently involved during acute and chronically painful conditions,[17] leading to different patterns of processing associated with central and cortical sensitization. Neuroplasticity allows the neurons in the brain to compensate for injury and adjust their activity in response to new situations or changes in their environment.[16] This cortical process of the nociceptive stimulus seems to be dependent on the behavioural components of the individual, but also on genetic characteristics[19] associated with factors such as greater basal pain sensitivity and reduced pain-inhibitory capacity, which may increase the risk of developing a chronic pain state.

Different descending pathways lying diffusely in the midbrain and spinal cord, such as the endogenous opioid system and the noradrenergic system, decrease nociceptive information in the spinal cord particularly at the level of the dorsal horn by presynaptic inhibition of the C-fibre neurotransmitter release (SP and CGRP). These descending pathways play a major role in the endogenous control of pain and in the process of central sensitization of pain. A dysfunction in the descending pathways leads to an increase in the noxious input by a decrease in the activity of the inhibitory interneurons. This enhances the peripheral sensitization.

Neuropathic pain

Unlike nociceptive pain, which initiates protective reflexes to limit further damage, pain from damaged neurological tissues, including nerve roots, plexi, peripheral nerves and the central nervous system, has no beneficial effect to the organism and is termed neuropathic pain.[26] Neuropathic pain is characterized by greatly reduced pain thresholds (mechanohyperalgesia or ther-

mal hyperalgesia) and sometimes by painful sensations caused by light touch (mechanical allodynia) or variations in temperature (thermal allodynia). Such pain may also occur spontaneously. While classification of neuropathic pain is frequently according to the type of underlying pathology, this distinction does not account for the possible mechanisms that may be present; for example, touch-evoked allodynia due to A-β fibre sensitization, static mechanoallodynia and hyperalgesia due to C-fibre sensitization, which may be associated with sympathetic hyperactivity.[27] In fact, despite the multiple lesions giving rise to neuropathic types of pain, many of these conditions are associated with a paradoxical combination of sensory loss and hyperalgesia in the painful area, causing paroxysms of pain and a gradual increase of pain following repetitive stimulation.

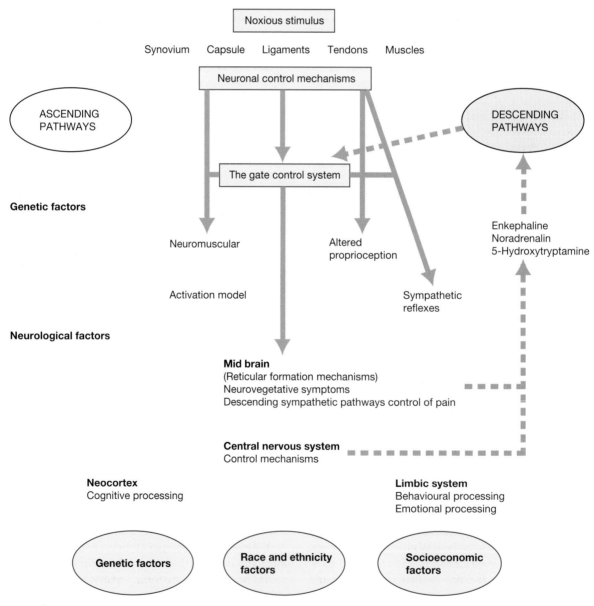

Figure 14.1. The pain process.

These painful phenomena may be explained by *hyperexcitability* of the peripheral and central nervous systems. This hyperexcitability is due to abnormalities of the ion channels leading to abnormal input (ectopic input or ectopia). These abnormal impulses occur in the absence of any permanent lesion. Moreover, it has been observed that abnormal sensitivity of peripheral nociceptors to catecholamines associated with an increase in the adrenergic innervations of the dorsal horn ganglia[3, 26, 27] leads to adrenosensitivity and sympathetically maintained pain. In the dorsal ganglia, it has been observed that some neurons with A-β fibres begin to express SP/CGRP after a peripheral injury which may be induced by nerve growth factor. In the dorsal horn rearrangements may be found. There is sprouting of A-β and A-δ fibres with postsynaptic structures that normally receive C-fibre input, and sympathetic sprouting that may induce coupling between sympathetic efferents and sensory neurons. These mechanisms may provoke *disinhibition*. The release of SP or CGRP may favour local sensitization. These compensatory responses in neuropathic pain evoke *fail-safe mechanisms*.

A reorganization of the cortical areas occurs as part of neuropathic pain. These changes make it impossible for the diffuse analgesic system to control endogenously the rate of inputs, leading to central disinhibition of pain.

Motor alterations

Due to synaptic connections with the motor neurons at different and adjacent spinal levels, motor alterations may occur very early in the course of a musculoskeletal disorder through changes in the myotonic reflexes, modifications of motor organization, modifications of the proprioceptive innervation of the muscles and tendons, and reorganization of the motor cortex associated with behaviour processing. In neuropathic pain, lipid atrophy of muscle fibres may be observed due to modifications of motor neuron tone, changes in the sympathetic system, modifications of vascular tone or genetic factors.

Aberrant movement patterns and postures are often seen in patients with nociceptive musculoskeletal pain. Both increases and decreases in muscle activity have been shown, along with alterations in neuronal mechanisms, proprioception and local muscle morphology. Muscle activation and recruitment are altered in the presence of noxious stimulus (neuromuscular activation model). These changes affect the ability of muscles to perform synergistic functions related to maintaining joint stability and control.[28] Tonic muscle pain can inhibit the motor system. Motor cortex inhibition is followed by a reduction in the excitability of both cortical and spinal motor neurons.[29]

The *pain adaptation model* is characterized by a decrease in motor activity from the spinal cord and the cortex in the agonist muscles and an increase in the antagonist muscles. These changes may be associated with altered patterns of motor recruitment, altered muscle coordination and proprioceptive deficits. In low back pain patients, for example, different abnormalities have been found, including a decrease in the recruitment of the multifidus during coordination exercises, delay in the recruitment of the trunk muscles during standing anticipation, absence of 'flexion relaxation' of the erector spinae during a total flexion movement, asymmetric muscle activation in smaller forward movements that seems to be driven by asymmetric contraction of the erector spinae and rectus abdominus muscles, and inhibition of the recruitment of the knee extensors. In wrist arthropathies, some patients demonstrate coactivation of the muscles that facilitates the fixation and immobilization of the hand and inhibits any muscular stretching. This phenomenon occurs in patients with pain from tendons and muscles and at rest. Some subjects coactivate muscles just at the end of the movement near to the painful position. In osteoarthritis of the knee, an early inhibition of the extensors has been found to be associated with alterations of proprioception of the knee. Muscle atrophy not correlated with pain is often observed, and in some cases fasciculations are seen.

Weakness and wasting of the muscles acting around a joint may be seen. This phenomenon, sometimes called 'arthrogenous muscle weakness', is associated with motor reflex inhibition, with immobilization, with reduction of voluntary muscle activation and with modification of proprioceptive feedback. All these modifications of the motor control of movement may be observed during the physical examination.

Muscle fatigue is another important manifestation frequently associated with musculoskeletal pain. In RMP, muscle fatigue is often localized but may be generalized. Muscular fatigue is a failure to maintain force at an expected level and is perceived both physically and mentally.[30] It derives from three mechanisms: from muscle itself, when it is due to accumulation of byproducts such as hydrogen ions, and phosphate and lactic acid accumulation; from changes in anterior horn cell performance, due to slowing of anterior horn cell discharges, sensory feedback from muscle spindles and abnormalities in the neuromuscular junction; and from central nervous system pathways, due to a sense derived from the cortical and somatosensory cortical areas that increased effort is required to maintain the same force. Modifications leading to muscle fatigue can arise both from noxious inputs and from neuropathic disorders.

CLINICAL EVALUATION OF REGIONAL MUSCULOSKELETAL PAIN

Taking the history of the pain and associated conditions is the first and fundamental step in making the diagnosis. The past history of the subject indicates diseases that may be associated with nervous system lesions, including trauma, spinal surgery, radiotherapy, metabolic causes (e.g. diabetes mellitus) and alcoholism. In the acute stage, the words used to describe the pain allow a distinction to be made between nociceptive and neuropathic pain (Table 14.2).

Nociceptive pain

Nociceptive pain, arising from tendons, ligaments or capsular structures, is fairly well localized.[31] Other signs may coexist, including stiffness, swelling and creaking or cracking (Figure 14.2). Pain that is worse in the morning or during the second part of the night suggests an inflammatory component,

Table 14.2. Words used when describing pain

	Joint or soft-tissue pain	Neuropathic pain
Functional terms	Deep pain	Dysaesthesia
	Burning	Neuralgia
	Cramps	Spontaneous
	Localized	Diffuse
		Fasciculations
Physical terms	Hyperalgesia	Hyperpathia
		Hyperalgesia
		Causalgia
		Hypoalgesia
		Hypoaesthesia

(1) History of the pathologic process of pain: 'How? When? Where? Duration?'

Nociceptive pain	Neuropathic pain	All
Stiffness	Electric shock/	Fatigue
Swelling	shooting type	Weakness
Cracking, clicking	Numbness/	
or creaking	paraesthesia	
Deformity	Neuropathic	
Non-neuropathic	referred pain	
referred pain		

(2) Associated with systemic diseases ('red flags'):
Fever
Night sweats
Weight loss

(3) Previous medical history ('red flags'):
Cancer
Infection
Inflammatory rheumatic disorders
Radiotherapy
Metabolic diseases

(4) Disability

(5) Emotional distress ('yellow flags')

Figure 14.2. Clinical diagnosis of RMP.

including neurogenic inflammation, as does pain occurring without any activity or movement. Even including referred pain, nociceptive pain does not affect the whole of a limb.[32]

In non-inflammatory RMP, noxious stimuli occur during physical activity or 1–3 hours after that activity. Periarticular pain arising from tendons is often induced by a specific type of activity, particularly leisure or occupational activities. Pain arising from ligaments often follows a traumatic event. Post-exertional muscle pain may occur 1–2 days after the activity, and is described as fatigue, weakness, stiffness or tightness in the area of the muscle.[30]

Neuropathic pain

Many patients describe persistent or paroxysmal pains that are independent of any mechanical stimulus. Neuropathic pain is more diffuse than nociceptive pain, and is characterized by paraesthesia distally to the causative neurological lesion and in the field of the nerve or root or plexus affected. Dysfunction of the nervous system gives rise to spontaneous excitation causing burning, pins and needles, or numbness, typically but not always in a neurological distribution.

Paraesthesiae are often masked by more severe sensations, such as electric-shock-like, shooting or burning pains. Some sensations are typical. For example, the sensation of wearing a tight wristband is typical of a median nerve lesion and the sensation of wearing a tight ankle band suggests a lesion of the L5 nerve root. Paraesthesiae are the main and typical subjective sensations of neuropathic pain and must be carefully searched for.

Typically, there is no 'time signal' in neuropathic pain, but emotions, fatigue or physical activity may enhance the neuropathic symptoms. Pain that radiates distally below the elbow when associated with shoulder pain suggests a neurological cause.[33] In the case of neurological lesions associated with musculoskeletal disorders, neuropathic pain occurs at the same moment as the musculoskeletal pain. In an entrapment neuropathy, patients may notice a worsening of symptoms at night, in relation to the sleeping position or related to postural ischaemia of the neural structures (see Figure 14.2). A constant and severe pain, without any variation with activity, is more likely to be of neuropathic or psychogenic origin than to arise from a nociceptive cause.

Some words are not specific. 'Weakness', 'fatigue' and the 'sensation of swelling' may be associated with rheumatic nociceptive or neuropathic pains.

General evaluation

When taking the history of pain it is essential to search for the 'red flags': fever, loss of weight, sweating, a previous history of cancer, infection and systemic diseases, loss of control of the sphincters and severe motor loss. RMP may be associated with neurological disorders.[34] This does not mean that the pain is neuropathic, but that the neurological disorder may have provoked a musculoskeletal disorder. Disorders such as Parkinson's disease, multiple sclerosis and lateral amyotrophic sclerosis must be searched for specifically.

The psychological background of the patient must be evaluated, looking for emotional distress, anxiety or a past history of depression. This background should be systematically evaluated, both in typical nociceptive pain due to inflammatory or non-inflammatory disorders, and in neuropathic pain. The 'yellow flags' in painful conditions include anxiety, fear of pain and depression. The relationship between reported pain intensity and the peripheral stimulus that evokes it depends on many factors, such as the level of arousal, anxiety, depression, attention, expectation and anticipation.[17] Understanding of these mechanisms is supported by the functional and anatomical pathways of the nociceptive or neuropathic stimulus in the subcortical and cortical regions of the brain. Two systems are activated by a nociceptive stimulus. Firstly, the lateral system (S1, S2 areas of the cortex) plays a role in the analysis of the location and the intensity of the stimulus. In contrast, the medial system (anterior cingulated cortex) is involved in the affective components of pain.[35] An increase of activity in the medial system is associated with 'hyperattention' or 'hypervigilance' and anticipation of pain and empathy for pain (our ability to experience another's pain). As the insula is now considered to be the link between the lateral and medial systems, activation of the insula may produce activations in the sensory discriminative system and in the descending pathways.[36]

In RMP associated with occupational activities, a rapid screening of the patient's work-related satisfaction is essential.

PHYSICAL EXAMINATION

This part of the chapter does not aim to list all the tests for each of the rheumatological conditions causing RMP, but to check the fundamental elements of the physical examination appropriate to all causes of RMP.[37] The physical examination must include a careful examination of the skin and joints and of the muscle structures around the joint, palpation of precise anatomical sites over ligaments and tendons, assessment for the presence of a joint effusion, and range of motion testing.

Inspection

The physical examination of a subject with RMP starts when the patient enters the room. Examine the way they walk and the posture of the trunk, and of the head in cases of occipitocervical pain. Also examine the automatic movements of the cervical spine during the interview, and the posture of the upper limb if the patient is complaining of upper limb pain. Any abnormalities are mainly associated with nociceptive pain and with either motor or proprioceptive changes related to the nociceptive pain or a fear-induced inhibition of movement from the cognitive and behavioural components of pain. The latter occur in both nociceptive and neuropathic pain.

In musculoskeletal disorders, different abnormalities may be found by inspection: bony swelling due to osteophytes in all superficial joints, deformity, an effusion, pitting oedema and overlying skin changes. Periarticular oedema may suggest underlying neurogenic inflammation. In areas such as the olecranon or patella, localized periarticular swelling may suggest a bursitis. Deformity of the joint is sometimes observed in the knee (varus, valgus, recurvatum) or the elbow (valgus, recurvatum). Muscle wasting is not specific to any particular pain, but it is a good marker of an organic lesion. Fasciculations may be seen in a radiculopathy, but also in tense, underrested or highly stressed patients. When fasciculations are confined to the territory of a peripheral nerve or a nerve root, they suggest a neuropathic cause of the pain.[30]

Palpation

Warmth, tenderness and crepitus are always signs of nociceptive pain and of inflammation. Careful palpation of specific anatomical sites is of great importance, especially for pain arising from bursae, tendons and the articular zone of a superficial joint.[37] In superficial joints, palpation may demonstrate joint swelling due to synovitis or an effusion (hydrarthrosis).

The threshold at which the palpation induces pain is important to note. Pressing any anatomical site is potentially painful, but certain areas are more sensitive, for example the trapezius, the long head of the biceps and the lateral epicondyle. Light touch or brushing is not usually painful.

The joint structures are covered by the skin, and primary or secondary sensitization of neurological structures creates superficial hyperpathic skin sensitivity that is seen in both nociceptive and neuropathic pains. This may occur in inflammatory disorders of the joint and also in inflammatory disorders of soft tissues, such as bursitis, tendonitis and tendon sheath inflammation. In the absence of visible skin changes, superficial pain may be neuropathic in origin. Findings may include a decreased threshold to noxious stimuli, increased pain from suprathreshold stimuli and spontaneous pain in a typical neurological distribution. Pain caused by light touch may be observed in psychogenic pain, and it is one of the non-organic signs described by Waddell for the lumbar spine, but also useful for the cervical spine.[38] Such a response has the same characteristics as neuropathic pain but without a defined neurological anatomical distribution. A 'hypervigilant' state during palpation may be observed in neuropathic pain due to hyperpathia, but may be associated with the fear of pain due to increased attention.

In pain of muscular origin the physical examination may find trigger points in the muscle. Trigger points are discrete, focal, hyperirritable points in a taut band of skeletal muscle. They produce pain locally and in a referred pattern. Palpation of a hypersensitive bundle, or of a nodule of muscle fibre, using moderate pressure is the typical physical finding of a trigger point. There may also be an associated abnormal motor response, but this does not distinguish between neuropathic or nociceptive inputs.

Joint movement

Analysis of the joint movement helps the differential diagnosis of pain arising from the joint itself and from other structures around the joint (Figure 14.3). Theoretically, pain provoked by a passive joint movement originates from the joint itself and is related to the disability caused by joint disease. There is a high correlation between the level of pain and physical disability during movement in RMP in any acutely painful condition.[39, 40] This is not usually the case in chronic pain, when primary and secondary local sensitization and sensitization of the central nervous system are prominent.

Pain provoked only by active movement or during resisted movement is usually associated with painful stimuli from active structures, such as muscle, tendon and the tendon–osseous junction or enthesis. This explains why the best tests for disorders of the rotator cuff tendons and in subacromial impingement are active tests,[41, 42] even if the precise anatomical lesion of the rotator cuff tendinopathy is not thereby clarified.[41] A clinical test should discriminate unwell from healthy people if it is to be called a diagnostic test. More than 20 clinical diagnostic tests exist for the subacromial impingement syndrome.[41] When compared with magnetic resonance imaging (MRI) findings, the tests with the highest specificity were the drop arm test (97.2%), the Yergason test (86.1%) and the painful arc test (80.5%). However, when the MRI findings were strongly suggestive, the sensitivity and the specificity of the Hawkins' and drop arm tests were found to be 100%. When several clinical tests were combined, the sensitivity was greater but the specificity less. The active Hawkins' and Neer's tests seem to be positive both with subacromial bursitis and with rotator cuff tears.[43]

In upper limb disorders associated with soft tissue lesions the recommended tests are those that produce local pain on resisted movements.[44] In lateral epicondylitis, lateral elbow tenderness is associated with pain in the lateral elbow on resisted wrist extension (sensitivity 73%, specificity 97%). In flexor and extensor peritendinitis or tenosynovitis of the forearm–wrist region, the best test seems to be the self-reported resisted wrist-extension test.[44] The occurrence of paraesthesia or of an electric-shock-like pain during the resisted flexion test is suggestive of neuropathic pain, although this may be seen in combination with nociceptive pain.

In neck pain, palpation of a facet joint has the highest sensitivity (82%), and the upper limb tension test has the highest specificity (94%).[45] Pain occurring during passive rotation of the neck had a sensitivity of 77% and a specificity of 92%, and was significantly correlated with the number of sick-leave days.[45] Trapezius tenderness is associated with local motor dysfunction but it has a weak specificity in cervical disorders (65%).

Limitation of passive flexion and internal rotation of the hip suggest an articular lesion of the hip.

Pathological changes in the knee are difficult to diagnose specifically. Thus, in anterior knee pain chondromalacia is often diagnosed, and many clinical tests have been described to detect this. In a study of 85 knees in which clinical tests were compared with the arthroscopic findings, the sensitivity and specificity, the predictive values and the accuracy of the tests were all low.[46] A combination of inspection and palpation is essential when looking for muscular dysfunction around the

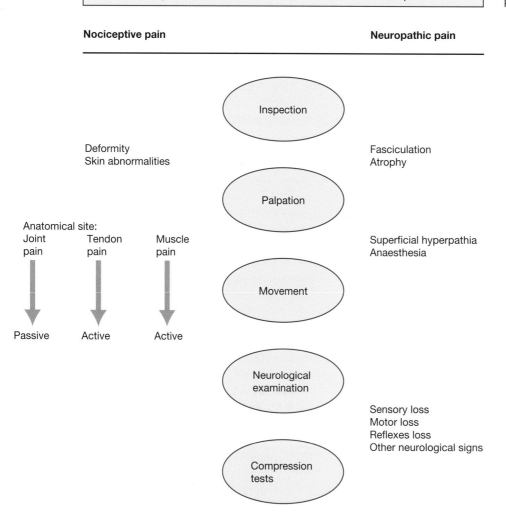

Figure 14.3. Clinical diagnosis of RMP: physical examination.

knee. Patients with patellofemoral syndrome may be classified by the presence or absence of patellar misalignment, the presence or absence of quadriceps wasting, selective vastus medialis obliquus wasting, or a timing dysfunction and altered reaction pattern between the vastus medialis and the vastus lateralis that is visible by inspection during an isometric contraction of the quadriceps with the knee in full extension.[47] The combination of clinical and physical examination in predominantly nociceptive knee pain may help to distinguish mechanical joint pain, using such features as age greater than 50 years, morning stiffness lasting less than 30 minutes, pain only on movement and the bony swelling, and crepitus associated with osteoarthritis, from pain due to inflammation, wherein it is more common to find palpable synovitis, morning stiffness lasting more than 15 minutes and pain in the second part of the night. In acute knee pain, the clinical criteria for an exacerbation of osteoarthritis are 89% sensitive and 88% specific.[48]

A major problem remains that the diagnostic value of clinical tests for most types of nociceptive pain has been poorly evaluated. For example, a meta-analysis of the accuracy of physical diagnostic tests for assessing meniscal lesions of the knee found that of 402 studies identified only 13 met the inclusion criteria. The authors concluded that these tests are of little value in clinical practice.[49] In another study it was found that for meniscal tears joint-line tenderness is sensitive (75%) but not specific (27%), while the MacMurray test is specific (97%) but not sensitive (52%).[48]

In conclusion, active and passive joint examination can differentiate the origin of the nociceptive pain as arising from the joint or from the soft tissues, but is of little value in diagnosing the actual aetiological lesion.

Neurological examination

With neuropathic pain a systematic neurological examination is essential, looking carefully for weakness, reflex loss and sensory impairment. In general, agreement rates between observers for neurological signs are high.

In RMP the diagnosis of nerve entrapment is likely when a test that produces traction on the nerve (a provocation test), for example the straight-leg raising test in sciatica, reproduces the pain. It cannot, however, distinguish the underlying lesion causing the neuropathic pain. In sciatica due to disc herniation, a meta-analysis found that the pain distribution seemed to be the only useful item from the history, and the straight-leg raising test was the most sensitive test on examination.[50]

In upper limb nerve entrapment there are certain common findings on clinical examination. Dysaesthesia and paraesthesia are more prominent at rest than during activity and often occur during the night. Dysaesthesia is localized to the sensory distribution of the nerve, and Tinel's sign is frequently positive when percussion of the nerve at the site of compression elicits dysaesthesia in the sensory distribution of the nerve. Traction or compression tests have been described for each upper limb nerve entrapment syndrome. In carpal tunnel syndrome (CTS), nine tests have been proposed. A review of the literature found 57 clinical studies of the sensitivity and specificity of these tests,

but only 21 met the required quality criteria. From these studies, it appears that in carpal tunnel compression, Durkan's test had the best sensitivity (49–87%) and specificity (90–99%), and Tinel's sign had a sensitivity of 45–63% and a specificity of 40–67%.[51, 52] Despite this, Durkan's test is not used as a specific test for CTS in the consensus statement from the Southampton UK Workshop.[44] In ulnar nerve compression at the elbow the best tests are a combination of local pressure over the nerve at the elbow and a full flexion test with the elbow held flexed for 30 seconds (sensitivity 91%, specificity 97%), provoking paraesthesia in the ulnar border of the hand. In a radial nerve compression in the radial tunnel, the best tests are tenderness in the supinator area evoked by palpating the radial nerve 4–7 cm distal to the epicondyle, and either pain provoked by resisted forearm supination or resisted middle-finger extension (specificity of 96%).[44]

SUMMARY

The clinical management of RMP starts with taking a careful history of the pain and of the past history of pain in the patient. Without this simple but fundamental step, and particularly in non-inflammatory diseases of the musculoskeletal system, the diagnosis is often inaccurate. In order to distinguish nociceptive from neuropathic pain typical clinical characteristics, such as the mode of onset of the pain, the words used to describe the

PRACTICE POINTS

- Noxious inputs are provoked by mechanical, chemical and thermal stimuli and cause pain.

- Central sensitization is responsible for a larger zone of noxious inputs and resultant secondary pain, and referred pain occurring later in the course of the musculoskeletal disorder.

- Connections to the reticular system are responsible for the systemic effects associated with the noxious stimuli.

- Neuropathic pain short-circuits the sensory pathways of pain regulation.

- Muscular atrophy and disuse, excessive rest and central changes may lead to deconditioning early in the course of RMP.

- Integration of noxious stimuli in the cortex is related to the sensation of pain.

- Soft-tissue disorders are associated with precisely localized tenderness.

- Passive painful movements are usually related to lesions of the joint.

- Painful active movements are associated with a muscular or tendinous nociceptive stimulus.

- Paraesthesiae are the best indicator of neuropathic pain.

- Severe muscle wasting in acute pain suggests a neuropathic cause.

pain, the distribution of pain and its radiation pattern, and neurological abnormalities on physical examination are all helpful. Diagnosis is not made easy, however, by the poor sensitivity and specificity of many of the clinical tests, and is further complicated when there is associated psychological distress. Unfortunately, physical tests for specific lesions, particularly those causing upper-limb pain where neuropathic and nociceptive pain may coexist, and clinical tests in pain around the knee and in the cervical spine, have not been standardized and lack good methodological criteria of reproducibility and validity. Indeed, it seems that the more difficult it is to diagnose a problem physically, the more tests have been described! Further research in this field is essential to improve the validity of the clinical examination in RMP syndromes.

RESEARCH AGENDA

- Validation is needed of the best physical signs in each RMP syndrome, in terms of both sensitivity and specificity.
- The best criteria for a rapid and complete musculoskeletal health screen in primary care should be evaluated.

REFERENCES

1. International Association for the Study of Pain. 1979.
2. Portenoy R. Mechanisms of clinical pain. *Neurol Clin* 1989; **7**: 205–229.
3. Lundeberg T, Ekholm J. Pain from periphery to brain. *Disabil Rehab* 2002; **24**: 402–406.
4. Janssen SA. Negative affect and sensitization to pain. *Scand J Psychol* 2002; **43**: 131–137.
5. Hadler NM. Workers with disabling back pain. *New Engl J Med* 1997; **337**: 341–343., Palmer K
6. Linaker CH, Walker-Bone K et al. Frequency and impact of regional musculo-skeletal disorders. *Baillères Best Practice Res Clin Rheumat* 1999; **13**: 197–215.
7. Grossi G, Soares JJ, Angesleva J et al. Psychosocial correlates of long-term sick-leave among patients with musculoskeletal pain. *Pain* 1999; **80**: 607–619.
8. Vahtera J, Kivimaki M, Pentti J. Effect of organisational downsizing on health of employees. *Lancet* 1997; **350**: 1124–1128.
9. Brekke M, Hjortdahl P, Kvien TK. Severity of musculoskeletal pain: relations to socioeconomic inequality. *Soc Sci Med* 2002; **54**: 221–228.
10. Kivimaki M, Vahtera J, Ferrie JE et al. Organizational downsizing and musculoskeletal problems in employees: a prospective study. *Occup Environ Med* 2001; **58**: 811–817.
11. Rollman GB, Lautenbacher S. Sex differences in musculoskeletal pain. *Clin J Pain* 2001; **17**: 20–24.
12. Hagen KB, Bjorndal A, Uhlig T et al. A population study of factors associated with general practitioner consultation for non-inflammatory musculoskeletal pain. *Ann Rheumat Dis* 2000; **59**: 788–793.
13. Edwards CL, Fillingim RB, Keefe F. Race, ethnicity and pain. *Pain* 2001; **94**: 133–137.
14. Gibson SJ, Farrel M. A review of age differences in the neurophysiology of nociception and the perceptual experience of pain. *Clin J Pain* 2004; **20**: 227–239.
15. Renn CL, Dorsey SG. The physiology and processing of pain: a review. *AACN Clin Issue* 2005; **16**: 277–290.
16. Katz WA, Rothenberg R. Section 3: The nature of pain: pathophysiology. *J Clin Rheumatol* 2005; **11**(Suppl 2): S11–S15.
17. Brooks J, Tracey I. From nociception to pain perception: imaging the spinal and supraspinal pathways. *J Anat* 2005; **207**: 19–33.
18. Dubner R. The neurobiology of persistent pain and its clinical implications. *Clin Neurophysiol* 2004; **57**(Suppl): 3–7.
19. Edwards RR. Individual differences in endogenous pain modulation as a risk factor for chronic pain. *Neurology* 2005; **65**: 437–443.
20. Kidd BL. What are the mechanisms of regional musculoskeletal pain? *Baillière's Clin Rheumatol* 1999; **13**: 217–230.
21. Coutaux A, Adam F, Willer JC et al. Hyperalgesia and allodynia: peripheral mechanisms. *Joint Bone Spine* 2005; **72**: 359–371.
22. Kang YM, Choi WS, Pickar JG. Electrophysiologic evidence for an intersegmental reflex pathway between lumbar paraspinal tissues. *Spine* 2002; **27**: E56–E63.
23. Schaible HG, Ebersberger A, Von Banchet GS. Mechanisms of pain in arthritis. *Ann NY Acad Sci* 2002; **966**: 343–354.
24. Leffler AS, Kosek AS, Hansson P. The influence of pain intensity on somatosensory perception in patients suffering from subacute/chronic lateral epicondylalgia. *Eur J Pain* 2000; **4**: 57–71.
25. Glosh P, Cheras PA. Vascular mechanism in osteoarthritis. *Best Pract Res Clin Rheumatol* 2001; **15**: 693–710.
26. Koltzenburg M, Scadding J. Neuropathic pain. *Curr Opin Neurol* 2001; **14**: 641–647.
27. Schwartzman RJ, Maleki J. Postinjury neuropathic pain syndromes. *Med Clin North Am* 1999; **83**: 597–626.
28. Sterling M, Jull G, Wright A. The effect of musculoskeletal pain on motor activity and control. *J Pain* 2001; **2**: 135–145.
29. Le Pera D, Graven-Nielsen T, Oliviero A et al. Inhibition of motor system excitability at cortical and spinal level by tonic muscle pain. *Clin Neurophysiol* 2001; **112**: 1633–1641.
30. Kincaid JC. Muscle pain, fatigue, and fasciculations. *Neurolog Clin* 1997; **15**: 697–709.
31. Rice JR, Pisetsky DS. Pain in the rheumatic diseases. Practical aspects of diagnosis and treatment. *Rheum Dis Clin North Am* 1999; **25**: 15–30.
32. Moll JMH. Clinical assessment. In: *Rheumatology in Clinical Practice*. Blackwell Scientific, Oxford, 1987, pp. 193–256.
33. Manifold SG, McCann PD. Cervical radiculitis and shoulder disorders. *Clin Orthopaed Relat Res* 1999; **368**: 105–113.
34. Collange C, Burde MA. Musculoskeletal problems of neurogenic origin. *Baillière's Best Practice and Res Clin Rheumatol* 2000; **14**: 325–343.
35. Apkanian AV, Bushnell MC, Treede RD et al. Human brain mechanisms of pain perception and regulation in health and disease. *Eur J Pain* 2005; **9**: 463–484.
36. Singer T, Seymour B, O'Doherty J et al. Empathy for pain involves the affective but not the sensory components of pain. *Science* 2004; **303**: 1157–1162.
37. Grahame R. Examination of the patient. In: Klippel JH, Dieppe A (eds), *Rheumatology*, 2nd edn. Mosby, London, 1997, pp. 2.1–2.15.
38. Sobel JP, Sollenberger P, Robinson R et al. Cervical nonorganic signs: a new clinical tool to assess abnormal illness behavior in neck pain patients: a pilot study. *Arch Phys Me Rehab* 2000; **81**: 170–175.
39. Hermann KM, Reese CS. Relationships among selected measures of impairment, functional limitation, and disability in patients with cervical spine disorders. *Phys Ther* 2001; **81**: 903–914.
40. Kaergaard A, Andersen JH, Rasmussen K et al. Identification of neck–shoulder disorders in a 1 year follow-up study. Validation of a questionnaire based method. *Pain* 2000; **86**: 305–310.
41. Calis M, Akgun K, Birtane M et al. Diagnostic values of clinical diagnostic tests in subacromial impingement syndrome. *Ann Rheumat Dis* 2000; **59**: 44–47.
42. Naredo E, Aguado P, De Miguel E et al. Painful shoulder: comparison of physical examination and ultrasonographic finding. *Ann Rheumat Dis* 2002; **61**: 132–136.
43. MacDonald PB, Clark P, Sutherland K. An analysis of the diagnostic accuracy of the Hawkins and Neer subacromial impingement signs. *J Shoulder Elbow Surg* 2000; **9**: 299–301.
44. Palmer K, Walker-Bone K, Linaker C et al. The Southampton examination schedule for the diagnosis of musculoskeletal disorders of the upper limb. *Ann Rheumat Dis* 2000; **59**: 5–11.
45. Sandmark H, Nisell R. Validity of five common manual neck pain provoking tests. *Scand J Rehab Med* 1995; **27**: 131–136.
46. Viikari-Juntura E, Takala E, Riihimaki H et al. Predictive validity of symptoms and signs in the neck and shoulders. *J Clin Epidemiol* 2000; **53**: 800–808.
47. Niskanen RO, Paavilainen PJ, Jaakkola M et al. Poor correlation of clinical signs with patellar cartilaginous changes. *Arthroscopy* 2001; **17**: 307–310.
48. Witvrouw E, Werner S, Mikkelsen C et al. Clinical classification of patellofemoral pain syndrome: guidelines for non-operative treatment. *Knee Surg Sports Traumatol Arthrosc* 2005; **13**: 122–130.
49. Jackson JL, O'Malley PG, Kroenke K. Evaluation of acute knee pain in primary care. *Ann Intern Med* 2003; **139**: 575–588.

50. Scholten RJ, Deville WL, Opstelten W et al. The accuracy of physical diagnostic tests for assessing meniscal lesions of the knee: a meta-analysis. *J Fam Pract* 2001; **50**: 938–944.

51. Vroomen PC, De Krom MC, Knottnerus JA. Diagnostic value of history and physical examination in patients suspected of sciatica due to disc herniation: a systematic review. *J Neurol* 1999; **246**: 899–906.

52. Massy-Westropp N, Grimmer K, Bain G. A systematic review of the clinical diagnostic tests for carpal tunnel syndrome. *J Hand Surg (Am)* 2000; **25**: 120–127.

Chapter 15
Limb pain

Michael Shipley

INTRODUCTION

Limb pain is common. Shoulder pain, for example, affects up to 50% of the population in a year, and is commoner still in the elderly. People with regional pain are more likely to have recurrences of the same pain, or pain elsewhere.[1] In most cases it is the result of an injury, sometimes recalled, sometimes not. Such pain may be severe or mild but commonly settles without intervention – some studies suggest that under half of affected individuals present to a clinician.[2] Forearm pain in workers is usually short-lived and recovers with or without treatment but is often followed by more pain in the same place or elsewhere.[3] More widespread pain affecting the limbs may be part of a generalized arthritis or other systemic disease that needs appropriate diagnosis and treatment.

The evidence base for accurate diagnosis and effective treatment of many of these syndromes is inadequate but improving. The Cochrane Collaboration[4] is a helpful source of information about reliable studies. A useful source of information for patients can be found at MedlinePlus.[5] Some of the complex non-pharmaceutical interventions used in the treatment of pain may not be best assessed by randomized, double-blind, controlled trials. To use a placebo control the interventions must be divided into characteristic or specific elements and incidental elements (placebo or non-specific). This may not be appropriate for such complex interventions, as has been recently pointed out by Paterson and Dieppe.[6] The elements of treatment regarded as incidental in a drug trial may be integral to non-pharmaceutical interventions. For most pharmaceutical interventions the biomedical diagnosis determines eligibility for the trial. In complex interventions the process of diagnosis is interwoven with the initial treatment and response and may be modified at any stage. Standard trial designs may effectively underestimate the effectiveness of such complex interventions. Pragmatic or randomized cluster study designs may be more appropriate.

Early diagnosis, explanation to the patient and effective treatment are important. However, in Chapter 16 in this book, Croft argues cogently that, at least at the first visit to a general practitioner, it may be best to treat shoulder pain, for example, as a non-specific regional pain problem, without investigating it or trying to determine a specific underlying cause. This is the approach that has been taken with low back pain for quite a while, as long as the 'red flags' (trauma, infection and malignancy) have been ruled out. To quote Croft: 'The general principle remains that regional musculoskeletal pain can be seen as both (i) a local problem with an underlying pathological cause and (ii) a pain syndrome that shares characteristics common to pain syndromes elsewhere in the body, regardless of location.' The question is whether making a specific diagnosis will help determine the best treatment. The dilemma is the lack of good evidence for the commonest forms of treatment of many limb pain problems. There must be a balance – diagnosing lateral epicondylitis does inform the advice and treatment given, as does a diagnosis of a rotator cuff syndrome, as compared with shoulder girdle pain (see below). The discussion will go on. Whatever the case, in many situations initial treatment is conservative – what might be called guided self-management. The patient is advised to continue normal activity and work but to avoid activities that produce acute exacerbation of the pain and to use simple over-the-counter analgesics (paracetamol (acetaminophen) or a non-steroidal anti-inflammatory drug (NSAID), which can also be applied locally). In some situations where more support is needed physical therapies have a role, but the aim should still be to maintain normal activity and work through the pain. Medical intervention may be necessary if the pain is severe or does not settle. Prescribed NSAIDs or compound analgesics or local corticosteroid injections are often used and may produce more rapid pain relief. They may not alter the longer term outcome, however. Certain jobs are associated with an increased risk of specific local problems, and affected individuals may be entitled to or seeking workers' compensation.[7] The process of pursuing a claim may add to the stress and distress. In some circumstances the nature of the problem is associated with a predictably poor outcome and warrants earlier specialist referral and more active intervention.

The role of various imaging techniques in the diagnosis of limb pain is controversial. Accuracy relies on the experience of the clinician interpreting the images and the clinical skills of the primary and secondary clinician in understanding whether the observed abnormalities are a relevant and likely cause of pain or coincidental to it. There have been very few studies that have dealt with the cost-effectiveness of clinical examination versus imaging. X-rays are inexpensive but of limited value, except to exclude bony lesions, fractures or tumours. Ultrasound scanning allows for imaging during movement, which is important in diagnosing shoulder pain, for example, but is highly dependent on the skills of the operator. Magnetic resonance imaging (MRI) and computed tomography (CT) are expensive and best reserved for specialist practice. They should only be undertaken when it is clear that the results are likely to alter management strategies significantly. Arthroscopy and other surgical techniques are invasive and are usually, and probably appropriately, reserved for individuals in whom other treatments have failed. There may be a role for early arthroscopic intervention in the knee, for example, especially in elite athletes with meniscal tears.

The early recognition and appropriate treatment of such localized pain syndromes is important and will probably help to avoid the development of more severe, generalized chronic limb pain syndromes in susceptible individuals. The early recognition and treatment of lateral epicondylitis or carpal tunnel syndrome in someone who works at a keyboard, in an instrumental performing artist or in an individual whose work involves a great deal of lifting, carrying or working with the arms above the head may prevent the development of what is best called a chronic (work-related) upper limb pain syndrome (previously termed 'repetitive strain injury'). Such syndromes are associated with the development of more widespread pain, sometimes affecting the whole of the limb, and eventually present not only with use but at rest. This may occur in the context of a generalized pain syndrome – chronic widespread pain (fibromyalgia) and other associated syndromes, such as tension headaches, irritable bowel syndrome or chronic fatigue syndrome. Central 'wind-up' and the added impact of anxiety, stress, sleep disturbance and a threat to the individual's employment all compound the situation and make the pain both more difficult to treat and more difficult to explain by simple anatomical or pathological mechanisms. Prevention is the key, early recognition essential and sometimes a brief period of rest from work or use should be advised. The patient's employer may have to be involved and asked to make adjustments to the workplace or to the nature of the job. The person affected will often need support and reassurance, as well as help to control the pain. Sleep disturbance is common and may need treating.

Psychological factors and taking time off work are poor prognostic predictors for some localized pain problems and probably for the development of generalized pain syndromes. Workers' compensation cases may be being contemplated or pending, and this complicates and sometimes appears to prolong the recovery.[8]

Asymmetrical limb pain may be part of a seronegative spondyloarthropathy, which occasionally presents as a monarthritis. Rheumatoid arthritis may present also as a monarthritis, but less commonly. Systemic symptoms, malaise, weight loss, or skin or bowel disease may suggest a systemic illness. Morning exacerbation of pain and stiffness may suggest an inflammatory arthritis, or polymyalgia rheumatica in a patient over 55 years old. Some paraneoplastic syndromes present with limb pain. A brief general symptom enquiry is important, even when seeing a patient with an apparently localized problem.

UPPER LIMB PAIN

Shoulder pain

Definitions of shoulder pain are difficult and controversial.[9] Practically it is useful to distinguish two patterns:

- *shoulder pain* – pain felt predominantly around the shoulder joint and radiating into the deltoid region (occasionally also in a C6 distribution, when the pain is severe but without neurological symptoms or signs)
- *shoulder girdle pain* – pain between the base of the neck and the shoulder.

Shoulder girdle pain may be referred from the neck, localized (muscular, and often posture- or stress-related) or a secondary phenomenon to severe shoulder pain when the shoulder is held elevated and adducted as a protective manoeuvre. It is best to ask the patient to point to the site when they complain of a painful shoulder. The examination of the shoulder has been well reviewed by Brox.[10] Shoulder pain, as opposed to shoulder girdle pain, is most commonly due to rotator cuff tendinopathy in primary care, and is associated with significantly reduced health. Prevention and earlier intervention is warranted.[11] Pins and needles, numbness, muscle weakness or wasting make it likely that the pain arises from the nerve root compression in the neck or nerve compression at the thoracic outlet. Pain, weakness and wasting, without other sensory symptoms, is due to brachial neuralgia.

Shoulder girdle pain is the commonest cause of shoulder pain. It is usually proximal to the shoulder and not significantly worsened by shoulder or arm movements. Neck movements may be painful or feel tight. There are tender trigger points in the trapezius muscle, around the C7 spinous process and at the upper medial edge of the scapula. It may be unilateral or bilateral. The patient complains of burning pain and discomfort in the muscle, which is often tense and contracted. They may describe the muscle as swollen. Not infrequently, the patient himself or herself recognizes that the pain is worsened by carrying, by working at a computer or instrument, and by anxiety or stress. The workplace may not be ideal with, for example, the relative height of desk, keyboard and chair such that the arms need to be elevated or are unsupported. There is probably an association with radiological evidence of cervical spondylosis, although it is not clear if this relationship is causal or coincidental, and with associated muscular neck pain and occipital headaches. Postural advice, workstation review and relaxation classes are helpful, and simple analgesics are appropriate to try to stop the build up of pain and the development of a vicious circle of pain and muscular spasm. Some people respond to dry needling (acupuncture) or trigger-point injections with small doses of local anaesthetic and/or corticosteroids. Treatment of shoulder girdle pain is not well researched and the evidence base for this, as for many localized pain syndromes, remains inadequate. This does not necessarily mean that treatment does not work, merely that its efficacy is unproven.[12]

Applied anatomy of the shoulder joint

The shoulder joint is a complex structure with a large range of movement. There are three synovial joints (the shallow glenohumeral, the acromioclavicular and the sternoclavicular joints), which act together during normal shoulder movements. Shoulder abduction is initiated by a 'force couple' between the deltoid pulling up and out and the supraspinatus pulling down and in. A turning moment holds the head of the humerus down, and it glides under the acromion and coracoacromial ligament without impingement. The subacromial/subdeltoid bursa is interposed between the acromion and rotator cuff. The first 90° of abduction occur at the glenohumeral joint, and the scapula then rotates across the posterior rib cage. This normal scapulothoracic rhythm is altered in individuals with rotator cuff syndromes. Weakness of the rhomboid muscles leads to winging of the scapula when the arms are held forwards. The acromioclavicular and sternoclavicular joints also move.

Shoulder pain may arise from an inflammatory arthritis or osteoarthritis. The latter is uncommon unless there has been a severe prior injury or it is part of generalized osteoarthritis. In the elderly it may be due to polymyalgia rheumatica, although this is usually symmetrical and affects the trapezius and neck muscles as well as the pelvic girdle, buttocks and thighs. The commonest origin of shoulder pain is the rotator cuff mechanism. It is typified by pain that is worse on abduction and elevation, lifting with the arm outstretched or reaching behind the back. The pain is felt predominantly in the deltoid region and is usually worse at night, especially when lying on the affected arm. It presents as an active painful arc syndrome, with pain worse in the midrange of abduction. Passive elevation and abduction of the arm are less painful, except when the pain is very severe and there is marked muscle spasm. The severity of the painful arc may be altered by abducting the arm first in internal and then in external rotation. All these signs suggest a problem arising from the rotator cuff, but it is often difficult clinically to judge whether it is *rotator cuff tendinopathy*, a *partial tear or small complete tear* of the rotator cuff or *subacromial bursitis*. All may coexist.

There is evidence that rotator cuff pathology is due to direct injury, working with the hands above the head, impingement of the rotator cuff against the lower surface of the acromion, and an osteoarthritic or unstable acromioclavicular joint. Weakness or inactivity of the supraspinatus muscle probably increases this impingement. The weakness may be due to pain or disuse or

neurological causes. The function of the supraspinatus is to depress and rotate the humeral head as the deltoid pulls up and out. *Calcific tendonitis* is visible on x-rays as a radio-opaque deposit lying in the rotator cuff adjacent to its insertion into the greater tuberosity. *Calcific bursitis*, due to release of the crystalline deposit into the subacromial bursa, is exquisitely painful, causes local swelling and inflammation and is also visible on x-rays as cloudy radio-opacity in the bursa. An ultrasound scan is probably the best way of specifically diagnosing the underlying cause(s) and of devising a treatment strategy, but such scans are difficult to interpret by the inexperienced.[13]

Whether specific differential diagnosis of these different pathologies affects the decision to treat or the outcome is unclear.[14] As long as the pain is mild, simple analgesia, sedative analgesia at night and/or NSAIDs suffice. If the pain persists or is very severe, a local corticosteroid injection under low pressure into the subacromial bursa is effective in reducing pain rapidly in around 70% of patients. There is a theoretical, and possibly actual, risk of converting a partial rotator cuff tear into a complete tear by injecting corticosteroid. This may also occur occasionally without treatment, however (see below). Calcific tendonitis responds to a local corticosteroid injection, but may need to be aspirated under ultrasound guidance. Calcific bursitis should be aspirated and injected with corticosteroid.

In a full thickness, major *rotator cuff tear*, the arm cannot be actively abducted as the deltoid pulls up unopposed and the head of the humerus impinges on the acromion. The only elevation then occurs at the scapulothoracic joint. Passive elevation is relatively well maintained, unless inhibited by pain. In young people it is possible to repair a traumatic tear surgically. In older people this is more difficult and the outcome less certain because the tissue is more friable. Retraining the remaining muscles of the rotator cuff may help to restore some function. If pain is severe in the older patient, occasional corticosteroid injections are acceptable, as long as resultant pain relief is significant and relatively long lasting.

Acromioclavicular joint instability or *secondary osteoarthritis* causes pain that is localized to the site of the joint. The patient points specifically to the joint, which may be tender. The pain is increased by reaching behind the back or across the chest. Trauma is the usual initial cause. Osteoarthritis leads to osteophytes which, if on the undersurface, contribute to impingement. Rest and analgesia help. Occasionally, a corticosteroid injection is necessary. Surgery is rarely required.

Adhesive capsulitis (frozen shoulder) causes intense, diffuse shoulder pain and is uncommon.[15, 16] The joint stiffens over a few weeks and there is complete loss of all movements, including rotation. This loss of rotation also occurs in shoulder arthritis, but is rare in rotator cuff syndromes unless pain is severe. Adhesive capsulitis may develop after rotator cuff tendinopathy, injury, stroke or myocardial infarction, or spontaneously. It is associated with poorly controlled insulin-dependent diabetes. Adhesions form in the joint and the capsule contracts during the stiff phase with only minimal synovial inflammation. The aetiology and cause of the fibrosis is not clear. The pain resolves gradually over a few months but the stiffness persists for up to 18 months. A full range of movement is rarely restored but there is little long-term disability in most. Joint arthrography shows contraction of the axillary capsule extension and this is a diagnostic feature of adhesive capsulitis. Capsulitis is poorly visualized on MRI. High doses of NSAIDs and analgesics are used but the pain is difficult to control. The early use of oral corticosteroids reduces pain but does not prevent stiffening or speed recovery. Intra-articular local anaesthetic combined with corticosteroid has been advocated. In a recent study the use of both an intra-articular injection and a subacromial lateral injection plus physiotherapy appeared to be more effective at 6 weeks in reducing pain and improving range of movement than either subacromial or intra-articular injection plus physiotherapy. It was also more effective than physiotherapy plus sham injection or sham injection alone. The outcomes at 16 weeks were the same but there was a high dropout rate.[17] Manipulation under anaesthetic during the fibrotic phase occasionally has been advocated for the restoration of function but arthroscopic release of the fibrous tissue in the rotator interval is also advocated. Referral to an expert in upper-limb surgery is appropriate.

Proximal bicipital tendinopathy is uncommon but may occur in isolation or coexist with a rotator cuff syndrome. It is usually traumatic and causes pain in front of the humeral head. It is worsened by flexion combined with supination of the elbow against resistance. Rest, pain relief and a corticosteroid injection alongside the tendon in its groove help. Rupture of the tendon is due to trauma in younger athletes or manual workers and warrants surgical repair. In older patients a spontaneous tear of the long head of biceps causes sudden shoulder pain and bruising anteriorally extending to the elbow. Subsequently the muscle contracts and causes a painless swelling in the mid-upper arm. There is little residual disability.

Brachial neuralgia is uncommon and causes diffuse burning pain in the trapezius and upper arm when the upper brachial plexus is involved. Its cause is unknown. Pain decreases but muscle wasting develops. The weakness causes difficulty in abducting the arm. Winging of the scapula develops if the scapulothoracic nerve is affected. Suprascapular nerve involvement leads to wasting of the supraspinatus and infraspinatus muscles. The nerves become demyelinated. Nerve-conduction studies are diagnostic and may demonstrate reinnervation, an indicator of potential recovery. Weakness persists for several months but recovery is usual. A short course of oral corticosteroids during the painful phase and rest in a sling may help.

The *shoulder–hand syndrome (complex regional pain syndrome)* is discussed later in this chapter.

Elbow pain

Pain around the elbow arises most commonly from extra-articular structures, and occasionally from inflammatory arthritis or osteoarthritis.

Applied anatomy of the elbow

The elbow comprises a stable hinge joint between the humerus and ulna, and the proximal radiohumeral and radioulnar joints.

Lateral epicondylitis (tennis elbow) causes pain at the insertion of the common extensor tendon at the lateral epicondyle and is an enthesitis. It is common and often self-limiting. Pain is felt at the lateral epicondyle, which is tender. A variant causes pain and tenderness where the common extensor tendon crosses the radiohumeral joint, about 1 cm distal to the epicondyle. The pain often radiates to the proximal wrist extensor muscles. Gripping hard with the wrist dorsiflexed worsens the pain. Pain may occur at rest. Radial tunnel syndrome due to compression of the posterior interosseous nerve as it passes through the supinator muscle occasionally mimics lateral epicondylitis – dorsiflexion of the middle finger reproduces the pain. *Medial epicondylitis (golfer's elbow)* is less common, causing pain and tenderness over the medial epicondyle at the insertion of the common wrist flexor muscles. Holding a heavy object with the hands and forearms supinated (e.g. carrying a tray) worsens the pain of medial epicondylitis, as does resisted flexion of the wrist with the elbow straight. The clinical diagnosis is clear-cut and investigation is rarely necessary. If epicondylitis does not settle with rest and analgesia a local corticosteroid injection helps speed recovery. There is some evidence that acupuncture also relieves painful lateral epicondylitis.[18] *Distal bicipital tendinopathy* is usually due to trauma and causes pain and tenderness in the antecubital fossa. *Triceps tendonitis* causes pain and tenderness at the olecranon process.

Olecranon bursitis arises from trauma and leads to localized swelling, pain and tenderness over the tip of the elbow. Elbow flexion is uncomfortable. Aspiration produces clear, slightly cloudy or blood-stained fluid. Bursitis is occasionally due to an inflammatory arthritis or gout. Aspirated fluid is then cloudy. Infective bursitis is usually associated with local cellulitis. The fluid is purulent and there may be lymphadenitis. Aspiration relieves the pain but corticosteroid must not be injected. Cloudy fluid should be examined by polarized light microscopy for urate crystals, and Gram staining and culture undertaken. If infection is excluded, a local corticosteroid injection helps. Infective bursitis requires antibiotics.

Forearm pain

Anterior interosseous syndrome is due to anterior interosseous nerve entrapment proximal to the pronator teres, and causes forearm aching and weakness of pronation and wrist flexion. *Posterior interosseous syndrome* is due to posterior interosseous nerve entrapment just distal to the elbow, and causes forearm aching. It mimics medial epicondylitis but the tenderness is more distal. *Pronator teres syndrome* is due to compression of the median nerve at the elbow, and causes forearm aching and symptoms of carpal tunnel syndrome, which are not relieved by a resting wrist splint.

Worked-related forearm pain is a common complaint of keyboard workers and instrumental musicians, in whom it occurs in isolation or develops into a more generalized arm-pain syndrome, often also producing shoulder-girdle pain. The aetiology of diffuse, chronic forearm pain is controversial.[3, 19] Early diagnosis and treatment of local problems, such as epicondylitis, carpal tunnel syndrome or tenosynovitis, helps to avoid it. Work-related pain is associated with a sudden increase in workload, changed working practices and poor management of these changes. Dissatisfaction with levels of support from colleagues or middle managers leading to workplace disharmony is common. Work-related mechanical causes are important. Poor posture, inadequate workplace design and failure to adhere to recommendations about rest periods all contribute. Affected individuals show high levels of psychological distress and illness behaviour, and complain of other somatic disorders. The threat of, or worries about, dismissal or the patient threatening litigation add to the stress and the pain becomes self-perpetuating. The patient, their coworkers, managers and the occupational health team all become anxious, and more workers in the office are affected unless the situation is managed appropriately. Eventually the pain does not simply occur at work but affects the individual at weekends and when on holiday.

Diagnosis is essentially clinical – the way in which the problem develops and is described by the patient is typical. Although rarely necessary to do so, it has been demonstrated that there is increased temperature of the affected arm on thermography and also changes in the sensitivity to vibration.[20]

Treatment of specific lesions is important, as is adequate pain control. Sleeplessness is helped by nocturnal low doses of tricyclic antidepressants such as amitriptyline. It is sometimes best for the individual to have a short break from work and then to return, but working shorter hours. Regular breaks to change posture and relax the affected muscles are recommended by workplace legislation and should be required. Postural advice, relaxation techniques and ergonomic assessment of the workplace are important. It is often necessary to address office stresses and working practices as well. Changing work practices and the way compensation was paid led to less public discussion, and all combined to reduce the high incidence of this problem in Australian industries.[21] Studies have indicated similar risk factors in other shoulder and back regional pain syndromes.[22]

Wrist and hand pain

Pain in the wrist and hand is common and often a cause of great anxiety. It affects 5–10% of working-age individuals and is more commonly reported in older patients.[3] It is caused by trauma, overuse, inflammatory arthritis or osteoarthritis. It may be caused by more proximal problems.

Applied anatomy of the wrist and hand

The wrist joint comprises the distal radius and triangular cartilage which articulate with the proximal carpal bones (scaphoid, lunate and triquetral). The synovial cavity is contiguous with the intercarpal joints. Forearm muscles work together to perform movements, and stabilize them by opposition. The arch of carpal bones and the flexor retinaculum form the carpal tunnel, which contains the superficial and deep finger flexor tendons and the median nerve. These tendons lie in a common synovial tendon sheath, which extends from just proximal to the wrist to mid-palm. The flexor pollicis longus and flexor carpi ulnaris have individual sheaths. The finger extensor tendons

also share a synovial sheath lying under the extensor retinaculum. The extensor pollicis longus and abductor pollicis brevis share a compartment that crosses the radial styloid. Thumb movements occur at the first carpometacarpal and trapezoschaphoid joints, which are prone to osteoarthritis. The flexor pollicis brevis attaches to the base of the proximal phalanx of the thumb by a tendon containing a sesamoid bone. During finger flexion, five fibrous bands or pulleys hold down the flexor tendons in their sheaths. The lumbrical and interosseous muscles produce complex movements essential to fine hand functions, such as writing, and movements involving extension of the interphalangeal joints and flexion at the metacarpophalangeal joints.

Carpal tunnel syndrome is the commonest peripheral nerve entrapment syndrome. It is caused by flexor tenosynovitis. It occurs in the third trimester of pregnancy. Repetitive wrist and hand activity increases the risk of developing it. Its status as a work injury is controversial.[23] Pain, tingling and numbness affect the thumb, index, middle and radial side of ring fingers (median nerve distribution), and typically wake the patient or are present on waking. There is intense aching in the forearm and the fingers feel, but do not usually look, swollen. Holding a book or newspaper may precipitate the symptoms. When it is severe or of long-standing, thenar eminence wasting affecting the flexor pollicis and opponens pollicis and numbness cause clumsiness. The patient's description of the symptoms is often diagnostic.[24] Tapping the median nerve in the carpal tunnel (Tinel's sign) or holding the wrist in forced dorsiflexion (Phalen's test) causes tingling in the fingers. There is weakness of abduction of the thumb when it is adducted towards the fifth digit. Ultrasound scan or MRI demonstrates the carpal tunnel and median nerve well, but such investigations are rarely necessary. A diagnostic and therapeutic first approach is to use a wrist splint at night. If this relieves or reduces the symptoms its use for a few weeks may suffice. If not, a corticosteroid injection into the carpal tunnel is indicated, but recurrence is common and some opt for surgery. It is usual to perform nerve-conduction studies if the diagnosis is in doubt and to check for nerve damage. Slowing of median nerve conduction at the wrist suggests demyelination due to compression. In long-standing carpal tunnel syndrome the action potential is reduced or absent due to nerve fibre loss or damage, and needle electromyography detects denervation. If the changes are mild, a needle is inserted just to the ulnar side of the palmaris longus tendon, or about 0.5 cm to the ulnar side of flexor carpi radialis at the distal wrist skin crease, and at an angle of 45° pointing towards the middle finger. Local anaesthetic is injected superficially, but not into the carpal tunnel before the needle is advanced. A small test injection of corticosteroid may cause finger pain, indicating that the needle is in the nerve and needs repositioning. Then 1 mL of corticosteroid (hydrocortisone acetate 25 mg) is injected slowly. This may precipitate the symptoms initially due to a volume effect in the already tight carpal tunnel. Techniques differ, but this is an effective approach when the symptoms are mild and there is no permanent numbness or thenar muscle wasting.[25] Recurrent daytime symptoms, symptoms unrelieved by splinting or injection, or the presence of significant nerve damage need day-case surgical decompression or endoscopic surgery.[26] Pins and needles often worsen briefly postoperatively as the nerve recovers. Limited or no recovery of sensation and/or strength occurs if the lesion is severe and of long-standing.

Flexor tenosynovitis at the wrist is caused by unaccustomed or repetitive use. It also occurs in inflammatory arthritis. There is volar swelling and tenderness just proximal and distal to the wrist. The wrist feels stiff, painful and swollen, especially in the morning. Rest in a splint helps. Gripping and manual work cause *finger flexor tenosynovitis*. There is palpable finger flexor tendon thickening and nodularity, and tendon sheath synovitis. The affected finger(s) are stiff in the morning and there is pain in the palm and along the dorsum of the finger(s), which is reproduced by passive finger extension. Dactylitis may be due to psoriatic or reactive arthritis. Nodular flexor tenosynovitis is more common in diabetic individuals and less responsive to treatment.[27] A nodule catching at one of the pulleys overlying the metacarpophalangeal joint in the palm causes *trigger finger* – the patient wakes with the finger flexed and has to force it straight with a painful or painless click. Gripping also causes triggering. The nodule and the 'catch' in movement are felt in the palm. A low-pressure corticosteroid injection (hydrocortisone acetate 12.5 mg) alongside the tendon nodule in the palm helps. If persistent or recurrent, surgical release is necessary.

Thumb flexor tenosynovitis and *trigger thumb* is often due to local injury (e.g. opening a tight jar). The thumb interphalangeal joint sticks in flexion and snaps straight or cannot be bent. The sesamoid bone is tender on the volar surface of the thumb metacarpophalangeal joint. A corticosteroid injection adjacent to the sesamoid bone at the site of maximal tenderness helps.

Extensor tenosynovitis at the wrist affects the common extensor compartment and causes a well-defined typical hourglass shaped swelling proximal and distal to the wrist. The extensor retinaculum causes the constriction. By comparison, wrist joint synovitis causes diffuse swelling distal to the radius and ulna. Repetitive wrist and finger movements with the wrist in dorsiflexion cause extensor tenosynovitis, and this is one of the causes of forearm and wrist pain in keyboard workers. Rest helps, as does a corticosteroid injection into the tendon sheath. Wrist supports for the keyboard and mouse help prevent the problem.

De Quervain's stenosing tenosynovitis affects the tendon sheath of abductor pollicis longus and extensor pollicis brevis at the radial styloid. It is common in young parents, presumably due to holding a baby, and results from excessive use of the thumb with a computer mouse. Pain is felt around the styloid. By contrast, first carpometacarpal osteoarthritis causes pain at the base of the thumb. There is local tenderness and swelling. There may be crepitus or a tendon nodule causing triggering. Pressing the thumb into the palm (Finkelstein's test) increases the pain at the styloid. A low-pressure corticosteroid injection (hydrocortisone acetate 12.5 mg) alongside the tendon may help.[28]

First carpometacarpal osteoarthritis causes pain at the base of the thumb and is often associated with nodal osteoarthritis. It is due to inflammation of the ligament insertions around the joint, and causes swelling, local inflammation and pain. Initially, the pain may limit hand function, but over several months pain reduces in most as the joint stiffens and adducts, giving the hand a squared appearance. Conservative management is usual but a corticosteroid injection helps severe pain. Surgical replacement is rarely warranted. *Nodal osteoarthritis* is familial and most commonly involves the distal or, less often, proximal interphalangeal joints. The pain usually reduces over a few months, leaving bony swellings. Most patients manage without treatment once they know the prognosis is good. Local NSAID gels may help. The swelling, and occasionally joint instability, sometimes cause distress. Surgical fusion of the index distal or thumb interphalangeal joint in slight flexion improves pinch gripping. Proximal interphalangeal joint involvement may be mistaken for early rheumatoid arthritis; it often compromises the grip and impairs hand function significantly.

LOWER LIMB PAIN

Pain in the leg arises locally, is referred from the back, or is part of a generalized condition (rheumatoid arthritis, seronegative spondyloarthritis, polymyalgia rheumatica or a chronic pain syndrome). Spinal pain is common, and is discussed elsewhere. Facet joint osteoarthritis produces pain radiating from the buttock to the posterior thigh. It is worsened by back extension and may be uni- or bilateral. There may be a short or long history of back pain. Pain in the leg due to nerve-root impingement from a disc prolapse, from a spondylolisthesis or from spondylosis causing root or spinal canal narrowing is sharp or burning and usually associated with pins and needles or numbness and loss of power or reflexes. The pain may worsen with walking causing spinal claudication or nerve-root claudication. A disc prolapse causes acute low back pain and stiffness, and there is often a scoliosis when standing or bending forwards. These features are important in deciding the differential diagnosis of pain in the leg.

'Hip' pain

Great care is needed to identify the site and origin of pain around the hip. It is best to ask the patient to point to where they mean by the 'hip'. They may mean the iliac crest, buttock, trochanter, groin or anterior thigh. True hip pain is usually felt in the groin, anterior thigh and lower buttock. Buttock pain may be referred from the lumbar spine, or arise from the sacroiliac or hip joint or the ischiogluteal bursa. Trochanteric pain arises from the trochanteric bursa, gluteus medius muscle insertions or the thoracolumbar spine. It may be due to a disc prolapse at L1/2 or L2/3. Hip-joint pain radiates to the anterolateral thigh, buttock or anterior knee, and rarely to the shin or trochanteric region. It is worse when weight bearing and walking. Osteoarthritis is the commonest cause of hip arthritis in adults. Inflammatory arthritis is less common, but may present in younger people with seronegative spondyloarthropathy. Associated sacroiliitis causes buttock and posterior thigh pain. Persistent and unexplained hip pain, especially in elite athletes, warrants MRI to establish an accurate diagnosis.[29] 'Hip' pain in children and adolescents has different causes, such as Perthe's disease and slipped capital femoral epiphysis.[30]

Applied anatomy of the hip joint

The hip is a large ball-and-socket joint and is important in standing, walking, running and swimming. It is highly stable but has a wide range of movement. The femoral head is covered in hyaline cartilage, which is thickest at its upper weight-bearing pole. It is inserted deep into the acetabulum, which is extended by a fibrocartilaginous rim or labrum. The fibrous joint capsule is strong and lined by synovium. The joint is stabilized by powerful muscles. The upper surface of the acetabulum is normally horizontal and bears maximum load. A shallow acetabulum (dysplasia) and a more angulated upper surface predispose to early osteoarthritis. The acetabular cartilage lies in a horseshoe shape in the upper, medial and lateral surfaces. The hyaline cartilage of the femoral head is thickest at the upper pole and covers its surface, except at the point where the ligamentum teres inserts into the fovea, a small notch in the bony head. There is a break in the cartilage at the ligamentum teres that carries blood vessels to the femoral head. The femoral head is mounted on the femoral neck at an angle of 125–140° to the femoral shaft. The normal relationship of the femoral neck and shaft increases the leverage of the muscles inserting into the proximal femur. The greater trochanter is the site of insertion of the gluteal muscles. The lesser trochanter is the site of insertion of the hip flexors. The iliotibial band runs across the greater trochanter from the iliac crest to the lateral tibial tubercle and is part of the fascia lata. It is separated from the greater trochanter by the trochanteric bursa. A second bursa lies between the trochanter and the deep surface of the gluteus maximus. The iliopsoas bursa is anterior to the joint capsule, deep to the psoas tendon and just lateral to the femoral vessels. The ischiogluteal bursa lies between the gluteus maximus and the ischial tuberosity. Hip movements rely on the complex interaction of several muscles around the joint. The main extensors are the gluteus maximus and the hamstrings, and the main flexor is the iliopsoas muscle. The adductor longus, magnus and brevis muscles adduct and the gluteus medius and minimus abduct the hip.

Causes of anterior hip and groin pain

The commonest cause of anterior thigh pain that radiates to the anterior thigh and lower buttock is osteoarthritis or an inflammatory arthritis of the hip joint. There is pain and restricted flexion and reduced rotation of the hip, especially when the joint is held in flexion. X-ray, and occasionally MRI, aids diagnosis. In osteoarthritis the initial treatment should be conservative, with analgesia and NSAIDs. Eventually, in most patients total hip replacement, or a resurfacing procedure in younger patients, is a necessary and highly effective solution. Inflammatory arthritis warrants specialist referral for treatment, but may also eventually require surgery.

Causes of hip joint pain

Congenital dislocation and *severe hip dysplasia* are usually diagnosed in infants or young children, but minor dysplasia may present later in life, causing hip pain. On x-ray the normally horizontal upper surface of the acetabulum slopes upwards and laterally. The femoral head is less well covered than usual. This leads to increased stress on the upper, outer portion of the acetabulum and on the adjacent labrum, which becomes stressed and may tear. An *acetabular labral tear* causes repeated, sudden, painful, giving way in young physically active adults. The x-ray may show mild dysplasia, but the labral tear is demonstrated only by MRI arthrography. Dysplasia also leads to early osteoarthritis. These young people should be referred for a specialist surgical opinion. Osteotomy may be warranted to prevent pain and delay the onset of osteoarthritis.

Osteonecrosis of the femoral head may be caused by a fracture that disrupts the blood supply to the femoral neck. It occurs also in adults on corticosteroids, in alcoholics and in deep-sea divers and tunnellers. The hip pain is often extremely severe and worse with weight bearing. X-rays are normal in the early stages, but if this condition is suspected MRI is the best non-invasive diagnostic approach. Although the pain may settle, most patients need a surgical referral for femoral head resurfacing or replacement.

Groin injuries are common sporting injuries in men and women, particularly soccer players, gymnasts and horse riders. *Adductor enthesopathy* produces medial groin pain. Tears occur at the tendon insertion into the pubic tubercle or about 1 cm distal to this. There is local tenderness. Pain is caused by forced abduction and resisted adduction of the hip, and makes intercourse uncomfortable for women. Rest, local ultrasound and NSAIDs are all used initially, and occasionally a local corticosteroid injection alongside the tendon at the point of tenderness is helpful, but must be followed by a period of rest.

Iliopsoas bursitis presents as a painful swelling lateral to the neurovascular bundle in the groin deep to the point where the iliopsoas tendon runs under the inguinal ligament. The bursa separates the tendon from the anterior surface of the hip and may communicate with the joint cavity. The iliopsoas is a hip flexor and inserts into the lesser trochanter. The pain is worsened by hyperextension and resisted flexion of the hip. It can be aspirated and injected with corticosteroid under ultrasound guidance. The swollen bursa is clearly demonstrated on MRI.

Pubic symphysitis (osteitis pubis) is a rare inflammatory condition that develops after childbirth, pelvic surgery or athletic trauma. It is occasionally septic but usually sterile. The cause is unknown but the condition is possibly a type of algodystrophy. Pain and tenderness in the midline over the symphysis is worsened during the stance phase of walking. X-rays show lysis of the bony surfaces and widening. Aspiration and culture are essential to exclude infection. The condition settles after a period of rest, and pain is relieved by NSAIDs. A local corticosteroid injection into the symphysis is occasionally helpful.

Rectus femoris enthesitis is caused by blocked kicks and sprint starts. The muscle flexes the hip and extends the knee. Pain arises at the insertion into the anterior superior iliac spine, which is tender, and the pain is worsened by resisted hip flexion. *Rectus abdominis enthesitis* is a cause of groin strain in athletes. The pain is felt over the tender upper pubic ramus and in the lower abdomen. Both are clearly seen on MRI. Rest and NSAIDs help. The tendon may rupture close to its insertion, and in athletes requires surgical repair.

Causes of lateral hip and thigh pain

Trochanteric bursitis and *greater trochanteric pain syndrome* are usually due to direct local trauma or unaccustomed walking or other weight-bearing exercise. They are associated with ipsilateral hip arthritis and obesity, and with rheumatoid arthritis. A tight iliotibial band crossing the greater trochanter causes a painful 'snapping' hip. There is deep, aching pain over the trochanter that may radiate down the lateral thigh to the knee. Pain is worsened by walking, going down stairs, squatting or lying on the affected side. Tenderness over the trochanter is best localized with the patient lying on the unaffected side. Resisted hip abduction is painful, but hip movements are full unless the pain is severe. Rest and analgesia or NSAIDs help, but a local corticosteroid injection onto the surface of the trochanter at the point of maximum tenderness helps more persistent pain. The condition may recur in a physically active, middle-aged patient.[31] Weight loss and iliotibial band stretching exercises help to reduce recurrence. MRI is justifiable if the response to injection is poor or the symptoms atypical. This may demonstrate a bursitis, but more recently it has been recognized that tendinopathy or a tear of gluteus medius at its insertion into the greater trochanter may cause similar symptoms.[32] The optimal management of these lesions is not yet clear. Persistent and proven trochanteric bursitis can be managed by surgical excision of the bursa[33] or by lengthening a tight iliotibial band (Z-plasty).

Meralgia paraesthetica is due to an entrapment neuropathy of the lateral femoral cutaneous nerve (LFCN). It causes severe burning pain, dysaesthesia, pain in response to light touch (allodynia) and numbness of the anterolateral thigh from the trochanter to just above the knee. The dysaesthesia and numbness distinguish it from trochanteric bursitis. The pain is made worse by sitting, lying or tight clothing. There is no loss of power or muscle wasting. Pelvic or inguinal surgery, prone positioning for surgery or a direct injury are sometimes identified as the cause. The course of the nerve is highly variable, but it usually runs under the lateral inguinal ligament close to the anterior superior iliac spine. If the nerve is more superficial to the anterior iliac wing or passes through the sartorius muscle it can be compressed more readily. Nerve compression also occurs as it emerges through the fascia lata about 10 cm distal to the anterior superior iliac spine. A lateral L2/3 disc compressing the L3 nerve root mimics the syndrome, although there is usually also back pain and there may be wasting of the vastus lateralis. Management is usually conservative. Rest and avoidance of local causes of pressure are helpful. Many people cope with the symptoms once they understand that the condition is rarely progressive or disabling. Electrostimulation to localize the nerve precisely and its site of compression helps more accurate injection of local corticosteroid if the dysaesthesia is severe.[34]

Knee pain

The commonest cause of knee pain in a young adult is injury, usually arising from sport. As we age, radiological osteoarthritis increases in frequency but its severity does not correlate well with the severity of pain. Indeed, poor quadriceps muscle tone, obesity and clinical depression are more common correlates – an observation that is highly relevant when deciding on a management course. Knee pain may arise from the ligaments, tendons and bursae that lie around the knee, from bone, from intra-articular mechanical derangements (torn menisci or cruciate ligaments), or from osteoarthritis or inflammatory arthritis. The hip is a potential source of knee pain and must always be examined.

Applied anatomy of the knee joint

The knee is the largest and most complex joint in the body. It comprises the medial and lateral tibiofemoral and patellofemoral compartments. The synovial cavity is large and extends into the suprapatellar bursa, which produces a typical crescentic swelling around and about 5 cm proximal to the patella when distended with synovitis and synovial fluid. The menisci are fibrocartilagenous, half-moon-shaped structures that lie between the outer margins of the rounded femoral and flatter tibial articular surfaces. They attach in front and behind to the intercondylar area of the tibia and circumferentially to the joint capsule. They alter shape to maintain congruity of the adjacent joint surfaces during movement and are important in weight bearing. Their inner margins are avascular and liable to tears and irreversible damage.

The knee is a complex hinge joint that rotates into a locked position in full extension. There is normally a valgus angle of around 7° between the femur and the tibia. When this angle is increased (valgus) or decreased (varus) the joint is more stressed, and this may predispose to osteoarthritis and to periarticular lesions. The patella is a sesamoid bone in the quadriceps tendon and its medial and lateral facets articulate with the femoral intercondylar groove. The quadriceps muscle normally pulls towards the anterior superior iliac spine at an angle of 15° to the tibia. If this angle is greater than 20° lateral dislocation of the patella is possible, especially when the vastus medialis muscle is weak or the patient is hypermobile. Little muscular effort is required when standing if the lower limb is correctly aligned.

Increasing flexion is associated with increasing instability of the joint and more dependence on periarticular structures and muscles. The capsule is strong, with areas of more condensed fibres creating the medial and lateral collateral ligaments. The medial collateral ligament runs from the medial femoral condyle to the medial tibia deep to the pes anserinus. The lateral collateral ligament runs from the lateral aspect of the lateral condyle down and back to the biceps femoris tendon, and inserts into the fibula. The internal cruciate ligaments maintain tension at various angles of flexion and contribute to anteroposterior joint stability. The anterior cruciate ligament prevents anterior displacement of the tibia on the femur, and the posterior cruciate ligament prevents posterior displacement. The knee is highly dependent on strong muscles for its stability and movements. The quadriceps extends the knee, acting through the patella and inserting at the tibial tubercle. The vastus medialis component holds the patella in the intercondylar groove and locks the knee in extension. The 'hamstrings' act across the knee as flexors and the hip as extensors. They also help pull the trunk up from flexion. The semimembranosus and semitendonosus insert into the medial and the biceps femoris into the lateral tibial plateau, and help pull the trunk up by extending the hip. They also control medial and lateral rotation of the knee. The gastrocnemius, sartorius and gracilis flex the knee. There are several bursae around the knee. The prepatellar bursa is subcutaneous and lies in front of the patella. The infrapatellar bursa is also subcutaneous and lies over the patellar tendon and tibial tubercle. There is a large bursa in the medial popliteal fossa between the insertions of the semi-membranosus and the medial head of gastrocnemius. This is often connected to the joint cavity and can become distended to form a popliteal cyst. The anserine bursa lies between the medial collateral ligament and the tendons of sartorius, gracilis and semitendonosus as they merge to insert into the medial tibia as the pes anserinus.

Arthritis of the knee

The knee is commonly affected by osteoarthritis. This increases with age. There is a relationship between early injury of the menisci and cruciate ligaments and the earlier development of osteoarthritis when the joint is managed surgically,[35] and probably when surgery is not undertaken. Knee pain may be medial, lateral or retropatellar, according to the site of maximum involvement. When there is an effusion, the pain tends to be more diffuse and there is a sense of fullness or stiffness when bending the knee. Flexion is usually limited if the effusion is significant. All types of inflammatory arthritis affect the knee. Pseudogout is the cause of a hot, painful swollen knee in older people when chondrocalcinosis is evident on an x-ray and crystals of pyrophosphate are found in the fluid. Gout may also affect the knee. Aspiration of fluid from the knee is relatively easy to perform and is helpful diagnostically and therapeutically. It is often combined with the injection of corticosteroid unless joint infection is suspected or proven.[36]

Intra-articular injuries of the knee

The knee is a common site of injury, particularly during sports. The medial and lateral menisci are fibrocartilagenous structures that are resilient in the young but readily damaged by twisting injuries with the knee partly flexed. Ageing leads to loss of resilience and degeneration. These all predispose to osteoarthritis of the knee. In the younger person, during sport meniscal tears cause immediate acute pain initially and medial or lateral joint pain. The knee then swells and the pain is more diffuse. Full extension of the knee is limited. There is localized joint-line tenderness that persists. The acute episode may settle. In most cases episodic swelling occurs and the knee may lock in flexion. MRI is the best non-invasive investigation, and clearly demonstrates the lesion. There may be an associated cruciate injury. Arthroscopic trimming of the meniscus is helpful if problems persist

and for continuing active sports, but may not prevent later development of osteoarthritis in the affected compartment.[37] The value of meniscectomy in the older patient with degenerate menisci is unclear, particularly when there is established osteoarthritis.

Cruciate ligament tears are usually the result of a major knee injury and lead to a haemarthrosis in the young. The anterior cruciate is more commonly injured. The patient complains of severe pain, and the knee shows anteroposterior instability, which is best seen with the foot fixed and the knee at 45°. The acute phase is assessed by MRI, but is often managed conservatively. A specialist knee orthopaedic opinion is best obtained. Later the knee may be unsteady and painful. The anterior cruciate is more commonly torn. The knee hyperextends and the tibia can be drawn forwards abnormally.

Plica syndrome is associated with a congenital abnormality of the knee. It causes anteromedial knee pain, a sensation of snapping, pain and localized swelling. It is an arthroscopic diagnosis and removal of the plica may help.

In *osteochondritis dessicans* of the knee a fragment of bone and overlying cartilage detach. The fragment may form a loose body and cause pain and locking in flexion, or remain in situ. In younger patients the lateral femoral condyle is the usual site. A similar problem affecting the medial femoral condyle is seen in older patients. The cause is unknown, but the pathology is that of osteonecrosis. The lesion is seen best on a tunnel anteroposterior X-ray or MRI. Loose fragments can be reattached or removed.

Pigmented villonodular synovitis is rare but most commonly affects the knee. It may follow injury but the cause is unknown. Localized proliferative synovitis becomes nodular and brown due to haemosiderin deposition. Any effusion is also deep brown. The diagnosis is usually made on MRI and confirmed by biopsy. It is prone to invade bone locally, so it is best removed arthroscopically.

Causes of anterior knee pain

Prepatellar bursitis causes anterior knee pain, with superficial swelling and inflammation. It often follows trauma. *Infrapatellar bursitis* causes pain, swelling and tenderness superficial to the patellar tendon. Rest, icing and sometimes a corticosteroid injection are helpful. Patellar tendonitis is common in jumpers. The tendon is tender and may be swollen. This is seen clearly on MRI. Rest helps, but a steroid injection is best avoided. *Anterior knee pain syndrome* without abnormal patellar tracking is often bilateral and occurs in adolescent women. *Chondromalacia patellae* is an arthroscopic diagnosis. The patellar cartilage is thin and fibrillated. It occurs with *patellar maltracking*, which presents in adolescence or early adult life and is associated with a valgus knee deformity, lateral displacement of the patella and a tendency to lateral dislocation. The patella rides high on the lateral femoral condyle on a skyline x-ray. Rest, avoiding wearing high heels and isometric quadriceps exercises help. The role of surgery is unproven. Pain may arise at the insertion of quadriceps into the proximal patella or at the insertion of the patellar tendon distally.

Causes of medial knee pain

Medial ligament insertion pain produces local pain and tenderness over the medial tibia just distal to the joint line. It is caused by a valgus strain injury and occurs in overweight women with fat thighs. Pain is reproduced by exerting a valgus stress on the knee. Clinically it is difficult to distinguish from *anserine bursitis*, which produces pain and tenderness behind the medial ligament and more distally. *Pellegrini–Stiega disease* is caused by an injury to the medial ligament at its insertion into the medial femoral condyle. It causes medial femoral condylar pain and tenderness, and leads to linear calcification, probably in a haematoma, that is seen overlying the medial femoral condyle on an anteroposterior x-ray. Rest helps all these conditions, but occasionally a local corticosteroid injection is necessary. A medial meniscal tear or medial compartment osteoarthritis also cause medial knee pain

Causes of lateral knee pain

Iliotibial band syndrome is due to overuse in runners. Knee flexion causes friction between the iliotibial band as it crosses the lateral collateral ligament and the lateral femoral condyle. The pressure is greatest at about 30° of flexion. The band is painful and tender at the knee. Lateral synovial recess inflammation may lead to bursa formation. MRI is the investigation of choice to demonstrate changes deep to the iliotibial band. Rest followed by retraining is effective for most.[37] A lateral meniscal tear or lateral compartment osteoarthritis also cause lateral knee pain.

Causes of posterior knee pain

The semimembranosus bursa becomes distended by a knee effusion in patients in whom there is a valve-like connection, leading to a *popliteal cyst (Baker's cyst)*. Fluid enters the bursa but cannot return, and the pressure increases during walking, standing from sitting and climbing stairs. A *ruptured popliteal cyst* causes sudden pain behind the knee and in the upper calf, followed by upper calf tenderness and swelling, and ankle oedema. The knee effusion may reduce in size. The patient may present to the accident and emergency department. The condition mimics a deep venous thrombosis, although this causes pain and tenderness lower in the calf. Doppler ultrasound examination confirms the diagnosis and excludes a deep venous thrombosis. Rest and NSAIDs help and a compression stocking should be applied, but anticoagulation is contraindicated. Aspiration and injection of the knee is necessary if there is an inflammatory arthritis. Occasionally a slow leak of fluid from a ruptured popliteal cyst causes a painless cystic swelling in the calf and may require surgery. The medial or lateral hamstring insertions may be injured by overuse and produce localized pain and tenderness at their insertion.

Lower leg pain

Compartment syndromes occur in athletes and are due to increased pressure leading to ischaemia in the confined anatomical compartments of the lower leg. The commonest is *anterior compartment syndrome*, which affects the tibialis anterior, extensor digitorum longus and extensor hallucis longus muscles, the deep peroneal nerve and the anterior tibial artery and vein. The pain is diffuse, feels like cramp and follows exercise. It resolves with rest but recurs with further exertion. The compartment is swollen and is tender. It is an important cause of exercise-related anterior leg pain. Intracompartmental pressures are measured before and after exercise prior to surgical decompression. An acute compartment syndrome is a surgical emergency and usually follows trauma. Muscle necrosis and permanent nerve damage may occur if the pressure is not relieved. Compartment syndromes occur in the other compartments of the leg and in the volar compartment of the forearm.

Fibular tunnel syndrome is due to compression of the lateral popliteal nerve just distal to the head of the fibula. It is caused by compression from a walking cast, sitting cross-legged or injury. There are pins and needles or numbness of the lateral calf and foot, and occasionally a foot drop develops. The site of the lesion is localized by nerve-conduction studies to distinguish it from an L5 nerve-root lesion.

Stress fractures of the tibia or fibula are caused by fatigue failure in normal bone in dancers, runners and jumpers. Women athletes with amenorrhoea are particularly at risk. Stress fractures occur spontaneously in older people with osteoporosis. The metatarsal bones are also affected (a 'march' fracture). The pain is worse with weight bearing, and there is local tenderness and swelling. Initially x-rays are normal, but MRI or a technetium bone scan is diagnostic. Early diagnosis, rest for up to 6 weeks and exercise in water help maintain fitness in elite athletes and others. Assessment for osteoporosis is obligatory.

Ankle and foot pain

The ankle and foot are frequently injured or the site of osteoarthritis or inflammatory arthritis. Pain is usually worse when moving from rest to weight bearing.

Applied anatomy of the ankle and foot

The foot and ankle absorb the weight of the body during standing and walking. During jumping, six times the body weight is transmitted through the feet. The ankle complex comprises the ankle (a semistable hinge), subtalar and midtarsal joints. The medial and lateral malleoli, the deltoid ligament medially and the collateral ligament laterally contribute to joint stability. The joint capsule is lax in front and behind but powerfully strengthened medially and laterally. There is a shock-absorbing fibrofatty pad under the calcaneum. The subtaloid joint between the talus and calcaneum has a complex surface shape and aids walking on uneven surfaces. There is limited but important movement at the tarsometatarsal joints between the three cuneiform bones and the bases of the metatarsal bones. The metatarsophalangeal joints and the first interphalangeal joint are important during walking. The first metatarsophalangeal joint requires around 60° of dorsiflexion during normal walking. The lateral toes help control fine balance. The plantar fascia is thick centrally and becomes broader and thinner distally. It inserts into the medial tubercle of the calcaneum proximally and divides in the mid-foot to merge with the flexor tendons distally. It is elastic for shock absorption but stabilizes the longitudinal arch of the foot. The medial arch is high and flexible, and acts as a resilient spring during standing and walking. The metatarsal heads are protected by a shock-absorbing fibrofatty pad. Hammer toes pull this pad forward and cause painful metatarsalgia.

The muscles that control standing and walking comprise extrinsic muscles in the three compartments of the lower leg, the tendons of which are enclosed in synovial sheaths as they cross the ankle joint, and the intrinsic foot muscles. The powerful ankle plantar flexors are in the calf and insert into the posterior calcaneum through the Achilles tendon. The dorsiflexors in the anterior compartment have tendons, each in its own sheath, which change direction in front of the ankle under the extensor retinaculum. The foot everters are in the lateral compartment and their tendons change direction in a single sheath behind the lateral malleolus. The toe plantar flexors are deep in the calf and their tendons change direction in individual sheaths in the tarsal tunnel behind the medial malleolus. The intrinsic foot muscles lie under and between the tarsal and metatarsal bones and are virtually inactive during standing. As weight is transferred to the forefoot during walking and running these muscles become active and hold the foot rigid during toe off.

Pain in the medial ankle

Tibialis posterior tendinopathy causes medial pain and swelling behind the medial malleolus. The tibialis posterior muscle stabilizes the hind foot and limits eversion; it is under greatest tension during running and dancing. It is often associated with a flat or pronated foot. Longitudinal splits develop in the tendon (tendinopathy) and may progress to full tears. Synovitis of the tendon sheath near the medial malleolus also occurs. Rest helps and a surgical boot may be needed. Once it has settled, any inversion deformity requires an arch support. Ultrasound scan or MRI demonstrates the lesion. A synovitis can be treated with a local corticosteroid injection, but this is best avoided if there is significant tendon splitting, to reduce the risk of a full tear. In severe tendinopathy and in athletes, an expert surgical opinion is best.

Tarsal tunnel syndrome is an entrapment neuropathy of the posterior tibial nerve in the tunnel as it turns around the medial malleolus. The patient wakes with burning pain and pins and needles in the toes, sole and heel. There may be weakness of toe flexion. Tinel's sign is positive behind the medial malleolus, where there may be swelling. Nerve-conduction studies are diagnostic. Treatment of the cause of compression is necessary if rest and an arch support do not help.

Pain in front of the ankle

Tibialis anterior tenovaginitis (also involving the extensor digitorum longus and extensor hallucis longus) produces pain and crepitus in front of the ankle and over the dorsum of the foot. The swelling extends across the joint, distinguishing it from synovitis of the ankle joint, which bulges to either side of the extensor tendons. The condition arises from unaccustomed walking or running or tight shoes. Rest and looser shoes help. A corticosteroid injection is sometimes necessary.

Pain in the lateral ankle

Peroneus longus and *brevis tendinopathy* cause pain and tenderness where tendons in their sheaths run posterior to the lateral malleolus. The longus tendon runs under the sole to insert into the base of the first metatarsal bone. The brevis tendon inserts into the base of the fifth metatarsal, and may be affected by an enthesitis causing pain and tenderness at the fifth metatarsal base. Rest helps and corticosteroid injections are occasionally necessary.

Pain under the heel

Plantar fasciitis[38] is an enthesitis of the fascia at its insertion into the medial calcaneum. It is seen in sports that involve a heavy heel strike and in overweight, middle-aged joggers. A flat arch may be present. There is weight-bearing pain under the heel, particularly when getting up from bed or a chair. Walking eases the pain initially, but worsens it with distance. Tenderness is localized to the anterior calcaneum. In around 30% of cases a bony spur is seen at the origin of the plantar fascia on x-ray. Such spurs may be asymptomatic and bilateral, but increase the risk of injury. Younger patients occasionally develop plantar fasciitis due to seronegative arthritis.

Subcalcaneal bursitis produces pain under the heel pad, but is difficult to diagnose clinically. In older patients the normal fat-packed fibrous septa of the subcalcaneal pad may rupture after direct trauma and in the obese, and cause heel pain. A heel cup, an arch support and thick-soled shoes help. MRI is rarely necessary, but demonstrates inflammation of the plantar fascia, bursitis or diffuse signal change in the heel pad. Stretching exercises reduce shortening of the plantar fascia, and some advise a nocturnal dorsiflexion splint. Injections of local anaesthetic and corticosteroid are commonly employed and relieve the pain, although these interventions are painful and it is suggested that they can cause damage. The evidence base for such treatments is weak.[39]

Pain behind the heel

The Achilles tendon is the body's strongest tendon but is prone to injury during sports or when changing from heeled shoes to walking barefoot. *Achilles tendinopathy*[40] is due to overuse and probably involves microtrauma of the tendon. The pain, tenderness and swelling occur about 1–2 cm proximal to the insertion into the calcaneum. It is worse when walking. Rest and a heel raise in the shoe are usually sufficient, and stretching when the pain has reduced prevents recurrence. Local corticosteroid injections are contraindicated as they may precipitate rupture of the tendon.

Achilles tendon rupture occurs usually in the middle-aged or older patient during sports. In the younger, active patient the tear is repaired surgically, but in the older patient, conservative management in a cast is usual.[41] Pain at the insertion of the tendon is due to overuse or, occasionally, a seronegative arthritis. Rest, a heel raise and NSAIDs help, but an adjacent low-pressure corticosteroid injection may be appropriate.

Retrocalcaneal bursitis is uncommon, but occurs in runners and dancers. Pain, tenderness and swelling lie between the tendon and the ankle joint. It can be safely injected with corticosteroid. High-backed training shoes are rarely available now because they caused pain and a subcutaneous bursitis superficial to the Achilles tendon.

Arch disorders and foot pain

A flat longitudinal arch is often asymptomatic but may produce local midtarsal pain, or pain in the medial or lateral ankle when standing and walking. The foot flattens and everts in the stance phase of walking. Weight is borne along the lateral border of the foot. As weight is taken off the heel it transfers to the metatarsal heads. A flat foot may be congenital or acquired, and reversible or irreversible. Congenital flat foot is more common, and may be rigid or reversible and due to hypermobility. Congenital flat foot is familial and asymptomatic until adolescence or adulthood. Bridging between the talus and calcaneous or navicula and calcaneous (tarsal coalition) causes a rigid flat foot with a complete loss of the medial longitudinal arch in all positions. Severe flat foot deformities are common in rheumatoid arthritis. Arch supports and exercises to strengthen inversion help the painful mobile flat foot. Untreated the condition may lead to a spastic flat foot, with painful peroneal muscle spasm. Chronic flat foot increases the risk of inflammation of the tibialis posterior tendon. If this tendon ruptures the foot flattens suddenly. Eventually, a flat foot becomes rigid and a moulded semi-rigid insole can be helpful.

A high-arched foot (pes cavus) and toe clawing is congenital and often hereditary. There is pain in the arch due to poor shock absorption and loss of eversion of the foot during the stance phase. Shoes with high arch supports and metatarsal pads are helpful.

Generalized leg pain

Generalized leg pain is much less common than generalized arm pain. Causes of leg pain include claudication due to poor circulation, nerve compression in the spine from a disc prolapse or spondylosis (usually unilateral), claudication arising from spinal canal stenosis (usually bilateral), or spinal root canal stenosis (often unilateral and in a nerve root distribution). Peripheral neuropathy causes symmetrical burning leg pain in a stocking distribution.

COMPLEX REGIONAL PAIN SYNDROME

Complex regional pain syndrome (CRPS) types 1 and 2 (previously called Sudek's atrophy or reflex sympathetic dystrophy)[42] affects either the arm or leg. It has a cumbersome definition: 'a complex disorder or group of disorders that may develop as a consequence of trauma affecting the limbs, with (type 2) or without (type 1) obvious nerve lesions'. The nomenclature is complex. CRPS is uncommon but usually follows some form of injury or surgical intervention (type 1). In the arm it may follow what appears to be a typical rotator cuff tendinopathy, previously usually called a shoulder–hand syndrome. When associated with neurological damage, for example after a

nerve injury, it is called type 2. With nerve injury it was previously called 'causalgia'.

Usually only one limb is affected. It is more common in women than men and after the age of 40 years. The typical pattern of pain and other sensory abnormalities is diffuse, more widespread than the pain originating from the site of initial injury, and does not fit usual neurological or anatomical patterns. The pain often appears disproportionate to the initial injury. The initial symptom complex includes often severe, burning pain, hyperaesthesia, allodynia (pain felt on light touch) and autonomic dysfunction (increased temperature, increased sweating and colour changes). Initially the area is swollen and oedematous. The early phase is probably reversible, but is difficult to recognize. Over a few weeks to several months the pain persists but dystrophic changes develop. The joint(s) become stiff, the skin thin and cold, and there is local hair loss. There is usually underlying osteoporosis. A late phase may develop, with pain, joint contractures, and muscle and skin atrophy. Movement of the affected limb may be limited. The pathological cause is unclear. There are often psychosocial complications, but psychogenic factors have never been shown to be the cause of CRPS.[43] Abnormal pain behaviour, guarding

PRACTICE POINTS

- At the initial visit most individuals with limb pain can be reassured that the pain will settle with simple treatment and the passage of time – appropriate rest, simple analgesia are often used first. Physical treatments may help if the pain does not settle.

- A more specific diagnosis may subsequently be appropriate and clues to the differential diagnosis of these clinical syndromes are described in this chapter.

- This process may then suggest more specific and targeted treatments. The evidence base for some treatments is limited, but there is evidence that the patient can be helped to remain at work and functioning normally.

- Imaging as a means of investigating limb pain should be limited to patients in whom there is a high risk of a more serious underlying cause or when the pain persists despite initial treatment. Interpretation of the findings is not always easy.

- It is important to keep people at work and functioning normally, or suggest a brief period of rest, so as not to jeopardize their long-term employment.

- Early recognition of the diagnosis, good pain control and appropriate advice may reduce the risk of developing a chronic pain syndrome.

- There may be important psychological or social factors that need to be considered in the management of limb pain.

- Management of work-related limb pain is best undertaken with the help and support of the employer, and may involve a period of rest and/or reduced activity.

and immobility are often seen in the later phases. The most severely affected individuals will always need psychological support as part of the management of this extremely distressing problem. However, it is important to note that most often there are less dramatic forms of this enigmatic condition, and in one group of patients with the diagnosis of CRPS of an upper extremity, 70% were still working after 5.5 years.[43]

Diagnosis is difficult, partly because CRPS has not been well known among doctors outside the group of pain specialists.[43] It is important to recognize the unusual nature and distribution of the pain, the associated skin changes (warm, red and oedematous) and osteoporosis (as seen on x-rays or as patchily increased activity on an isotope bone scan), although this is a late sign. Adequate pain control is difficult but important and it is essential that the patient is persuaded to move the limb and to weight bear if a leg is affected in the early painful phase. Mild forms are probably common (perhaps 75% of the total[43]) and may go unrecognized, recovering fully, but early referral to a pain management clinic is advisable. The evidence base for treatment is poor. Recently, trials have included the use of calcitonin and bisphosphonates in the early phase.[44] Evidence of sympathetically maintained pain may be adduced from a positive response (pain reduction) to an intravenous infusion of phentolamine. If positive, a stellate ganglion block for upper-limb pain or a block of the sympathetic chain for lower-limb involvement is used. Regional infusions of lignocaine or the alpha blocker guanethedine, with a tourniquet, are also used. The evidence base for such treatments is poor. Psychological and physiotherapy support are essential to help the severely affected patient keep active and move the affected limb despite the pain. In the later stages, the outlook is poor and chronic disability usual.

RESEARCH AGENDA

- Studies of interventions for limb pain are often underpowered and poorly designed. The Cochrane Collaboration and other such evidence-based organizations provide information about the studies that are available and their reliability.

- More carefully designed studies would help, but the evidence base for many interventions may remain unsatisfactory. No evidence from randomized, controlled trials does not necessarily mean that there is no beneficial effect; rather the treatment is, to use the Scottish legal term, 'unproven'.

- Many individuals with localized limb pain turn to alternative or complementary approaches before reporting to their healthcare professional. These techniques may be helpful or may simply allow the problem to settle by the passage of time. These therapies are not easily amenable to the standard randomized, placebo-controlled trial, which was developed to test drugs. In studies of acupuncture and other non-pharmacological therapies the diagnosis and treatment may vary; and the effects that are seen may be the result of such interactions as talking and listening, which are integral to rather than incidental parts of the treatment. The use of controlled placebo or sham trials for such complex interventions may lead to false-negative results.

- For complex non-pharmacological interventions, randomized pragmatic designs or randomized cluster designs may be more appropriate than studies that use explanatory designs.

REFERENCES

1. Croft P. The epidemiology of pain: the more you have the more you get. *Ann Rheum Dis* 1996; **55**: 859–860.
2. Lock C, Allgar V, Jones K et al. Prevalence of back, neck and shoulder problems. *Physiother Res Intl* 1999; **4**:161–169.
3. MacFarlane GJ, Hunt MH, Silman A. Role of mechanical and psychosocial factors in the onset of forearm pain: prospective population-based study. *BMJ* 2000; **321**: 676–679.
4. Cochrane Collaboration. Available at: http://www.cochrane.org (accessed 27 August 2006).
5. MedlinePlus. Available at: http://www.nlm.nih.gov/medlineplus (accessed 27 August 2006).
6. Paterson C, Dieppe P. Characteristic and incidental (placebo) effects in complex interventions such as acupuncture. *BMJ* 2005; **330**: 1202–1204.
7. Palmer KT. Pain in the forearm, wrist and hand. *Best Pract Res Clin Rheumatol* 2003; **17**: 113–135.
8. Hadler NM, Carey TS, Garrett J. The influence of indemnification by workers' compensation insurance on recovery from acute back pain. *Spine* 1995; **15**: 2710–2715.
9. van der Heijden GJMG. Shoulder disorders: a state of the art review. *Ballière's Clin Rheumatol* 1999; **13**: 287–309.
10. Brox JI. Shoulder pain. *Best Pract Res Clin Rheumatol* 2003; **17**: 33–56.
11. Oestoer AJK, Richards CA, Prevost AT et al. Diagnosis and relation to general health of shoulder disorders presenting to primary care. *Rheumatology* 2005; **44**: 800–805.
12. Green S, Buchbinder R, Glazier R et al. Systematic review of randomised controlled trials of interventions for the painful shoulder: selection criteria, outcome and assessment. *BMJ* 1998; **316**: 354–360.
13. Roberts CS, Walker JA, Seligson D. Diagnostic capabilities of shoulder ultrasonography in the detection of complete and partial rotator cuff tears. *Am J Orthopaed* 2001; **30**: 159–162.
14. Speed C, Hazleman B. Shoulder pain. *Clin Evidence* 2002; **7**: 1122–1139.
15. Warner JJ. Frozen shoulder; diagnosis and management. *J Am Acad Orthopaed Surg* 1997; **5**: 130–140.
16. Hay EM, Paterson SM, Lewis M et al. Pragmatic randomised controlled trial of local corticosteroid injection and naproxen for treatment of lateral epicondylitis of elbow in primary care. *BMJ* 1999; **319**: 964–968.
17. Ryans I, Montgomery A, Galway R et al. A randomized controlled trial of intra-articular triamcinolone and/or physiotherapy in shoulder capsulitis. *Rheumatology* 2005; **44**: 529–535.
18. Trinh KV, Phillips SD, Ho E et al. Acupuncture for the alleviation of lateral epicondyle pina: a systematic review. *Rheumatology* 2004; **43**: 1085–1090.
19. Helliwell P. The elbow, forearm, wrist and hand. In: Croft P, Brooks PM (eds), *Clinical Rheumatology: Regional Musculoskeletal Pain.* Ballière Tindall, London, 1999, pp. 311–328.
20. Greening J, Lynn B. Vibration sense in the upper limb in patients with repetitive strain injury and a group of at-risk office workers. *Int Arch Occup Environ Health* 1998; **71**: 29–34.
21. Feuerstein M, Miller VL, Burrell LM et al. Occupational upper extremity disorders in the federal workforce. *Occup Environ Med* 1998; **40**: 546–555.
22. Macfarlane GJ. Generalised pain, fibromyalgia and regional pain: an epidemiological view. *Ballière's Clin Rheumatol* 1999; **13**: 403–414.
23. Yagev Y, Carel RS, Yagev R. Assessment of work-related risk factors for carpal tunnel syndrome. *Isr Med Assoc J* 2001; **3**: 569–571.
24. Pal B, O'Gradaigh D, Merry P. Diagnosis of carpal tunnel syndrome. *Rheumatology* 2001; **40**: 595–597.
25. Singh VAR, Sachdev A, Shekhar WS et al. A prospective study of the long term efficacy of local methyl prednisolone acetate in the management of mild carpal tunnel syndrome. *Rheumatology* 2005; **44**: 647–650.
26. Trumble TE, Gilbert M, McCallister WV. Endoscopic versus open surgical treatment of carpal tunnel syndrome. *Neurosurg Clin North Am* 2001; **12**: 255–266.

27. Stahl S, Kanter Y, Karnelli E. Outcome of trigger finger treatment in diabetes. *J Rheumatol* 1997; **24**: 931–936.

28. Rankin ME, Rankin EA. Injection therapy for management of stenosing tenosynovitis (de Quervain's disease) of the wrist. *J Natl Med Assoc* 1998; **90**: 474–476.

29. De Paulis F, Cacchio A, Michelini O et al. Sports injuries in the pelvis: diagnostic imaging. *Eur J Radiol* 1998; **27**(Suppl 1): S49–S59

30. Zacher J, Gursche A. 'Hip' pain. *Best Pract Res Clin Rheumatol* 2003; **17**: 71–85.

31. Shbeed MI, O'Duffy JD, Michet CJ Jr et al. Evaluation of glucocorticosteroid injection for the treatment of trochanteric bursitis. *J Rheumatol* 1996; **23**: 2104–2106.

32. Kingzett-Taylor A, Tirman PF, Feller J et al. Tendonosis and tears of gluteus medius and minimus muscles as a cause of hip pain: MR imaging findings. *Am J Roentgenol* 1999; **173**: 1123–1126.

33. Slawski DP, Howard RF. Surgical management of refractory trochanteric bursitis. *Am J Sports Med* 1997; **25**: 86–89.

34. Grossman MG, Ducey SA, Nadler SS et al. Meralgia paraesthetica: diagnosis and treatment. *J Am Acad Orthop Surg* 2001; **9**: 336–334.

35. Neyret P, Donell SD, Dejour H. Osteoarthritis of the knee following meniscetomy. *Br J Rheumatol* 1994; **33**: 267–268.

36. Shipley M, Black C, Compston J et al. Rheumatology and bone disease. In: Kumar P, Clark M (eds), *Clinical Medicine*, 5th edn. WB Saunders, London, 2002, pp. 511–586.

37. Biundo JJ, Irwin RW, Umpierre E. Sports and other soft tissue injuries, tendinitis, bursitis and occupation-related syndromes. *Curr Opin Rheumatol* 2001; **13**: 146–149.

38. Buchbinder R. Plantar fasciitis. *N Engl J Med* 2004; **350**: 2159–2167.

39. Crawford F, Atkins D, Edwards J. *Interventions for Heel Pain.* Cochrane Review. Cochrane Database Systematic Review 2000; *CD000416.*

40. Maffulli N, Sharma P, Luscombe KL. Achilles tendinopathy: aetiology and management. *J R Soc Med* 2004; **97**: 472–476.

41. Jarvinen TAH, Kannus P, Paavola M et al. Achilles tendon injuries. *Curr Opin Rheumatol* 2001; **13**: 150–155.

42. Raja S, Grabow TS. Complex regional pain syndrome I (reflex sympathetic dystrophy). *Anesthesiology* 2002; **96**: 1254–1260.

43. Geertzen JH, Dijkstra PU, Groothof JW et al. Reflex sympathetic dystrophy of the upper extremity: A 5.5 year follow-up: II. Social life events, general health and changes in occupation. *Acta Orthop Scand* 1998; **279**(Suppl):19–23.

44. Manicourt DH, Brasseur JP, Boutsen Y et al. Role of alendronate therapy for post-traumatic complex regional pain syndrome type I of the lower extremity. *Arthritis Rheum* 2004; **50**: 3690–3697.

Chapter 16

Diagnosing regional pain: the view from primary care

Peter Croft

INTRODUCTION

The view from primary care is little changed since the original version of this chapter appeared in 1999. The general principle remains that regional musculoskeletal pain can be seen as both (i) a local problem with an underlying pathological cause and (ii) a pain syndrome that shares characteristics common to pain syndromes elsewhere in the body, regardless of location.

The diagnostic approach to the local problem can be based on triage:

1. Is there evidence for a serious cause?
2. If not (1), is there an important cause to be identified that might help to guide or otherwise influence effective management?
3. If not (1) or (2), treat it as a 'non-specific' pain syndrome, which does not so much require a regional diagnostic label but rather more general approaches to pain management (such as those reviewed by Main and Williams[1]).

There has been criticism of the 'non-specific' label as it is used in back pain[2] because of the implication that such a label carries – that treatments targeted at local causes of the pain are irrelevant. New research, for example, has suggested that there are clinical subgroups of back pain sufferers who might selectively respond to different treatments.[3, 4] Furthermore, primary care practitioners themselves appear to believe that non-specific low back pain is not one condition, and that in practice they are identifying subgroups and treating them differently.[5] However, this does not mean that the 'triage' approach is wrong, but rather that we should be prepared to expand stage (2) of triage ('important cause') when effective treatments for clinically distinct subgroups are identified. Equally, we should continue to question whether apparently important diagnoses do actually result in more effective treatment. Lumping together different shoulder-pain presentations in primary care is, for example, guaranteed to raise the hackles of the mildest musculoskeletal

diagnostician, and yet there remains surprisingly little hard evidence that subclassifying shoulder pain in primary care makes any difference to outcome.

THE PARADIGM OF LOW BACK PAIN

National consensus, guideline or evidence review bodies support the idea of diagnostic triage for low back pain, emphasizing the need first to identify serious red-flag diagnoses. The arguments remain in favour of using clinical symptoms and signs as the method to raise suspicion of red-flag problems and as the basis for further investigation. The crucial diagnostic step is to rule out serious underlying conditions that may need urgent attention. Cancer, infection, spinal cord compression, aneurysm and systemic inflammatory disease are considered to be such red-flag diagnoses. This approach has two crucial advantages from the point of view of the primary care clinician. First, the suspicion of a red-flag diagnosis is triggered by the presence of red-flag characteristics (e.g. pain with an unusual and progressive pattern, fever or weight loss). Second, epidemiological evidence indicates a very low frequency of serious underlying pathological diagnoses in populations of low back pain sufferers who present in primary care.[6] In other words the primary care physician does not need to hunt for such conditions in the absence of suspicious characteristics and can be encouraged to make a positive diagnosis of 'simple low back pain' as the key to sensible general pain management approaches.

Is 'simple low back pain' simply an expression of our ignorance about the underlying cause of back pain? Although there is randomized controlled trial evidence that spinal radiographs used as a routine investigation for low back pain in primary care do not result in improvement in the back problem,[7] it may be that they are simply not picking up relevant pathology. However, imaging that provides more detail than radiographs about abnormalities of spinal and paraspinal structures and tissues does not appear to provide 'useful' or 'important' diagnoses either. In a randomized, controlled trial of the use of magnetic resonance imaging (MRI) in the investigation of back pain, Jarvik et al.[8] demonstrated that, although the number of diagnoses made was higher and led to more interventions in the MRI group, the clinical outcomes were no better than in a control group who had no MRI. It is important to emphasize that radiography, computed tomography (CT) scans and MRI all have their place in those patients whose clinical features raise the suspicion of a red flag or an important diagnosis, but the Jarvik paper provides further justification for not pursuing diagnosis in the absence of such clinical pointers.

Recent evidence from treatment trials has shed a different light on the blanket assumption that all non-specific back pain can be lumped together in one diagnostic category. The general idea of these trials has been to match specific treatments to different clinical subgroups in order to enhance the effectiveness of the interventions. Whether we buy in to the pathological mechanism that is being proposed by these classifications may be less important than the demonstration of the additional effectiveness of such targeted treatment. The two trials each used a method of selecting treatment on the basis of the patient's response to pain in clinical examination, and showed improved outcomes in the group whose treatment had been targeted compared with those who received treatment without the diagnostic selection.[3, 4] The problem for primary care is that such combined diagnostic and intervention approaches tend to involve rather specialized groups of therapists (in this case physiotherapists trained in the McKenzie method) and the diagnostic principles are not widely accepted or understood in the medical community. Further evidence from trials of the effects of classification on outcome is needed before this situation is likely to change.

Other trials continue to support the notion that simple principles of pain management can safely and effectively be applied by a range of primary care clinicians and therapists, after triaging, on the basis of a label of 'simple' undifferentiated regional pain ('back' or 'neck' or 'shoulder' pain) without the need for more detailed diagnosis.[9]

The 1999 version of this chapter drew attention to the introduction of yellow flags – psychosocial characteristics that may accompany low back pain and other regional pains. There is increasingly strong evidence that such characteristics are the strongest predictors of long-term pain and disability in patients presenting with low back pain in primary care. Attention has tended to focus away from 'distress' factors (anxiety, depression) towards 'thought' factors (ideas, knowledge and attitudes (cognitions) about pain). Patients who catastrophize about their pain (e.g. think it will not get better) are more likely than non-catastrophizers to develop chronic pain and not recover.[10, 11] This suggests the need for a new approach to diagnosis. Rather than using complex categories of local tissue pathology, such a 'classification-based' approach would emphasize a simple separation of patients into those with or without social or psychological risks for persistence, or into those with or without multiple regional pains.[12]

However, there are some concerns about such an approach. First, although evidence continues to accumulate that psycho-social factors are strong predictors of outcome of regional pain syndromes, it is not clear whether subgrouping patients on this basis (e.g. 'diagnosing' a catastrophizing patient) leads to more effective treatment and better outcomes. So the caveat in the 1999 article (that the value of identifying psychosocial characteristics in everyday clinical practice has yet to be empirically established) still holds. This question (If back pain sufferers with psychological problems are separated out, will it improve clinical outcome?) is similar to the question about physical classifications of low back pain. There is too little evidence for the superior effectiveness of targeted psychological interventions in low back pain in primary care (as distinct from their undoubted efficacy in secondary care subgroups) to assume their diagnostic usefulness in primary care. Once again best evidence supports the idea of simple low back pain as the diagnostic category of choice and of using clinical flags and other cues for the application of general principles of pain management (including physical, psychological and social interventions).

Is there any evidence that clinical subgrouping and targeted treatment may be beneficial in sorting out other regional musculoskeletal pain presenting in primary care? Walker-Bone et al.[13] have reviewed attempts to establish the validity of clinical classifications of neck and upper-limb pains, and concluded that systematic critical evaluation of clinical classifications is still in its infancy. Although there is general agreement that rotator cuff syndromes are the commonest pathological diagnostic group among shoulder problems seen in primary care,[14] and that ultrasound scanning can help in establishing the 'important' diagnosis of rotator cuff tears,[15] systematic reviews of diagnostic and prognostic studies on the shoulder have identified the lack of studies in primary care settings. The good-quality studies that have been done emphasize that the most useful prognostic feature is the severity of pain at presentation in primary care for both shoulder[16] and neck.[17]

A different angle involves the distinction between 'isolated' regional pain (treated as a local problem) and 'regional pain with pain elsewhere' (treated as a general pain syndrome irrespective of the actual locations involved). Low back pain provides an example. Natvig et al.[18] have suggested that the two groups represent different syndromes. Thomas et al.[19] have identified that the presence of 'pain elsewhere' is the most important predictor of outcome in patients with low back pain presenting in primary care. In Raspe's scheme,[12] pain elsewhere is one stage of 'amplified' back pain, in which other comorbidities, somatization and psychological distress feed into other stages. All these approaches have clear links with the idea of 'flags', which signal risk of poor outcome. This suggests that, if empirical evidence emerges that such classifications improve treatment selection and outcomes, we can move beyond 'simple' or 'non-specific' regional pain to a classification system based on a much wider range of characteristics than traditional pathoanatomical features.

Another observation moving us beyond the back pain paradigm is that these sorts of models are highly unlikely to be exclusive to low back pain. Similar risks for persistence in relation to the presence of other pains and psychosocial features are found in prospective studies of neck pain and shoulder pain (e.g. Bot et al.[20]). Each syndrome itself gives rise to higher than expected future rates of other musculoskeletal pain. General characteristics (pain duration, previous pain episodes, psychological and social factors) are more important predictors of the chronicity of any regional pain than the location of the pain.

All of this means that even the traditional mode of approach of minimal classification by region may be rather obsolete for primary care. The diagnostic triage might eventually be (1) red flags (some, but not all, of which will be regional-specific symptoms and signs, some of which will indicate systemic disease, and some of which could be psychiatric), (2) important regional diagnoses, and (3) the rest (the majority) subclassified by psychological factors or by the severity or extent of pain irrespective of location.

Other aspects of the triage approach remain controversial. Observational studies suggest that systematic triage in primary care may be difficult to achieve (e.g. the necessity for a neurological examination of all low back pain sufferers), while studies of the application of the guidelines suggest that more, rather than fewer, low back pain sufferers may be referred to secondary care if the guidelines are applied too rigidly. Furthermore, the individual clinician wants to retain the capacity to interpret a particular patient's problem in the light of experience or a wider knowledge of the patient, rather than assuming a formulaic approach dictated by absolute rules such as 'never x-ray the back unless specific additional characteristics are present'. Some clinicians continue to be concerned about an approach that consigns most low back pain and other regional pains in primary care to a 'black box' in terms of diagnosis and classification. They wish to retain the possibility that helpful and useful subclassifications of simple regional musculoskeletal pain can be identified that will guide treatment and predict outcome. This seems reasonable, but it has to be remembered that strong empirical evidence in favour of new classifications (with the possible exception of the yellow flags) has yet to appear. Finally, it is important to emphasize that the usefulness of any classification has to take into account its own possible therapeutic influence when it is applied. For example, if chiropractic manipulation is shown to be effective, is the chiropractic diagnostic procedure, which accompanies and precedes the manipulation, part of the 'effective package'?[21] The evidence has yet to accrue.

Despite all these concerns, the basic triage approach has gained in authority and forms the basis, for example, of the section on back pain in *Current Medical Diagnosis and Treatment*,[22] with its marked refusal to use diagnostic labels other than those of the main red flags. The increasing rationale for such an approach to be applied to other syndromes of regional musculoskeletal pain is apparent in the latest edition of that textbook, in which the chapter on arthritis and musculoskeletal syndromes is organized around symptoms and not diagnoses. The American College of Rheumatology expert consensus publication on diagnosis[23] uses the term 'red flags' and provides a list of characteristics indicating the need for

urgent evaluation similar to that seen in back pain guidelines: significant trauma, constitutional symptoms and signs, and neurological symptoms and signs, as well as a hot swollen joint raising the possibility of infection or systemic inflammatory disease. The list published by the *American Journal of Medicine*[24] is similar, although it does not use the term 'red flags' but instead adds the time dimension, which is often the key diagnostic element in primary care: 'lack of response during 2 to 6 weeks of treatment'. The evidence base for these schemes goes back to earlier non-consensus expert clinical opinion, such as that of Fries and Mitchell.[25]

TESTING THE PARADIGM: NECK PAIN IN PRIMARY CARE

One source of evidence is that of the primary care expert. In 1997, a group of UK primary care physicians met together, each with a declared interest in musculoskeletal problems as evidenced by their membership of the Primary Care Rheumatology Society in the UK. The purpose of the meeting was to consider whether the 'low back pain' paradigm could be applied to other pain syndromes in primary care. Neck pain was the chosen example.

The first conclusion of this group was that neck pain did fit satisfactorily into the model of triage developed for low back pain. As with low back pain, the first priority for the patient and the primary care practitioner was to identify those cases of neck pain accompanied by red-flag characteristics, indicating a possible serious underlying diagnosis. There was broad agreement on the red flags: age (the young and the old); the presence of systemic symptoms, such as fever or weight loss; pain that was progressive and severe or sudden and severe in onset; neurological symptoms and signs; a history of recent trauma; a history of systemic inflammatory disease (rheumatoid arthritis or ankylosing spondylitis) or bone disease (osteoporosis); and a previous diagnosis of cancer or treatment with oral steroids. The diagnoses to be ruled out in this scheme include fracture, tumours, infection, subarachnoid haemorrhage and complications of rheumatoid arthritis or ankylosing spondylitis. Such a list is not exhaustive but reflects the concerns of the primary care physician.

Having ruled out the red flags, the next branch of the triage was tackled. Here, the consensus group of primary care practitioners identified a group of diagnoses that they characterized as 'important' (i.e. there are important reasons actively to consider them as possibilities in the primary care setting): nerve root pain (potentially serious), whiplash syndrome (medico-legal issues) and migraine (treatment potential).

Once these have been considered, the group regarded it as reasonable to lump all other cases together as simple undifferentiated neck pain. However, they did feel that there was a set of 'useful diagnostic labels' for practical use in the primary care setting, 'useful' in the sense that they could be used optimistically because they implied an absence of red flags and a good prognosis. Their diagnostic labels were neck sprain or strain, mechanical neck pain and acute torticollis. Also included in this was the presence of psychological problems (yellow-flag features) on the basis that this feature would early on guide the primary care physician in how to manage the problem.

The group contrasted their 'important' and 'useful' diagnostic groups and labels with the wide range of pathological terms that could be selected. Many of these were considered 'harmful' because they did not contribute to the management of the symptom and because they might be counterproductive to an active optimistic approach to treatment. This point is taken up again below.

THE EVIDENCE BASE FOR DIAGNOSIS

What type of evidence other than that of the 'clinical expert' can help in determining the usefulness of diagnostic classifications? The elegant experiments of Bogduk and his colleagues[26] are one example. In these, a highly specific mode of pain relief accompanied by randomized placebo treatments provides evidence of regional pathology in the neck of chronic whiplash sufferers as a source of their pain.[27] This is convincing work, but the primary care clinician has to ask about the setting in which the diagnosis is needed – Do such tests apply to the average patient with musculoskeletal pain who walks through the front door of the general practice surgery?

The issue of the setting in which diagnosis is to be made is crucial to judging diagnostic 'usefulness'. A study of different 'diagnostic expert systems' applied to a set of 1254 cases of acute abdominal pain, for example, indicated that a diagnostic bias towards the ordinary and the common performed better than expert medical knowledge.[28] In primary care, knowing that 'common things occur commonly' is an aid to diagnosis. The point of the red flag approach is to create a group in which the probability of a serious problem is higher than in the 'average run of cases' in primary care. This then justifies further investigation or referral and the application of specialist 'expert' knowledge as well as safeguards against assuming that rarities never occur. Thus, one systematic review of diagnostic tests for the evaluation of back and neck pain concluded that 'advanced anatomical and physiological tests within the first month should be reserved for patients with red flags for serious pathological conditions on clinical examination'.[29]

Applying algorithms

The evidence base for most decisions not to investigate every regional pain, when such a base exists, is usually derived from large case series demonstrating the low likelihood of a serious problem. Such case series might emerge from clinical experts or from formal observational studies in less selected populations than are found in the specialist clinic. An example of the output of such a combination of expert and research 'evidence' is the *American Journal of Medicine*'s set of algorithms for the diagnosis and management of musculoskeletal complaints.[24] The essential separation arrived at by this large consensus group was into 'articular' versus 'non-articular', followed by decisions about whether the problem is inflammatory or not, and whether it is acute or chronic.

Applying these algorithms from the Lipsky article to a regional pain syndrome presented in primary care can be described as follows:

- *Acute, non-inflammatory and articular.* We arrive at red-flag questions similar to those listed above for neck and low back pain, and based on published expert clinical evidence.
- *Chronic, non-inflammatory and articular.* The algorithms take us first to low back pain and once again the red-flag approach, based on observational studies and expert consensus detailed in earlier publications; the second route goes to osteoarthritis: this will be considered in detail below under 'regional pain syndromes in older people'.
- *Non-articular; local or widespread.*

Taking the non-articular route, the algorithms first ask us to consider whether we are dealing with a local or a widespread problem. This was discussed above and is a theme which also emerges from Helliwell's useful distinction between specific and non-specific arm pain.[30]

Taking the route to the local disorders, we reach again the red-flag questions as the key to whether further investigation is needed. In the absence of red flags, however, the *American Journal of Medicine* algorithms end up with a large table of diagnostic labels. Just how useful are these? There is plenty to contemplate as evidence for or against particular classification systems of regional non-articular musculoskeletal pain. Van der Heijden[31] and Hay et al.[32] both quote evidence to suggest that going beyond a distinction between 'pain and restricted movement' and 'pain with no restricted movement', when dealing with most shoulder pain, has no great benefits because it will not affect treatment or outcome. Many clinicians will quarrel with this view on the basis of personal experience – particularly those who use, for example, the Cyriax method of diagnosis to guide highly specific treatments. From the point of view of controlled trial evidence, however, the Cyriax system has not been tested in terms of its effectiveness in influencing clinical outcomes. Tunks and Crook's review[33] similarly highlights the absence of empirical evidence of a randomized or controlled variety to back up the popular clinical classification of myofascial pain syndromes. In contrast, some small amount of evidence is beginning to emerge about what may or may not help 'regional pain, unspecified other than by its location and the absence of red flags' in the reviews of treatment evidence presented in Chapter 18. So why worry about whether diagnosis is pursued beyond the red flags or not?

MIGHT DIAGNOSIS BE HARMFUL?

'Romantic diagnoses' is the term applied in Germany to labels, usually having a superficially attractive and specific pathological content, for which there is no empirical evidence to justify their use.[34] There are two varieties: one in which it is entirely possible that the pathology is present but the link with pain may be weak or non-existent (e.g. moderate radiographic osteoarthritis), and one in which there may be very little actual evidence that the pathology is present, but the symptoms and signs are assumed to represent it (e.g. tenosynovitis).

An extreme example of recent romantic labelling in the literature is 'carotidynia'.[35] This label rose to prominence in various journals in the late 1960s as a description for a syndrome of unilateral neck pain accompanied by tenderness over the carotid artery; it could be acute or chronic, but no structural abnormality of the carotid artery or surrounding territory was described. In some publications, tenderness over the carotid artery did not have to be present. By 1989, the term and the diagnosis were falling into disrepute, although it still appears in the latest editions of prominent rheumatology textbooks.

A different category of label is one that mixes the external cause into the name: 'repetitive strain injury' or 'cumulative trauma disorder', for example. The problem for research of labelling a set of symptoms by its presumed cause is clear: How can cause be studied without a definition of the problem that can be applied equally to those who are and those who are not exposed to the cause in question? It is of dubious value in clinical practice as well. A survey of social security doctors in Britain[36] showed that half of the experts thought 'repetitive strain injury' was a genuine organic disease entity and the other half did not; the survey concluded that the terms should not be used. Both Helliwell[30] and Linaker[37] refer to the British consensus on upper limb pain definitions for occupational physicians, which avoids any use of such terms.[38]

The romantic diagnoses are what the primary care consensus group regarded as potentially 'harmful' labels. One general practitioner (GP) in the group had imposed a ban on using the term 'cervical spondylosis' in his own practice as a diagnostic label. This was not simply because of the finding, highlighted by Bogduk[26], that degenerative changes in the neck are common in the general population and seem no more common in those with neck pain than in those without. This GP had banned it because of the erroneous implication that radiographic investigation should guide management of the neck pain and because the use of the label in itself transmitted wrong messages of chronic disease and future incapacity to the patient. Roland and van Tulder[39] have discussed this in relation to the reporting of spinal radiographs. These authors point to the terminology of 'degeneration' and the implications it carries about the state of the spine, which may be neither true nor helpful to the patient. They highlight the figure from published studies that there is a 40–50% false-positive rate for all degrees of spinal degeneration reported on radiography; i.e. 40–50% of people, if they had such a radiographic report, would not have pain. The term 'degenerative disease', they point out, may promote patterns of belief and behaviour contrary to current guidelines on treatment; MRI is likely to be worse in this respect, as it identifies an even higher prevalence of structural abnormality. Empirical evidence of the usefulness or otherwise of imaging in other regional syndromes is less complete, but there are similar suggestions from imaging series of the shoulder,[40] for example, that indiscriminate use will not improve clinical outcome.

Yet, for all the common sense of this primary care view, it is only right to point out that it is not based on strong scientific evidence about the harm of labels, the undesirability of radiographs and so on. Indeed, many primary care practitioners argue that radiographs serve a purpose in reassurance that may be therapeutic in itself. As we move into an era where safer, but more expensive, imaging is becoming available, the need remains for empirical evidence (both qualitative and quantitative) about the advantages and disadvantages of investigation beyond the role of supplying a handy diagnosis. It is ironic that the expert consensus publications, despite their use of diagnostic labels, conclude that current evidence suggests that neither radiographs nor scans nor blood tests add to the management of regional pain unless there is clinical suspicion of a red flag.

WHAT EXACTLY IS REGIONAL MUSCULOSKELETAL PAIN?

There is no evidence that the common regional pain syndromes seen in primary care are about specific regional inflammation. This is a rheumatological view and reflects the idea that inflammation is the organizing feature of these problems. Once again, the setting in which this information is to be applied becomes crucial. The list of 'common localized non-articular musculoskeletal complaints' in primary care will not be restricted to inflammatory syndromes.

Example: chest pain

Consider chest pain. This rarely rates an entry in musculoskeletal texts and does not make the *American Journal of Medicine* list of common regional complaints. Surely its place is in the cardiology chapter. What is the evidence?

A study in primary care by Svavarsdottir et al.[41] identified all patient contacts for chest pain and followed them up 3–4 years later. Heart disease was diagnosed in 18% of cases, and the chest pain remained undiagnosed in 9.5%. The most common diagnostic category by far was a musculoskeletal problem: 49% of all patients presenting with chest pain were considered to have such a problem. Nor, so the authors claimed, was this a label of exclusion: 'the history was the main diagnostic tool for musculoskeletal problems'. No serious disease had been missed, but those with heart disease had been examined and investigated more thoroughly, suggesting that the red-flag method is in place here. However, the red flag in this case is heart disease, which is rather more common than red flags at other musculoskeletal sites.

Klinkman et al.[42] reported that 20% of all episodes of care for chest pain in primary care were diagnosed as musculoskeletal in origin, oesophagitis being the next most common; again heart disease represented 10% of cases but consumed most of the investigation/treatment resources. Fruergaard et al.[43] reported on the investigation of 204 patients with acute chest pain presenting to the accident and emergency department and not caused by myocardial infarction; most were ischaemic heart disease of some sort, the main alternative diagnoses being gastro-oesophageal disease and chest-wall syndromes, the latter being identified in 25% of the cases, with 'careful examination of the chest wall' given as the basis of diagnosis.

Another study of non-cardiac chest pain was reported by Chambers and Bass,[44] who reported that chest pain is frequent in the community and is usually benign. However, because of the serious implications of coronary heart disease, 'overinvestigation is frequent'. They identify problems parallel to those discussed above in relation to 'harmful' diagnoses: investigation may entrench the idea of cardiac disease, so chronic pain and disability are common in those referred for coronary investigations, even when the latter prove to be normal. These authors mention in their discussion of differential diagnosis that obvious musculoskeletal problems can be treated with non-steroidal anti-inflammatory drugs (NSAIDs). It is not clear what the basis is for an 'obvious' diagnosis of musculoskeletal chest-wall pain and whether the recommendation to use NSAIDs is evidence based or not.

Chest pain is thus an intriguing example from the musculoskeletal point of view. Because, understandably, the focus is on a non-musculoskeletal red flag, the clinical and investigative pathways are very different from those of other regional pain syndromes, and this is presumably why it does not figure prominently as a rheumatologist's problem. Yet the evidence suggests that the same problem of chronic pain in the absence of a clear-cut regional pathology is present and that the same difficulty exists in arriving at a positive diagnosis of musculoskeletal problems as affects other areas. From a primary care perspective, it is predominantly a musculoskeletal problem in terms of frequency, even if the red-flag diagnostic concern is diverted to other possibilities.

Regional pain in older people

The traditional view of regional pain in older people is provided by the work of Sternbach[45] in the 1960s, namely that most regional pains in older people decline in prevalence, except for joint pain which increases in frequency. Harris[46] conducted a systematic review of pain in older people, which suggested that milder, less persistent regional pain episodes do get less frequent with age, whereas chronic more severe pain increases. Thomas et al.[47] confirmed this in a population sample of older people, showing that, while overall pain prevalence changes little in older age, pain that interferes with life becomes more frequent. Disability is the issue in the older age group, and it is osteoarthritis that is the dominant diagnosis in the older age groups.

So, do we here have the exception to all the generalizations above about regional pain, i.e. that most regional pain in older people is caused by a specific local pathology in the joint? The first stage of triage still applies to joint pain in older people – there are red-flag symptoms, signs and diagnoses for joint pain in older people just as much as the young. But is the third stage redundant – is the bulk of 'simple chronic joint pain in older people' dominated by a specific diagnosis of 'osteoarthritis'?

It all depends what is meant by 'osteoarthritis'. The proposal from an international workforce is that a diagnosis of osteoarthritis is made on a combination of pain and radiographic changes.[48] The problem for primary care is that this leaves out a large number of older people who have joint pains labelled as 'osteoarthritis' but in whom there is no evidence of definite radiographically shown osteoarthritis. The alternative proposal from McAlindon,[49] is that we should regard knee pain, for example, as a chronic pain syndrome, some of which is linked to radiographic changes. There is good reason to think this is reasonable – a radiograph is not needed to select simple primary care treatments for joint pain (they would be the same whether radiographic changes were seen or not); psychological and social factors are as influential as in other regional pain syndromes,[50] and treating depression in older patients with knee pain is effective in reducing their knee-related disability;[51] and pain elsewhere has the same impact on the severity and level of disability of knee pain as it has for other regional pains.[52, 53] The conclusion is that the triage can operate in older people with joint pain as well. First, consider red flags. Second, consider important diagnoses, which will include the need to diagnose the presence of radiographically shown osteoarthritis if this will affect management (e.g. if the problem is severe enough to be considered for referral for joint replacement or steroid injection). Third, consider the remaining cases as belonging to a chronic pain syndrome, which might be labelled 'osteoarthritis' but is actually 'non-specific chronic joint pain' for which a range of local and general primary care treatments can be considered.[54, 55]

Osteoarthritis is, however, both a pathological diagnosis and a clinical syndrome. Returning to the *American Journal of Medicine* approach, osteoarthritis is the first diagnosis reached after red flags have been ruled out. Once this diagnosis has been made, the emphasis is on the assessment and management of pain and restricted function. However, the approach also highlights the need to determine 'whether the pain and disability are caused by osteoarthritis', which is the first step after red flags concerned with finding a formal diagnosis for non-inflammatory regional musculoskeletal pain. As McAlindon[49] points out, there is not a great deal of empirical evidence to support this need, unless we are dealing clinically with the minority who have severe pain and disability from their chronic joint problem, at which point radiographically shown severity may be an important influence on management. Hadler[56] has laid down the challenge to consider osteoarthritis as a clinical problem of regional pain and disability rather than as an important pathological diagnosis to make. McAlindon[49] has reviewed empirical evidence that supports the view that muscle strength and psychosocial factors are more important determinants of pain and disability in chronic non-inflammatory joint pain than are radiographic changes. This has implications for how we manage such patients. However, Lane and Thompson's systematic review of the evidence concerning the management of osteoarthritis in primary care[55] comes to the conclusion that 'Before considering therapeutic options for osteoarthritis of the knee, it is essential to establish that a patient's knee pain is attributable to osteoarthritis', which is in direct contrast to the conclusion drawn by Hadler. It seems unlikely that the actual treatment will vary greatly wherever doctors place themselves on this diagnostic and investigational spectrum, but for the clinician faced with the individual patient, epidemiological evidence must be tempered by the knowledge that there is a group of patients who will benefit from a radiological diagnosis and an orthopaedic procedure. Even for this group, however, empirical studies have highlighted the absence of consensus about the indications for referral of the patient with hip or knee pain for a surgical opinion. In a Canadian study, family practitioners disagreed on the status of 28 of 32 patient factors that might affect referral to orthopaedic surgeons, and similar disagreements were observed among rheumatologists.[57] Such variation is paralleled by the disagreements observed between orthopaedic surgeons themselves in Canada and America about the indications for and the choice of treatments for knee osteoarthritis.[58] Recent work from Peat et al.[59] has identified the importance of measuring pain severity and persistence and the severity of disability when managing knee pain in older people. It seems justified, therefore, to highlight the lack of evidence about which classification of chronic non-inflammatory articular pain will most effectively guide and influence management to the benefit of the patient.

The suggestion that both clinical features and radiographic changes need to be present to constitute a diagnosis of osteoarthritis[48] is unsatisfactory for primary care, since much joint pain will be excluded. Diagnosis of the subgroup of older people with chronic joint pain who have radiographically shown osteoarthritis is important for research (because we need to know how symptoms might progress and what relationship this has to progression seen on radiography), but in clinical practice the reality is that most patients with chronic joint pain will be treated on the basis of their clinical presentation, pain severity and disability, regardless of the radiographic features.

In the terminology of the World Health Organization International Classification of Function, the prevalence of the impairment (pain) may decline with age, but the consequences of regional pain in terms of disability and handicap become more severe.[60] Clinical, psychological and social factors, such as the widespread nature of pain or the presence of depression, are potentially as important for classifying pain in older people as they are in younger age groups. Despite the importance of defining subgroups with red flags and important diagnoses such as osteoporosis, it may be that an approach that concentrates on severity of pain and functional restriction is the diagnostic step in older people to the extent that diagnosis 'tells us what to do'.

CONCLUSION

There are no common 'need to knows' in what we usually incorporate under the heading of regional musculoskeletal pain. Red flags in primary care patients are rare and depend on other features (e.g. weight loss or fever). There are also non-specific influences on the need to know ('This is how mother's cancer started', 'I remember a patient who presented just like this last year'). Once red flags have been identified, treatments are often so non-specific that the precise diagnosis seems not to matter, but research is emerging that is testing how far treatment targeting based on specific classifications and diagnoses might improve outcome. Investigations, such as laboratory tests, are generally not helpful in the absence of clinical symptoms

---

PRACTICE POINTS

- Regional musculoskeletal pain represents characteristics of both local pathology and a general problem of pain.

- Triage asks: 'Is there a serious or important cause of the pain to be identified?' or 'Can this be treated as a problem of pain management?'

- Serious causes of regional pain are rare in primary care.

- All regional pain, regardless of cause, deserves proper assessment of biological, psychological and social influences on pain persistence, and a broad approach to its treatment.

- Although older people report less pain, they have a higher prevalence of troublesome disabling pain.

RESEARCH AGENDA

- New and creative approaches are needed to classifying regional pain and targeting treatment.

- Evidence is required about the advantages of classifying and diagnosing common regional pain syndromes in order to improve outcome.

- The long-term advantages of pain relief and functional improvement in older people with joint pain should be investigated.

---

and signs beyond the pain itself because of their low predictive value in a primary care setting. Current evidence-based guidelines for diagnosis incorporate advice against indiscriminate investigation but also provide diagnostic algorithms that represent 'best evidence' for diagnostic approaches based on expert consensus, and evidence suggests that this approach is likely to be useful for neck and shoulder pain and for chronic joint pain in older people.

ACKNOWLEDGEMENTS

The author is indebted to the Primary Care Rheumatology Society's Neck Pain Consensus Group for their insights: John Dickson, Gillian Hosie, Stan Hill, Pamela Brown, Graham Davenport and Peter Lanyon. Also to the McKenzie physiotherapy faculty worldwide, for their insight that clinicians who believe in diagnosis may be more help to patients in pain than epidemiologists who philosophise about it.

REFERENCES

1. Main CJ, Williams AC. Musculoskeletal pain. *BMJ* 2002; **325**: 534–537.
2. Waddell G. Subgroups within 'non-specific' low back pain. *J Rheumatol* 2005; **32**: 395–396.
3. Long A, Donelson R, Fung T. Does it matter which exercise? A randomized control trial of exercise for low back pain. *Spine* 2004; **23**: 2593–2602.

4. Fritz JM, Delitto A, Erhard RE. Comparison of classification-based physical therapy with therapy based on clinical practice guidelines for patients with acute low back pain. A randomized clinical trial. *Spine* 2003; **28**: 1363–1372.

5. Kent P, Keating J. Do primary care clinicians think that nonspecific low back pain is one condition? *Spine* 2004; **29**: 1022–1031.

6. Deyo RA, Rainville J, Kent DL. What can the history and examination tell us about low back pain? *JAMA* 1992; **268**: 760–765.

7. Kerry S, Hilton S, Dundas D et al. Radiographs for low back pain: a randomized controlled trial and observational study in primary care. *Br J Gen Pract* 2002; **52**: 534–535.

8. Jarvik JG, Hollingworth W, Martin B et al. Rapid magnetic resonance imaging vs radiographs for patients with low back pain: a randomized controlled trial. *JAMA* 2003; **289**: 2810–2818.

9. Dziedzic K, Hill J, Lewis M et al. Effectiveness of manual therapy or pulsed shortwave diathermy in addition to advice and exercise for neck disorders: a pragmatic randomized controlled trial in physical therapy clinics. *Arthritis Rheum* 2005; **53**: 214–222.

10. Picavet HS, Vlaeyen JW, Schouten JS. Pain catastrophising and kinesiophobia: predictors of chronic low back pain. *Am J Epidemiol* 2002; **156**: 1028–1034.

11. Burton AK, Tillotson KM, Main CJ et al. Psychosocial predictors of outcome in acute and subchronic low back trouble. *Spine* 1995; **20**: 722–728.

12. Raspe H. How epidemiology contributes to the management of spinal disorders. *Best Pract Res Clin Rheumatol* 2002; **16**: 9–21.

13. Walker-Bone K, Palmer KT, Reading I et al. Criteria for assessing pain and nonarticular soft-tissue rheumatic disorders of the neck and upper limb. *Semin Arthritis Rheum* 2003; **33**: 168–184.

14. Ostor AJ, Richards CA, Prevost AT et al. Diagnosis and relation to general health of shoulder disorders presenting in primary care. *Rheumatology* 2005; **44**: 800–805.

15. Dinnes J, Loveman E, McIntyre L et al. The effectiveness of diagnostic tests for the assessment of shoulder pain due to soft tissue disorders: a systematic review. *Health Technol Assess* 2003; **7**(iii): 1–166.

16. Kuipers T, van der Windt DAWM, van der Heijden GJMG et al. Systematic review of prognostic cohort studies on shoulder disorders. *Pain* 2004; **109**: 420–431.

17. Viikari-Juntura E, Takala E, Riihimaki H et al. Predictive validity of symptoms ands signs in the neck and shoulders. *J Clin Epidemiol* 2000; **53**: 800–808.

18. Natvig B, Bruusgaard D, Eriksen W. Localized low back pain and low back pain as part of widespread musculoskeletal pain: two different disorders? A cross-sectional population study. *J Rehab Med* 2001; **33**: 21–25.

19. Thomas E, Silman AJ, Croft PR et al. Predicting who develops chronic low back pain in primary care: a prospective study. *BMJ* 1999; **318**: 1662–1667.

20. Bot SD, van der Waal JM, Terwee CB et al. Predictors of outcome in neck and shoulder symptoms: a cohort study in general practice. *Spine* 2005; **30**: E459–E470.

21. Paterson C, Dieppe P. Characteristics and incidental (placebo) effects in complex interventions such as acupuncture. *BMJ* 2005; **330**: 1202–1205.

22. Tierney LM Jr, McPhee SJ, Papadakis MA (eds). *Current Medical Diagnosis and Treatment*, 44th edn. McGraw-Hill, New York, 2005.

23. American College of Rheumatology Ad Hoc Committee on Clinical Guidelines. Guidelines for the initial evaluation of the adult patient with acute musculoskeletal symptoms. *Arthritis Rheum* 1996; **39**: 1–8.

24. Lipsky P. Algorithms for the diagnosis and management of musculoskeletal complaints. *Am J Med* 1997; **103**: 1S–85S.

25. Fries JF, Mitchell DM. Joint pain or arthritis. *JAMA* 1976; **235**: 199–204.

26. Bogduk N. The neck. *Best Pract Res Clin Rheumatol* 1999; **13**: 261–285.

27. Lord SM, Barnsley L, Wallis BJ et al. Chronic cervical zygapophyseal joint pain after whiplash. A placebo-controlled prevalence study. *Spine* 1996; **21**: 1737–1745.

28. Puppe B, Ohmann C, Goos K et al. 1995 Evaluating four diagnostic methods with acute abdominal pain cases. *Method Inform Med* 1995; **34**: 361–368.

29. Haldeman S. Diagnostic tests for the evaluation of back and neck pain. *Neurol Clin* 1996; **14**: 103–117.

30. Helliwell PS. The elbow, forearm, wrist and hand. *Best Pract Res Clin Rheumatol* 1999; **13**: 311–328.

31. van der Heijden GJMG. Shoulder disorders: a state-of-the-art review. *Best Pract Res Clin Rheumatol* 1999; **13**: 287–309.

32. Hay EM, Dziedzic K, Sim J. Treatment options for regional musculoskeletal pain: what is the evidence? *Best Pract Res Clin Rheumatol* 1999; **13**: 243–259.

33. Tunks E, Crooks J. Regional soft tissue pains: alias myofascial pain? *Best Pract Res Clin Rheumatol* 1999; **13**: 345–369.

34. Leibbrand W. *Die Spekulative Medizin der Romantik*. Claassen, Hamburg, 1956.

35. Biousse V, Bousser MG. The myth of carotidynia. *Neurology* 1994; **44**: 993–995.

36. Diwaker HN, Stothard J. What do doctors mean by tenosynovitis and repetitive strain injury? *Occupat Med* 1995; **45**: 97–104.

37. Linaker CH, Walker-Bone K, Palmer K et al. Frequency and impact of regional musculoskeletal disorders. *Ballière's Best Pract Res Clin Rheumatol* 1999; **13**: 197–221.

38. Harrington JM, Carter JT, Birrell L et al. Surveillance case definitions for work related upper limb pain syndromes. *Occupat Environ Med* 1998; **55**: 264–271.

39. Roland M, van Tulder M. Should radiologists change the way they report plain radiography of the spine? *Lancet* 1998; **352**: 229–230.

40. Tallroth K. Shoulder imaging. A review. *Ann Chirurg Gynaecol* 1996; **85**: 95–103.

41. Svavarsdottir AE, Jonasson MR, Gudmundsson GH et al. Chest pain in family practice. Diagnosis and long-term outcome in a community setting. *Can Family Phys* 1996; **42**: 1122–1128.

42. Klinkman MS, Stevens D, Gorenflo DW. Episodes of care for chest pain: a preliminary report from MIRNET (Michigan Research Network). *J Family Pract* 1994; **38**: 345–352.

43. Fruergaard P, Launbjerg J, Hesse B et al. The diagnoses of patients admitted with acute chest pain but without myocardial infarction. *Eur Heart J* 1996; **17**: 1028–1034.

44. Chambers J, Bass C. Atypical chest pain: looking beyond the heart. *Q J Med* 1998; **91**: 239–244.

45. Sternbach R. Survey of pain in the US: the Nuprin Report. *Clin J Pain* 1986; **2**: 4.

46. Harris L. *Pain in Older People: A Systematic Review of the Literature.* Dissertation for Masters in Medical Science, Keele University, 2005.

47. Thomas E, Peat G, Harris L et al. The prevalence of pain and pain interference in a general population of older adults: cross-sectional findings from the North Staffordshire Osteoarthritis Project (NorStOP). *Pain* 2004; **110**: 361–368.

48. Felson DT, Lawrence RC, Dieppe PA et al. Osteoarthritis: new insights. Part 1: The disease and its risk factors. *Ann Intern Med* 2000; **133**: 635–646.

49. McAlindon TE. Regional muskuloskeletal pain. The knee. *Ballière's Best Pract Res Clin Rheumatol* 1999; **13**: 329–344.

50. O'Reilly SC, Muir K, Doherty M. Knee pain and disability in the Nottingham community. *Br J Rheumatol* 1998; **37**: 870–873.

51. Lin EH, Katon W, Von Korff M et al. Effect of improving depression care on pain and functional outcomes among older patients with arthritis: a randomised controlled trial. *JAMA* 2003; **290**: 2428–2429.

52. Bradley LA, Kersh BC, DeBerry JJ et al. Lessons from fibromyalgia: abnormal pain sensitivity in knee osteoarthritis. *Novartis Found Symp* 2004; **260**: 258–270.

53. Croft P Jordan K, Jinks C. 'Pain elsewhere' and the impact of knee pain in older people. *Arthritis Rheum* 2005; **52**: 2350–2354.

54. Peat G, McCarney R, Croft P. Knee pain and osteoarthritis in older adults; a review of the community burden and current use of primary health care. *Ann Rheum Dis* 2001; **60**: 91–97.

55. Lane NE, Thompson JM. Management of osteoarthritis in the primary care setting: an evidence-based approach to treatment. *Am J Med* 1997; **103**: 25S–30S.

56. Hadler NM. Knee pain is the malady – not osteoarthritis. *Ann Intern Med* 1992; **116**: 598–599.

57. Coyte PC, Hawker G, Croxford R et al. Variation in rheumatologists 'and family physicians' perceptions of the indications for and outcomes of knee replacement surgery. *J Rheumatol* 1996; **23**: 730–738.

58. Mancuso CA, Ranawat CS, Esdaile JM et al. Indications for total hip and total knee arthroplasties. Results of orthopaedic surveys. *J Arthroplasty* 1996; **11**: 34–46.

59. Peat G, Thomas E, Croft P. Brief assessment and staging of joint pain in older people: findings from the Clinical Assessment of Knee Pain (CAS-K) study. *Family Pract* 2005; **22**(Suppl 1): 116.

60. World Health Organization. *The Burden of Musculoskeletal Conditions at the Start of the New Millennium.* Report of a WHO Scientific Group. WHO Technical Report Series No. 919. WHO, Geneva, 2003.

Chapter 17
Injection therapies for soft-tissue disorders

Cathy Speed

INTRODUCTION

Local injection therapies include the local infiltration of substances such as corticosteroid, anaesthetic, sclerosants, dry needling and nerve blockade. Such treatments are used in the management of a spectrum of painful regional musculoskeletal complaints and have been used since several thousand years BC.[1]

Routes and injectates for local injection therapies in soft-tissue complaints are:

Routes
- intra-articular (capsulitis, facet joint)
- intrasheath (tenosynovitis)
- intrabursal (bursitis)
- local infiltration (carpal tunnel, trigger point, ligament, muscle)
- epidural (lumbar, caudal, transforaminal selective nerve root).

Injectates
- none (dry needling)
- local anaesthetic
- corticosteroids (with/without anaesthetic)
- sclerosants
- botulinum toxins
- heparin
- Traumeel
- Actovegin.

CORTICOSTEROID INJECTIONS

Steroid hormones were initially recognized as potent anti-inflammatory substances in the 1930s, and a flurry of activity during that decade resulted in the isolation of a number of steroids, most importantly compound E, later known as cortisone.[2] This was administered in 1948 to a patient with rheumatoid arthritis with dramatic results, and the evolution of steroid therapies for a spectrum of disorders swiftly followed.[2, 3] Administration of local corticosteroid injections for musculoskeletal complaints began in the 1950s. The administration of steroid through local, extra-articular infiltration or intra-articular injection is now the most commonly used procedure undertaken by rheumatologists.[4]

Most local corticosteroid injections for soft-tissue disorders are extra-articular, where the corticosteroid may be delivered into the lesion itself, such as in the case of an intrabursal injection, or around the lesion, as in peritendinous/tendon sheath infiltration. Steroid injections are also used for back pain and diagnostic blockades; these are described in more detail below.

Intra-articular injections are most commonly used in the presence of joint disease but are also used in the treatment of capsulitis (typically that of the shoulder). In such cases, the injection may be combined with additional hydrodistension of the joint.[5]

Rationale for use and mechanisms of action

Corticosteroids are used in most soft-tissue lesions to provide an anti-inflammatory effect. They exert their manifold effects on the inflammatory process through a number of mechanisms, including marked effects on transcription and translation and the inhibition of cytokines, chemokines, adhesion molecules, receptors, enzymes and other mediators.[6] Corticosteroids may also have some inducing effects on some cytokine receptors. Additional effects on alternative sources of pain in soft-tissue lesions have yet to be established, but may be important, as the origin of pain in soft-tissue disorders is highly complex and the existence of inflammatory changes in soft-tissue complaints – and their relative contribution to pain – appears to be variable. Although inflammation is clearly evident in cases of bursitis and in early capsulitis,[7, 8] its role in tendinopathies is less clear. With the exception of some cases of tenosynovitis, most histological studies of a range of chronic tendon lesions (such as Achilles, patellar, lateral elbow, wrist and rotator cuff tendinopathies) have demonstrated an absence of cellular evidence for inflammation.[9, 10] Degenerative features predominate, characterized by alteration in cellular and extracellular components of the tendon and paratenon or sheath.[9–11] It is for this reason that the term 'tendinosis' (degeneration) is preferred to 'tendinitis', which suggests inflammation.

The histopathological studies of tendon performed to date, however, have limitations. Notably, the presence or absence of biochemical features of inflammation has been largely ignored, although normal levels of prostaglandin have been shown in painful Achilles' tendon lesions.[12] In addition, most studies have involved end-stage, non-healing lesions; it is not clear whether the degenerative features are primary or whether they are preceded by an inflammatory phase. Other mechanisms of tendon pain have been proposed, including irritation of mechanoreceptors by vibration, traction or shear forces. Triggering of nociceptive receptors by neurotransmitters, such as substance P, and biochemical irritants, such as chondroitin sulphate, extravasated by damaged tendon may also play roles.[13, 14] The influences of corticosteroid on such processes are undefined.

General indications for corticosteroid injections in soft-tissue lesions

Corticosteroid injections are rarely used in isolation in soft-tissue complaints. Other issues must be addressed, including correction of causative and provocative factors and appropriate rehabilitation.[15] Ideally, local corticosteroid injections should be considered when there is an excessive or chronic inflammatory response, and where rehabilitation is inhibited. They have little or no role to play in most acute injuries, where inflammation is present as a vital component of the healing response, and inhibiting this process may potentially result in a suboptimal outcome. They are also not indicated in the management of ligament and muscle injuries, and do not appear to offer any advantage over dry needling in myofascial pain.[16]

Clinical evidence for the use of corticosteroid injections in soft-tissue lesions

Although studies and reports relating to the use of corticosteroid injections in soft-tissue disorders span the last five decades, the quality of many studies is limited and good evidence for benefit in many soft-tissue disorders is scant. The literature relating to some of the most common soft-tissue conditions can be used to illustrate this point.

Tendinopathies

Trigger finger   Trigger finger is a condition where evidence strongly supports the use of corticosteroids in its management. In a double-blind placebo-controlled trial of methylprednisolone acetate 20 mg (0.5 mL) with lignocaine versus 1% lignocaine 0.5 mL in 41 subjects with trigger finger, Lambert et al.[17] found a significant improvement in 60% of the treatment group compared with 16% in the control group at 1 month follow-up. Similar findings have been noted by others. In another randomized controlled trial (RCT) involving 127 trigger thumbs in 115 adults, Maneerit et al.[18] demonstrated that percutaneous trigger

thumb release combined with steroid injection has a higher success rate than that of steroid injection alone. Corticosteroid injections in trigger finger appear to be less effective in diabetic patients, in whom soft-tissue lesions are frequently more resistant to most therapies, for reasons that are not fully understood.[19]

Tennis elbow   A systematic overview of corticosteroid injections for lateral epicondylitis identified 12 RCTs with an adequate methodological score for consideration, although the median score of 40/100 indicated overall poor to moderate quality of trials on this subject. Pooled analysis indicated short-term (2–6 weeks) effectiveness only, with a pooled odds ratio of 0.15 (95% confidence interval (CI) 0.1–0.23) and a χ^2 value of 13.3 (5 degrees of freedom), indicating statistical heterogeneity. Studies of better methodological quality had more favourable results. No conclusions could be made with respect to the most suitable corticosteroid, dose, injection interval or injection volume.[20]

The same group performed a multicentre pragmatic RCT comparing the clinical effectiveness of local corticosteroid injection, standard non-steroidal anti-inflammatory drugs (NSAIDs), and simple analgesics for the early treatment of lateral epicondylitis.[21] Local corticosteroid injection was effective at 4 weeks' follow-up, but the outcome at 1 year was good in all groups and was not influenced by early treatment.

Rotator cuff tendinopathy   Injection of corticosteroids by the subacromial approach is considered to be the most suitable route when treating rotator cuff lesions. A Cochrane Review of interventions for shoulder complaints concluded that there is some evidence for short-term (4 weeks) benefit of subacromial corticosteroid injections in rotator cuff tendinosis with respect to range of motion, but not pain.[22, 23] Effectiveness over the longer term and in other shoulder complaints is unknown, as there are insufficient data of adequate quality upon which to base a recommendation for practice.

Achilles' tendinopathy   The sole prospective, double-blind RCT in the literature addressing the effectiveness of corticosteroid injections in Achilles' paratenonitis involved 28 active patients with three lesions, and showed no benefit of peritendinous methylprednisolone and marcaine over marcaine injections alone.[24]

Corticosteroid injections for other disorders

Plantar fasciitis   Corticosteroid injections, with or without additional local anaesthetic, are commonly used in the management of pain in plantar fasciitis. However, systematic reviews have found no significant long-term benefit of corticosteroid injection versus placebo, and there is evidence that symptoms resolve spontaneously in most cases.[25] In a systematic review of treatments for heel pain, Atkins et al. identified only one small RCT of 19 people with recalcitrant heel pain, comparing local injection of hydrocortisone acetate 25 mg with saline; no significant difference in pain relief (relative risk (RR) 0.52, 95% CI 0.15–1.79) was noted.[26] The same systematic review and a subsequent RCT[27] found no evidence of significant long-term benefit from corticosteroid plus local anaesthetic injections versus alternative treatments, and only limited evidence of a short-term (1 month) benefit.

Local corticosteroid injections for plantar heel pain can be painful, and the pain of injection does not appear to be reduced by local anaesthesia or tibial nerve blockade.[27] Plantar fascial rupture after injection has also been reported to occur in up to 33% of patients, although these reports relate to clinical observations unconfirmed by imaging.[28] Infection, subcutaneous fat atrophy, skin pigmentation changes, fascial rupture, peripheral nerve injury and muscle damage are all reported unwanted effects.[29]

Adhesive capsulitis   Histological and histochemical studies indicate that adhesive capsulitis (frozen shoulder) is a cytokine-driven inflammatory process resulting in synovitis, where chemotactic and cellular responses and synovitis occur, followed by fibroplasia and capsular contracture.[7, 30] Hence, an anti-inflammatory approach may be indicated in the early stages, although there is little basis for this approach in the later restrictive phases of the condition.

Two systematic reviews (involving the same two RCTs)[22, 31–33] of the use of local injections in frozen shoulder, plus one subsequent RCT,[33] found no clear evidence of benefit from intra-articular corticosteroid injection versus control treatment. In the reviews, no reduction in pain or improved range of movement with intra-articular corticosteroid was noted in either the first RCT (24 people with shoulder pain, 4 weeks of follow-up)[32] or in the second RCT (30 people with frozen shoulder, 24 weeks of follow-up).[33] The subsequent RCT compared three intra-articular injections of triamcinolone versus three intra-articular injections of saline, and also found no significant difference in pain score, change in mobility or function.[34]

Combined intra-articular and subacromial corticosteroid injections have not been demonstrated to be superior to placebo.[22, 23, 35] Hydrodistension may be useful, at least in the short term. In a study of 22 subjects with adhesive capsulitis recruited from a rheumatology clinic, Gam et al.[5] demonstrated that distension of the glenohumeral joint with 0.5% lignocaine 19 mL, in addition to intra-articular steroid injection, given weekly for 6 weeks was superior to weekly intra-articular corticosteroid injection alone in increasing the range of movement and reducing analgesic use at 12 weeks, although no significant reduction in subject-rated function or pain at rest was noted. Both groups received intra-articular steroid, so the effect of the hydrodistension itself is not known. Hydrodistension is more painful than injection alone.

A further RCT of arthrographic glenohumeral joint distension in 48 subjects with frozen shoulder compared normal saline and corticosteroid with placebo (arthrogram) in 48 subjects. Excluding four withdrawals from the placebo group, the between-group differences for disability and pain measures significantly favoured distension over placebo at 6 weeks. At 12 weeks, a significantly greater improvement in a patient preference measure (problem-elicitation technique) score for the distension group was noted.[36]

Facet joint injections   Facet joint injections with steroid and anaesthetic into the joint itself are performed under fluoroscopic control and are commonly used in the management of chronic back pain considered to be arising from this source. Reported success rates for lumbar and cervical facet joint injections vary from 16% to 86%.[37] Overall, there is little sound evidence to indicate that these injections have long-term benefit. Two systematic reviews of the use of facet joint injections in people with chronic back pain found no significant difference in pain relief with facet joint injections (intra-articular corticosteroid) versus placebo (intra-articular saline), or versus facet joint nerve blocks.[38, 39] Adverse effects included pain at the injection site, infection, haemorrhage, neurological damage and chemical meningitis.

There have been no RCTs of facet joint injections in the management of chronic neck pain.

Implications of the existing literature

The limited evidence to support the use of local corticosteroid injections in many chronic soft-tissue conditions may be related to methodological issues relating to the research to date or to a true lack of effect. Trigger finger is notably one of the few tendon lesions where there is evidence of chronic inflammation;[11] this may explain the improvement demonstrated with local corticosteroids. Relevant methodological issues include study design and accuracy of both diagnosis and injection. Inadequacies of study design include small sample sizes and heterogeneous study populations, unsuitable outcome measures, short-term follow-up, inadequate blinding and lack of a true placebo. The increasing availability of imaging in the form of magnetic resonance imaging (MRI) and ultrasound scanning should improve diagnostic reliability.

Injection accuracy

In a case–control study, Eustace et al.[40] demonstrated that, even in the hands of musculoskeletal specialists, only a minority of injections for shoulder pain are performed accurately (29% of subacromial and 42% of intra-articular injections), and that outcome is significantly correlated with the accuracy of injection. Zhingis et al.[41] demonstrated similar results in subjects with de Quervain's tenosynovitis. Another case–control study found that only 10% of intra-articular injections were placed correctly, even by experienced operators.[42] For this reason, the use of ultrasound-guided injection is becoming popular. Further research is needed to evaluate the efficacy of injections under ultrasound guidance.

Potential adverse effects

The overall incidence of side-effects after local corticosteroid injections for soft-tissue complaints is unknown, and the relevance of factors such as the steroid used, the tissue involved, the extent of the injury, the phase of healing at the time of injection and postinjection events (particularly loading of the tissue) has not been established. The vast majority of unwanted effects of local corticosteroid injections are minor, such as short-term local pain after injection, a postinjection flare, facial flushing, local skin lesions, temporary menstrual irregularity and postmeno-pausal haemorrhage.[43] Complete tendon rupture with loading after steroid injection is recognized, although the literature on this subject is limited to case reports.[44, 45] Sepsis is reported in 1/14,000 to 1/50,000 intra-articular/soft-tissue injections.[4] Other commonly reported side-effects include tissue atrophy and hypersensitivity reactions.[43] Resuscitation facilities should be available in the event of a rare severe reaction. Corticosteroid arthropathy and osteonecrosis are rare (0.8%) and seem to affect mostly weight-bearing joints after intra-articular injections.

Practical suggestions for use

Many of the recommendations for the use of local corticosteroid injections are based on anecdote. For both local and intra-articular injections there is no consensus with respect to environment (operating theatre, treatment room, clinic), the skin preparation, the wearing of gloves, use of local anaesthetic, the safe number of injections at one site, or the appropriate interval between injections.[4, 15]

Agents differ with respect to their potency and solubility, the latter inversely correlating with the duration of action (Table 17.1).[44] There are few data on the absorption of corticosteroids from peritendinous injections, but methylprednisolone acetate remains in plasma for a mean of 16 days after peri-articular injection.[46] Short- or moderate-acting, more soluble preparations (e.g. hydrocortisone, methylprednisolone) are recommended for soft-tissue injections on the theoretical basis of likelihood of fewer side-effects; agents with low solubility should not be used for this purpose.[22]

Local anaesthetic mixed with the corticosteroid is usually used in soft-tissue injections with the aim of improving patient comfort and increasing the volume of the injection for wider dispersion.[4, 15, 47] Although this is a common practice, some manufacturers advise against mixing agents because of the theoretical risk of clumping and precipitation of steroid crystals. There is no evidence that injection of local anaesthetic in advance of the corticosteroid is beneficial, or of a difference in outcome between the addition of long-acting versus short-acting anaesthetic.[47]

Local steroid injections in the vicinity of the Achilles' or patellar tendon, and in the circumstances of a tear, are frequently discouraged owing to the concerns with respect to rupture of heavily loaded tendons and/or impairment of tissue repair where disruption is already present.[48, 49] Although used by some in trigger-point injections, there appears to be no benefit of infiltration of corticosteroid over local anaesthetic or dry needling, and the potential side-effects are greater. These injections are therefore reserved for use in the resistant trigger point. The Practice Points at the end of this chapter list some suggestions for local corticosteroid injections for soft-tissue injuries in the face of a vacuum of evidence.

LOCAL ANAESTHETIC INJECTIONS AND DRY NEEDLING

Injections of local anaesthetic alone are used for both diagnostic and therapeutic purposes in soft-tissue conditions. Local anaesthetics reversibly block sodium channels and hence nociceptive impulses. In some cases, the duration of analgesia obtained can exceed the duration of action of the local anaesthetic, for reasons that are not fully understood.

Subacromial injection of short-acting local anaesthetic (e.g. 2% lignocaine 2–5 mL) was recommended by Neer[50] for the evaluation of the patient with rotator cuff tendinopathy. Neer proposed that the test allows differentiation between tears of the

Table 17.1. A comparison of injectable corticosteroids

Preparation	Potency*	Concentration (mg/mL)	Solubility (% wt/vol)	Onset of action	Dose
Hydrocortisone acetate (Hydrocortistab)	1	25	0.002	Variable	5–25 mg
Prednisolone acetate (Deltastab)	4	25	0.001	Variable	5–25 mg
Methylprednisolone acetate† (Depomedrone)	5	20, 40, 80	0.001	1–5 days	20–80 mg
Triamcinalone acetonide† (Adcortyl, Kenalog)	5	10, 40	0.004	Variable	5–40 mg
Betamethasone sodium phosphate/acetate	25	6	NA	2–24 hours	0.25–2 mg
Dexamethasone phosphate	25	4	0.01	2–24 hours	NA
Triamcinalone hexacetonide‡	5	20	0.0002	Variable	NA‡

NA, Not applicable.

*Hydrocortisone equivalents (per mg).

†Opinions differ as to the equivalent dose range between these two drugs; they may differ with mode and site of application.

‡Insolubility makes it unsuitable for use in soft-tissue injections.

rotator cuff and impingement syndrome/tendinosis. By injecting an analgesic medication into the subacromial space of the shoulder, the tendons of the rotator cuff will be effectively anaesthetized and weakness due to pain inhibition would be abolished, allowing detection of weakness due to a tear. The test, although popular, has not been validated.

Local injection of trigger points with anaesthetic or saline in the patient with myofascial pain aims to reduce symptoms and allow a stretching and exercise programme to proceed. Dry needling may be equally effective, although the use of local anaesthetic may reduce postinjection soreness.[51] Where multiple muscle groups are involved, the use of dry needling or acupuncture is preferable.

The mechanism of action of needling and anaesthetic injection appears to be mechanical disruption of the trigger point and, where local anaesthetic is used, desensitization of the area.[52] It has been proposed that pain relief, increased range of motion and improved exercise tolerance are achieved with this therapeutic approach.[52] Careful localization of the trigger point is first necessary, and several techniques have been described to achieve this, including manual palpation and percussion with a tendon hammer. Stretching the area locally prior to injection/needling is also usually recommended. On inserting the needle parallel to the muscle fibres, the clinician should feel resistance as the needle encounters the taut band and the patient may report a dull ache at the site or a full reproduction of their symptoms, including pain in the zone of referral (Figures 17.1 and 17.2). A local twitch response is also anticipated during the procedure. After needling or injection of the band, the needle can be redirected to other local bands.

There is evidence to suggest that trigger point injection and ligamentous injections are beneficial in the control of back pain. Trigger point injection using methylprednisolone or triamcinolone plus lignocaine versus lignocaine alone is reported to increase the number of people obtaining pain relief after 3 months (60–80% versus 20%).

Side-effects of local anaesthetic injection are rare. Injection of large volumes into a highly vascular area may theoretically result in systemic effects. Adrenalin is not recommended in local anaesthetics for procedures involving the appendages because of the risk of ischaemic necrosis.[53]

OTHER AGENTS

A number of other substances are used in local injections of soft-tissue complaints.

Sclerosants (prolotherapy)

Injection of various solutions, such as a mixture of dextrose 12.5%, glycerin 12.5%, phenol 1.25% and lidocaine 0.25%, with the goal of producing a sclerosing effect to reduce pain and disability, has long been used to treat soft-tissue injuries and

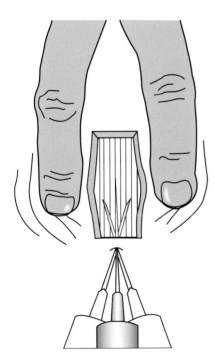

Figure 17.1. Trigger point injection. After needling the trigger point, the needle is redirected into other taut muscle bands without being withdrawn from the skin. Reproduced with permission from Simons DG, Travell JG, Simons LS, Cummings BD, *Travell Simons' Myofascial Pain and Dysfunction: The Trigger Point Manual*, 2nd edn, pp. 63–158. Lippincott Williams & Wilkins, Baltimore, OH, 1999.

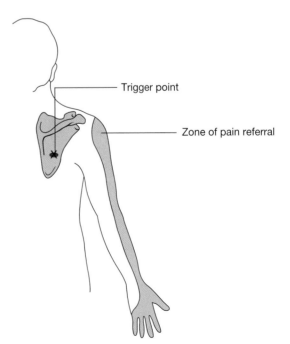

Trigger point

Zone of pain referral

Figure 17.2. A trigger point and its zone of referral. Reproduced with permission from: Speed CA, Dalton S, Hazleman BL, *Fast Facts: Soft-Tissue Rheumatology*, p. 87. Oxford University Press, Oxford, 2001.

spinal pain. The evidence base is limited and treatment protocols are varied. Postinjection pain and stiffness are the most common side-effects.[54]

Botulinum toxins

Botulinum toxins (BTX) are purified proteins, produced by the anaerobic bacterium *Clostridium botulinum*, which block the presynaptic release of the neurotransmitter acetylcholine. There are as many as seven antigenically distinct botulinum neurotoxins, but only types A and B are in clinical use. This increasingly popular group of agents is used in the treatment of a number of painful conditions, including myofascial pain, muscular low back pain, spasticity, headache and various other neurological disorders.[55, 56] Clinical effects are typically seen between 3 and 10 days after injection. Pain relief is usually temporary, lasting weeks to months, and repeat administration is usually necessary. As with other injection therapies for soft-tissue conditions, stretching and exercise therapy are important components for a successful outcome. However, when administered properly, the procedure is usually very safe, although the long-term side-effects of regular injections are not known. Reported side-effects include injection-site pain, muscle soreness, headache, fever, abdominal symptoms, a flu-like illness, rash and antibody formation. The development of immunoresistance results in inefficacy of the treatment, but can be limited by using the smallest possible effective dose and extending the interval between treatments as long as possible. Those who do develop resistance may in the future benefit from the use of other botulinum toxin serotypes. Muscle paralysis can occur with misplaced injections or excessive doses.

Studies of BTX in myofascial disorders imply similar results to injection of saline or local anaesthetic, and therefore BTX should be reserved for resistant cases. In an RCT of 132 patients with cervical or shoulder myofascial pain or both and active trigger points, Ferrante et al.[57] noted no significant differences between saline and BTX-A groups with respect to visual–analogue pain scale scores, pressure algometry or rescue medication. In a small study comparing dry needling with lidocaine injection and BTX-A injection, lidocaine or BTX-A appeared superior in achieving reduced visual–analogue pain scale scores, and lidocaine resulted in higher pain thresholds than the other two groups.[58]

Other agents

Low-dose heparin has been used in the management of Achilles' tendinopathies, with the aim to limit the formation of adhesions. However, there is some evidence that there is no beneficial effect,[59] and it has been suggested that heparin may, in itself, cause a degenerative tendinopathy.

A calf-derived deproteinized haemodialysate, Actovegin, has been suggested to be useful in the management of Achilles' paratenonitis, but a large, high-quality trial is needed.[59]

Traumeel is a mixture of diluted extracts from minerals and medicinal plants, including *Arnica*, that is proposed to have anti-inflammatory properties. It is increasingly popular in the treatment of soft-tissue injuries, but trials are lacking.

NEURAL BLOCKADE IN THE MANAGEMENT OF SOFT-TISSUE DISORDERS

Neural blockade is used for the diagnosis and treatment of a variety of chronically painful conditions. Such procedures aim to reduce nociceptive input into the dorsal horn on the hypothesis that, if a nerve is quiescent for some time, peripheral sensitization can be reduced or reversed.[60] Techniques can be divided into peripheral somatosensory nerve blocks and neuraxial blockade.

Peripheral somatosensory nerve blockade

Peripheral somatosensory nerve blocks are also used in the management of pain in soft-tissue complaints. Common examples include carpal tunnel injection, suprascapular nerve block in the management of shoulder pain, and ilioinguinal nerve blocks for posthernia pain.

Carpal tunnel syndrome

Local corticosteroid injection into the carpal tunnel significantly improves symptoms in the short term. Two randomized, placebo-controlled trials (one using methylprednisolone 40 mg and one betamethasone 1.5 mg) demonstrated significantly more people with symptom improvement at 1 month after corticosteroid injection than with placebo injection.[61, 62] Another study of steroid injection in 48 patients with mild carpal tunnel syndrome (CTS) demonstrated improvement in nerve-conduction parameters, symptom severity and functional scores in 79% of cases at a median follow-up of 16 months.[63]

A comparison of the effects of local steroid injection versus surgical decompression in new-onset CTS of at least 3 months' duration in 163 wrists with CTS showed local steroid injection is better than surgical decompression for the symptomatic relief of CTS over the short term.[64] At 1 year, local steroid injection is as effective as surgical decompression for the symptomatic relief of CTS.

Shoulder pain

The suprascapular nerve supplies sensory nerves to the posterosuperior aspect of the shoulder, including major portions of the rotator cuff. There is some evidence to suggest that suprascapular nerve block using steroid/bupivacaine is temporarily effective in reducing pain in rotator cuff tendinitis and tears, and improves movement range in tendinitis. The procedure can be done in an outpatient setting with little or no risk of complication.[65] The benefit of using steroid and lignocaine over anaesthetic alone is questionable.

Different techniques for suprascapular nerve blockade have been described, including needle tip guided by superficial bony landmarks, and a near-nerve electromyographically guided technique.[66]

Dahan et al.[67] performed a double-blind RCT examining the efficacy of suprascapular nerve blockade in 34 subjects with frozen shoulder, comparing a series of three suprascapular nerve blocks using 0.5% bupivacaine 10 mL, versus saline 10 mL, delivered over a 7-day period. A 64% reduction in pain

PRACTICE POINTS

Corticosteroid injection in soft-tissue lesions

Indications

- Reserve for chronic injuries, after a failure of intensive use of other approaches for at least 2 months.
- Use when rehabilitation is inhibited by symptoms.

Contraindications

- If pain relief and anti-inflammatory effects can be achieved by other methods.
- Local or systemic infection.
- Coagulopathy.
- Tendon tear.
- Local corticosteroid injections are often unnecessary and should be avoided in the younger patient.

Potential unwanted effects

- Hypersensitivity (local or systemic).
- Tissue atrophy.
- Tendon rupture.
- Infection (local or systemic).
- Postinjection 'flare' of symptoms.
- Osteonecrosis/steroid arthropathy (intra-articular injections, weight-bearing joints).

Local steroid injections in tendinopathies

- Informed consent should be obtained from the patient, who must be willing to follow postinjection guidelines.
- The practitioner should have full knowledge of the local anatomy.
- Select the finest needle that will reach the lesion.
- The practitioner's hands and the patient's skin should be cleansed and a no-touch technique used.
- Use short/medium-acting corticosteroid preparations in most cases, with local anaesthetic.
- Injection should be peritendinous; avoid injection into tendon substance.
- The minimum interval between injections should be 6 weeks.
- Use a maximum of three injections at one site.
- Soluble preparations may be useful in those patients who have had a hypersensitivity/local reaction to previous injection.
- Details of the injection should be carefully recorded.
- Do not repeat if two injections do not provide at least 4 weeks' relief.
- Warn the patient of early postinjection local anaesthesia, to avoid initial overuse.
- Advise a minimum postinjection rest of 2 weeks and avoidance of heavy loading for 6 weeks.
- The patient should inform the doctor if there is any suggestion of infection or other significant adverse event.

RESEARCH AGENDA

- A number of sources of soft-tissue pain have been identified: the mechanism of action of local injections in such conditions is uncertain and need to be elucidated.
- Recent systematic reviews have highlighted the methodological limitations in clinical studies relating to the efficacies of such techniques.
- Well-designed clinical studies for assessing the use of most injection therapies in clearly defined soft-tissue disorders under image guidance are warranted. Under ideal conditions (including image guidance), what are the comparative efficacies of different injection therapies?

in the treatment group versus 13% in the placebo group was observed at 1 month. There was a non-significant 15.8% improvement in shoulder function in the treatment group versus 4% in the placebo group ($p = 0.24$), but no improvement in shoulder mobility was noted. No side-effects other than transient vagal symptoms and local tenderness at the injection site were reported.

Neuraxial blockade

The epidural space is easily accessible for performing blockade for musculoskeletal pain. Epidurals are most commonly done in the caudal or lumbar space for sciatica. The evidence suggests that epidural steroids may be of short-term benefit in recent-onset radicular leg pain,[68] but there is no evidence of efficacy in back pain without nerve root irritation.[69] Prolonged symptomatology, previous back surgery and spinal stenosis are associated with lower rates of success.[70–73] Readers are referred to more extensive texts on this subject.

SUMMARY

A number of local injection therapies are available for the management of soft-tissue mediated pain. They should be reserved for the treatment of chronic soft-tissue lesions and as part of a programme that includes identification and correction of provocative factors. Although an increasing number of techniques and injectates are available, the current evidence for the use of many is scant. Accuracy of diagnosis and injection appears to be important for maximum benefit to be achieved.

REFERENCES

1. Dorfer L, Moser M, Bahr F et al. A medical report from the stone age? *Lancet* 1999; **354**: 1023–1025.
2. Bernsten CA, Lin AN. History of corticosteroid therapy. In: Lin AN, Paget SA (eds), *Principles of Corticosteroid Therapy*. Arnold, New York, 2002, pp. 3–5.
3. Hench PS, Kendall EC, Slocumb CH et al. The effect of a hormone of the adrenal cortex (17-hydroxy-11-dehydrocorticosteroine: Compound E) and of pituitary adrenocorticotrophic hormone on rheumatoid arthritis: preliminary report. *Proc Staff Meet Mayo Clin* 1949; **24**: 181–197.
4. Haslock I, Macfarlane D, Speed C. Intra-articular and soft-tissue injections: a survey of current practice. *Br J Rheumatol* 1995; **34**: 449–452.

5. Gam AN, Schydlowsky P, Rossel I et al. Treatment of frozen shoulder with distension and glucocorticoid compared with glucocorticoid alone. *Scand J Rheumatol* 1998; **27**: 425–430.

6. Paget SA. Clinical use of corticosteroids: an overview. In: Lin AN, Paget SA (eds), *Principles of Corticosteroid Therapy*. Arnold, New York, 2002, pp. 6–16.

7. Rodeo SA, Hannafin JA, Tom J et al. Immunolocalization of cytokines and their receptors in adhesive capsulitis of the shoulder. *J Orthopaed Res* 1997; **15**: 427–436.

8. Sakai H, Fujita K, Sakai Y et al. Immunolocalization of cytokines and growth factors in subacromial bursa of rotator cuff tear patients. *Kobe J Med Sci* 2001; **47**: 25–34.

9. Riley GP, Harrall RL, Constant CR et al. Tendon degeneration and chronic shoulder pain: changes in collagen composition of the human rotator cuff tendons in rotator cuff tendinitis. *Ann Rheum Dis* 1994; **53**: 359–366.

10. Chard MD, Cawston TD, Riley GP et al. Rotator cuff degeneration and lateral epicondylitis: a comparative histological study. *Ann Rheum Dis* 1994; **53**: 30–34.

11. Josza J, Kannus P. Overuse injuries of tendons. In: Josza J, Kannus P (eds), *Human Tendons*. Human Kinetics, New York, 1997, pp. 164–253.

12. Alfredson H. In situ microdialysis in tendon tissue: high levels of glutamate, but not prostaglandin E2 in chronic Achilles tendon pain. *Knee Surg Sport Traumatol Arthrosc* 1999; **7**: 378–381.

13. Gotoh M, Hamada K, Yamakawa H et al. Increased substance P in subacromial bursa and shoulder pain in rotator cuff disease. *J Orthopaed Res* 1998; **16**: 618–621.

14. Khan KM, Cook JL, Maffulli N et al. Where is the pain coming from in tendinopathy? It may be biochemical, not only structural in origin. *Br J Sport Med* 2000; **34**: 81–83.

15. Speed CA. Fortnightly review: corticosteroid injections in tendon lesions. *BMJ* 2001; **323**: 382–386.

16. Speed CA. Local injections for soft tissue lesions. In: Hazleman BL, Riley GP, Speed CA (eds), *The Oxford Textbook of Soft Tissue Rheumatology*. Oxford University Press, Oxford, 2002.

17. Lambert MA, Morton RJ, Sloan JP. Controlled study of the use of local steroid injection in the treatment of trigger finger and thumb. *J Hand Surg* 1992; **17B**: 69–70.

18. Maneerit J, Sriworakun C, Budhraja N et al. Trigger thumb: results of a prospective randomised study of percutaneous release with steroid injection versus steroid injection alone. *J Hand Surg (Br)* 2003; **28**: 586–589.

19. Murphy D, Failla JM, Koniuch MP. Steroid versus placebo injection for trigger finger. *J Hand Surg* 1995; **20A**: 628–631.

20. Assendelft WJ, Hay EM, Adshead R et al. Corticosteroid injections for lateral epicondylitis: a systematic overview. *Br J Gen Pract* 1996; **46**: 209–216.

21. Hay EM, Paterson SM, Lewis M et al. Pragmatic randomised controlled trial of local corticosteroid injection and naproxen for treatment of lateral epicondylitis of elbow in primary care. *BMJ* 1999; **319**: 964–968.

22. Green S, Buchbinder R, Glazier R et al. Interventions for shoulder pain. *Cochrane Database of Systematic Reviews* 2000; **2**: CD001156.

23. Speed CA, Hazleman BL. Shoulder pain. *Clin Evid* 2004; **12**: 1735–1754.

24. DaCruz DJ, Geeson M, Allen MJ et al. Achilles paratendonitis: an evaluation of steroid injection. *Br J Sport Med* 1988; **22**: 64–65.

25. Crawford F. Plantar heel pain (including plantar fasciitis). *Clin Evid* 2002; **7**: 1091–1100.

26. Atkins D, Crawford F, Edwards J et al. A systematic review of treatments for the painful heel. *Rheumatology* 1999; **38**: 968–973.

27. Crawford F, Atkins D, Young P et al. Steroid injection for heel pain: evidence of short term effectiveness. A randomised controlled trial. *Rheumatology* 1999; **38**: 974–977.

28. Sellman JR. Plantar fascial rupture associated with corticosteroid injection. *Foot Ankle Intl* 1994; **15**: 376–381.

29. Fadale PD, Wiggins MD. Corticosteroid injections: their use and abuse. *J Am Acad Orthopaed Surg* 1994; **2**: 133–140.

30. Nevasier RJ, Nevasier TJ. The frozen shoulder. Diagnosis and management. *Clin Orthopaed Related Res* 1987; **223**: 59–64.

31. van der Windt DAWM, van der Heijden GJMG, Scholten RJPM et al. The efficacy of non-steroidal anti-inflammatory drugs (NSAIDs) for shoulder complaints. A systematic review. *J Clin Epidemiol* 1995; **48**: 691–704.

32. Berry H, Fernandes L, Bloom B et al. Clinical study comparing acupuncture, physiotherapy, injection and oral anti-inflammatory therapy in the shoulder. *Curr Med Res Opinion* 1980; **7**: 121–126.

33. Rizk T, Pinals R, Talaiver A. Corticosteroid injections in adhesive capsulitis: investigation of their value and site. *Arch Phys Med* 1991; **72**: 20–22.

34. Snels IA, Beckerman H, Twisk JW et al. Effect of triamcinolone acetonide injections on hemiplegic shoulder pain: a randomized clinical trial. *Stroke* 2000; **31**: 2396–2400.

35. Richardson AT. The painful shoulder. *Proc R Soc Med* 1975; **68**: 11–16.

36. Buchbinder R, Green S, Forbes A et al. Arthrographic joint distension with saline and steroid improves function and reduces pain in patients with painful stiff shoulder: results of a randomised, double blind, placebo controlled trial. *Ann Rheum Dis* 2004; **63**: 302–309.

37. Hogan QH, Abram SE. Neural blockade for diagnosis and prognosis. *Anesthesiology* 1997; **86**: 216–241.

38. Bigos S, Bowyer O, Braen G et al. *Acute Low Back Problems in Adults*. Clinical Practice Guideline No. 14. AHCPR Publication No. 95–0642. Agency for Health Care Policy and Research, Public Health Service, US Department of Health and Human Services, Rockville, MD, 1994.

39. Nelemans PJ, de Bie RA, de Vet HCW et al. *Injection Therapy for Subacute and Chronic Benign Low Back Pain*. The Cochrane Library, Issue 2, Update Software, Oxford, 2001.

40. Eustace JA, Brophy DP, Gibney RP et al. Comparison of the accuracy of steroid placement with clinical outcome in patients with shoulder symptoms. *Ann Rheum Dis* 1997; **56**: 59–63.

41. Zhingis C, Failla JM, van Holsbeeck M. Injection accuracy and clinical relief of de Quervain's tendinitis. *J Hand Surg* 1998; **23A**: 89–96.

42. Jones A, Regan M, Ledingham J et al. Importance of placement of intra-articular steroid injections. *Br Med J* 1993; **307**: 1329–1330.

43. Consumers Association. Articular and periarticular corticosteroid injections. *Drug Ther Bull* 1995; **33**: 67–70.

44. Unverfirth LJ, Olix ML. The effect of local steroid injections on tendon. *J Bone Joint Surg* 1973; **55-A**: 1315.

45. Gottlieb NL, Riskin WG. Complications of local corticosteroid injections. *JAMA* 1980; **240**: 1547–1548.

46. Mattila J. Prolonged action and sustained serum levels of methylprednisolone acetate. *Clin Trial J* 1983; **20**: 18–23.

47. Kannus P, Jarvinen M, Niittymaki S. Long- or short-acting anesthetic with corticosteroid in local injections of overuse injuries? A prospective, randomised, double-blind study. *Intl J Sport Med* 1990; **11**: 397–400.

48. Benazzo F, Stennardo G, Valli M. Achilles and patellar tendinopathies in athletes: pathogenesis and surgical treatment. *Bull Hosp Joint Dis* 1996; **54**: 236–240.

49. Josza J, Kannus P. Treatment principles in tendon injuries and other tendon disorders. In: Josza J, Kannus P (eds), *Human Tendons*. Human Kinetics, New York, 1997, pp. 491–525.

50. Neer CS. Impingement lesions. *Clin Orthop Relat Res* 1983; **173**: 70–77.

51. Jaeger B, Skootsky SA. Double blind controlled study of different myofascial trigger point injection techniques. *Pain* 1987; **4**(Suppl): 560.

52. Mense S, Simons DG, Russell IJ. *Muscle Pain. Understanding its Nature, Diagnosis and Treatment*. Lippincott, Williams &Wilkins, Philadelphia, 2001, pp. 205–288.

53. McCauley WA, Gerace RV, Scilley C. Treatment of accidental digital injection of epinephrine. *Ann Emerg Med* 1991; **6**: 665–668.

54. Dagenais S, Haldeman S, Wooley JR. Intraligamentous injection of sclerosing solutions (prolotherapy) for spinal pain: a critical review of the literature. *Spine* J 2005; **5**: 310–328.

55. Figgitt DP, Noble S. Botulinum toxin B: a review of its therapeutic potential in the management of cervical dystonia. *Drugs* 2002; **62**: 705–722.

56. Foster L, Clapp L, Erickson M et al. Botulinum toxin A and chronic low back pain. A randomized, double-blind study. *Neurology* 2001; **56**: 1290–1293.

57. Ferrante FM, Bearn L, Rothrock R et al. Evidence against trigger point injection technique for the treatment of cervicothoracic myofascial pain with botulinum toxin type A. *Anesthesiology* 2005; **103**: 377–383.

58. Kamanli A, Kaya A, Ardicoglu O et al. Comparison of lidocaine injection, botulinum toxin injection, and dry needling to trigger points in myofascial pain syndrome. *Rheumatol Int* 2005; **25**: 604–611.

59. McLauchlan GJ, Handoll HH. Interventions for treating acute and chronic Achilles tendinitis. *Cochrane Database of Systematic Reviews* 2001; **2**: CD000232.

60. Abram SE. Neural blockade for neuropathic pain. *Clin J Pain* 2000; **16**: 56–61.

61. Marshall S, Tardiff G, Ashworth N. *Local Corticosteroid Injection for Carpal Tunnel Syndrome*. Cochrane Library, Issue 1. Update Software, Oxford, 2001.

62. O'Gradaigh D, Merry P. Corticosteroid injection for the treatment of carpal tunnel syndrome. *Ann Rheum Dis* 2000; **59**: 918–919.

63. Ly-Pen D, Andreu JL, de Blas G et al. Surgical decompression versus local steroid injection in carpal tunnel syndrome: a one-year, prospective, randomized, open, controlled clinical trial. *Arthritis Rheum* 2005; **52**: 612–619.

64. Agarwal V, Singh R, Sachdev A et al. A prospective study of the long-term efficacy of local methyl prednisolone acetate injection in the management of mild carpal tunnel syndrome. *Rheumatology (Oxford)* 2005; **44**: 647–650.

65. Vecchio PC, Adebajo AO, Hazleman BL. Suprascapular nerve block for persistent rotator cuff lesions. *J Rheumatol* 1993; **20**: 453–455.

66. Karatas GK, Meray J. Suprascapular nerve block for pain relief in adhesive capsulitis: comparison of 2 different techniques. *Arch Phys Med Rehab* 2002; **83**: 593–597.

67. Dahan TH, Fortin L, Pelletier M et al. Double blind randomized clinical trial examining the efficacy of bupivacaine suprascapular nerve blocks in frozen shoulder. *J Rheumatol* 2000; **27**: 1464–1469.

68. Cousins MJ, Walker S. Chronic pain: management strategies that work. *Anesthes Analges* 2001; **V92**(3S): 15–25.

69. Koes BW, Scholten RJ, Mens JM et al. Efficacy of epidural steroid injections for low back pain and sciatica: a systematic review of randomised clinical trials. *Pain* 1995; **63**: 279–288.

70. Abram SE. Treatment of lumbosacral radiculopathy with epidural steroids. *Anesthesiology* 1999; **91**: 1937–1941.

71. van Tulder MW, Koes BW, Bouter LM. Conservative treatment of acute and chronic nonspecific low back pain: a systematic review of randomized controlled trials of the most common interventions. *Spine* 1997; **22**: 2128–2156.

72. Koes BW, Scholten RJPM, Mens JMA et al. Epidural steroid injections for low back pain and sciatica: an updated systematic review of randomized clinical trials. *Pain Digest* 1999; **9**: 241–247.

73. Watts RW, Silagy CA. A meta-analysis on the efficacy of epidural corticosteroids in the treatment of sciatica. *Anaesth Intens Care* 1995; **23**: 564–569.

Chapter 18

Treatment options for regional musculoskeletal pain: what is the evidence?

Krysia Dziedzic, Joanne L. Jordan, Julius Sim and Elaine M. Hay

ASSESSMENT OF REGIONAL MUSCULOSKELETAL PAIN

The classification and assessment of patients with regional musculoskeletal pain are problematical. Specific issues relating to each of the anatomical regions are covered in the following chapters. Here, we address problems broadly grouped into three categories:

- case definition
- measurement of outcome
- prediction of chronicity.

Case definition

Regional musculoskeletal pain syndromes have been traditionally divided into periarticular and articular disorders. Periarticular complaints include capsulitis, tendinitis, bursitis, enthesitis, fasciitis and ligamentous lesions. Cartilage, ligaments, locking and degeneration are thought to be responsible for articular problems. Making a precise clinical diagnosis is at the heart of the practice of medicine so that the clinician can decide upon appropriate treatment and give guidance to the patient on the probable outcome. In research terms, uniformity of case definition is important to describe the study population and to control for possible predictors of prognosis. In regional musculoskeletal pain, however, there is a problem. Classification criteria are either non-existent or have been shown to have poor reproducibility when formally tested.[1] There is a lack of agreement about how specific diagnoses are defined and an absence of gold-standard diagnostic tests based on clinical,

radiographic or pathological criteria. Furthermore, in order to develop models of management, the professions have developed their own specific approaches to classifying disorders, leading to the inability of doctors, physiotherapists, chiropractors and osteopaths, among others, to communicate using common terms.

This lack of diagnostic uniformity results in confusion for researchers, clinicians and patients alike. Inconsistent messages (e.g. neck pain being variously called 'cervical spondylosis', 'wear and tear', 'osteoarthritis' and 'degeneration') may lead to increased anxiety and fear among individuals with regional musculoskeletal pain. For researchers, it leads to problems in deciding to which groups of patients the findings from clinical studies can be applied. Careful studies are needed to investigate the clinical epidemiology of regional musculoskeletal pain syndromes in both primary and secondary care settings. In this way, it may be possible to document the natural history of these disorders in order to establish whether 'splitting' into either clinical or pathological diagnostic groups offers useful information in terms of prognosis and response to treatment.

Measurement of outcome

The management of regional musculoskeletal pain, especially medical treatment, is usually directed at the pathology or impairment level, and its effectiveness can be measured at this level as, for example, a reduction in swelling or an increase in range of movement. There is an assumption that this will in turn improve function (activity limitation and participation restriction). In general terms, function is a more important outcome from a patient's point of view, but it is difficult to measure. There is a lack of reliable and valid outcome measures for measuring disability and participation restriction resulting from regional musculoskeletal pain. Questionnaires have been developed by a number of research groups to measure functional outcome in, for example, shoulder pain and neck pain. However, it is often not clear exactly which dimension these are measuring, whether they are all measuring the same thing, and how a score on a questionnaire relates to how a patient functions in real life.[2] In as much as it indicates whether individual patients perceive their life to be restricted or diminished in some way by their condition, handicap is the most patient-focused outcome, yet it is frequently neglected.

Prediction of chronicity

Most soft-tissue regional musculoskeletal pain problems are self-limiting. Others will wax and wane over months and possibly years before spontaneously settling, and a small proportion will become chronic. The challenge for the researcher is to identify the features (risk factors) at presentation or early in the course of an episode of regional pain that predict which patients are likely to follow a chronic course. Risk factors fall into two broad groups: those that can be modified (e.g. everyday activities) and those that cannot (e.g. length of history and comorbidity). The modification of risk factors may allow treatment to be targeted appropriately. To date, length of history appears to be a consistent predictor of chronicity but is clearly of little help to the clinician in terms of being amenable to modification. However, it does raise the possibility that early intervention in regional pain syndromes might offer the best chance of avoiding persisting problems. This hypothesis needs to be tested in randomized controlled trials (RCTs).

Psychological distress and a lack of social support have been shown to be important predictors of poor functional outcome in subjects with spinal pain and work-related soft-tissue musculoskeletal injury.[3] This is an important area for ongoing research. The role of psychological factors in predicting functional outcome and the use of healthcare resources in other regional musculoskeletal pain syndromes needs to be established. Studies continue to be needed to determine the extent to which modification of psychological factors using, for example, cognitive–behavioural approaches results in a reduction of disability and participation restriction in these disorders.

These three issues (case definition, outcome measurement and the prediction of chronicity) need to be considered when reviewing the evidence available to help the clinician to practise effective evidence-based healthcare. In this chapter the sources of evidence and their strengths and weaknesses are summarized, and the current systematic review evidence for various modalities used for treating regional musculoskeletal pain is considered.

THE NATURE OF EVIDENCE-BASED PRACTICE

In recent years there has been increasing demand for evidence-based healthcare, defined as 'the conscientious, explicit and judicious use of current best evidence in making decisions about the care of individual patients'.[4] Although clinical judgement has an important role to play in evidence-based practice, on its own it is an unreliable basis for effective professional practice and may perpetuate unfounded or mistaken practices.[5] A large proportion of current practice in healthcare has not yet been subjected to critical evaluation. Consequently, clinical practitioners often lack a firm evidential basis for decisions about treatment modalities or approaches to management. Increasing stringency in the allocation of healthcare resources, and the development of clinical governance, have created a greater need for justification and accountability, which has increased the demand for objective evidence of treatment effectiveness.[6]

Sources of evidence

Clinicians have at their disposal a range of sources of evidence – both formal and informal – on the effectiveness of various treatment or management approaches. It is important that clinical decisions should be based not on 'any' evidence but on the best available evidence. The evidence needed to support evidence-based practice should be up to date, objective, verifiable or auditable, relevant and generalizable to practice, and above all intelligible, so that it can be readily disseminated to clinical practitioners. In practical terms, evidence-based practice means 'integrating individual clinical expertise with the best available external clinical evidence from systematic research'.[4]

Although the RCT is considered by many to be the gold-standard source of evidence, good-quality RCTs are often lacking in the field of musculoskeletal pain. Furthermore, although the RCT is, in principle, the optimum means of establishing the clinical effectiveness of an intervention, its practical feasibility as a research design differs between clinical specialities. The RCT is perhaps more readily applied to areas such as oncology than it is to clinical rheumatology, 'where diagnosis is uncertain, outcome non-specific, understanding poor, and the mechanism of many interventions unexplained'.[7] In addition, the results of an RCT conducted on groups of patients in highly controlled experimental settings do not necessarily answer the question of how to treat the individual patient presenting in the clinic,[8] where issues such as diagnostic uncertainty, differential responsiveness to treatment and suboptimal adherence come into play. It is important for the clinician to remember that the findings from RCTs have to be interpreted in a specific clinical context, with the aid of clinical judgement and other sources of information.[7]

Despite their methodological strength, RCTs are not the only source of information available to the discerning clinician. In the rest of this section the sources of evidence available to the clinician when making decisions about treatment options are briefly reviewed in approximately ascending order of their quality and robustness.

Clinical experience

Clinical experience is the practitioner's cumulative knowledge, gained during his or her professional practice, about the most effective ways in which to manage particular clinical presentations. It is, however, an informal and non-systematic process, prone to a range of heuristic and other biases. Although personal clinical experience is a potentially unreliable guide to effective clinical decision-making,[5] it may be all that the clinician has at his or her disposal when dealing with rare clinical presentations. Moreover, the clinical judgement that derives from professional experience plays a role in applying evidence from RCTs and other studies to the management of individual patients.[4]

Case studies and series

These are detailed descriptions of the progression and/or treatment of a particular patient or groups of patients.[9, 10] Their descriptive nature, with no experimental control or manipulation, means that changes in the patient's disease or clinical status cannot be unambiguously attributed to the treatment received. Case studies are susceptible to various biases in interpretation, and are difficult to generalize from. However, they generate hypotheses that can subsequently be tested through one of the designs described below.

Quasi-experimental trials

A quasi-experiment usually differs from a true experiment by the absence of randomization to treatment groups.[10] Random allocation may be difficult when seeking to compare, for example, two or more systems of treatment, each of which is specific to a clinical centre. In such a situation, it is not possible to randomize patients to different systems of treatment within a centre, and it may also not be feasible, for administrative or geographical reasons, to randomize patients between centres. Accordingly, the investigator is obliged to work with predetermined treatment groups. As a result, this design cannot ensure the comparability of treatment groups and is therefore prone to the influence of confounding variables.[11] Quasi-experimental designs therefore possess less internal validity than do true experimental designs such as the RCT.[12]

A single-system ($n = 1$) study applies the principles of experimental manipulation and control to a single patient.[13] The patient is put through at least two consecutive phases in which the treatment under investigation is administered alternately with 'baseline' phases in which either no treatment or another treatment is applied. The patient serves as his or her own control, and inferences on treatment effect are made when changes in outcome measures coincide with the transition between phases. Single-system studies allow the responses of individual patients to be analysed intensively and can counter many threats to internal validity.[12] They do, however, present certain difficulties in terms of generalizing findings from a single subject.[8]

Randomized controlled trials

Of all the designs available to investigate questions of clinical effectiveness, the RCT approximates most closely to the ideals of a true experiment and is regarded as the gold-standard approach for such questions. The random allocation of patients to groups is undertaken to ensure that, in the long run, potential confounding variables – both known and unknown – are distributed equally across each group.[14] The greater the sample size, the greater the equalizing effect of randomization. Any inequalities between groups that survive the randomization process are chance, rather than systematic, differences and are therefore taken into account by inferential statistical testing. Hence, the only non-random difference between groups is the specific treatment received, and any difference in outcome can be attributed to this factor alone. An RCT may take one of two forms: explanatory or pragmatic.[15] An explanatory trial seeks to establish whether or not an intervention works in an absolute sense; it addresses the efficacy of that intervention. In this connection, 'efficacy' is the extent to which a treatment does more good than harm in the context of 'optimal diagnostic accuracy and compliance of both health providers and patients'.[16] Explanatory trials often compare a single intervention with a placebo in carefully controlled, double-blind experimental conditions. New pharmaceutical agents are usually tested using this design. This design does not, however, lend itself to the testing of broader treatment packages (e.g. exercise programmes), in which tight experimental control and blinding of practitioner and patient are often impossible. In these circumstances, a pragmatic trial may be preferable. This design assesses whether an intervention works in a relative sense, i.e. in relation to one or more alternative interventions. In this case, the trial seeks to determine the effectiveness of the intervention. Effectiveness differs from efficacy in that it represents the benefit of an intervention in relation to other such interventions in the context of everyday clinical practice, in which diagnosis, compliance and overall experimental control may be less adequately controlled than in a more structured experimental setting.

The choice of whether to adopt a pragmatic or an explanatory approach will depend on the exact question that is being addressed and will clearly influence the choice of 'control' group. For example, an explanatory trial of acupuncture might compare 'true' acupuncture with 'sham' acupuncture, whereas a pragmatic trial might compare 'true' acupuncture with an alternative treatment such as painkillers. The former design would assess the efficacy of acupuncture in terms of the specific effects resulting from a needle placed at a particular site. The latter design would investigate the effectiveness resulting from a patient–acupuncturist interaction but would not establish whether it was the needles, the acupuncturist or the non-specific effect of spending time with another person that was the important ingredient of the intervention package.

The realities of clinical practice are reflected by the pragmatic trial design, so that, having been randomized, patients within a pragmatic RCT may not experience the interventions being tested in precisely the way in which they are prescribed in the study protocol. Some patients may fail to adhere to their allocated treatment, drop out of the study or even come to receive an intervention other than the one to which they were assigned. This phenomenon, referred to as 'protocol deviation',[17] raises the question of how the data relating to such patients should be analysed. One approach is to conduct a per protocol analysis, which is restricted to those patients who remain on, and complete, their assigned treatment, protocol deviators being excluded from the analysis. The disadvantage of this approach is that groups of patients at the point of analysis are likely to differ – in both size and nature – from those at the point of randomization. For example, if one intervention has moderate-to-major side-effects, patients in whom the condition has been less severe, or who are experiencing below-average pain relief, may be more inclined to drop out of this arm of the trial because the benefits of the treatment do not sufficiently outweigh the costs. These same categories of patient are, however, less likely to drop out of an alternative intervention with fewer or less severe side-effects. The result is that the comparability of the two groups produced by the process of randomization has now been undermined. An intention-to-treat analysis addresses this criticism. In this approach, all subjects are analysed according to the groups to which they were randomized, irrespective of whether or not they actually received the assigned treatment.[18] Even if some patients dropped out of the study, received a non-assigned treatment or turned out to be ineligible for the treatment assigned to them, they are still retained in their original treatment arm for the purposes of analysis.[19] In this way, randomization is preserved. An intention-to-treat analysis reflects more accurately the realities of clinical practice. Unlike a per protocol analysis, it takes into account the issues of non-compliance, drop-out and contamination that are prone to occur in everyday practice.[18] The price that is paid for this in a comparative trial is that the absolute effect of an intervention is underestimated, as those patients who did not receive a treatment, or received it incompletely, are treated as though they received it as prescribed in the study protocol.

Sometimes, it is not feasible, or not desirable, to randomize patients individually to different treatments. It may be, for instance, that an intervention has to be delivered at the level of a practice rather than that of the individual patient (e.g. a system of patient management that cannot realistically apply to only certain patients within a practice). Alternatively, if patients from a given practice are likely to be in close contact or communication with one another, there may be a danger of contamination, whereby patients allocated to one treatment come to receive an alternative treatment. Finally, if one treatment within a trial involves the practitioner learning a diagnostic or clinical skill, the practitioner cannot be expected to 'unlearn' that skill when faced with patients randomized to an alternative intervention.[14] In each of these situations, a possible solution is to randomize groups, or 'clusters', of patients to the study interventions. Cluster randomized trials present particular challenges in terms of sample size and data analysis.[20, 21] More particularly, they are susceptible to a number of biases, and require careful design.[22]

Systematic reviews

In the past, reviews of treatment effectiveness were neither rigorous nor systematic and were prone to subjective and idiosyncratic influences on the part of the reviewer. How the sources to be included in the review were selected, and the manner in which those included were analysed, were often not explicit.[23] Hence, the conclusions reached in the review might reflect not so much the merits of the treatments being examined as conscious or unconscious bias in selecting studies for inclusion.[23, 24] The systematic review is now advocated as the approach of choice in place of the traditional 'narrative' literature review. In contrast with the traditional approach, the systematic review is conducted according to a strict set of objective methodological standards and procedures. The methodological strengths and weaknesses of individual studies are normally assessed according to a set of agreed criteria,[25, 26] so that findings can be interpreted in the light of the methodological strength, or otherwise, of the individual studies concerned. Given that studies revealing statistically significant findings are more likely to be published in the academic and professional literature than those where the findings were non-significant,[27] rigorous and conscientious attempts are made to identify all relevant studies. This may involve going beyond the usual peer-reviewed journals to the 'grey' literature, such as conference proceedings, unpublished trial reports, theses and dissertations. Failure to accomplish a comprehensive search of relevant sources will undermine the conclusions of an otherwise rigorous systematic review.[28, 29]

Meta-analytic systematic reviews

The process of meta-analysis plays an important key role in systematic reviewing.[30, 31] It involves the statistical analysis of results from a number of individual studies, so as to synthesize their findings and form conclusions across these studies.[32] A systematic review that incorporates meta-analysis does not merely assimilate the conclusions of individual studies, but aggregates the data on which these conclusions were based. In this way, it provides a more precise, and therefore more trustworthy, estimate of the true effect of a treatment. Trials that, taken individually, may have insufficient statistical power to provide credible information can contribute meaningfully to the conclusions derived from aggregated data. Furthermore, trials that are in some sense atypical – in terms of patient inclusion, diagnosis or outcome assessment – can be identified and their findings subjected to critical scrutiny.[33] In this way, inclusion and exclusion criteria can be identified for studies in a meta-analysis just as they are for patients in a clinical trial.[34] The use of meta-analysis also permits treatment effects to be examined over a range of settings and populations, whereas the findings of an individual RCT may be restricted to a particular context.[35]

Meta-analysis has its critics. It tends, for example, to focus on a single outcome measure, whereas Eysenck[36] argues that 'effects are often multivariate rather than univariate'. Meta-analysis is hard to perform on studies of different design. It is not normally feasible to include data from quasi-experimental studies along with those from RCTs, as the subsequent aggregate analysis will assume that all patients have been randomized to the interventions being tested. Moreover, although a meta-analysis will provide a more precise estimate of a treatment effect – as evidenced by a narrower confidence interval than that of any of the individual studies[37] – it cannot in itself detect or correct for bias or confounding arising from poor study design. Meta-analyses can be prone to a number of biases.[38] Publication bias, as outlined above in relation to systematic reviews, is a major concern, and should be investigated carefully.[39] It is also important to explore heterogeneity in the results of individual studies, and where it is found its source should be determined.[33] Finally, studies included in a meta-analysis are prone to conscious or unconscious selection bias in relation to the anticipated outcome of the analysis.[40]

EVIDENCE FOR THE EFFECTIVENESS OF TREATMENT OPTIONS IN REGIONAL MUSCULOSKELETAL PAIN

Despite the commonly held belief that there is little evidence to support seemingly useful interventions in common self-limiting regional pain disorders, a large number of reviews now exist that inform the experienced clinician on the treatment options. As well as summarizing the evidence that exists to manage a particular condition, systematic reviews also identify areas warranting further research. The aim of this chapter is to present an overview of the evidence and highlight gaps where more research is still needed. This is not a systematic review, but a systematic search of the literature and a summary of the best, most recent systematic reviews evaluating non-surgical interventions for regional musculoskeletal pain.

A systematic search of MEDLINE, AMED, The Cochrane Database of Systematic Reviews, Database of Reviews of Effectiveness (DARE), the Health Technology Assessment Database and PsycINFO was conducted from 1998 (the date of the previous version of this chapter[41]) to July 2005. The search strategy was developed to capture all systematic reviews of the effectiveness of any non-surgical interventions for managing regional musculoskeletal pain. Reviews were considered to be systematic if a comprehensive search strategy and an assessment of the quality of the included trials had been carried out. Only systematic reviews of controlled clinical trials, preferably randomized controlled trials, were included in this overview of the evidence. Systematic reviews of secondary publications, such as other systematic reviews, were excluded to avoid additional interpretation of the primary studies.

A total of 1200 unique references were downloaded from the electronic databases. The titles and abstracts were examined and those that were not systematic were excluded, leaving 170 papers to be reviewed. The most up to date, rigorous and comprehensive systematic reviews were selected for each intervention and condition to provide an overview of the evidence. Eighty-three systematic reviews are included in the updated version of this chapter. For the purpose of this overview, interventions are considered in four categories: general approaches, non-pharmacological treatments, pharmacological treatments, and other treatments.

General approaches (Table 18.1)

Systematic reviews of non-surgical interventions for musculoskeletal pain conclude that insufficient evidence exists for the benefit of many interventions. However, in certain syndromes specific treatments have been shown to be useful – e.g. carpal tunnel syndrome (oral steroids, mobilizations) and shoulder pain (non-steroidal anti-inflammatory drugs (NSAIDs), acupuncture, subacromial steroid injections). Manipulation and some electrotherapies (pulsed electromagnetic energy (PEME) and transcutaneous electrical nerve stimulation (TENS/TNS)) are beneficial for neck pain.

Non pharmacological treatments (Table 18.2)
General management
There is inconclusive evidence for multidisciplinary biopsychosocial rehabilitation, chiropractic spinal manipulation and manual therapy due to conflicting results or poor-quality studies.

Physiotherapy general approaches
Ice-massage and cold packs have been shown to be beneficial for pain and functional disability in osteoarthritis.[42] Two systematic reviews on impingement syndrome suggest that therapeutic exercise and mobilizations are beneficial. Green et al.[43] demonstrated that exercise with or without mobilization was helpful for rotator cuff problems. The use of other therapies appears dependent on the site of treatment. For example, ultrasound was shown to be beneficial for lateral epicondylitis[44, 45] and yet to be ineffective for shoulder pain, except with calcific tendinitis. Laser treatment was found to be ineffective for lateral epicondylitis and mechanical neck disorders but helpful for adhesive capsulitis of the shoulder. There is insufficient and/or poor quality evidence for physical interventions for patellofemoral pain, shoulder instability and temporomandibular joint pain.

Balneotherapy
There is some evidence that combination baths have short-term benefits for pain relief and function in knee osteoarthritis over single bath treatments.

Electrotherapy
There are seven systematic reviews of electrotherapy in knee osteoarthritis. Overall, there are inconclusive findings because of poor-quality studies and insufficient or conflicting evidence. However, there is evidence of a benefit for acupuncture-like TNS and TNS in osteoarthritis of the knee in relieving pain and stiffness.[46] There is also a suggestion that laser and ultrasound treatment may provide some benefit in the relief of pain in specific conditions, e.g. epicondylitis (ultrasound) and chronic joint disorders (laser).

Acupuncture
Seven systematic reviews of acupuncture for musculoskeletal pain were identified. Overall, there was insufficient evidence for the effectiveness of acupuncture, except for knee osteoarthritis, where acupuncture was beneficial for pain relief.[47] There were two reviews on lateral elbow pain, which came to different conclusions, although the most recent review concluded that acupuncture was beneficial.[48]

Exercise

There have been a number of large systematic reviews on the benefits of exercise, the majority of which have been conducted for lower-limb osteoarthritis. Where there is sufficient evidence, a benefit of exercise on pain and disability can be demonstrated for exercise including strengthening exercise, aerobic exercises, quadriceps strengthening and aerobic walking. There is insufficient evidence for the effectiveness of exercise in upper-limb conditions and systematic reviews in this area are generally lacking.

Orthoses

There is no evidence for the effectiveness of splinting or braces in lateral epicondylitis or knee osteoarthritis. There may be some benefit for orthoses in patellofemoral pain, although this overall conclusion is based on low-quality studies.

Pharmacological treatments (Table 18.3)
Analgesics

Paracetamol (acetaminophen) is beneficial for hip and knee pain in osteoarthritis in the short term, and has a better side-effect profile than NSAIDs. Paracetamol (acetaminophen) is not beneficial for reducing disability in knee and hip osteoarthritis.

Oral NSAIDs and Cox-2 inhibitors

NSAIDs appear to be beneficial for patellofemoral pain syndrome in the short term. There is inconclusive and conflicting evidence for the benefit of NSAIDs in lateral elbow pain. There appears to be some benefit in knee osteoarthritis in the short term for pain relief, but with possible adverse events, especially in the elderly. NSAIDs have not been demonstrated to be sufficiently effective in neck disorders. Cox-2 inhibitors are not superior to NSAIDs in arthritis, but have fewer gastrointestinal

Table 18.1. Summary of evidence from systematic reviews of the effectiveness of interventions in musculoskeletal regional pain: general approaches

Intervention	Condition	Study	No. of trials (No. of people)	Overall conclusion*
Various interventions	Rotator cuff tears	Ejnisman et al.[59]	8 studies (455)	Inconclusive: insufficient evidence
Various treatments	Heel pain	Atkins et al.[60]	11 RCTs (465)	Inconclusive: insufficient evidence
Various interventions	Achilles tendinitis	McLauchlan and Handoll[61]	9 trials (697)	Inconclusive: insufficient evidence
Therapies	Hand OA	Towheed[62]	31 RCTs (2648 in 30 RCTs)	Inconclusive: insufficient evidence
Non-surgical treatments	Carpal tunnel syndrome	O'Connor et al.[63]	21 studies (884)	Positive for oral steroids, splints, yoga and mobilizations to carpus
Various interventions	Shoulder pain	Green et al.[64]	31 RCTs (1437 in 29 RCTs)	Inconclusive: insufficient evidence Positive for NSAIDs and subacromial steroid injections for abduction in rotator cuff tendinitis
Non-surgical treatments	Patellofemoral pain syndrome	Bizzini et al.[65]	20 RCTs (not reported)	Positive for acupuncture, quadriceps strengthening, brace, exercise with patellar taping and biofeedback
Various treatments	Complex regional pain syndrome type 1/RSD	Forouzanfar et al.[66]	26 RCTs (788)	Inconclusive: insufficient evidence
Physical therapies (physiotherapy, chiropractic)	Neck pain	Kjellman et al.[67]	27 RCTs (not reported)	Inconclusive: conflicting evidence Positive for PEME, manipulation and TNS (acute)
Various interventions	Subacromial pain	Johansson et al.[68]	40 studies (not reported)	Positive for corticosteroid injection in short term and acupuncture Negative for ultrasound

*Unless otherwise stated, conclusions are given for the outcomes pain and disability. Terms are used as follows:

Positive: one or more interventions favoured over other intervention or placebo.

Negative: one or more interventions unfavourable compared with other interventions or placebo.

Inconclusive: for various reasons, such as poor-quality studies, studies give conflicting results or insufficient evidence, no definite conclusion can be drawn.

OA, osteoarthritis; PEME, pulsed electromagnetic energy; RSD, reflex sympathetic dystrophy; TNS, transcutaneous nerve stimulation.

Table 18.2. Summary of evidence from systematic reviews of the effectiveness of interventions in musculoskeletal regional pain: non-pharmacological treatments

Intervention	Condition	Study	No. of trials (No. of people)	Overall conclusion*
General management				
Multidisciplinary biopsychosocial rehabilitation	Neck or shoulder pain	Karjalainen et al.[69]	1 RCT (70), 1 CCT (107)	Inconclusive: poor-quality studies
Chiropractic spinal manipulation	Neck pain	Ernst[70]	4 RCTs (419)	Inconclusive: poor-quality studies
Manual therapy	Neck pain	Sarigiovannis and Hollins[71]	12 RCTs (1407)	Inconclusive: conflicting results
Manual therapy in myofascial trigger point treatment	Myofascial pain syndrome	de las Penas et al.[72]	5 RCTs (375), 2 CCTs (40)	Inconclusive: conflicting results
Physiotherapy general approaches				
Rehabilitation	Subacromial impingement syndrome	Michener et al.[73]	12 trials (599)	Positive for exercise and mobilizations
Rehabilitation	Lateral epicondylitis	Trudel et al.[45]	31 RCTs	
Ultrasound			6 RCTs (332)	Positive
Acupuncture			5 RCTs (308)	Positive
Exercise			4 RCTs (125)	Positive
Mobilization			2 RCTs (42)	Positive
PEME			1 RCT (30)	Negative
Laser			6 RCTs (294)	Negative
Non-operative management	Shoulder instability	Gibson et al.[74]	19 trials (782) – 14 higher quality trials	Inconclusive: insufficient evidence and poor quality
Physical interventions	Patellofemoral pain syndrome	Crossley et al.[75]	16 CCTs (867)	Inconclusive: insufficient evidence
Physical interventions Exercise + mobilizations Laser Ultrasound PEME	Shoulder pain	Green et al.[43]	26 RCTs (median sample size 48; range 14–180)	Positive for rotator cuff Positive for adhesive capsulitis Negative; except positive for calcific tendinitis Positive for calcific tendinitis
Physical therapies (biofeedback, acupuncture, TNS)	Temporomandibular joint	Jedel and Carlsson[76]	7 CCTs (369)	Inconclusive: poor quality
Therapeutic exercise and orthopaedic manual therapy	Impingement syndrome	Desmeules et al.[77]	7 trials	Positive
Physical therapy	Lateral epicondylitis	Smidt et al.[44]	23 RCTs	Inconclusive: insufficient evidence, poor quality and conflicting, except positive for ultrasound
Ice massage and cold packs	OA	Brosseau et al.[42]	3 RCTs (179)	Positive
Balneotherapy	Knee OA	Brosseau et al.[78]	3 RCTs (160)	Positive initially for disability Negative for pain Positive combination bath vs single bath treatments for pain at 1 month

Continued

Table 18.2. *Continued*

Intervention	Condition	Study	No. of trials (No. of people)	Overall conclusion*
Electrotherapy				
Electromagnetic fields	Knee OA	Marks et al.[79]	11 studies (815)	Inconclusive: poor quality
	Knee and neck OA	Hulme et al.[80]	3 RCTs (259)	Inconclusive: insufficient evidence
Ultrasound	Patellofemoral pain	Brosseau et al.[81]	1 RCT (53)	Inconclusive: poor quality
	Musculoskeletal disorders	van der Windt et al.[82]	38 studies (not reported)	Inconclusive: insufficient evidence
	Epicondylitis			Positive for pain
	Ankle			Negative
	Soft tissues, shoulder disorders			Negative
	Rheumatic conditions			Inconclusive: poor quality
	Temporomandibular joint			Inconclusive: poor quality
	Knee OA	Marks et al.[83]	5 RCTs (673)	Inconclusive: poor quality
	Knee OA	Welch et al.[84]	3 RCTs (294)	Inconclusive: poor quality
Laser	Tendinitis	Abdulwadud.[85]	3 RCTs (89)	Inconclusive: insufficient evidence
	Musculoskeletal	de Bie et al.[86]	21 RCTs (811)	Inconclusive: poor quality
	OA	Brosseau et al.[87]	7 RCTs (345)	Inconclusive: conflicting
	Chronic joint disorders (knee, temporomandibular, zygoapophyseal)	Bjordal et al.[88]	11 RCTs (565)	Positive
TNS, AL-TENS	Knee OA	Osiri et al.[46]	7 RCTs (294)	Positive: over ≥ 4 weeks, effective pain control and relieved stiffness
Electrical muscle stimulation	Knee OA	Marks et al.[89]	7 studies (230)	Inconclusive: poor quality
Acupuncture	Temporomandibular joint	Ernst and White[90]	3 RCTs (205)	Inconclusive: insufficient evidence
	Neck pain	White and Ernst[91]	14 RCTs (724)	Inconclusive: conflicting
	Lateral elbow pain	Green et al.[92]	4 RCTs (239)	Inconclusive: insufficient evidence
	Lateral epicondyle pain	Trinh et al.[48]	6 RCTs and quasi-RCTs (282)	Positive
	Shoulder pain	Green et al.[93]	9 RCTs and quasi-RCTs (525)	Inconclusive: insufficient evidence
	Knee OA	Ezzo et al.[47]	7 RCTs and quasi-RCTs (393)	Positive for pain
	Myofascial trigger point pain	Cummings and White[94]	23 RCTs (1279)	Inconclusive: insufficient evidence
Exercise				
Strengthening	OA	Pelland et al.[95]	22 RCTs (2325)	Positive for strengthening in knee OA
	Knee and hip OA	Fransen et al.[96]	Hip: 2 RCTs (100)	Inconclusive for hip OA: insufficient evidence
			Knee: 17 RCTs (2562)	Positive for knee OA, exercise classes = individual exercises

Continued

Table 18.2. *Continued*

Intervention	Condition	Study	No. of trials (No. of people)	Overall conclusion*
Exercise – *continued*				
	OA	Brosseau et al.[97]	Knee: 1 RCT (39)	Inconclusive: insufficient evidence
Aerobic exercises	OA	Brosseau et al.[98]	12 RCTs (1363)	Positive
Quadriceps strengthening	Patellofemoral pain syndrome	Heintjes et al.[99]	12 trials (754)	Inconclusive for disability: conflicting Positive for pain, open = closed kinetic chain exercises
Exercise	Mechanical neck disorders	Sarig-Bahat[100]	16 studies (1332)	Inconclusive: poor quality
Aerobic walking or strengthening exercises	Knee OA	Roddy et al.[101]	20 RCTS (13 pooled (2304))	Positive for aerobic walking Aerobic walking = strengthening exercises
Orthoses	Lateral epicondylitis	Borkholder et al.[102]	11 RCTs (362)	Inconclusive: poor quality
	Lateral epicondylitis	Struijs et al.[103]	5 RCTs (300 randomized; 242 analysed)	Negative
	Knee OA	Brouwer et al.[104]	4 RCTs (444)	Inconclusive
	Patellofemoral pain	D'hondt et al.[105]	5 RCTs (362)	Positive: poor quality

*Unless otherwise stated conclusions are given for the outcomes pain and disability. Terms are used as follows:

Positive: one or more interventions favoured over other intervention or placebo.

Negative: one or more interventions unfavourable compared with other interventions or placebo.

Inconclusive: for various reasons, such as poor-quality studies, studies give conflicting results or insufficient evidence, no definite conclusion can be drawn.

A > B: intervention A was more effective than intervention B.

A = B: intervention A was equivalent to intervention B.

AL-TENS, acupuncture-like TNS; CCT, controlled clinical trial; OA, osteoarthritis; PEME, pulsed electromagnetic energy; RCT, randomized controlled trial; TNS, transcutaneous nerve stimulation.

side-effects. Recent concerns have been raised about the cardiovascular safety profile of these agents.[49–51]

Topical NSAIDs

There is evidence that topical NSAIDs are more beneficial than placebo in the first 2 weeks for reduction of pain and disability in osteoarthritis and chronic musculoskeletal pain, and have fewer side-effects than oral NSAIDs. Topical application is as effective as oral NSAIDs in chronic musculoskeletal pain, but not in knee osteoarthritis.

Topical preparations

There seems to be sufficient evidence to confirm the effectiveness of rubefacients and capsaicin for musculoskeletal and rheumatic diseases.

Other pharmacological treatments

Pharmacological interventions for chronic temporomandibular joint pain and reflex sympathetic dystrophy have insufficient evidence for their benefit, except in reflex sympathetic dystrophy where calcitonin appears to be of some benefit. Nandrolone appears to be beneficial for patellofemoral pain in the short term, but is considered a controversial treatment. Muscle relaxants have not been demonstrated to be sufficiently effective in neck disorders and botulinum toxin A is ineffective.

Corticosteroid injections and local anaesthetics

The evidence is inconclusive for lateral epicondylitis, shoulder pain and knee osteoarthritis, except in the first few weeks in knee osteoarthritis where injections are beneficial for pain relief.

For mechanical neck disorders, local anaesthetics and corticosteroid injections appear to provide some pain relief.

Hyaluronate (Hyaluronan)

There seems to be evidence of the benefit of Hyaluronan for osteoarthritis of the knee but insufficient evidence on its safety. There is inconclusive evidence for its use in temporomandibular disorders. Mild transient reactions (e.g. pain at the injection site) have been identified.[52]

Table 18.3. Summary of evidence from systematic reviews of the effectiveness of interventions in musculoskeletal regional pain: pharmacological treatments

Intervention	Condition	Study	No. of trials (No. of people)	Overall conclusion*
Analgesics				
Paracetamol	OA	Zhang et al.[106]	10 RCTs (1712)	Positive for pain Negative for disability NSAIDs > paracetamol for pain and disability Positive vs NSAIDs for gastro-intestinal side-effects
NSAIDs				
Oral NSAIDs	Lateral elbow pain	Green et al.[107]	14 RCTs (725 (not reported in 2 RCTs))	Inconclusive: conflicting
Including Cox-2	Knee OA	Bjordal et al.[108]	23 RCTs (10,845)	Positive in short term Inconclusive in long term Positive for adverse effects
Cox-2 inhibitors				
Celecoxib	OA and RA	Deeks et al.[109]	9 RCTs (15,187 (3 RCTs; 1947 people with OA))	Positive NSAIDs = Celecoxib Positive vs NSAIDs for gastro-intestinal side-effects
Valdecoxib	OA and RA	Edwards et al.[110]	9 RCTs (5726)	Positive NSAIDs = Valdecoxib Positive vs NSAIDs for gastro-intestinal side-effects
Rofecoxib	OA	Garner et al.[51]	26 RCTs (15,647)	Positive Negative vs other Cox-2 inhibitors, NSAIDs or paracetamol *Controversial* – this drug was withdrawn in September 2004
Topical NSAIDs	OA	Lin et al.[111]	13 RCTs (1983)	Positive in short term for pain and function Negative vs oral NSAIDs Positive vs oral NSAIDs for adverse effects
	Chronic musculo-skeletal pain	Mason et al.[112]	14 RCTs (1502)	Positive in short term Topical NSAIDs = placebo for side-effects Topical = oral NSAIDs Positive vs oral NSAIDs for adverse effects
Topical preparations				
Rubefacients containing salicylates	Pain	Mason et al.[113]	Acute pain: 3 RCTs (182) Chronic pain: 6 RCTs (429)	*Acute pain* Positive *Chronic pain* Inconclusive: insufficient evidence Positive for rheumatic disease
Capsaicin	Chronic pain	Mason et al.[114]	Neuropathic: RCTs (656) Musculoskeletal: 3 RCTs (368)	*Neuropathic* Positive Local adverse events *Musculoskeletal* Positive Local adverse events

Continued

Table 18.3. *Continued*

Intervention	Condition	Study	No. of trials (No. of people)	Overall conclusion*
Corticosteroid injection	Lateral epicondylitis	Smidt et al.[115]	13 RCTs (1028)	Inconclusive: poor quality
	Knee OA	Bellamy et al.[116]	26 RCTs (1721)	Positive for pain inconclusive for function in short term. Inconclusive for pain and function in longer term (4–24 weeks). Negative vs hyaluronic acid
	Shoulder	Buchbinder et al.[117]	26 RCTs (1455 (1 RCT not reported))	Inconclusive: poor quality
Hyaluronate (Hyaluronan)				
Hyaluronate	Temporo-mandibular joint disorders	Shi et al.[52]	7 trials (364)	Inconclusive: insufficient evidence. Mild transient reactions
Viscosupplementation (Hyaluronan)	Knee OA	Bellamy et al.[118]	63 trials (not reported)	Positive. Insufficient evidence on safety
Other pharmacological treatments				
Pharmacotherapy	Patellofemoral pain syndrome	Heintjes et al.[119]	8 trials (354)	Positive for NSAIDs for short-term pain. *Positive for nandrolone Controversial*. Inconclusive: conflicting glucos-aminoglycan polysulphate
Medicinal and injection therapies	Mechanical neck disorders	Peloso et al.[120]	32 RCTs (approx. 3200)	Positive for local anaesthetics for chronic pain. Positive for epidural corticosteroid injections for chronic neck and arm pain. Inconclusive for NSAIDs and muscle relaxants. Negative for botulinum toxin A
Pharmacological interventions	Chronic temporo-mandibular joint	List et al.[121]	11 RCTs (368)	Inconclusive: insufficient evidence
Medicinal treatments	Reflex sympathetic dystrophy	Perez et al.[122]	21 RCTs (not reported)	Inconclusive: insufficient evidence and poor quality. Positive for calcitonin

*Unless otherwise stated conclusions are given for the outcomes pain and disability. Terms are used as follows:

Positive: one or more interventions favoured over other intervention or placebo.

Negative: one or more interventions unfavourable compared with other interventions or placebo.

Inconclusive: for various reasons, such as poor-quality studies, studies give conflicting results or insufficient evidence, no definite conclusion can be drawn.

A > B: intervention A was more effective than intervention B.

A = B: intervention A was equivalent to intervention B.

NSAIDs, non-steroidal anti-inflammatory drugs; OA, osteoarthritis; RA, rheumatoid arthritis.

Other treatments (Table 18.4)
Glucosamine and chondriotin preparations
We identified two systematic reviews of reasonable size. An earlier review by McAlindon et al.[53] suggested a benefit of glucosamine and chondriotin preparations on outcomes. However, a more recent review by Towheed et al.[54] suggests that gluco-samine is ineffective for pain relief for knee osteoarthritis, and that the evidence is conflicting for reduction of disability.

Dietary supplements
One systematic review reviewed 11 trials of *S*-adenosylmethionine (SAMe) in osteoarthritis (1442 patients) and found that

Table 18.4. Summary of evidence from systematic reviews of the effectiveness of interventions in musculoskeletal regional pain: other treatments

Intervention	Condition	Study	No. of trials (No. of people)	Overall conclusion*
Glucosamine and chondriotin preparations				
Glucosamine and chondroitin preparations	OA	McAlindon et al[53]	15 RCTs (1710)	Positive
Glucosamine	OA (mainly knee)	Towheed et al[54]	20 RCTs (2570)	Inconclusive for disability: conflicting Negative for pain
Complementary and alternative medicines				
Articulin-F	OA	Long et al[56]	1 RCT (42)	Positive for pain severity and disability
Avocado/soybean unsaponifiables	Hip or knee OA	Long et al.[56]	2 RCTs (327)	Inconclusive: conflicting Effects more evident in hip than knee OA
Eazmov	OA, non-specific arthritis or RA	Long et al.[56]	1 RCT (60)	Negative for pain and disability vs diclofenac
Ginger	Hip or knee OA	Long et al.[56]	1 RCT (67)	Ginger = placebo Negative for pain and function vs ibuprofen
Gitadyl	Mild to moderate OA	Long et al.[56]	1 RCT (35)	Gitadyl = ibuprofen
Reumalex	Chronic stable arthritic conditions	Long et al.[56]	1 RCT (82 (51 with OA))	Positive for pain Reumalex = placebo for disability and function
Stinging nettle	OA at base of thumb or index finger	Long et al.[56]	1 RCT (27)	Positive
Willow bark (plus standard physiotherapy)	Hip or knee OA	Long et al.[56]	1 RCT (78)	Positive for pain and overall assessment vs physiotherapy only Willow bark = physiotherapy only for function
Harpagophytum procumbens	Hip or knee OA	Gagnier et al.[123]	5 RCTs (385)	Inconclusive for ethanolic *Harpagophytum* (< 30 mg/day harpagoside): poor quality Positive for *Harpagophytum* powder (harpagoside 60 mg)

Continued

overall SAMe was beneficial in reducing disability in the short term and equivalent to NSAIDs.[55] Interestingly, it also had a beneficial effect on depression.

Complementary and alternative medicine

There is limited evidence for the benefit of complementary and alternative medicine in the treatment of regional musculoskeletal pain. A systematic review in osteoarthritis concluded that specific preparations are beneficial in some instances, but conclusions are drawn from small numbers of studies.[56]

Summary

We conducted a systematic search for systematic reviews published from 1998 to July 2005. We excluded invasive treatments such as surgery and extracorporeal shockwave therapy. We also excluded conditions that did not reflect specific regional pain problems (e.g. low back pain, fibromyalgia, chronic widespread pain and inflammatory arthritides).

Anyone contemplating a systematic review should consider targeting the review to a specific area and intervention, which would allow summaries of systematic reviews such as this to be conducted more easily. We found differing results between systematic reviews that had picked a condition of interest compared with those selecting a specific intervention.

We made no prior decision about selection of outcome measures, but the consensus work of OMERACT has become increasingly influential in primary outcome selection in trials,[57] and all included reviews used pain and/or disability as main outcomes. This allowed us to compare evidence from different systematic reviews with greater ease.

Table 18.4. *Continued*

Intervention	Condition	Study	No. of trials (No. of people)	Overall conclusion*
Phytodolor	Musculoskeletal pain	Ernst[124]	10 RCTs (1135)	Inconclusive: poor quality Pytodolor = synthetic drugs
Combined homeopathic remedies	OA	Long and Ernst[125]	4 RCTs (406)	Inconclusive: insufficient evidence
Massage	Lateral epicondylitis or iliotibial band friction syndrome	Brosseau et al.[126]	2 RCTs (60)	Inconclusive: poor quality
Dietary supplements				
S-Adenosylmethionine (SAMe)	OA	Soeken et al.[55]	11 RCTs (1442)	Positive for disability and depression in short term SAMe = NSAIDs

*Unless otherwise stated conclusions are given for the outcomes pain and disability. Terms are used as follows:

Positive: one or more interventions favoured over other intervention or placebo.

Negative: one or more interventions unfavourable compared with other interventions or placebo.

Inconclusive: for various reasons, such as poor-quality studies, studies give conflicting results or insufficient evidence, no definite conclusion can be drawn.

A > B: intervention A was more effective than intervention B.

A = B: intervention A was equivalent to intervention B.

OA, osteoarthritis; RA, rheumatoid arthritis.

PRACTICE POINTS

- Healthcare professionals should utilize up-to-date, high-quality evidence when reaching clinical decisions.

- Systematic reviews can inform clinical decisions by identifying and synthesizing a large volume of available research evidence.

- Clinical judgement should be used when applying evidence from RCTs and systematic reviews to the treatment of individual patients.

- There is a lack of high-quality evidence from RCTs in some areas of regional musculoskeletal pain.

- 'No evidence' for an intervention does not, however, imply 'no effect' and does not justify 'no action'.

- Practitioners should endeavour to generate clinical guidelines from the available research evidence.

When we first produced an overview of the evidence for regional pain problems (see Hay et al.[41]) there was a disappointing lack of high-quality evidence from randomized controlled trials in many areas of regional musculoskeletal pain. We now have an increasing body of evidence to draw upon and there are a number of evidence-based treatment options available to practitioners. The strength of evidence of non-pharmacological interventions is increasing in line with the research agenda for regional musculoskeletal pain.[58]

RESEARCH AGENDA

- There is a need for more, and better, RCTs in regional musculoskeletal pain, particularly for non-pharmacological therapies.

- Such trials should adopt pragmatic as well as explanatory approaches, and should consider cost-effectiveness as well as clinical effectiveness.

- Other methods should be used in situations where RCTs are inappropriate or impracticable.

- Clinical priorities should drive the research agenda.

REFERENCES

1. Liesdek C, Windt van der DAWM, Koes BW et al. Soft-tissue disorders of the shoulder. A study of inter-observer agreement between general practitioners and physiotherapists and an overview of physiotherapeutic treatment. *Physiotherapy* 1997; **83**: 12–17.
2. Croft P. Measuring up to shoulder pain. *Ann Rheum Dis* 1998; **57**: 65–66.
3. Crook J, Moldofsky H, Shannon H. Determinants of disability after a work related musculoskeletal injury. *J Rheumatol* 1998; **25**: 1570–1573.
4. Sackett DL, Gray JAM, Haynes RB et al. Evidence based medicine: what it is and what it isn't. *BMJ* 1996; **312**: 71–72.
5. Sim J. Sources of knowledge in physical therapy. *Physiother Theory Pract* 1995; **11**: 193–194.
6. Gray JAM. *Evidence-Based Healthcare: How to Make Health Policy and Management Decisions*, 2nd edn. Churchill Livingstone, Edinburgh, 2001.
7. Croft P. Admissible evidence. *Ann Rheum Dis* 1998; **57**: 387–389.
8. Sim J. The external validity of group comparative and single system studies. *Physiotherapy* 1995; **81**: 263–270.

9. Rothstein JM. The case for case reports. *Phys Ther* 1993; **73**: 492–493.

10. Portney LG, Watkins MP. *Foundations of Clinical Research: Applications to Practice*, 2nd edn. Prentice Hall, Upper Saddle River, NJ, 2000.

11. Brennan P, Croft P. Interpreting the results of observational research: chance is not such a fine thing. *BMJ* 1994; **309**: 727–730.

12. Sim J, Wright C. *Research in Health Care: Concepts, Designs and Methods*. Nelson Thornes, Cheltenham, 2000.

13. Barlow DH, Hersen M. *Single Case Experimental Designs: Strategies for Studying Behavior Change*, 2nd edn. Pergamon, Oxford, 1984.

14. Machin D, Campbell MJ. *Design of Studies for Medical Research*. Wiley, Chichester, 2005.

15. Schwartz D, Lellouch J. Explanatory and pragmatic attitudes in therapeutic trials. *J Chronic Dis* 1967; **20**: 637–648.

16. Linden van der S, Bouter L, Tugwell P. What are the minimal methodological requirements for a good trial? 1. The clinician's view. In: Schlapbach P, Gerber NJ (eds), *Physiotherapy: Controlled Trials and Facts*. Karger, Basel, 1991, pp. 1–8.

17. Matthews JNS. *An Introduction to Randomized Controlled Clinical Trials*. Arnold, London, 2000.

18. Wright CC, Sim J. Intention-to-treat approach to data from randomized controlled trials: a sensitivity analysis. *J Clin Epidemiol* 2003; **56**: 833–842.

19. Lewis JA, Machin D. Intention to treat – who should use ITT? *Br J Cancer* 1993; **68**: 647–650.

20. Kerry SM, Bland JM. Sample size in cluster randomisation. *BMJ* 1998; **316**: 549.

21. Kerry SM, Bland JM. Analysis of a trial randomised in clusters. *BMJ* 1998; **316**: 54.

22. Puffer S, Torgerson D, Watson J. Evidence for risk of bias in cluster randomised trials: review of recent trials published in three general medical journals. *BMJ* 2003; **327**: 785–789.

23. Mulrow CD. Rationale for systematic reviews. *BMJ* 1994; **309**: 597–599.

24. Collins R, Gray R, Godwin J et al. Avoidance of large biases and large random errors in the assessment of moderate treatment effects: the need for systematic overviews. *Stat Med* 1987; **6**: 245–250.

25. Moher D, Jadad AR, Nichol G et al. Assessing the quality of randomized controlled trials: an annotated bibliography of scales and checklists. *Control Clin Trials* 1995; **16**: 62–73.

26. Verhagen AP, de Vet HCW, de Bie RA et al. The art of quality assessment of RCTs included in systematic reviews. *J Clin Epidemiol* 2001; **54**: 651–654.

27. Easterbrook PJ, Berlin JA, Gopalan R et al. Publication bias in published research. *Lancet* 1991; **337**: 867–872.

28. Bjordal JM, Greve G. What may alter the conclusions of reviews? *Phys Ther Rev* 1998; **3**: 121–132.

29. Crombie IK, McQuay HJ. The systematic review: a good guide rather than a guarantee. *Pain* 1998; **76**: 1–2.

30. Light RJ. Accumulating evidence from independent studies: what we can win and what we can lose. *Stat Med* 1987; **6**: 221–228.

31. Egger M, Davey Smith G. Meta-analysis. Potentials and promise. *BMJ* 1997; **315**: 1371–1374.

32. Whitehead A. *Meta-Analysis of Controlled Clinical Trials*. Wiley, Chichester, 2002.

33. Higgins J, Thompson S, Deeks J, Altman D. Statistical heterogeneity in systematic reviews of clinical trials: a critical appraisal of guidelines and practice. *J Health Service Res Policy* 2002; **7**: 51–61.

34. LaValley M. A consumer's guide to meta-analysis. *Arthritis Care Res* 1997; **10**: 208–213.

35. Gøtzche PC. Why we need a broad perspective on meta-analysis. *BMJ* 2000; **321**: 585–586.

36. Eysenck HJ. Problems with meta-analysis. In: Chalmers I, Altman DG (eds), *Systematic Reviews*. BMJ Publishing, London, 1995, pp. 64–74.

37. Sim J, Reid N. Statistical inference by confidence intervals: issues of interpretation and utilization. *Phys Ther* 1999; **79**: 186–195.

38. Sterne JAC, Egger M, Davey Smith G. Investigating and dealing with publication and other biases in meta-analysis. *BMJ* 2001; **323**: 101–105.

39. Thornton A, Lee P. Publication bias in meta-analysis: its causes and consequences. *J Clin Epidemiol* 2000; **53**: 207–216.

40. West RR. A look at the statistical overview (or meta-analysis). *J R Coll Physicians Lond* 1993; **27**: 111–115.

41. Hay EM, Dziedzic K, Sim J. Treatment options for regional musculoskeletal pain: what is the evidence? *Ballière's Clin Rheumatol* 1999; **13**: 243–259.

42. Brosseau L, Judd MG, Marchand S et al. *Thermotherapy for treatment of Osteoarthritis*. Cochrane Review. The Cochrane Library, Issue 4. Wiley, Chichester, 2003.

43. Green S, Buchbinder R, Hetrick S. *Physiotherapy Interventions for Shoulder Pain*. Cochrane Review. The Cochrane Library, Issue 2. Wiley, Chichester, 2003.

44. Smidt N, Assendelft WJ, Arola H et al. Effectiveness of physiotherapy for lateral epicondylitis: a systematic review. *Ann Med* 2003; **35**: 51–62.

45. Trudel D, Duley J, Zastrow I et al. Rehabilitation for patients with lateral epicondylitis: a systematic review. *J Hand Ther* 2004; **17**: 243–266.

46. Osiri M, Brosseau L, McGowan J et al. *Transcutaneous Electrical Nerve Stimulation for Knee Osteoarthritis*. Cochrane Review. The Cochrane Library, Issue 4. Wiley, Chichester, 2000.

47. Ezzo J, Hadhazy V, Birch S et al. Acupuncture for osteoarthritis of the knee: a systematic review. *Arthritis Rheum* 2001; **44**: 819–825.

48. Trinh KV, Phillips SD, Ho E et al. Acupuncture for the alleviation of lateral epicondyle pain: a systematic review. *Rheumatology* 2004; **43**: 1085–1090.

49. Solomon SD, McMurray JJ, Pfeffer MA et al. Cardiovascular risk associated with celecoxib in a clinical trial for colorectal adenoma prevention. *N Engl J Med* 2005; **352**: 1071–1080.

50. Bresalier RS, Sandler RS, Quan H et al. Cardiovascular events associated with rofecoxib in a colorectal adenoma chemoprevention trial. *N Engl J Med* 2005; **352**: 1092–1102.

51. Garner SE, Fidan DD, Frankish RR et al. *Rofecoxib for Osteoarthritis*. Cochrane Review. The Cochrane Library, Issue 1. Wiley, Chichester, 2005.

52. Shi Z, Guo C, Awad M. *Hyaluronate for Temporomandibular Joint Disorders*. Cochrane Review. The Cochrane Library, Issue 1. Wiley, Chichester, 2003.

53. McAlindon TE, LaValley MP et al. Glucosamine and chondroitin for treatment of osteoarthritis: a systematic quality assessment and meta-analysis. *JAMA* 2000; **283**: 1469–1475.

54. Towheed TE, Maxwell L, Anastassiades TP et al. *Glucosamine Therapy for Treating Osteoarthritis*. Cochrane Review. The Cochrane Library, Issue 2. Wiley, Chichester, 2005.

55. Soeken K, Lee W, Bausell R et al. Safety and efficacy of S-adenosylmethionine SAMe for osteoarthritis. *J Family Pract* 2002; **51**: 425–430.

56. Long L, Soeken K, Ernst E. Herbal medicines for the treatment of osteoarthritis: a systematic review. *Rheumatology* 2001; **40**: 779–793.

57. Bellamy N, Kirwan J, Boers M et al. Recommendations for a core set of outcome measures for future phase III clinical trials in knee, hip, and hand osteoarthritis. Consensus development at OMERACT III. *J Rheumatol* 1997; **24**: 799–802.

58. Chard JA, Tallon D, Dieppe PA. Epidemiology of research into interventions for the treatment of osteoarthritis of the knee joint. *Ann Rheum Dis* 2000; **59**: 414–418.

59. Ejnisman B, Andreoli CV, Soares BGO et al. *Interventions for Tears of the Rotator Cuff in Adults*. Cochrane Review. The Cochrane Library, Issue 4. Wiley, Chichester, 2003.

60. Atkins D, Crawford F, Edwards J et al. A systematic review of treatments for the painful heel. *Rheumatology* 1999; **38**: 968–973.

61. McLauchlan GJ, Handoll HHG. *Interventions for Treating Acute and Chronic Achilles Tendinitis*. Cochrane Review. The Cochrane Library, Issue 2. Wiley, Chichester, 2001.

62. Towheed TE. Systematic review of therapies for osteoarthritis of the hand. *Osteoarthritis Cartilage* 2005; **13**: 455–462.

63. O'Connor D, Marshall S, Massy-Westropp N. *Non-surgical Treatment (Other than Steroid Injection) for Carpal Tunnel Syndrome*. Cochrane Review. The Cochrane Library, Issue 1. Wiley, Chichester, 2003.

64. Green SE, Buchbinder R, Forbes A et al. *Interventions for Shoulder Pain*. Cochrane Review. The Cochrane Library, Issue 2. Wiley, Chichester, 1999.

65. Bizzini M, Childs J, Piva S et al. Systematic review of the quality of randomized controlled trials for patellofemoral pain syndrome. *J Orthop Sports Phys Ther* 2003; **33**: 4–20.

66. Forouzanfar T, Koke AJ, van Kleef M et al. Treatment of complex regional pain syndrome type I. *Eur J Pain* 2002; **6**: 105–122.

67. Kjellman GV, Skargren EI, Oberg BE. A critical analysis of randomised clinical trials on neck pain and treatment efficacy: a review of the literature. *Scand J Rehab Med* 1999; **31**: 139–152.

68. Johansson K, Oberg B, Adolfsson L et al. A combination of systematic review and clinicians' beliefs in interventions for subacromial pain. *Br J Gen Pract* 2002; **52**: 145–152.

69. Karjalainen K, Malmivaara A, van TM et al. *Multidisciplinary Biopsychosocial Rehabilitation for Neck and Shoulder Pain among Working Age Adults*. Cochrane Review. The Cochrane Library, Issue 3. Wiley, Chichester, 2001.

70. Ernst E. Chiropractic spinal manipulation for neck pain: a systematic review. *J Pain* 2003; **4**: 417–421.

71. Sarigiovannis P, Hollins B. Effectiveness of manual therapy in the treatment of non-specific neck pain: a review. *Phy The Rev* 2005; **10**: 35–50.

72. de las Penas CF, Sohrbeck CM, Fernandez CJ et al. Manual therapies in myofascial trigger point treatment: a systematic review. *J Bodywork Mov Ther* 2005; **9**: 27–34.

73. Michener L, Walsworth M, Burnet E. Effectiveness of rehabilitation for patients with subacromial impingement syndrome: a systematic review. *J Hand Ther* 2004; **17**: 152–164.

74. Gibson K, Growse A, Korda L et al. The effectiveness of rehabilitation for nonoperative management of shoulder instability: a systematic review. *J Hand Ther* 2004; **7**: 229–242.

75. Crossley K, Bennell K, Green S et al. A systematic review of physical interventions for patellofemoral pain syndrome. *Clin J Sport Med* 2001; **11**: 103–110.

76. Jedel E, Carlsson J. Biofeedback, acupuncture and transcutaneous electric nerve stimulation in the management of temperomandibular disorders: a systematic review. *Phys Ther Rev* 2003; **8**: 217–223.

77. Desmeules F, Cote CH, Fremont P. Therapeutic exercise and orthopedic manual therapy for impingement syndrome: a systematic review. *Clin J Sport Med* 2003; **13**: 176–182.

78. Brosseau L, MacLeay L, Robinson V et al. Efficacy of balneotherapy for osteoarthritis of the knee: a systematic review. *Phys Ther Rev* 2002; **7**: 209–222.

79. Marks R, Ghassemi M, Duarte R et al. A review of the literature on shortwave diathermy as applied to osteo-arthritis of the knee. *Physiotherapy* 1999; **85**: 304–316.

80. Hulme JM, Judd MG, Robinson VA et al. *Electromagnetic Fields for the Treatment of Osteoarthritis*. Cochrane Review. The Cochrane Library, Issue 1. Wiley, Chichester, 2002.

81. Brosseau L, Casimiro L, Judd MG et al. *Therapeutic Ultrasound for Treating Patellofemoral Pain Syndrome*. Cochrane Review. The Cochrane Library, Issue 4. Wiley, Chichester, 2001.

82. van der Windt DA, van der Heijden GJ, van den Berg SG et al. Ultrasound therapy for musculoskeletal disorders: a systematic review. *Pain* 1999; **81**: 257–271.

83. Marks R, Ghanagaraja S, Ghassemi M. Ultrasound for osteo-arthritis of the knee: a systematic review. *Physiotherapy* 2000; **86**: 452–463.

84. Welch V, Brosseau L, Peterson J et al. *Therapeutic Ultrasound for Osteoarthritis of the Knee*. The Cochrane Library, Issue 3. Wiley, Chichester, 2001.

85. Abdulwadud O. *Does Laser Therapy Improve Healing and Function in Patients with Tendinitis Compared to no Treatment?* Evidence Centre Evidence Report 11. Centre for Clinical Effectiveness (CCE), 2001. Available at: http://www.mihsr.monash.org/cce/res/pdf/c/467.pdf (accessed 27 August 2006).

86. de Bie RA, Verhagen AP, Lenssen AF et al. Efficacy of 904 nm laser therapy in the management of musculoskeletal disorders: a systematic review. *Phys Ther Rev* 1998; **3**: 59–72.

87. Brosseau L, Gam A, Harman K et al. *Low Level Laser Therapy (Classes I, II and III) for Treating Osteoarthritis*. Cochrane Review. The Cochrane Library, Issue 3. Wiley, Chichester, 2004.

88. Bjordal JM, Couppe C, Chow RT et al. A systematic review of low level laser therapy with location-specific joint disorders (DARE provisional record). *Austr J Physiother* 2003; **49**: 107–116.

89. Marks R, Ungar M, Ghasemmi M. Electrical muscle stimulation for osteoarthritis of the knee: biological basis and systematic review. *NZ J Physiother* 2000; **28**: 6–20.

90. Ernst E, White AR. Acupuncture as a treatment for temporomandibular joint dysfunction: a systematic review of randomized trials. *Arch Otolaryngol Head Neck Surg* 1999; **125**: 269–272.

91. White AR, Ernst E. A systematic review of randomized controlled trials of acupuncture for neck pain. *Rheumatology* 1999; **38**: 143–147.

92. Green S, Buchbinder R, Barnsley L et al. *Acupuncture for Lateral Elbow Pain*. Cochrane Review. The Cochrane Library, Issue 1. Wiley, Chichester, 2002.

93. Green S, Buchbinder R, Hetrick S. *Acupuncture for Shoulder Pain. Cochrane Review*. The Cochrane Library, Issue 2. Wiley, Chichester, 2005.

94. Cummings TM, White AR. Needling therapies in the management of myofascial trigger point pain: a systematic review. *Arch Phys Med Rehabil* 2001; **82**: 986–992.

95. Pelland L, Brosseau L, Wells G et al. Efficacy of strengthening exercises for osteoarthritis (part I): a meta analysis. *Phys Ther Rev* 2004; **9**: 77–108.

96. Fransen M, McConnell S, Bell M. *Exercise for Osteoarthritis of the Hip or Knee*. Cochrane Review. The Cochrane Library, Issue 2. Wiley, Chichester, 2001.

97. Brosseau L, MacLeay L, Robinson VA et al. *Intensity of Exercise for the Treatment of Osteoarthritis*. Cochrane Review. The Cochrane Library, Issue 2. Wiley, Chichester, 2003.

98. Brosseau L, Pelland L, Wells G et al. Efficacy of aerobic exercises for osteoarthritis (part II): a meta-analysis. *Phys Ther Rev* 2004; **9**: 125–145.

99. Heintjes E, Berger MY, Bierma-Zeinstra SMA et al. *Exercise Therapy for Patellofemoral Pain Syndrome*. Cochrane Review. The Cochrane Library, Issue 4. Wiley, Chichester, 2003.

100. Sarig-Bahat H. Evidence for exercise therapy in mechanical neck disorders (DARE provisional record). *Man Ther* 2003; **8**: 10–20.

101. Roddy E, Zhang W, Doherty M. Aerobic walking or strengthening exercise for osteoarthritis of the knee? A systematic review. *Ann Rheum Dis* 2005; **64**: 544–548.

102. Borkholder C, Hill V, Fess E. The efficacy of splinting for lateral epicondylitis: a systematic review. *J Hand Ther* 2004; **17**: 181–199.

103. Struijs PA, Smidt N, Arola H et al. *Orthotic Devices for Tennis Elbow*. The Cochrane Library, Issue 2. Wiley, Chichester, 2001.

104. Brouwer RW, Jakma TSC, Verhagen AP et al. *Braces and Orthoses for Treating Osteoarthritis of the Knee*. Cochrane Review. The Cochrane Library, Issue 1. Wiley, Chichester, 2005.

105. D'hondt NE, Struijs PAA, Kerkhoffs GMMJ et al. *Orthotic Devices For Treating Patellofemoral Pain Syndrome*. Cochrane Review The Cochrane Library, Issue 2.Wiley, Chichester, 2002.

106. Zhang W, Jones A, Doherty M. Does paracetamol (acetaminophen) reduce the pain of osteoarthritis? A meta-analysis of randomised controlled trials (DARE provisional record). *Ann Rheum Dis* 2004; **63**: 901–907.

107. Green SE, Assendelft WJJ, Barnsley L et al. *Non-steroidal Anti-Inflammatory Drugs (NSAIDs) for Treating Lateral Elbow Pain in Adults*. Cochrane Review. The Cochrane Library, Issue 4. Wiley, Chichester, 2001.

108. Bjordal J, Ljunggren A, Klovning A et al. Non-steroidal anti-inflammatory drugs, including cyclo-oxygenase-2 inhibitors, in osteoarthritic knee pain: meta-analysis of randomised placebo controlled trials. *BMJ* 2004; **329**: 1317.

109. Deeks JJ, Smith LA, Bradley MD. Efficacy, tolerability, and upper gastrointestinal safety of celecoxib for treatment of osteoarthritis and rheumatoid arthritis: systematic review of randomised controlled trials. *BMJ* 2002; **325**: 619–623.

110. Edwards J, McQuay H, Moore R. Efficacy and safety of valdecoxib for treatment of osteoarthritis and rheumatoid arthritis: systematic review of randomised controlled trials. *Pain* 2004; **111**: 286–296.

111. Lin J, Zhang W, Jones A et al. Efficacy of topical non-steroidal anti-inflammatory drugs in the treatment of osteoarthritis: meta-analysis of randomised controlled trials (DARE provisional record). *BMJ* 2004; **329**: 324–326.

112. Mason L, Moore R, Edwards J et al. Topical NSAIDs for chronic musculoskeletal pain: systematic review and meta-analysis. *BMC Musculoskelet Disord* 2004; **5**: 28.

113. Mason L, Moore R, Edwards J et al. Systematic review of efficacy of topical rubefacients containing salicylates for the treatment of acute and chronic pain. *BMJ* 2004; **328**: 995.

114. Mason L, Moore R, Derry S et al. Systematic review of topical capsaicin for the treatment of chronic pain. *BMJ* 2004; **328**: 991.

115. Smidt N, Assendelft WJ, van der Windt DA et al. Corticosteroid injections for lateral epicondylitis: a systematic review. *Pain* 2002; **96**: 23–40.

116. Bellamy N, Campbell J, Robinson V et al. *Intraarticular Corticosteroid for Treatment of Osteoarthritis of the Knee*. Cochrane Review. The Cochrane Library, Issue 2. Wiley, Chichester, 2005.

117. Buchbinder R, Green S, Youd JM. *Corticosteroid Injections for Shoulder Pain*. Cochrane Review. The Cochrane Library, Issue 1. Wiley, Chichester, 2003.

118. Bellamy N, Campbell J, Robinson V et al. *Viscosupplementation for the Treatment of Osteoarthritis of the Knee*. Cochrane Review. The Cochrane Library, Issue 2. Wiley, Chichester, 2005.

119. Heintjes E, Berger MY, Bierma-Zeinstra SMA et al. *Pharmacotherapy for Patellofemoral Pain Syndrome*. Cochrane Review. The Cochrane Library, Issue 3. Wiley, Chichester, 2004.

120. Peloso P, Gross A, Haines T et al. *Medicinal and Injection Therapies for Mechanical Neck Disorders*. Cochrane Review. The Cochrane Library, Issue 2. Wiley, Chichester, 2005.

121. List T, Axelsson S, Leijon GR. Pharmacologic interventions in the treatment of temporomandibular disorders, atypical facial pain, and burning mouth syndrome A qualitative systematic review. *J Orofac Pain* 2003; **17**: 301–310.

122. Perez RS, Kwakkel G, Zuurmond WW et al. Treatment of reflex sympathetic dystrophy CRPS type 1: a research synthesis of 21 randomized clinical trials. *J Pain Symptom Manage* 2001; **21**: 511–526.

123. Gagnier J, Chrubasik S, Manheimer E. *Harpgophytum procumbens* for osteoarthritis and low back pain: a systematic review. *BMC Complement Alternative Med* 2004; **4**: 13.

124. Ernst E. The efficacy of phytodolor for the treatment of musculoskeletal pain: a systematic review of randomized clinical trials. *Natural Med Online* 3: 2000.

125. Long L, Ernst E Homeopathic remedies for the treatment of osteoarthritis: a systematic review. *Br Homoeopath J* 2001; **90**: 37–43.

126. Brosseau L, Casimiro L, Milne S et al. *Deep Transverse Friction Massage for Treating Tendinitis*. Cochrane Review. The Cochrane Library, Issue 4. Wiley, Chichester, 2002.

Chapter 19

Fibromyalgia: an interdisciplinary approach

Peter J. Keel

THEORETICAL BACKGROUND OF TREATMENT: PSYCHOPATHOLOGY AND FUNCTIONAL DEFICITS

Neuroticism and depression

Psychological profiles of fibromyalgia (FM) patients show much variation, but overall are within normal limits. The exception to this relates to scales assessing physical or depressive symptoms, which can cause elevated scores for neuroticism or somatization (psychosomatic disturbance), as well as false-positive scores for hypochondriasis and hysteria.[1, 2] These elevations are mainly due to the typical functional symptoms of FM, such as sleeping disorders, irritable bowel syndrome and headaches. The latter are associated with the onset of widespread body pain,[3] but are also a consequence of the disease (Figure 19.1). Patients usually become less productive, feel useless and fear the thought of becoming a burden to others. Insecurity about the origin of their problems and about prognosis can be another important stressor. One study[4] has confirmed a higher lifetime prevalence of mood and anxiety disorders in FM patients, as well as a higher number of medically unexplained physical symptoms across several organ systems.

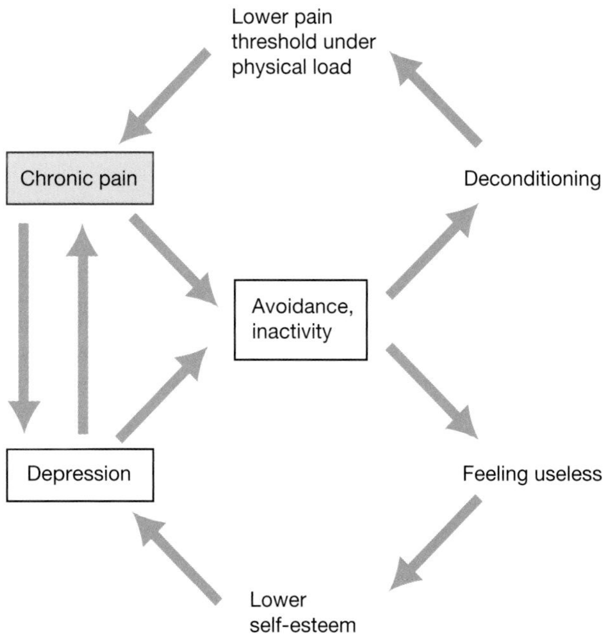

Figure 19.1. Vicious circles of persisting pain: interactions of pain, inactivity and depression.

Coping style

A passive coping style marked by pessimism, catastrophizing,[5] negative affect and helplessness can frequently be found.[6] Coping strategies predicted disability in patients with primary FM.[5] Patients with rheumatoid arthritis or systemic lupus erythematosus perceived higher control over their symptoms than did those with FM,[7] but this was changed in a positive direction by participation in a self-management programme. Pretreatment self-efficacy also predicted post-treatment physical activity after a training intervention.[8] Higher levels of self-efficacy were associated with better outcome, and seem to mediate the effectiveness of rehabilitation-based treatment programmes.

Acceptance of pain has a positive effect on mood and activity levels.[9] Turk et al.[10] have identified three subgroups of FM patients based on psychosocial and behavioural characteristics. These groups show substantial differences in clinical presentation of their symptoms, and suggest that FM should be seen as a heterogeneous disorder. In the view of Turk et al., treating patients as a homogeneous group may compromise research results, impede understanding of the mechanisms underlying the condition and deter development of effective treatment.

There is some evidence that frequent exposure to daily stressors mediates the high levels of psychological distress reported by FMS patients.[11] In addition, stressful life experiences, in combination with factors such as high levels of negative affect and pain, are highly related to seeking medical care for FM symptoms.[6] Recent and past highly stressful, emotionally traumatic events seem to play a role in the onset and course of the disorder.[6] Physical trauma can also influence the development of FMS.[6] Central sensitization may play an important role in this process, a mechanism that can explain the general hypervigilance of FMS patients (see below).

The conclusion from all these observations is that thorough information about the nature of the illness is an important basis for treatment. Teaching self-help strategies and stress-management techniques can help to change the patient's coping style and improve self-efficiency. This can help patients to cope with pain and reduce depression and anxiety.

Pain proneness and stress hypothesis

If FM is a psychosomatic disorder, then it would be expected that psychosocial problems might be a typical feature. However, patients tend to deny psychosocial conflicts, and in many cases such problems are not overtly present. What are found in the majority of cases are traits of the 'pain-prone personality'[12] (Box 19.1) or 'counterdependency'.[13] Some of these features, which are part of 'type-A behaviour', were identified in a sample of FM patients.[14] A lack of 'aggression towards others' and an excess of 'initiative for conflict resolution' could repeatedly be found.[15] However, these same traits can also be found in a broad spectrum of psychosomatic disorders as well as other conditions. A central hypothesis for treatment interventions is that this excessive striving for achievement, coupled with a deficient aggressive defence system, is responsible for a persistent elevated level of stress,[16, 17] which may lead to FM in susceptible individuals (Box 19.2). The resulting psychological distress can cause changes in sleep and endocrine rhythms, besides the psychological and behavioural perturbations mentioned above.

Parallel observations, about disturbances of sleep or growth-hormone production, have been made in relation to various traumatic experiences (e.g. motor vehicle accidents[18]). As long ago as 1975, Moldofsky et al.[19] observed that patients with FM have abnormal sleep patterns. As growth hormone is secreted predominantly during stages 3 and 4 of non-random eye movement (non-REM) sleep, it was hypothesized that FM may be associated with impaired secretion of growth hormone.[20] Growth hormone deficiency in adults has been associated with symptoms that are similar to those described by patients with FM: low energy, poor general health, reduced exercise capacity, muscle weakness, cold intolerance and dysthymia. Furthermore, growth hormone is important in maintaining muscle homeostasis, and it was theorized that suboptimal levels may be a factor in the impaired resolution of muscle microtrauma in FM. To determine whether suboptimal growth hormone production could be relevant to the symptomatology of FM, Bennett et al.[20] assessed the clinical effects of an experimental treatment with growth hormone (daily injections) in women with low IGF-1 levels. Significant improvements were found after 9 months, but after discontinuing the injections patients soon experienced a worsening of symptoms. Crofford et al.[16] also postulate that FM falls into the spectrum of 'stress-associated syndromes', since the onset of the illness frequently occurs after acute or chronic stress, and exacerbation of symptoms can be observed during periods of physical or emotional stress. Many clinical features of FM can be related to a hyporeactivity of the hypothalamic–pituitary–adrenal axis, which has been observed in FM: low basal cortisol levels, exaggerated adrenocorticotrophic hormone (ACTH) response and blunted cortisol response to increased ACTH. Similarly there is a hyporeactivity of the sympathetic nervous system. The changes may also be due to overstimulation (overactivity) caused by chronic stress.[21] The autonomic dysfunctions may explain the diverse clinical manifestations of FM, such as widespread pain, sleep disorder, fatigue, pseudo-Raynaud phenomenon, Sicca syndrome and intestinal irritability. Tests of heart rate variability and tilt-table testing have confirmed this hyporeactivity under stress.[21, 22]

These neuroendocrine dysfunctions caused by chronic hyperarousal might possibly explain the link of FM to some of the adverse childhood experiences that seem to play a role in the

---

Box 19.1. The pain-prone personality (counterdependency)

- Hard worker, high goals of achievement (strong work ethic)
- Excessive activity, compulsive perfectionism
- Inability to relax and enjoy life
- Self-reliance
- Caregiver role-identity
- Denial of emotional and interpersonal conflicts (emotional suppression and idealization of relationships)
- Inability to cope with anger and hostility
- Infantile, needs to be dependent and cared for

Box 19.2. Theoretical concept of fibromyalgia

- Functional disorder with non-specific psychological deficits
- Disturbance of coping with stress and conflicts (assertiveness)
- Lack of awareness of feelings of anger, sadness, pain, etc. (alexithymic)
- Unawareness of stressful life situation or situation seems unchangeable (persistent stress)
- Imprinted by childhood experiences (toughness, helpfulness; emotional neglect, physical or sexual abuse)
- Organ selection due to somatic factors (genetic predisposition, disuse, degeneration)

development of the disorder. Poverty, lack of affection, harshness, and physical or sexual abuse have generally been identified as potential influences on the development of chronic pain syndromes and depressive symptoms (dysthymia).[23, 24] Repetitive traumatic events and post-traumatic stress disorder (PTSD) are reported by many chronic pain patients (including those with FM), if insight-orientated psychotherapy can be established. A prevalence of 21% for FM was found in a sample of 29 patients with PTSD,[25] while none of the 37 controls was affected in this way.

Interventions aimed at reducing daily stress levels through behaviour change seem promising in view of these observations. They can also promote the motivation for insight-orientated psychotherapy. This may be indicated in order to address these issues thoroughly, when cognitive–behavioural interventions have failed to bring sufficient improvements (see below).

Perceptual changes: hypersensibility

Hypersensitivity to pain (secondary hyperalgesia) and hyperexcitability to other adverse stimuli can be observed in FM.[26, 27] Input to central nociceptive pathways is abnormally processed in patients with FMS.[28] These changes might be due to the persisting pain causing central sensitization through neuronal changes (increased excitability of spinal cord neurons, enlargement of the receptive fields of these neurons by neuroplasticity, reduction in pain threshold and recruitment of novel afferent inputs[28]). The N-methyl-D-aspartate (NMDA) and opioid receptor systems are considered central in nociception and antinociception. Activation of NMDA receptors has a permissive effect on release of substance P in the dorsal horn of the spinal cord. Substance P seems to be a major aetiological factor in central sensitization. Several studies have shown a three-fold increase of substance P in the cerebrospinal fluid of pain patients.[28] Further temporal summation of second pain or wind-up leads to pain amplification in the dorsal horn neurons of the spinal cord. The pain that is transmitted by unmyelinated C fibres is reported as dull, aching, or burning, sensations frequently reported by chronic pain patients.

One hypothesis is that these changes in pain perception are due to an initially or temporarily elevated pain threshold in phases of hyperactivity, which could be due to traumatic experiences, as postulated by PTSD researchers. Patient behaviours observed during therapy[29] support this view. Patients ignore the increasing pain when they are engaged in a strenuous activity until they have finished a perfect job. This triggers more severe pain than would be normal, forcing them to rest for a longer period of time. Nielson et al.[30] also observed such a tendency to alternate between overdoing and withdrawal from activities of daily living. Staud et al.[31] could demonstrate that isometric exercise has opposite effects in FM patients compared with normal controls, due to a widespread deficiency of central inhibition. Pain-management strategies based on the 'gate control' concept can partly help to reduce this hypersensitivity to pain. Cognitive–behavioural strategies, an insight-orientated analysis of this working style or activity pacing can induce behaviour change, helping to reduce pain.

Deconditioning

Physical deconditioning is another important feature of FM. While pain-induced inactivity and exaggerated fears of exacerbation of the pain through physical activity may induce deconditioning as a secondary phenomenon (see Figure 19.1), growth hormone production seems to play a role as well. But deconditioning and inactivity have only been observed in patients with a long duration of illness. In a small subgroup of patients with a shorter duration of illness,[29] hyperactivity was found. Fitness training can therefore be an important ingredient of therapy, but has to be integrated in a set of strategies, including information and methods to improve self-perception. Patients have to learn that excessive activity will increase pain drastically, whereas moderate activity can lead to a tolerable increase while fitness and activity tolerance are improved.

PSYCHOTHERAPEUTIC APPROACHES IN FM PATIENTS

General considerations

The features of 'pain proneness' or 'counterdependency' mentioned above (see Box 19.1) explain some of the difficulties encountered when treating FM patients. Initially, the pain tolerance of these patients seems to have been high, allowing them to engage in an abusive working style by ignoring painful stimuli in order to avoid depending on others. Eventually, however, an increasing intolerance for painful stimuli and a lower pain threshold develop. Other features are the repression or denial of traumatic experiences, which make it difficult to engage these patients in psychotherapy. They tend to idealize their partners in spite of obvious problems, while keeping a negative self-image. The motor for this overadaptive highly self-reliant behaviour seems to be the personality traits mentioned above, plus the secondary losses (productivity, helpfulness, physical fitness) that can reinforce this overadaptation through low self-esteem (see Figure 19.1).

While establishing insight-orientated psychodynamic therapy might prove difficult, due to these patients' lack of insight and motivation, an integrated cognitive–behavioural approach is promising. The treatment is focused on the pain and its consequences, especially the target symptoms listed in Box 19.3. Besides cognitive–behavioural pain-control strategies, physical exercises and relaxation can be integrated into the treatment (Box 19.4). The therapeutic team consists of psychologists or

---

Box 19.3. Target symptoms of integrated therapy

- Initial or partial hyperactivity, perfectionism
- Maladaptive stress-coping, lack of assertiveness
- Hypersensitivity to pain
- Inactivity due to pain in later stages
- Consecutive depression and sleep disturbance
- Fears and anxiety about nature of illness

psychiatrists, and physiotherapists, with occasional integration of a rheumatologist or a rehabilitation specialist.

COMPONENTS OF INTEGRATED TREATMENT PROGRAMMES

Information and education

Information and education are important components, as a well-informed patient 'is an essential member of a successful chronic illness management team'.[7] Patients should be informed about the nature and biopsychosocial background of their illness. They have to be confronted with the usually chronic but benign course, and the limited treatment possibilities in FM. This helps to reduce unrealistic expectations and improves motivation for self-help. In addition, the mechanisms and the 'psychology of pain' (gate-control concept, learning processes, psychosocial influences[32]) have to be explained in order to give patients a basis for understanding and application of self-control techniques. The medical aspects are best presented by a rheumatologist, whose topics may include the nature of the illness, pathophysiological concepts, effectiveness of treatments and the rationale of an integrative approach. Psychologists (or psychiatrists) and physiotherapists can provide additional information and introduce the treatment concept. It is important that all therapists clearly share a common concept.

Multimodal group approach

This is an interdisciplinary approach involving various therapists in teaching self-help strategies such as pain coping, stress inoculation, relaxation and physical exercises. The objective of the treatment is for patients to learn to accept the pain as something they have to live with, to get a better understanding about the pain and to gain a certain self-control over their pain (Box 19.5). Acceptance of chronic pain means abandoning the illusion that a medical authority, a miraculous drug or any other passive therapy might cure the illness. Better understanding is achieved through observation and registration of modulating factors. Pain diaries can help to discover positive or negative influences of environmental or personal factors. These observations are an important basis for the application of self-help strategies and stress management.

Such treatment can be offered on an outpatient or inpatient basis. In the outpatient group programme described below,[29] 15 weekly group sessions lasting 2 hours were offered. Every session consisted of the following elements, each lasting between 20 and 30 minutes (see Box 19.4): information, instruction in self-control strategies, physical exercises, relaxation and group discussion.

Cognitive–behavioural strategies

Stress inoculation and cognitive restructuring techniques[33] can be used, but should be tailored more specifically to the condition of FM patients. Patients can be asked, for example, to list activities that they can use to divert their attention from the pain as well as from the unpleasant thoughts associated with it. Most often, leisure activities, social engagements, physical exercises or relaxation are mentioned. Patients can also be told to monitor their thoughts and behaviours whenever pain sets in or increases, and to apply suitable strategies (see the example in Table 19.1).

Gymnastics and relaxation

Gymnastics include stretching and aerobic exercises for improvement of coordination, muscle strength, endurance and flexibility. Gymnastics should be conducted in a playful manner using instruments (balls, ropes, towels, feathers, etc.), games, dance and music. This helps divert patients from pain and makes them more relaxed, besides putting an element of fun into therapy. A standard programme for home use should be firmly introduced. The exercises have to be coordinated with information about the effects of physical activity and deconditioning on pain, pain tolerance and fitness. While some patients have to be encouraged to overcome their fear and passivity, others have to be taught to avoid excessive activity. Patients learn to assume responsibility and search out the right level of activity for themselves. They must understand the motives for their working style and become more aware of their own bodies. Body awareness can be practised in group sessions with guided self-observation (e.g. by miming emotions). As a relaxation technique, autogenic training[34] or the progressive relaxation technique of Jacobson[35] are recommended. Patients should practise relaxation and physical exercises at home daily and apply techniques of pain control.

Table 19.1. Example of a cognitive–behavioural strategy

Situation: *My neck and my shoulders hurt. I can hardly turn my head. It hurts a lot at night ....*

Maladaptive reactions (misbeliefs)	Favourable reactions (corrections)
It is a horrible pain	It is this neck pain again. It feels tense
Perhaps a nerve is trapped	It is the stress because of this trip tomorrow. I feel tense. I am afraid something might go wrong
It is getting worse and worse	If I manage to relax, the pain will decrease
I am helpless, I have to see a doctor	I can help myself: a warm bath and relaxation exercises will ease the tension
I have to avoid any strain to the neck	I will go swimming regularly. It will be good for my neck

Group discussions: motivation and resistance

In order to keep up motivation and adherence to the home exercise, its frequency and effects should be discussed during group sessions. Patients are encouraged to share their experiences. Individual examples can be used as models and analysed during group sessions. Hearing about the success of other group members is often more encouraging and convincing than recommendations coming from therapists. The amplifying effects of the group setting are useful, besides being more economical. If patients fail to exercise regularly, reasons have to be carefully checked. Lack of time due to hyperactivity, or poor motivation due to poor results or doubts might be reasons. Tackling these barriers is an essential part of rehabilitative therapy for musculoskeletal disorders, as described in the functional restoration concept.[36] The group discussions should be structured. An analysis of the circumstances that influence the pain can give patients some insight into its nature and modulating factors. These measures can give patients a better understanding of their illness. The therapist has to play an active role in this phase by asking questions and checking for certain behaviours (Box 19.6). Homework tasks, such as pain diaries and activity protocols, can improve self-observation. Talking about traumatic childhood experiences can encourage patients to engage in insight-orientated therapy. However, this has to be done with caution, and avoidance of certain topics has to be respected, as confrontation with present and past traum-

atic experiences or conflicts might be too painful. Fears of renewed traumatization by the therapist are frequent, but patients might also have experienced a lack of empathy and understanding, and covert or overt rejection (e.g. 'The pain is not real', 'I can't help you, you are a case for the psychiatrist').

Precautions for individual therapy

The individual therapist has to actively protect the therapy by addressing the issues and reassuring the patient of his or her acceptance of the patient's view of the situation. This includes accepting the initial denial of actual conflicts and past traumatic experiences, even if there is clear evidence of such circumstances. Goals might have to be modest, as there is often only a limited space for change. Patients might be trapped in long-standing conflicts that cannot be resolved. They might feel unable to break an unhappy partnership due to fears of loss or traumatization by an abusive partner. The inability to undertake such drastic changes may stem from the described personality traits (altruism, avoidance of conflict, and lack of self-esteem and self-confidence).

RESULTS OF INTERVENTION STUDIES

In a review of multidisciplinary group programmes Bennett[37] points out that:

> (1) FM is a complex chronic pain condition and current treatment is palliative rather than curative; (2) the major aim of treatment is to improve function, not abolish pain; and (3) a cycle of chronic pain, stress, and psychological arousal often generates a set of secondary symptoms. These secondary symptoms provide a positive feedback loop that is amenable to modification by cognitive–behavioural techniques. Multidisciplinary group treatment programs are especially suited to such techniques; their aim should be to maximize subsequent clinician–patient interactions. Thus, a current concept of optimal management is a blend of multidisciplinary group therapy and individualized clinician-based treatment.

There is growing evidence that at least in subgroups of patients, lasting positive effects can be achieved with integrated treat-

---

Box 19.6. Topics for guided interviews

- Effects of pain on mood and behaviour: vicious circles (avoidance due to pain, fostering deconditioning and activity intolerance; inactivity due to pain, fostering depression with heightened pain perception)
- Achievement behaviour, perfectionism: pain-prone personality (see Box 19.1)
- Assertiveness, conflict avoidance: to be everything for everybody all the time
- Reactions of spouse, family, colleagues, etc.: Consideration? Attention?
- Role of past traumatic experiences: harshness, hardship, abuse

ment programmes. The various elements have been tested in a number of outcome studies. Combining at least the three elements of information, exercise and cognitive–behavioural therapy is advantageous for motivation and adherence.

Information and education

Information/education alone was tested by Goossens et al.[38] and Vlaeyen et al.[39] In a 3-year randomized clinical trial the effectiveness of a 6-week educational/cognitive intervention was compared with an educational-discussion intervention and a no-intervention control group. A total of 131 patients were randomly allocated to the three conditions. While the intervention groups were followed for 12 months, the control group was followed for only 6 weeks. At 6 weeks there was a significant difference in rating scale utilities between the three groups, caused by a significantly greater improvement in the educational-discussion intervention group compared with the control group. However, no significant differences in either rating scale or standard gamble utilities were found between the two intervention groups immediately after treatment, or at the 6- or 12-month follow-ups. The economic evaluation showed that the addition of a cognitive component to the educational intervention led to significantly higher healthcare costs and no additional improvement in quality of life compared with the educational intervention alone. Buckelew et al.[40] randomly assigned patients to one of four groups: education (attentional control group), biofeedback (cognitive and muscular relaxation), exercise (strength, mobility, endurance) and a combined treatment (biofeedback and exercise). The educational group not only failed to share the improvements of the three other groups but also deteriorated over time.

Nicassio et al.[41] compared a comprehensive behavioural intervention with an education/control group. The effects of the two interventions were evaluated across a 10-week treatment period and at 6-month follow-up, using measures of pain, depression, disability, pain behaviours and intervening variables. The behavioural intervention focused on the development of diverse pain coping skills, while the education/control group was presented with a range of health-related topics, without emphasizing skill acquisition. Although improvement across time was found in depression, self-reported pain behaviours, observed pain behaviours and myalgia scores, no differences in these outcomes were found between the behavioural and education/control groups. Burckhardt et al.[42] tested the effects of patient education alone and in combination with physical training in a randomized controlled trial. Both groups improved significantly in comparison to the control group, after 6 weeks and after 4–8 months according to the outcome criteria of quality of life and self-efficacy.

Fitness training

The effects of various types of fitness training alone were evaluated in several controlled studies. McCain[43] demonstrated that cardiovascular fitness training was more effective than flexibility classes. Martin et al.[44] compared the utility of an exercise programme, which included aerobic, flexibility and strengthening elements, in a controlled trial with 60 patients, using relaxation as a control condition. Each group met three times per week for 6 weeks for 1 hour of supervised exercise or relaxation. Only 38 patients (18 exercise and 20 relaxation) completed the study. Post-study assessments showed a significant improvement in the exercise group compared with the relaxation group. Similar improvements were also found when the pre- and post-study assessments of the exercise group were compared. The authors concluded that FM patients can undertake an exercise programme without adverse effects and that this is a helpful treatment in the short term. However, the high dropout rate of 37% raises doubts about the external validity of these results.

Wigers et al.[45] reported positive short-term effects of aerobic exercise and a stress-management treatment in a 4.5-year prospective study. 'Treatment as usual' was used as a control condition. Sixty patients were included. Aerobic exercise was the most effective intervention after completion of treatment. At 4-year follow-up there was no obvious group difference in symptom severity, which for aerobic exercise the authors considered to be due to poor compliance.

More recently a variety of different types of exercise regimens have been shown to be helpful for treating FM and related syndromes.[46] Individuals who are able to adhere to exercise long term almost always derive benefit, both with respect to improvements in symptoms as well as improvements in function. The largest challenge for research in this area is to develop programmes that target adherence and compliance. Exercise programmes that are combined with cognitive–behavioural approaches offer promise in this regard.[46]

Cognitive–behavioural interventions

Cognitive–behavioural interventions alone were found to be effective in a series of studies. Since information and education play an important role in this concept, it is perhaps not surprising that no difference was found between the two treatments investigated separately in the studies already mentioned above.[39, 41] Stress management alone seems to be less effective than an exercise treatment.[45] A successful controlled study using operant behavioural techniques is mentioned below.[47]

Other psychotherapeutic interventions

Other techniques have been evaluated in controlled trials. Ferraccioli et al.[48] reported positive effects with electromyographic biofeedback training. Haanen et al.[49] evaluated the effects of hypnotherapy using physical therapy as the control condition. The patients in the hypnotherapy group showed a significantly better outcome on a number of parameters.

Integrated approach

An integrated approach, as described above, has been used in a number of controlled outcome studies. White and Nielson[50] did a follow-up assessment of their multimodal treatment programme (including cognitive–behavioural methods, physical exercises, relaxation, pacing and enhancement of pain tolerance, and family education) with 25 subjects who had completed the original intervention study.[30] Twenty-two subjects participated at a mean of 30 months after discharge. The short-term improvement that had been observed in all ten target variables was maintained. A pooled index of these ten variables showed statistically significant improvement from baseline.

Bennett et al.[51] evaluated the impact of a 6-month group therapy programme consisting of formal lectures, group sessions emphasizing behaviour modification, stress-reduction techniques, strategies to improve fitness and flexibility, and support sessions for spouses or significant others. The groups met once a week for 6 months and the average session lasted 90 minutes. Patients were followed for 2 years and compared with a group of patients outside the programme. Out of 170 evaluated patients, 104 finally completed the programme, 70% of them had fewer than 11 tender points, and scores on the FM Impact Questionnaire (FIQ) had improved by 25%. Thirty-three patients, followed for 2 years after the programme had finished, continued to show improvement. A control group of 29 patients who never entered the programme showed no significant improvement. The authors conclude that the group treatment shows promise, but a more formal controlled study is needed to confirm this impression. A major weakness of this study was the high attrition rate.

Mason et al.[52] evaluated a multimodal treatment programme in a quasi-experimental design. Laboratory and self-report pain measures, together with psychological measures, were obtained from patients who were tested up to 6 months after treatment. Comparison data were also obtained from FM patients who failed to qualify for the treatment programme because of insurance coverage. Immediate and long-term treatment effects were evident in the psychological measures and subjective pain measures, but not in the laboratory pain measures. Participants who attended the month-long multimodal programme achieved significant and positive changes on most of the outcome measures, but long-term results were less favourable due to a high number of relapses. It seems that the intervention was too short to achieve lasting results.

Thieme et al.[47] compared a multidisciplinary inpatient programme with a standard medical programme emphasizing physical therapy. The operant behavioural techniques aimed at changing activity levels, medication schedules and social factors. Sixty-five per cent of the cognitive–behavioural therapy group showed clinically significant improvements, whereas the control group showed evidence of deterioration.

Mannerkorpi et al.[53] combined aquatic-based exercises with education (cognitive–behavioural therapy). Compared with standard medical care the results were quite positive, with significant improvements in physical and psychological measures. However, 24% of the exercise/education group dropped out of the study.

We have evaluated the efficacy of an integrated treatment programme as presented above in a controlled study involving 27 patients.[29] The experimental treatment programme consisted of the elements already described. Control groups were instructed in autogenic training only. At the end of the treatment, seven patients from the experimental group and two from the control group showed significant clinical improvement on three of six parameters. However, there was no significant difference between the two treatment groups. At follow-up 4 months after termination, the improvement was still present in five experimental cases but in none of the controls. This difference was statistically significant. Successful patients had been sick for a shorter period of time, and were less impaired by their condition.

Topical, complementary and alternative medicine interventions

Heat, cold, balneotherapy, massages and ultrasound are traditional therapies for musculoskeletal pain, but so far the scientific evidence for their long-term effectiveness in FM is inconclusive, with exception for balneotherapy. The same applies for many complementary and alternative medicine interventions. Acupuncture probably has positive effects. For a review see Wallace and Clauw.[54] In view of the importance of behavioural change these approaches should only be supplementary for temporary pain relief.

Drug treatment

Pharmacological therapy is most effective for improving the symptoms associated with FM, especially the sleep disturbance and anxiety-related symptoms. A trial of antidepressants is indicated if such symptoms or a history of major depressive disorder or anxiety disorders are present.

Antidepressants that have an effect on both serotonin and norepinephrine are most effective.[55] The drug of first choice is a low-dose (10–25 mg) tricyclic antidepressant (TCA) given as a single dose 1–2 hours before bedtime. This can then be titrated to antidepressant therapeutic doses (75–150 mg). However, such high doses are rarely necessary or tolerated. A meta-analysis[56] of nine placebo-controlled trials with sufficient statistical data for effect size computations showed that the overall effects of TCAs and related drugs (amitriptylin, dotiepin, cyclobenzaprine) were moderate. The largest effect was found in measures of sleep quality. There is some evidence that selective serotonin reuptake inhibitors (SSRIs) are also efficacious at higher doses, but this evidence is controversial.[57, 58] Recently, trials have focused on selective serotonin and norepinephrine reuptake inhibitors (SNRIs). While results for venlafaxin were discrepant, two randomized, placebo-controlled studies with duloxetin provide evidence that this relatively new drug is safe and effective in the treatment of fibromyalgia in women (still uncertain for men).[57] Anticonvulsants (e.g. gabapentin) can also be used as monotherapy or in combination with a TCA.[57] Paracetamol (acetaminophen), non-steroidal anti-inflammatory drugs (NSAIDs) and opioids can reduce pain but are not recommended as monotherapy.[57]

SUMMARY

Although the pathogenesis of FM remains unclear, there is growing evidence that it represents a stress-related functional disorder, comparable with other chronic pain syndromes such as migraine headache or irritable bowel syndrome. While a distinct pathology of peripheral muscles cannot be detected, physical deconditioning and abnormalities of the pain-control system, as well as of several neuroendocrine systems, point in the direction of altered pain tolerance and an altered stress response. Outstanding findings are disturbances on the hypothalamic–pituitary–adrenal axis, in growth-hormone production and of the autonomic nervous system, which can explain many of the symptoms observed. However, many of these abnormalities seem to be a consequence of elevated levels of pain and stress leading to non-restorative sleep and reduced activity.

PRACTICE POINTS

- Establish the diagnosis on the basis of diagnostic criteria (rheumatological) as well as additional functional symptoms (sleep disturbance, headache, irritable bowel syndrome, etc.).
- Check for signs of neuroticism, depression, anxiety, pain-prone personality and passive coping style.
- Search for psychological stressors or traumatization: family, work, finances in view of above personality traits and coping style.
- Be aware of secondary effects: deconditioning, depression, anxiety, loss of productivity, side-effects of drugs (NSAIDs, opioids).
- Inform and educate the patient.
- Low risk methods for pain reduction are:
  - paracetamol, amitriptyline
  - simple (inexpensive) treatment with heat, cold, massages
  - encourage self-treatment
  - cognitive–behavioural pain and stress management, relaxation.
- Integrate psychotherapy into medical treatment.
- Avoid secondary effects.

RESEARCH AGENDA

- Neuroendocrine and sympathetic dysregulation.
- Pain perception: hypo- and hypersensibility.
- Psychological markers: coping style, personality traits versus secondary effects.
- Distinct subgroups of patients, early versus late stages of illness.
- Evaluation of multimodal treatment programmes:
  - controlled outcome studies
  - sufficient follow-up (minimum 1 year)
  - tolerable dropout rates (maximum 30%)
  - identify effective ingredients.

Recent observations confirm that interdisciplinary treatment concepts, which have been used for various pain conditions for many years, have long-term efficacy, at least in some patient subgroups. The combination of education, cognitive–behavioural strategies and physical exercises seems to bring better long-term results than any one of these techniques alone. The cognitive–educational component seems to be important for the maintenance of progress and for adherence to the exercise programme. More controlled studies with sufficient follow-up over several years are necessary to confirm the long-term effectiveness of such approaches and to identify specific strategies for certain subgroups of patients.[59]

Mechanisms of improvement might be better understood when changes in biological and endocrine measures that seem to be involved have also been assessed. Research into the role of traumatic experiences and their effect on pain perception and pain tolerance also seems promising. As in the case of low back pain, early interventions seem important, as secondary effects such as inactivity, deconditioning, higher levels of pain, depression and anxiety all seem to have a negative impact on outcome.[60]

REFERENCES

1. Goldenberg DL. An overview of psychologic studies in fibromyalgia. *J Rheumatol* 1989; **19**: 12–14.
2. Celiker R, Borman P, Oktem F et al. Psychological disturbance in fibromyalgia: relation to pain severity. *Clin Rheumatol* 1997; **16**: 179–184.
3. McBeth J, MacFarlane GJ, Benjamin S et al. Features of somatisation predict the onset of chronic widespread pain: results of a large population–based study. *Arthritis Rheum* 2001; **44**: 940–946.
4. Walker EA, Keegan D, Gardner G et al. Psychosocial factors in fibromyalgia compared with rheumatoid arthritis: I. Psychiatric diagnoses and functional disability. *Psychosom Med* 1997; **59**: 565–571.
5. Martin MY, Bradley LA, Alexander RW et al. Coping strategies predict disability in patients with primary fibromyalgia. *Pain* 1996; **68**: 45–53.
6. Bradley LA, Alarcon GS. Psychosocial factors in fibromyalgia. In: Wallace DJ, Clauw DJ (eds), *Fibromyalgia & Other Central Pain Syndromes*. Lippincott Williams & Wilkins, Philadelphia, 2005, pp. 165–176.
7. Burckhardt CS, Bjelle A. Perceived control: a comparison of women with fibromyalgia, rheumatoid arthritis, and systemic lupus erythematosus using a Swedish version of the Rheumatology Attitudes Index. *Scand J Rheumatol* 1996; **25**: 300–306.
8. Buckelew SP, Huyser B, Hewett JE et al. Self–efficacy predicting outcome among fibromyalgia subjects. *Arthritis Care Res* 1996; **9**: 97–104.
9. McCracken LM, Carson JW, Eccleston C et al. Acceptance and change in the context of chronic pain. *Pain* 2004; **109**: 4–7.
10. Turk DC, Okifuji A, Starz TW et al. Effects of type of symptom onset on psychological distress and disability in fibromyalgia syndrome patients. *Pain* 1996; **68**: 423–430.
11. Uveges JM, Parker JC, Smarr KL et al. Psychological symptoms in primary fibromyalgia syndrome: relationship to pain, life stress, and sleep disturbance. *Arthritis Rheum* 1990; **33**: 1279–1283.
12. Blumer D, Heilbronn M. The pain-prone disorder: a clinical and psychological profile. *Psychosomatics* 1991; **22**: 395–402.
13. Gregory RJ, Manring J, Berry SL. Pain location and psychological characteristics of patients with chronic pain. *Psychosomatics* 2000; **41**: 216–220.
14. Mau W, Danz-Neeff H, Raspe H et al. Typ-A-Verhalten und Kontrollambitionen bei Patienten mit einem primären fibromyalgischen Syndrom. In: Müller W (ed.), *Generalisierte Tendomyopathie (Fibromyalgie)*. Steinkopff, Darmstadt, 1991, pp. 211–213.
15. Perini CH, Battegay R, Müller W et al. Vergleichende testpsychologische Untersuchungen bei verschiedenen rheumatischen Erkrankungen und der Hypertonie. *Z Rheumatol* 1982; **41**: 80–88.
16. Crofford LJ, Engleberg NC, Demitrack MA. Neurohormonal perturbations in fibromyalgia. *Baillière's Clin Rheumatol* 1996; **10**: 365–378.
17. Pillemer SR, Bradley LA, Crofford LJ et al. The neuroscience and endocrinology of fibromyalgia. *Arthritis Rheum* 1997; **40**: 1928–1939.

18. Moldofsky H. The contribution of sleep–wake physiology to fibromyalgia. *Adv Pain Res Ther* 1990; **17**: 227–241.

19. Moldofsky H, Scarisbrick P, England R. Musculoskeletal symptoms and non-REM-sleep disturbance of patient with 'fibrositis syndrome' and healthy subjects. *Psychosom Med* 1975; **37**: 341–351.

20. Bennett RM, Clark SC, Walczyk J. A randomized, double-blind, placebo-controlled study of growth hormone in the treatment of fibromyalgia. *Am J Med* 1998; **104**: 227–231.

21. Martinez Lavin M. Dysfunction of the autonomic nervous system in chronic pain syndromes. In: Wallace DJ, Clauw DJ (eds), *Fibromyalgia & Other Central Pain Syndromes*. Lippincott Williams & Wilkins, Philadelphia, 2005, pp. 81–87.

22. Friederich H-C, Schellberg D, Mueller K et al. Stress und autonome Dysregulation bei Patienten mit einem Fibromyalgiesyndrom. *Der Schmerz* 2005; **19**: 185–194.

23. Imbierowicz K., Egle UT. Childhood adversities in patients with fibromyalgia and somatoform pain disorder. *Eur J Pain* 2003; **7**: 113–119.

24. Toomey TC, Seville JL, Mann JD et al. Relationship of sexual and physical abuse to pain description, coping, psychological distress, and health-care utilization in a chronic pain sample. *Clin J Pain* 1995; **11**: 307–315.

25. Amir M, Kaplan Z, Neumann L et al. Posttraumatic stress disorder, tenderness and fibromyalgia. *J Psychosom Res* 1997; **42**: 607–613.

26. McDermid AJ, Rollman GB, McCain GA. Generalized hypervigilance in fibromyalgia: evidence of perceptual amplification. *Pain* 1996; **66**: 133–144.

27. Sorensen J, Graven Nielsen T, Henriksson KG et al. Hyperexcitability in fibromyalgia. *J Rheumatol* 1998; **25**: 152–155.

28. Staud R. The neurobiology of chronic musculoskeletal pain. In: Wallace DJ, Clauw DJ (eds), *Fibromyalgia & Other Central Pain Syndromes*. Lippincott Williams & Wilkins, Philadelphia, 2005, pp. 45–62.

29. Keel PJ, Bodoky C, Gerhard U et al. Comparison of integrated group therapy an group relaxation training for fibromyalgia. *Clin J Pain* 1998; **14**: 232–238.

30. Nielson WR, Walker C, McCain GA. Cognitive behavioral treatment of fibromyalgia syndrome: preliminary findings. *J Rheumatol* 1992; **19**: 98–103.

31. Staud R, Robinson ME, Price DD. Isometric exercise has opposite effects on central pain mechanism in fibromyalgia patients compared to normal controls. *Pain* 2005; **118**: 176–184.

32. Sternbach RA. *The Psychology of Pain*. Raven, New York, 1978.

33. Turk DC, Meichenbaum DH. A Cognitive–behavioural approach to pain management. In: Wall PD, Melzack R (eds), *Textbook of Pain*. Churchill Livingstone, Edinburgh, 1989, pp. 1001–1009.

34. Schultz JH, Luthe U. *Autogenic Training*, Vol. I. Grune and Stratton, New York, 1969.

35. Bernstein DA, Borkovec TD. *Entspannungstraining: Handbuch der progressiven Muskelentspannung*. Pfeiffer, Munich, 1975.

36. Mayer TG, Gatchel RJ. *Functional Restoration for Spinal Disorders: The Sports Medicine Approach*, 1st edn. Lea Febiger, Philadelphia, 1988.

37. Bennett RM. Multidisciplinary group programs to treat fibromyalgia patients. *Rheum Dis Clin North Am* 1996; **22**: 351–367.

38. Goossens ME, Rutten van Molken MP, Leidl RM et al. Cognitive–educational treatment of fibromyalgia: a randomized clinical trial. II. Economic evaluation. *J Rheumatol* 1996; **23**: 1246–1254.

39. Vlaeyen JW, Teeken Gruben NJ, Goossens ME et al. Cognitive–educational treatment of fibromyalgia: a randomized clinical trial. I. Clinical effects. *J Rheumatol* 1996; **23**: 1237–1245.

40. Buckelew SP, Conway J, Parker JC et al. Biofeedback/relaxation training and exercise interventions for fibromyalgia: a prospective trial. *Arthritis Care Res* 1998; **11**: 196–209.

41. Nicassio PM, Radojevic V, Weisman MH et al. A comparison of behavioral and educational interventions for fibromyalgia. *J Rheumatol* 1997; **24**: 2000–2007.

42. Burckhardt CS, Mannerkorpi K, Hedenberg L et al. A randomized, controlled clinical trial of education and physical training for women with fibromyalgia. *J Rheumatol* 1994; **21**: 714–720.

43. McCain GA. Role of physical fitness training in the fibrositis/fibromyalgia syndrome. *Am J Med* 1986; **81**(Suppl 3A): 73–77.

44. Martin L, Nutting A, MacIntosh BR et al. An exercise program in the treatment of fibromyalgia. *J Rheumatol* 1996; **23**: 1050–1053.

45. Wigers SH, Stiles TC, Vogel PA. Effects of aerobic exercise versus stress management treatment in fibromyalgia. A 4.5 year prospective study. *Scand J Rheumatol* 1996; **25**: 77–86.

46. Mannerkorpi K, Iversen MD. The use of exercise and rehabilitation regimens. In: Wallace DJ, Clauw DJ (eds), *Fibromyalgia & Other Central Pain Syndromes*. Lippincott Williams & Wilkins, Philadelphia, 2005, pp. 329–342.

47. Thieme K, Gromnica-Ihle E, Flor H. Operant behavioral treatment of fibromyalgia: a controlled study. *Arthritis Rheum* 2003; **49**: 314–320.

48. Ferraccioli G, Ghirelli L, Scita F. EMG–biofeedback training in fibromyalgia syndrome. *J Rheumatol* 1987; **14**: 820–825.

49. Haanen HCM, Hoenderdos HTW, van Romunde LKJ et al. Controlled trial of hypnotherapy in the treatment of refractory fibromyalgia. *J Rheumatol* 1991; **18**: 72–75.

50. White KP, Nielson WR. Cognitive behavioral treatment of fibromyalgia syndrome: a followup assessment. *J Rheumatol* 1995; **22**: 717–721.

51. Bennett RM, Burckhardt CS, Clark SR et al. Group treatment of fibromyalgia: a 6 month outpatient program. *J Rheumatol* 1996; **23**: 521–528.

52. Mason LW, Goolkasian P, McCain GA. Evaluation of multimodal treatment program for fibromyalgia. *J Behav Med* 1998; **21**: 163–178.

53. Mannerkorpi K, Nyberg F, Ahlmen M et al. Pool exercise combined with an education program for patients with fibromyalgia syndrome. A prospective randomized study. *J Rheumatol* 2000; **27**: 2473–2481.

54. Wallace DJ, Clauw DJ. *Fibromyalgia & Other Central Pain Syndromes*. Lippincott Williams & Wilkins, Philadelphia, 2005.

55. White KP, Harth M. An analytical review of 24 controlled clinical trials for fibromyalgia syndrome (FMS). *Pain* 1996; **64**: 211–219.

56. Arnold LM, Keck PE Jr, Welge JA. Antidepressant treatment of fibromyalgia. A meta-analysis and review. *Psychosomatics* 2000; **41**: 104–113.

57. Arnold LM. New therapies in fibromyalgia. *Arthritis Res Ther* 2006; **8**: 212–231.

58. Jung AC, Staiger T, Sullivan M. The efficacy of selective serotonin reuptake inhibitors for the management of chronic pain. *J Gen Intern Med* 1997; **12**: 384–389.

59. Turk DC, Okifuji A, Sinclair JD et al. Pain, disability, and physical functioning in subgroups of patients with fibromyalgia. *J Rheumatol* 1996; **23**: 1255–1262.

60. Waddell G. Low back pain: a twentieth century health care enigma. *Spine* 1996; **21**: 2820–2825.

Chapter 20

Efficacy of rehabilitative therapy in regional musculoskeletal conditions: an update

Edwin Y. Hanada

INTRODUCTION

Rehabilitation of regional musculoskeletal conditions is a time-limited, goal-orientated, interdisciplinary process that embraces the biopsychosocial approach to patient-centred care. The primary goals are to decrease symptoms, optimize daily function and participation, and minimize disability. Although both active (person participates in) and passive (individual has performed on them) modalities for rehabilitation are often utilized in the clinical setting, the emphasis of treatment should be on active participation, both in the physical and psychological realms.

While many of the conventional therapeutic modalities have a tenuous foundation of scientific evidence supporting their efficacy as treatment options, exercise appears to be the one physical modality with a growing scientific basis to support its utilization in the treatment of regional musculoskeletal disorders. Furthermore, although there has been some improvement in scientific rigour, for the most part there is a paucity of high-quality clinical trials that support less conventional therapies such as acupuncture, massage therapy and yoga. As clinicians, it is important to be familiar with the best evidence pertaining to both conventional and alternative treatment modalities, in order to be able to offer the full spectrum of evidence-based treatment choices to the individual. Synthesizing the best evidence for successful translation into multimodal rehabilitation of regional musculoskeletal disorders is the pre-eminent challenge for the clinician.

OVERVIEW OF RELEVANT THERAPEUTIC MODALITIES

Exercise

Exercise remains the foundation of the rehabilitation of regional musculoskeletal disorders, and may include activities to improve aerobic conditioning, strength, flexibility, proprioception and balance and, ultimately, to enhance function. These activities are often prescribed as an adjunct to medications or physical modalities. Evidence for the role of exercise as an intervention for regional musculoskeletal disorders may be further categorized into those studies pertaining either to pain in the spinal region or to pain in the extremities. This chapter is an update to an article published in 2003,[1] and reviews the evidence for the efficacy of different treatment modalities in the rehabilitation of regional musculoskeletal disorders.

Physical modalities
Thermotherapy

The most common physical modality employed for musculoskeletal disorders is thermotherapy, in the form of heat, either superficial or deep, and cold, or cryotherapy. Moist hot packs are commonly used for treating musculoskeletal disorders, and are usually applied for only 15- to 20-minute intervals, to avoid scalding, to heat the superficial tissues. Heat has been demonstrated to increase blood flow to the skin and to the joint, while decreasing joint stiffness.[2, 3] Also, it has been theorized that increasing the joint temperature, especially above 41°C, may subsequently decrease the activity of the cartilage-degrading enzymes. Furthermore, increased muscle temperature may reduce muscle spasm[4] and decrease inflammatory compounds known to sensitize and activate primary afferent fibres by increasing blood flow.[4]

For deep tissue heating, ultrasound therapy may be utilized. Ultrasound waves consist of alternating compression and rarefactions, require a medium for transmission, and emit energy with the ability to penetrate tissue, allowing them to be utilized for deep heating at tissue interfaces. The delivery of ultrasound therapy may be by continuous-wave beam with limited intensities to deliver thermal energy, or by brief pulses of high-intensity ultrasound waves separated by no power, which have no direct thermal effects and may aid in reduction of inflammation during acute phases of inflammation.[5]

Local application of cold therapy, in the form of ice packs, ice massage, cold baths or vapocoolant sprays to the skin, has been commonly utilized to decrease musculoskeletal pain and swelling. Topical use of cold has been shown to reduce skin, subcutaneous tissue, muscle and joint temperatures,[6] decrease blood flow, slow metabolic activity, reduce muscle tone, inhibit spasticity and increase joint stiffness.[4] Furthermore, cooling may produce analgesia,[7] through slowing of nociceptive nerve fibres so that the transmission of noxious stimulus is delayed to the spinal cord, or by serving as a counter-irritant by bombarding central pain pathways with painful cold stimulus, activating the descending inhibitory pathways in the spinal cord.[8]

Electrotherapy

Electrotherapy is commonly used for pain modulation in musculoskeletal disorders, most commonly in the form of transcutaneous electrical nerve stimulation (TENS),[9] which is a pulse generator that can be administered at high (> 50 Hz), low (< 10 Hz) or burst frequencies, for stimulation of peripheral nerves via skin-surface electrodes. TENS may act according to the gate-control theory of pain, and may activate peripheral A-δ fibres, thereby modulating pain-carrying A-δ and C-fibres at the level of the dorsal horn.[10] In addition, counter-irritation may activate neurons in the rostral ventral medulla, which in turn inhibits the activity of dorsal horn nociceptive neurons.[11] More recent studies have demonstrated the release of endorphins, at both low[12] and high frequency.[13]

Although it is desirable to keep patients as active as possible throughout their rehabilitation, these passive modalities are still often used as an adjunct to allow the patient to participate in their exercise therapy.

Alternative therapies
Acupuncture
Acupuncture has its roots in traditional Asian medicine and is gaining greater favour in western medicine, particularly for musculoskeletal pain disorders. Fine-calibre, sterile needles are inserted at predetermined acupuncture points, and it has been hypothesized that this stimulates endogenous opioid pathways.[14] More recently, treatment has also included the flow of electrical current through needles – electroacupuncture – for reducing pain.

Manipulative therapy
Manipulative therapy requires trained individuals to manually deliver a high-velocity thrust, with the aim of reducing spinal (and other joint) discomfort and increasing the range of motion.[15] The thrust may be applied either through a long or short lever arm, depending on whether the force is applied either distant from or close to the joint, respectively. It has been reported to contribute to pain modulation through the transient stretching of joint capsules, resetting the position of the nervous system to function optimally, and also by improving the body's biomechanical function.[15]

Yoga
Yoga arises from Indian culture, and has been adapted in western civilization as a therapy to increase flexibility, strength and stamina, while also fostering self-awareness, emotional stability and peace of mind.[16] Yoga implements controlled postures, breathing and meditation to achieve these goals. There are many different 'schools' of yoga, but further explanation of their different ideological backgrounds and theory is beyond the scope of this chapter.

Cognitive–behavioural therapy
Along with physical therapy, cognitive–behavioural therapy is important in the interdisciplinary rehabilitation setting for patients with regional musculoskeletal conditions. This may involve operant, cognitive or respondent treatments. Operant treatments include positive reinforcement of healthy behaviours and removal of attention towards pain behaviours, emphasizing time-contingent versus pain-contingent pain management, and encouraging the involvement of the spouse. Cognitive treatment emphasizes imagery and diverting attention to modify maladaptive thoughts, feelings and beliefs. Finally, respondent treatment aims to directly alter the physiological response to pain, such as through methods to promote relaxation and biofeedback to reduce muscular tension.

Summary
The rehabilitation of regional musculoskeletal conditions should be based on the biopsychosocial model, implementing the aforementioned therapeutic modalities, including exercise, physical modalities and cognitive–behavioural therapy, with special emphasis on patient-centred care in a supportive environment.

EVIDENCE FOR THE EFFICACY OF MODALITIES IN REGIONAL MUSCULOSKELETAL CONDITIONS

Exercise
Spinal pain
A variety of exercise therapies have been utilized in the treatment of individuals with spine pain, ranging from aerobic conditioning to progressive resistance exercises (PRE). A recent review of systematic reviews by Taylor et al.[17] on the efficacy of PRE in the rehabilitation of chronic spinal pain outlined the results of three systematic reviews. For the studies in the three reviews that focused on either chronic low back or neck pain, the majority of participants ranged in age from 30 to 65 years which reflects the typical age range for these disorders. The two reviews on back pain scored moderate to high on the evaluation of quality of studies that were included. Generally, the reviews found that PRE was associated with increased trunk extensor and flexor force production, reduced pain and improved activity.[18, 19] Similarly, Sarig-Bahat's review[20] on participants with chronic neck pain showed that PRE led to increased muscle

force production, increased range of motion, reduced pain and improved activity.

Although past studies support the view that exercise therapy is more effective than usual care by a general practitioner, there still exists conflicting evidence on the effectiveness of exercise therapy compared with placebo,[21] and whether flexion or extension exercises are more effective.[21] Despite the often confusing data, there is evidence to support utilizing exercise as an adjunct to other therapeutic modalities in the rehabilitation of spinal pain. A more recent study by the UK Back Pain Exercise and Manipulation Trial Group on 1334 patients consulting their general practitioner about low back pain found that all groups improved over time, but that there was additional improvement at 3 months and at 12 months with manipulation followed by exercise.[22]

The fundamental limitations of the randomized, controlled trials (RCTs) reviewed include the heterogeneity of the aetiology of the acute or chronic low back pain in the subjects participating in the majority of trials. The prescribed therapy in each trial was similar despite different aetiologies for the low back pain, although the frequency and duration of therapy in some cases were individualized. Generalized exercise therapy for non-specific back pain may not be as effective as specific exercises for specific spinal disorders.[23] The importance of determining the directional preference for each patient with back pain prior to initiating exercise treatment in that preferential plane has been well documented.[24–26] Furthermore, targeting specific muscles in the lower back may be more useful than a global strengthening regimen.

Hides et al.[27, 28] further delineated the importance of specific exercises for acute, first-episode, low back pain in their RCT that targeted the co-contraction of the multifidi and transversus abdominis, two muscles that have a recognized important role in spinal stabilization. Both the treatment and control groups showed significantly decreased pain after 4 weeks. More importantly, the recurrence rates at 1 and 3 years of follow-up was reduced by more than 50% in the exercise group compared to the control group.[28]

Future research should focus on determining the efficacy of specific exercise programmes for specific causes of low back pain in the acute and chronic stages, and to delineate the best prescription for the exercises, namely the mode, intensity, frequency, duration and repetition. Future research may also target the effect on spinal pain and function of activating the 'core muscles' (i.e. the muscles that contribute to spine stabilization), including the multifidus posteriorly, the transversus abdominis anteriorly, pelvic floor muscles inferiorly, and the diaphragm superiorly in a cylindrical manner.

The difficulty in translating this evidence into practice lies in the heterogeneity of the exercise prescriptions, including the technique, mode, frequency, number of repetitions, intensity and duration. More precise guidelines for the most effective exercise prescription for improving function in persons with chronic spinal pain are required. Typically, the participants in the studies that were reviewed trained for 10–12 weeks, two or three times per week.[18, 19] In addition, the nature of the aetiology of the chronic spinal pain differed in individual participants, and may have responded differently to the various exercise treatments. Finally, it is unclear whether the improvements in pain reduction, truncal strength and activity level are maintained for a sustained period of time. Therefore, further high-quality longitudinal studies are required.

Pain in the extremities

Shoulder   A systematic review by the Philadelphia Panel identified previous studies on the efficacy of thermotherapy, therapeutic exercise, massage, electrical stimulation and mechanical traction in the treatment of shoulder pain.[29] They concluded that only ultrasound provided clinically important pain relief, compared to controls, in the short term (< 2 months) in participants with calcific tendonitis. However, the efficacy of the interventions was not stratified to the presence of shoulder pain of specific aetiology.

More recently, in an RCT by Carette et al.[30] on 93 subjects with adhesive capsulitis of less than 1 year duration, the efficacy of a single intra-articular corticosteroid injection, a supervised physiotherapy programme and a combination of the two was determined compared to placebo. Results of this study demonstrated that a single intra-articular injection conducted under fluoroscopic guidance, combined with a simple home exercise programme, was effective in improving shoulder pain and decreasing disability, but that adding supervised physiotherapy for 12 sessions provided faster improvement in shoulder range of motion.[30] Results from another RCT[31] support these findings. In this study 80 patients with adhesive capsulitis who were randomized to receive intra-articular corticosteroids experienced a significant improvement in function, while those subjects who received supervised physiotherapy reported improved shoulder range of motion, particularly in external rotation, at 6 weeks. However, at follow-up at 16 weeks both groups had improved to a similar extent in both function and range of motion.[31]

For chronic shoulder pain of non-specific 'mechanical' origin, Geraets et al.[32] demonstrated that a graded exercise programme in 176 individuals led to greater improvements in the performance of daily activities than usual care, with only small to moderate effect sizes. However, this effect was smaller in those participants who demonstrated a painful arc during the initial physical examination.[32] A recent study by Zheng et al.[33] also found that patients with persistent shoulder pain had quicker symptomatic improvement with intra-articular injections, and those that seemed to be at high risk for disability after 52 weeks of follow-up were female and more than 60 years old.

Clearly, further longitudinal studies must be performed to determine further prognostic factors for successful intervention in shoulder pain, so that appropriate therapy can be tailored to the individual needs of patients, and to maximize its effectiveness. Furthermore, in those adults who do not get better in a timely fashion, new techniques must be developed in the realm of therapeutic modalities, to maximize their outcome.

Knee   Consensus guidelines supported by a systematic review and meta-analysis[34] suggest that strengthening and, to a lesser extent, aerobic conditioning exercises, in participants with knee osteoarthritis led to improvements in pain levels and function. However, the main limitations in extrapolating these findings again involve the heterogeneity of the exercise programmes, the extent of knee osteoarthritis and the variation in outcome measures. Despite these limitations, there is strong evidence supporting strengthening exercises in patients with knee osteoarthritis, with particularly positive effects on pain, disability and health status.[34]

The results of one RCT suggest that supplementing the home exercise programme with a class-based exercise programme can lead to improvement in locomotor function, and a decrease in pain while walking at 12 months of follow-up.[35] A recent trial suggests that a water-based exercise class in those older patients with hip and/or knee osteoarthritis may lead to improvements in pain and function, although the benefits were demonstrated only for a short period after the start of the intervention, partly due to the participants' high rate of non-adherence to the water-exercise classes.[36] One explanation for the benefits behind exercise may be found in a clinical trial of 4 months of moderate exercise designed to improve neuromuscular control and strength, three times a week, in 45 subjects who were susceptible to knee osteoarthritis.[37] The participants in this study had a high mean body mass index and had undergone partial medial meniscectomy 3–5 years previously.[37] The exercise intervention was associated with a significantly increased quantity of glycosaminoglycan content in the knee cartilage in the intervention group.[37]

Despite convincing benefits of exercise on improving function and decreasing pain in those with knee osteoarthritis, the best exercise prescription, including mode, frequency, duration and number of repetitions, remains to be determined. Future research requires these parameters to be resolved, to maximize function while preventing further harm to the knee joint, especially in preventing further loss of glycosaminoglycan.

Physical modalities
Superficial heat
The use of heat for low back pain has been studied previously, in a randomized, single-blinded study that compared the efficacy of continuous low-level heat-wrap therapy for 8 hour/day with that of ibuprofen and paracetamol (acetaminophen) in subjects with acute non-specific low back pain.[38] The extent and duration of pain relief, lateral trunk flexibility, muscle stiffness and disability were all improved in the heat-wrap group compared to the control groups.[38] However, there was an unequal distribution of patients in the treatment and control groups. Also in the setting of acute low back pain, the use of active warming with a carbon-fibre electric heating blanket compared to passive 'warming' with a woollen blanket during transfer to hospital was associated with a significantly higher reduction in pain.[39] These results were supported by a recent study of 100 individuals with low back pain of less than 3 months' duration that were randomized either to a group that received a low-level heat wrap with directionally preferential exercise, or to a group that received a single intervention such as heat-wrap therapy or exercise, or to a

control group that consisted of receiving a booklet with information on the management of low back pain.[40] In the group that received both the heat wrap and exercise, participants had a significantly higher level of function and a lower level of pain, and a greater number of these subjects returned to their pre-injury level of function.[40] Treatment was continued for only 5 days consecutively, which would not allow for the assessment of the long-term efficacy of this modality.

Longer term prospective studies should be conducted to determine the long-term efficacy of thermal therapy for musculoskeletal conditions. The difficulty in blinding the patients to thermotherapy, and the lack of consistently valid and reliable outcome measures in these studies, are shortcomings that need to be addressed in future investigations.

Deep tissue heating
The use of ultrasound for deep tissue heating is a common modality in the treatment of regional musculoskeletal disorders, but has tenuous evidence to support its widespread use in the rehabilitation setting. In an RCT involving 40 patients with a periarticular soft-tissue disorder of the shoulder who were randomly assigned to either a group that received true ultrasound therapy or a sham, along with superficial heat, electrical stimulation and an exercise programme for 5 days/week for 3 weeks, there was no statistically significant difference in outcomes such as pain, range of motion, Shoulder Disability Questionnaire scores and Health Assessment Questionnaire scores in the intervention group receiving true ultrasound compared to the control group.[41] In a study of 120 subjects with bilateral knee osteoarthritis (Altman grade II), the group receiving pulsed ultrasound with isokinetic exercises had significant gains in range of motion and strength, and improvements in ambulation speed after treatment, with a decrease in disability.[42] Generally, in these studies there was an inadequate reporting of trial methods, selection criteria, treatment parameters and outcome measures.

Cryotherapy
In a small RCT of patients with acute gouty arthritis, those subjects who were randomized to receive a local application of ice to the affected joints in addition to oral prednisone and colchicine reported significant pain reduction compared to the group that did not receive cryotherapy.[43] A systematic review concluded that in knee or hip osteoarthritis patients ice massage had a statistically significant beneficial effect on knee range of motion, quadriceps strength and knee function compared to control, but no significant effect on pain relief.[44] However, higher quality studies are needed, with standardized protocols and outcome measures, and with adequate numbers of subjects to convincingly evaluate the efficacy of cryotherapy in regional musculoskeletal disorders.

Transcutaneous electrical nerve stimulation (TENS)
A recent systematic review on the use of TENS for chronic low back pain demonstrated conflicting results on the efficacy of TENS in subjects with this disorder.[45] In one of the RCTs that

met the methodological quality criteria, there was significantly greater pain relief demonstrated in those subjects who received TENS treatment for their low back pain.[45] However, the other study that was included showed no statistically significant differences between treatment and control groups in the outcome measures.[45] An RCT involving 62 patients with chronic knee pain secondary to osteoarthritis who were randomized to receive either 60 minutes of TENS, isometric exercise training, or a combination of TENS and exercise 5 days/week for 4 weeks, did not show between-group differences in reduction of pain on a visual–analogue scale.[9] Generally speaking, there are conflicting results regarding the effect of TENS on musculoskeletal pain disorders. Comparisons between studies have been difficult because of the lack of standardization of the stimulation parameters and the type of TENS stimulation, the control for other simultaneous modalities, the use of outcome measures and the homogeneity of the patient population.

Larger RCTs with standardized outcome measures and parameters of application for the TENS modality need to be conducted to study its efficacy more definitively in the rehabilitation of musculoskeletal disorders.

EVIDENCE FOR THE EFFICACY OF ALTERNATIVE THERAPIES

Acupuncture

In a meta-analysis of RCTs to assess the efficacy of acupuncture in those subjects with low back pain, the evidence indicates that there is some short-term pain relief of chronic pain, but the data are inconclusive in acute low back pain.[46] However, the quality of the studies that were included in this review was variable, and the parameters used for the acupuncture also varied between studies. In a recent systematic review of the use of acupuncture in shoulder pain, further evidence for the variability in methodological quality, with small sample sizes and insufficient details of the intervention utilized, made it difficult to derive firm conclusions about the efficacy of this modality.[47] However, it was concluded that there may be short-term benefit in improving pain and function.[47]

Important future research questions include determining the optimal treatment dose, frequency and duration, and the effect of acupuncture as an adjunct to other therapies, as well as the role of maintenance treatments.

Manipulation

In one systematic review of 39 RCTs involving manipulative therapy for low back pain for those individuals with either acute or chronic spinal pain, manipulative therapy had no statistically or clinically significant effect on the improvement of symptoms over general practitioner care, analgesics, physical therapy, exercises or back school.[48] However, another systematic review to evaluate treatment modalities for mechanical neck disorders concluded that there was strong evidence of benefit favouring a multimodal care approach, involving exercises combined with manipulation or mobilization, for subacute and chronic neck pain, with short-term and long-term relief.[49]

Future RCTs are required to determine the optimal dose and duration of manipulative therapy, its duration of clinical effects, and its effects in relation to other modalities for various musculoskeletal disorders, with larger sample sizes. The reason for its efficacy in cervical spine rather than lumbar spine pain in a multimodal approach to rehabilitation has yet to be determined.

Yoga

There are very few well-designed studies exploring the efficacy of yoga on improving pain and function in musculoskeletal disorders. However, a study by Sherman et al.[50] on 101 adults with chronic low back discomfort randomized to a 12-week course of yoga classes, conventional therapeutic exercise classes, or a self-care book showed improvements in back-related function in the yoga group compared to the other two groups at 26 weeks. Furthermore, pain was improved significantly at 26 weeks in the yoga group compared to the book group, although this was not significantly different from the therapeutic exercise group.[50] In support of the potential benefits of yoga, an RCT involving 60 subjects with chronic low back pain randomized to a yoga group for 16 weeks or an education group demonstrated significant reductions in pain intensity, functional disability and pain medication usage in the yoga group compared to the control group, both immediately post-intervention and 3 months later.[51]

Further studies must be conducted with larger sample sizes, and longer follow-up to determine the long-term effects of yoga.

COGNITIVE–BEHAVIOURAL THERAPY

In their review, Vlaeyen and Linton[52] describe 'fear-avoidance' as the act of evading movements or activities based on being afraid of anticipated pain. This may arise from negative appraisals about pain and its consequences, and catastrophic thinking, which may in turn precipitate fear. This fear is characterized by avoidance behaviours, leading to a disabling cycle, such that daily activities are no longer performed, leading to functional disability, and subsequent deconditioning, both on the cardiovascular and musculoskeletal systems, which may further contribute to pain.[52] Pain-related fear is one of the most powerful predictors of observable physical performance and self-reported disability levels.[52] Therefore, one of the treatment goals should be to reduce these anticipatory fears in a clinical setting, and to positively reinforce favourable actions such as confrontation of these fears.

In one study the use of cognitive–behavioural techniques to decrease fear avoidance in a multimodal treatment regimen compared to physical treatments in participants with non-specific low back pain of less than 12 weeks' duration led to comparable improvements in disability scores in both groups after 12 months.[53] The cognitive–behavioural techniques included positive coping strategies, overcoming fear of 'hurt versus harm' and an implementation of a graded return to usual activities by increasing function, pacing strategies, fear-avoidance techniques, adhering to treatment, and recognizing

PRACTICE POINTS

- Rehabilitation of regional musculoskeletal conditions should be multimodal and patient centred.

- Exercise therapy should be the mainstay when possible, with physical modalities utilized as an adjunct.

- Cognitive–behavioural strategies should also be utilized as part of the rehabilitation plan, especially when 'fear-avoidance' is a barrier to participation and improvement during the rehabilitation process.

RESEARCH AGENDA

- High-quality RCTs are required to further assess the efficacy of physical modalities, alternative therapies and cognitive–behavioural interventions.

- Trials with larger numbers of subjects are required that have well-explained therapeutic parameters (mode, frequency, duration, number of repetitions) and standardized outcome measures.

and eliminating barriers to recovery.[53] Further studies are needed to explore the effects of these cognitive–behavioural techniques and to determine the best strategies to optimize their positive impact.

SUMMARY

This chapter has reviewed some recent evidence for the rehabilitation of regional musculoskeletal conditions. The efficacy of various modalities for the treatment of musculoskeletal pain according to the most recent scientific evidence has been presented. Included in the holistic approach to patient-centred management are exercise therapy, thermotherapy and TENS, and alternative therapies such as acupuncture, manipulative therapy and yoga. Cognitive–behavioural strategies in pain management have also been briefly reviewed. The need for further longitudinal studies to further specify the optimal parameters for each of these modalities was emphasized.

REFERENCES

1. Hanada E. Efficacy of rehabilitative therapy in regional musculoskeletal conditions. *Best Pract Res Clin Rheumatol* 2003; **17**: 151-166.
2. Castor CW, Yaron M. Connective tissue activation: VIII. The effects of temperature studied in vitro. *Arch Phys Med Rehab* 1976; 57: 5–9.
3. Harris EDJ, McCroskery PA. The influence of temperature and fibril stability on degradation of cartilage collagen by rheumatoid synovial collagenase. *N Engl J Med* 1974; 290: 1–6.
4. Wright A, Sluka KA. Nonpharmacological treatments for musculoskeletal pain. *Clin J Pain* 2001; **17**: 33–46.
5. Welch V, Brosseau L, Peterson J et al. *Therapeutic Ultrasound for Osteoarthritis of the Knee*. Cochrane Review. The Cochrane Library, Issue 2. Update Software, Oxford, 2002.
6. Oosterveld F, Rasker JJ, Jacobs JW. The effect of local heat and cold therapy on the intraarticular and skin surface temperature of the knee. *Arthritis Rheum* 1992; **35**: 146–151.
7. Basford JR. Physical agents. In: Delisa JA, Gans BM (eds), *Rehabilitation Medicine: Principles and Practice*, 3rd edn. Lippincott-Raven, Philadelphia, 1998, pp. 483–503.
8. Williams J, Harvey J, Tannenbaum H. Use of superficial heat versus ice for the rheumatoid arthritis shoulder: a pilot study. *Physiotherapy (Canada)* 1986; **38**: 8–13.
9. Cheing G, Hui-Chan C, Chan K. Does four weeks of TENS and/or isometric exercise produce cumulative reduction of osteoarthritic knee pain? *Clin Rehab* 2002; **16**: 749–760.
10. Melzack R, Wall PD. Pain mechanism: a new theory. *Science* 1965; **150**: 171–179.
11. Bushnell MC, Marchand F, Tremblay N et al. Electrical stimulation of peripheral and central pathways for the relief of musculoskeletal pain. *Can J Physiol Pharmacol* 1991; **69**: 697–703.
12. Clement-Jones V, McLoughlin L, Tomlin S. Increased beta-endorphin but not met-enkephalin levels in human cerebrospinal fluid after acupuncture for recurrent pain. *Lancet* 1980; **2**: 946–948.
13. Han JS, Chen XY, Sun SL. The effect of low- and high-frequency TENS on Met-enkephalin-Arg-Phe and dynorphin A immunoreactivity in human lumbar CSF. *Pain* 1991; **47**: 295–298.
14. Ha H, Tan EC, Fukunaga H et al. Naloxone reversal of acupuncture analgesia in the monkey. *Exp Neurol* 1981; **73**: 298–303.
15. Stevinson C, Ernst E. Risks associated with spinal manipulation. *Am J Med* 2002; **112**: 566–571.
16. Garfinkle M, Schumacher HRJ. Yoga. *Rheum Dis Clin North Am* 2000; **26**: 125–132.
17. Taylor N, Dodd K, Damiano D. Progressive resistance exercise in physical therapy: a summary of systematic reviews. *Phys Ther* 2005; **85**: 1208–1223.
18. Hubley-Kozey C, McCulloch T, McFarland D. Chronic low back pain: a critical review of specific exercise protocols on musculoskeletal and neuromuscular parameters. *J Manual Manip Ther* 2003; **11**: 78–87.
19. Liddle S, Baxter G, Gracey J. Exercise and chronic low back pain: what works? *Pain* 2004; **107**: 176–190.
20. Sarig-Bahat H. Evidence for exercise therapy in mechanical neck disorders. *Massage Ther* 2003; **8**: 10–20.
21. Tulder MW, Malmivaara A, Esmail R et al. *Exercise Therapy for Low Back Pain*. Cochrane Review. The Cochrane Library, Issue 2. Update Software, Oxford, 2000.
22. Team UBT. United Kingdom Back Pain Exercise and Manipulation (UK BEAM) randomised trial: effectiveness of physical treatments for back pain in primary care. *BMJ* 2004; **329**: 1377.
23. O'Sullivan P, Twomey L, Allison G. Evaluation of specific stabilizing exercise in the treatment of chronic low back pain with radiologic diagnosis of spondylolysis or spondylolisthesis. *Spine* 1997; **22**: 2959–2967.
24. Donelson R, Grant W, Kemps C et al. Pain response to sagittal end-range spinal motion. A prospective, randomized, multicentered trial. *Spine* 1991; **16**: S206–S212.
25. Delitto A, Cibulka M, Erhard R et al. Evidence for an extension-mobilization category in acute low back syndrome: a prescriptive validation pilot study. *Phys Ther* 1993; **73**: 216–228.
26. Kopp J, Alexander AH, Turocy R et al. The use of lumbar extension in the evaluation and treatment of patients with acute herniated nucleus pulposus, a preliminary report. *Clin Orthoped* 1986; **202**: 211–8.
27. Hides J, Richardson C, Jull G. Multifidus muscle recovery is not automatic after resolution of acute, first-episode low back pain. *Spine* 1996; **21**: 2763–2769.
28. Hides J, Jull G, Richardson C. Long–term effects of specific stabilizing exercises for first-episode low back pain. *Spine* 2001; **26**: E243–E248.
29. Philadelphia Panel. Philadelphia Panel evidence-based clinical practice guidelines on selected rehabilitation interventions for shoulder pain. *Phys Ther* 2001; **81**: 1719–1730.
30. Carette S, Moffett H, Tardif J et al. Intraarticular corticosteroids, supervised phyiosotherapy, or a combination of the two in the treatment of adhesive capsulitis of the shoulder: a placebo-controlled trial. *Arthritis Rheum* 2003; **48**: 829–838.
31. Ryans I, Montgomery A, Galway R et al. A randomized controlled trial of intra-articular triamcinolone and/or physiotherapy in shoulder capsulitis. *Rheumatology (Oxford)* 2005; **44**: 529–535.
32. Garaets JJ, Goossens ME, de Groot IJ et al. Effectiveness of a graded exercise therapy program for patients with chronic shoulder complaints. *Austr J Physiother* 2005; **51**: 87–94.

33. Zheng X, Simpson JA, van der Windt DAWM et al. Data from a study of effectiveness suggested potential prognostic factors related to the patterns of shoulder pain. *J Clin Epidemiol* 2005; **58**: 823–830.

34. Roddy E, Zhang W, Doherty M et al. Evidence-based recommendations for the role of exercise in the management of osteoarthritis of the hip or knee – the MOVE consensus. *Rheumatology (Oxford)* 2005; **44**: 67–73.

35. McCarthy CJ, Mills PM, Pullen R et al. Supplementing a home exercise programme with a class-based exercise programme is more effective than home exercise alone in the treatment of knee osteoarthritis. *Rheumatology (Oxford)* 2004; **43**: 880–886.

36. Cochrane T, Davey R, Mathes Edwards S. Randomised controlled trial of the cost-effectiveness of water-based therapy for lower limb osteoarthritis. *Health Technol Assess* 2005; **9**: 1–114.

37. Roos E, Dahlberg L. Positive effects of moderate exercise on glycosamino-glycan content in knee cartilage. *Arthritis Rheum* 2005; **52**: 3507–3514.

38. Nadler SF, Steiner DJ, Erasala GN et al. Continuous low-level heat wrap therapy provides more efficacy than ibuprofen and acetaminophen for acute low back pain. *Spine* 2002; **27**: 1012–1017.

39. Nuhr M, Hoerauf K, Bertalanffy P et al. Active warming during emergency transport relieves acute low back pain. *Spine* 2004; **29**: 1499–1503.

40. Mayer J, Ralph L, Look M et al. Treating acute low back pain with continuous low-level heat wrap therapy and/or exercise: a randomized controlled trial. *Spine J* 2005; **5**: 395–403.

41. Kurtais Gursel Y, Ulus Y, Bilgic A et al. Adding ultrasound in the management of soft tissue disorders of the shoulder: a randomized placebo-controlled trial. *Phys Ther* 2004; **84**: 336–343.

42. Huang M, Lin Y, Lee C et al. Use of ultrasound to increase effectiveness of isokinetic exercise for knee osteoarthritis. *Arch Phys Med Rehab* 2005; **86**: 1545–1551.

43. Schlesinger N, Detry M, Holland B et al. Local ice therapy during bouts of acute gouty arthritis. *J Rheumatol* 2002; **29**: 331–334.

44. Brosseau L, Yonge K, Robinson V et al. *Thermotherapy for Treatment of Osteoarthritis.* Cochrane Database Systematic Reviews. CD004522Update Software, Oxford, 2003.

45. Khadilkar A, Milne S, Brosseau L et al. *Transcutaneous Electrical Nerve Stimulation (TENS) Chronic Low-Back Pain.* Cochrane Database Systematic Reviews. CD003008. Update Software, Oxford, 2005.

46. Manheimer E, White A, Berman B et al. Meta-analysis: acupuncture for low back pain. *Ann Intern Med* 2005; **142**: 651–663.

47. Green S, Buchbinder R, Hetrick S. *Acupuncture for Shoulder Pain.* Cochrane Database Systematic Review. CD005319. Update Software, Oxford, 2005.

48. Assendelft W, Morton S, Yu E et al. Spinal manipulative therapy for low back pain. Cochrane Database Systematic Review. CD000447. Update Software, Oxford, 2004.

49. Kay T, Gross A, Goldsmith C et al. Exercises for mechanical neck disorders. Cochrane Database Systematic Review. CD004250. Update Software, Oxford, 2005.

50. Sherman K, Cherkin DC, Erro J et al. Comparing yoga, exercise, and a self-care book for chronic low back pain: a randomized controlled trial. *Ann Intern Med* 2005; **143**: 849–856.

51. Williams K, Petronis J, Smith D et al. Effect of Iyengar yoga therapy for chronic low back pain. *Pain* 2005; **115**: 107–117.

52. Vlaeyen JWS, Linton SJ. Fear-avoidance and its consequences in chronic musculoskeletal pain: a state of the art. *Pain* 2000; **85**: 317–332.

53. Hay E, Mullis R, Vohora K et al. Comparison of physical treatments versus a brief pain-management programme for back pain in primary care: a randomized clinical trial in physiotherapy practice. *Lancet* 2005; **365**: 1987–1989.

SECTION 6
Chronic widespread pain

Chapter 21
The epidemiology of chronic generalized musculoskeletal pain

Jan T. Gran

INTRODUCTION

Unexplained musculoskeletal pain has been described for centuries, and was mentioned at the time of Hippocrates and in the Old Testament (Job 30:16–17).[1] Surprisingly, pain in the muscles, joints and bony prominences still represents a challenge to physicians, and mostly remains an enigma to modern medicine.

According to the American College of Rheumatology (ACR) 1990 criteria,[2] chronic widespread pain (CWP) is defined as pain both above and below the waist, involving both sides of the body and lasting for at least 3 months. Although the criteria do not distinguish between primary and secondary forms of such generalized pain syndromes, pain caused by malignant, metabolic or infectious disorders is usually not included in the CWP concept. In this chapter the term CWP will be used synonymously with primary or idiopathic CWP and, in spite of recent criticism,[3] the ACR 1990 criteria for CWP will be used as the reference criteria for generalized musculoskeletal pain syndromes.

Valuable information about CWP can also be obtained by reviewing studies on the fibromyalgia syndrome (FM). FM is a syndrome of unknown aetiology, which is characterized by widespread musculoskeletal pain, fatigue, poor sleep and tenderness on palpation at multiple sites called tender points.[4] Although CWP is the cardinal feature of FM, the relationship between these two clinical expressions of chronic pain is by no means clear. Many workers still favour the view that FM is a distinct clinical syndrome,[5] but the available epidemiological evidence[6] suggests that the distribution of key features is continuous and no clear population groups can be identified. Thus, CWP and FM appear as continuous variables on the spectrum of chronic idiopathic pain syndromes; for this reason, the inclusion of a brief review of the corresponding data on FM appears mandatory when addressing epidemiological aspects of CWP.

PREVALENCE OF CWP AND FM

When evaluating data on the prevalence of CWP and FM, one is confronted with several major problems. First, the scarcity of epidemiological surveys on chronic pain syndromes sharply contrasts with the rather intense research activity in other medical specialities. Until the 1990s, very few true population studies had been performed at all, allowing no firm conclusions to be drawn regarding the frequency, distribution and natural disease course of CWP and FM. The reason for the apparent paucity of studies was conceivably the preference for studying disorders exhibiting severe disease outcome rather than performing surveys on non-fatal disorders, even though they may exert a major impact on the health economy and patients' quality of life. Second, the problem of comparability of the results is further compounded by the fact that, at the time of the early studies, no commonly accepted gold standard was available for diagnosis and case identification. However, such problems were later largely overcome by the introduction of the ACR 1990 criteria,[2] which have been employed by most recent workers, thereby allowing reliable comparisons. Third, comparisons are also hampered by the variability in study design. Some population studies on chronic generalized musculoskeletal pain were performed as part of general health surveys, while other studies were designed to determine prevalence rates of FM and CWP, and specific criteria for the condition were applied. Another group of surveys was designed to determine the distribution of the critical elements of FM in the general population. Fourth, the selection of cases for study has varied, with some authors performing true population studies and others basing their estimates on patients attending hospitals or consulting general practitioners. Finally, neither CWP nor FM appear as invariable conditions, because, with time, patients frequently move across different categories of pain syndromes.[7, 8] These factors should not be ignored when interpreting the various estimates of prevalence, incidence, risk factors, clinical course and disease outcome in FM and CWP.

Population studies of CWP

A few early epidemiological studies were aimed at exploring the frequency of undifferentiated pain syndromes, such as CWP, in the general population. These studies indicated that 38–57% of the population reported musculoskeletal pain,[9–11] and thus clearly signalled a need for further investigation of a problem hitherto often ignored by health authorities and scientists.

During the last decade there have been numerous studies on the prevalence of CWP in the general population (Table 21.1). The overwhelming majority of surveys have been conducted in western European countries and North America. Unfortunately, few data exist regarding the occurrence of CWP in other regions. By comparing countries exhibiting differences in healthcare systems, disability compensation and organization of social welfare, as well as race, culture and climate, such studies could provide valuable information regarding the aetiopathogenesis of CWP. However, at present, information regarding the occurrence of CWP is available only for industrialized countries.

Of the 13 studies presented in Table 21.1, only four included clinical examinations of the subjects investigated; in the remaining studies the conclusions were based on information obtained exclusively through distribution of questionnaires. However, the studies may be compared in spite of differences in study design as, surprisingly, no great differences regarding estimates of prevalence seem to exist between the studies. In the study by Andersson et al.,[12] 90% of the individuals complaining of pain on initial examination reported similar complaints when interro-gated 6 months later. Moreover, it was also found that among individuals reporting chronic pain on questionnaires, 85% were assessed as having chronic pain at the examination. Such findings suggest that postal surveys may allow relatively reliable calculations of CWP. On the other hand, several studies have shown that subjects reporting pain on questionnaires deny such manifestations when presenting for clinical examinations. Thus, some precaution should be taken when comparing the various surveys. Finally, except for the investigations by Andersson et al.[13] and Hunt et al.,[14] all surveys required the fulfilment of the ACR 1990 criteria[2] for the definition of CWP, which evidently facilitates comparisons between the various studies.

The studies on the prevalence of CWP showed some differences (see Table 21.1). The highest prevalence of CWP was recorded in an epidemiological study among subjects aged 25–74 years in Bromølla and Simremarken in the most southern parts of Sweden.[13] Although using classification criteria that were conceivably less restrictive than the recommended ACR 1990 criteria for CWP, more than 50% of the subjects studied reported pain at multiple sites compatible with CWP. Somewhat surprising was the finding that rates of pain were distributed equally between genders. Most other studies have shown a significantly increased prevalence of widespread pain among women compared with men. Moreover, pain was found more often among blue-collar workers and farmers than in other professions.

A rather low prevalence of CWP was found among adult residents in England, Sweden and Canada, the frequency ranging from 4.2% to 7.3%. These figures contrasted with results of surveys in Norway, Sweden, Israel and England, yielding preva-

Table 21.1. Prevalence of chronic widespread pain

Study	Year	Country	Subjects examined	Criteria	Age group (years)	Prevalence (%)		
						Men	Women	Total
Forseth and Gran[36]	1992	Norway	214	ACR	20–50	–	15.3	–
Croft et al.[87]	1992	England	Postal study	ACR	20–85	–	–	13.2
Croft et al.[88]	1993	England	Postal study	ACR	18–79	9.4	15.6	11.2
Andersson[13]	1994	Sweden	165	–	25–74	–	–	55 (1) 49 (2)
Wolfe et al.[39]	1995	USA	391	ACR	18 +	–	–	10.6
Jacobsson et al.[15]	1996	USA (Pima)	Postal study	ACR	35–70	–	–	0.0
Abusdal et al.[89]	1997	Norway	Postal study	ACR	25–55	–	22	–
Mikkelsson et al.[19]	1997	Finland	Postal study	ACR	Pre-adolescents	–	–	7.5
White et al.[37]	1999	Canada	Postal study	ACR	18 +	–	–	7.3
Hunt et al.[14]	1999	England	Postal study	–[a]	18–65	3.7	5.3	4.7
Buskila et al.[90]	2000	Israel	Interview	ACR	18 +	3.0	14.0	9.9
Lindell et al.[91]	2000	Sweden	147	ACR	20–74	–	–	4.2
Bergman et al.[17]	2001	Sweden	Postal study	ACR	20–74	–	–	11.4

[a]Manchester definition of chronic widespread pain.

lence rates of CWP ranging from 9.9% to 13.2%. Besides variable perception of pain among residents, methodological variations and sociocultural differences not detected by the study design employed, no apparent explanation can be found to explain these discrepancies. A strikingly different factor to all these studies was found by Jacobsson et al.[15] investigating the occurrence of unexplained pain among Pima Indians. No subject in this population reported chronic generalized musculoskeletal pain. The extremely low prevalence of CWP among Pimas also contrasts with the prevalence of inflammatory rheumatic diseases observed in these native Americans. Such a difference in occurrence of inflammatory versus non-inflammatory disorders should also be studied in other regions. In conclusion, most epidemiological studies on CWP in North America and Europe have found that a significant proportion of the population report chronic pain syndromes that cannot be further classified. Most likely, approximately 10% of the inhabitants suffer from generalized musculoskeletal pain, indicating that such manifestations constitute a major health problem in the western world.

Almost unanimously, all studies have detected higher rates of CWP among women than men. The skewed gender ratio is not easily explained, and a recent study[16] aimed to explore possible explanations for the female dominance in CWP. A postal survey was carried out of 1178 female participants living in south-east Cheshire in the north-west of England. Among pre- and perimenopausal women, the risk of CWP was unrelated to the length of the menstrual cycle or the usual length of period reported by participants. The risk was similar in current users and non-users of the oral contraceptive pill, and among users there was no relationship with duration of use. Among postmenopausal women, CWP was not related to age at menopause. The study thus demonstrated no association between sex hormone factors and CWP. Evidently, the mechanisms of gender differences are still incompletely understood, but they are likely to involve an interaction between biology, psychology and sociocultural factors.[4]

Both CWP and FM predominantly affect middle-aged women and men, and the prevalence seems to increase up to the age of 50–59 years for both genders, and then slowly decreases.[13] Bergman et al.[17] found the highest prevalence of CWP in the age group 59–74 years. The peak prevalence in the older age groups can, to some extent, be explained by the nature of CWP, being a chronic but non-fatal disorder, resulting in an accumulation of cases in the older age groups. However, the possible effect of age on the development of CWP has been incompletely investigated, the occurrence among younger individuals in particular.

Although it has been noted that chronic pain syndromes among young athletes have become more common,[18] rather few studies have been designed to explore the occurrence of pain syndromes among adolescents and children. Mikkelsson et al.[19] studied 1756 third- and fifth-grade schoolchildren and found widespread pain in 7.5%. The study showed that about half of the pre-adolescents complaining of musculoskeletal pain at least once a week at baseline had persistent pain symptoms at follow-up. Although FM has been addressed in several studies on younger individuals (see later), further investigations of CWP in children and adolescents are clearly warranted.

In conclusion, epidemiological research has confirmed the alleged high frequency of CWP in the general population and found it to be significantly higher in women than men. The aetiopathogenesis of CWP remains obscure; a diagnosis with definite definitions, explaining the pain, will be found in less than half of cases.[13] However, some aspects of CWP can be further explored by reviewing the occurrence, distribution and nature of FM.

FM: studies prior to the ACR criteria and studies from general practitioners and rheumatology clinics

In the 1980s, FM was reported in 4–5% of patients attending general medical and family clinics,[20, 21] suggesting that this is a condition encountered rather frequently by general practitioners. In a recent study, however, Bazelmans et al.[22] mailed questionnaires to general practitioners and estimated a population prevalence of 0.16%. This figure most likely represented an underestimation, as only 60% of the general practitioners returned the questionnaire, and the estimates determined cannot be interpreted in favour of a declining incidence. Studies from rheumatology clinics further emphasized the importance of chronic pain syndromes such as FM.[23–27] In one study from an outpatient clinic of rheumatology, 3.7% and 10.9% of all new cases suffered from primary and secondary FM, respectively.[28] Also, in specialist clinics other than rheumatology, undifferentiated pain syndromes appear to be rather frequent. Buskila et al.[29] enrolled 522 patients hospitalized on internal medicine wards and found that 36% reported chronic regional pain, 21% reported CWP and 15% of all patients had FM. According to White et al.,[30] FM is perceived to be one of the three most common diagnoses among new patient consultations across Canada.

The frequency with which chronic pain syndromes are encountered in the clinic will evidently vary greatly depending on the organization of the healthcare system, medical traditions, and awareness of the diagnosis and importance of CWP and FM among physicians and the public. Although these early studies provided little insight into aetiopathogenetic and epidemiological aspects of various pain syndromes, they emphasized an urgent need for further research. The studies done in the 1980s made it clear that a substantial proportion of the patients attending specialist clinics and consulting general practitioners suffered from pain conditions that could not be classified into traditional diagnostic groups of inflammatory rheumatic diseases. An urgent need for improved classification and diagnosis of pain conditions emerged.

Prior to 1990, several diagnostic criteria for FM were available.[1] In addition, some studies on the prevalence of CWP and FM were not specifically aimed at detecting such disorders, but were part of a general health survey in which other diseases were primary targets. In a Swedish population study[11] among subjects aged 50–70 years, a prevalence of FM of 1.1% was found according to the Yunus et al. criteria.[31] Similar figures were found in a Finnish population study,[32] in which 7217 individuals were screened and 3434 persons examined. Among adults aged 30 years and older, a prevalence of 0.8% was calculated. Clearly, these calculations represented minimum estimates of the prevalence rates of chronic pain conditions and are also difficult to compare with recent surveys owing to lack of appropriate classification criteria. In 1992, a study specifically constructed to estimate the occurrence of FM was performed in Germany.[33] Altogether, 541 adult subjects aged 25–74 years were screened and 80 persons examined. In spite of an improper description of classification criteria, the prevalence calculated (1.6–4.4%) was remarkably similar to later estimates.

FM: studies using the ACR criteria
Population studies of FM

The prevalence of FM in the general population according to the studies listed in Table 21.2 ranged from 0.1% to 3.3%. All studies, except those by Farooqi and Gibson[34] and Clark et al.,[35] were performed in western countries and showed that women contracted FM significantly more often than men, the estimates ranging from 1.0% to 4.9% in women and 0.0% to 1.6% in men. The impression is that FM appears to be distributed throughout the western world, with rather small differences in frequency between various geographical regions. An interesting exception is the study done by Forseth and Gran in 1992,[36] which estimated a prevalence of FM among women aged 20–49 years of 8.6–10.5%. The minimum figure of 8.6% is the most likely estimate as, owing to the study design, the overwhelming majority of non-responders were free from chronic pain syndromes. Moreover, the prevalence of CWP in this population was more or less similar to that found in other surveys. Thus, the total number of sufferers of chronic generalized musculoskeletal pain was probably not much different from that seen in other regions, but the proportion of FM in CWP was much higher. The cause

of this anomaly remains unknown, but some characteristics of this population may suggest tentative explanations. One possible explanation is an increased frequency of risk factors for FM in this population. This municipality is situated in a county that ranks by far the highest in Norway with respect to the use of tranquillizers and antidepressants, thereby emphasizing the close relationship between psychological distress and FM. Moreover, the frequency of disability recipients and the rate of sick leave and early job retirements in that county also exceed those of the whole country (8.5% versus 11.1%), providing a link between social factors and the development of FM, which is discussed thoroughly later in this chapter.

Other studies have also detected rather high prevalence rates of FM, at least in certain age groups. White et al.[37, 38] studied a random community sample of 3395 non-institutionalized adults and identified 100 cases, of whom 86 were women. It was found that FM affected 4.9% of adult women and 1.6% of adult men. The prevalence reached almost 8% in women in the age group 55–64 years, emphasizing the effects of accumulating occurrence in non-fatal disorders having a chronic disease course. Similarly, Wolfe et al.,[39] studying 3006 persons in Wichita, USA, determined a prevalence of FM of 2.0%, again the highest incidence being between the ages of 60 and 79 years. Moreover, few workers have addressed the occurrence of FM in younger age groups, in particular among children and adolescents. Among schoolchildren (aged 9–15 years) studied by Clark et al. in 1998,[35] about 1.2% suffered from FM according to the ACR 1990 criteria. Other studies[40–43] have yielded prevalence rates ranging from 0% to 6.2%. Clearly, estimates of FM will vary depending on the age groups investigated and the proportion of subjects in each age group. Not infrequently, the age distribution among responders and non-responders will differ, most often over-representing younger and under-representing older people,[44] thus rendering the subjects examined not entirely

Table 21.2. Population studies on FM using the ACR 1990 criteria

Study	Year	Country	Age group (years)	No. of subjects screened	Prevalence (%)		
					Men	Women	All
Makela and Heliovaara[32]	1991	Finland	30 +	3434	0.5	1.0	0.8
Forseth and Gran[36]	1992	Norway	20–49	2498	–	8.6–10.5[a]	–
Lydell and Meyers[92]	1992	South Africa	35 +	1102	–	3.2	–
Prescott et al.[45]	1993	Denmark	18–79	1219	–	1.3	0.7
Wolfe et al.[39]	1995	USA	18 +	3006	0.5	3.4	2.0
Lindell et al.[91]	1996	Sweden	20–74	2425	–	–	1.3
White et al.[37]	1994–1996	Canada	18 +	3395	1.6	4.9	3.3
Farooqi and Gibson[34]	1997	Pakistan	15 +	2090	–	–	0.1–3.2[b]
Clark et al.[35]	1998	Mexico	9–15	548	0.0	2.5	1.2
Carmona et al.[93]	2001	Spain	20 +	2998	0.2	4.2	2.4

[a]Minimum and maximum prevalences.
[b]Rural districts, 2.6%; poor urban districts, 3.2%; affluent urban, 0.1%.

representative of the population of those with widespread pain. Also, the number of non-responders differs, and a non-response rate of up to 47% has been observed in studies aimed at determining prevalence rates of FM.[45, 46] However, in spite of the apparent differences in study design, the prevalence of FM in the western world most likely ranges from 2% to 3%.

The prevalence studies of FM have clearly shown that this clinical picture represents a major proportion of the CWP concept. Apart from a variety of accessory clinical symptoms, both sociocultural and psychological factors may contribute to the difference between FM and CWP. Most likely, FM can be regarded as one variant of CWP rather than a distinct clinical disease entity.

INCIDENCE AND MORTALITY

Extremely few studies have been undertaken to determine the incidence of chronic musculoskeletal pain syndromes in the general population. The actual incidence of CWP among various age groups remains to be specifically estimated. However, the impression of an increasing incidence of such syndromes has been put forward by several authors.[47] Whether or not the alleged increase in incidence is an expression of a true rise in frequency or is caused by an increased awareness among the public and physicians of the necessity to diagnose such syndromes remains to be investigated.

Also in FM, few prospective studies addressing incidence have been performed. A Norwegian survey during the years 1990–1995 investigated the number of new cases evolving in a female population over a period of 5.5 years.[48] In the age group 20–49 years, the annual incidence of new cases of FM was 583/100,000, or approximately 0.6%. If in these patients the condition were to evolve into a chronic life-long pain syndrome, such an incidence would result in an accumulation of a large number of FM and CWP within a few years. However, some remarks about the design of this incidence study should be made. First, the results deal with women only, and an age group perhaps particularly prone to develop CWP and FM. Second, a further analysis of the cases found to have CWP showed that a significant proportion of cases with both FM and CWP later ceased to report pain manifestations. Such a course of disease has been confirmed by subsequent studies.[8] Third, the high prevalence rates of pain syndromes found in the study may be due to certain population characteristics, as discussed earlier in this chapter, and it may not be possible to extrapolate these rates to the rest of the Norwegian or Scandinavian populations. The results indicated, however, that the number of new cases is rather high and poses a particular health economic problem to the society involved.

A recent study by Macfarlane et al.[49] addressed the mortality of CWP. In a prospective follow-up study over 8 years in northwest England, 6569 people took part in two pain surveys during the period 1991–1992. It was found that 15% of the participants had widespread pain and that mortality was higher in people with widespread pain than in those who reported no pain (stand-ard mortality rate 1.31). The excess mortality among people with regional and widespread pain was almost entirely related to deaths from cancer. The results were highly surprising, and possible causes for the findings were thoroughly discussed by the authors. Smoking is one of the most important risk factors for deaths from cancer, and it is also more common among people with widespread pain. Similarly, psychological distress has been reported as a predictor of future deaths from cancer and is also more common among people with widespread pain. However, after adjusting for these additional factors, an approximate doubling of risk of death from cancer was found among people with widespread pain. The possibility that pain in itself confers an increased risk of developing malignant disease remains to be explored by future surveys. However, the results may have been biased by other confounding variables that it was not possible to detect due to the study design. The rate of malignancy among non-responders and their prevalence of CWP should be explored.

Thus, rather few data exist on the incidence and mortality of CWP in the population and, at present, no firm conclusions can be drawn. However, although exact rates of incidence and mortality are yet to be determined, some information regarding the presence of risk factors for contracting chronic pain syndromes is available.

RISK FACTORS

The most obvious risk factor for contracting CWP and FM is female gender.[50, 51] As shown in Tables 21.1 and 21.2, all studies have concluded an increased risk in women over males, but the factors responsible for the skewed sex distribution remain to be found.

As no definite genetic marker has been associated with chronic musculoskeletal pain, most surveys aimed at exploring the aetiopathogenesis have addressed environmental factors. Bergman et al.[8] found that the risk of developing CWP among subjects having no pain or chronic regional pain showed a highly significant trend, with the presence of a family history of chronic pain, genetic factors or environmental factors representing possible explanations. A Finnish study of widespread musculoskeletal pain in twin pairs concluded, however, that environmental factors were much more important than genetic factors.[52]

Many studies have focused on the possibility of sociocultural factors as potential risk factors for the development of pain syndromes. Although a recent review[51] concluded that, in general, there was little evidence that pain reporting, particularly widespread pain, varies by social class, a number of studies have detected important sociocultural differences between patients and controls. A strong inverse gradient with level of education and development of CWP and FM has been observed in several studies.[32, 37, 38, 53, 54] Similarly, a low level of income appears to be associated with at least the development of FM;[38, 54] and being divorced,[38, 54] being disabled,[38] being an immigrant,[17] current smoking,[55] living in a socially compromised housing area,[17] and being an assistant, non-manual, lower-level employee or a manual worker[17] have been associated with chronic generalized musculoskeletal pain. Finally, Hagen et al.[53] found that the odds of consulting were significantly increased by being a pensioner or an individual on sick leave. The possibility still exists that these factors are secondary effects of long-standing chronic, often unattended, musculoskeletal disease and not primary events in the aetiopathogenesis of CWP and FM. Further epidemiological studies and, in particular, prospective follow-up of initially pain-free persons developing widespread pain may throw new light on these unsolved problems.

Much attention has also been paid to the possibility of psychological factors as risk factors for contracting chronic generalized musculoskeletal pain. In a recent study[56] of adults aged 18–65 years, it was found that subjects who were free of CWP were at increased future risk of its development if they displayed other aspects of the process of somatization. Moreover, Benjamin et al.[57] investigated 1953 persons aged 18–65 years and observed that the odds of having a mental disorder for subjects with, versus those without, CWP were 3.18. Approximately 17% of those with CWP were estimated to have a psychiatric diagnosis. Similar results were found by Macfarlane et al.,[58] who observed in a population survey that psychological distress was associated with CWP in addition to an effect on whether consultation was sought for symptoms. One-quarter of those consulting primary care services with CWP have a mental disorder. Another survey[59] showed that living in a less-affluent area was associated with strong and widespread pain, together with high levels of physical disability and mental distress. According to Hudson et al.,[60] patients with FM displayed high lifetime rates of major depression, panic disorder and familial major mood disorder. However, findings in FM should not automatically be regarded as representative for CWP without clinical evidence of FM. In one study,[61] patients with confirmed FM were compared with 48 patients with CWP who did not meet the 1990 ACR criteria for FM.[2] Compared with FM, the latter group was more symptomatic on virtually all measures of psychological distress. Furthermore, depression and anxiety were common and frequently severe, even among community cases of FM. Thus, CWP and FM appear to be differentiated by the degree of pain,[38] the frequency and persistence of complaints, the multisymptomatic character of manifestations and the magnitude of psychological distress.

In conclusion, there is a body of evidence correlating psychological factors and chronic musculoskeletal pain. As mentioned earlier, it may be argued that psychological distress represents a secondary phenomenon, but the frequency and consistency of such manifestations strongly suggest that psychological factors are true risk factors for developing chronic generalized musculoskeletal pain. Finally, Magni et al.[62] found a strong correlation between depression and subsequent chronic musculoskeletal pain, strongly indicating psychological factors as primary causes in at least some instances of CWP. To some extent, findings in disorders other than CWP and FM have contributed to the accumulation of evidence suggesting psychological distress as a major contributory factor in chronic generalized musculoskeletal pain.

COMORBIDITY

In systemic lupus erythematosus (SLE), particular attention has been paid to the occurrence of FM, while CWP without clinical features of FM has received much less attention. The prevalence of FM is reportedly 1–22%.[63–66] Except for the study by Ostuni et al.,[66] all investigations indicate an increased incidence of FM in SLE compared with controls. In one study,[64] the development of FM in SLE was associated with corticosteroid withdrawal, and dose reduction was the probable precipitating factor in nearly one-third of the cases. There are several possible explanations for this interesting finding. First, the musculoskeletal complaints may have contributed significantly to the level of distress that initially resulted in initiation of corticosteroid therapy, and when doses were reduced, such problems reappeared. A high dose of corticosteroids may also have had an impact on the patients' level of psychological well-being, masking a possible fundamental psychological distress. Yet another possibility is an association between disturbances in the hypothalamus–hypophysis axis and development of unexplained musculoskeletal pain. Clearly, these highly interesting findings warrant further research.

In the study by Ostuni et al.,[67] a much higher incidence of FM was found in primary Sjøgren's syndrome (22%) compared with other systemic rheumatic diseases. Similarly, Bonafede et al.[68] found an increased incidence of FM in Sjøgren's syndrome, and Pendarvis and Pillemer[69] observed that 7% of patients with Sjøgren's syndrome had CWP. A possible relationship between FM features, depression and Sjøgren's syndrome should be further evaluated.[70] Also, a high prevalence of FM has been found in rheumatoid arthritis.[71] Thus, increased prevalence of chronic undifferentiated musculoskeletal pain has been documented in several inflammatory rheumatic diseases. Whether or not such findings could be due to increased awareness of such conditions among rheumatologists or associated with the process of inflammation can be addressed by examining cases with inflammatory non-rheumatic diseases.

The findings in inflammatory bowel disease (IBD) are contradictory. Buskila et al.[72] found FM in 30 of 113 patients with IBD, the frequency being 49% in Crohn's disease and 19% in ulcerative colitis, compared with 0% among controls. In contrast, a population-based study by Palm et al.[73] diagnosed FM and CWP in only 3.5% and 7.3%, respectively, in patients with IBD. Interestingly, no correlation with the extent of the intestinal inflammation and the occurrence of FM and CWP was found. In infectious disorders, FM has been detected in 5–16% of patients with hepatitis C,[74, 75] in 11–29% of individuals with human immunodeficiency virus (HIV) infection,[71, 76] in 19% of those with acute viral infection[77] and in 8% of cases of Lyme disease.[78]

Interestingly, among patients with acute viral infection, Rea et al.[77] found that 19% exhibited clinical evidence of FM at presentation, whereas at 2 and 6 months, only 3% and 1%, respectively, suffered from FM. Consequently, there is no proof linking inflammation to chronic musculoskeletal pain, and persistence of such manifestations is conceivably, to a large extent, due to inherent characteristics of the host rather than the triggering external agent.

PRACTICE POINTS

- CWP is present in most western communities with a prevalence of 1.5–7.3%. There is little knowledge of its prevalence in developing countries. It is defined as 'pain both above and below the waist, involving both sides of the body and lasting for at least three months'. The definition of FM also includes the presence of at least 11 of 18 specified tender points and alters the group of patients to include more women.

- Symptoms include widespread musculoskeletal pain, chronic fatigue and poor sleep, and tenderness on palpation at multiple sites in FM.

- Women are more affected than men and the incidence is greatest in the age group 55–64 years.

- The ACR 90 criteria are of value in studies to define a population but they exclude a variety of commonly associated non-specific symptoms that are an important part of the syndrome. These include tension headache and migraine, irritable bowel syndrome, paraesthesia, subjective feeling of swelling, anxiety, depression and poor memory.

- FM and CWP are best regarded as part of a continuum, varying from chronic regional pain to CWP. Initially the pain is intermittent, and not all develop a chronic condition. Nonetheless, the greatest risk factor for chronicity is previous pain.

- Risk factors for CWP include injury, depression, perceived stress, substance abuse, poor coping resources, poor social support and perceptions on health. Psychological distress is a major factor.

- The cause of CWP is unclear, but there is good evidence for a mixture of somatic and psychosocial dysfunction and increasing evidence that central sensitization and dysfunction of pain-modulating pathways are important elements in the pathogenesis. It is no longer acceptable to consider CWP as an entirely physical or entirely psychosocial problem, but a combination of both. There may be a genetic element involving serotonin- and dopamine-related genes, but environmental elements are more important.

- Doctors need to recognize that, however comfortable a simple somatic explanation for CWP may be, it is not appropriate. Both physical and psychosocial symptoms must be managed together.

RESEARCH AGENDA

- FM needs to be recognized as a defined chronic pain syndrome and investigated as such.

- The aetiology remains an enigma, but central sensitization and dysfunctional pain modulation are contributing factors and need to be better defined in order to develop more targeted treatment. Further investigation of aetiology and the changes in central nervous dysfunction is essential.

- The role of physical and psychosocial risk factors and their interaction needs to be better understood. In this context genetic aspects warrant further study.

- The long-term outcome of individuals with limited, chronic pain ought to be focused on in order to detect risk factors for the development of widespread pain in this particular group.

- Better constructed studies of different treatments are necessary.

Several studies on chronic musculoskeletal pain in non-inflammatory disorders have been performed. Between 20% and 32% of patients with irritable bowel syndrome have been found to suffer from FM and 4.2–11% from CWP.[79–82] Also, a high prevalence of FM has been found in diabetes.[83]

In summary, these findings do not suggest that inflammation is important in the pathogenesis of undifferentiated musculoskeletal pain. One may wonder what factor these disorders have in common that predisposes to development of CWP and FM. Among several potential candidates, all these disorders have in common chronicity and a rather unpredictable course of disease, and, in some disorders, a lack of curative therapy and an unknown aetiopathogenesis may represent contributory factors. This again emphasizes the possibility that psychological distress, in one way or another, is associated with aetiopathogenic mechanisms in CWP and FM. The findings of an increased incidence of chronic musculoskeletal pain syndromes among war veterans further strengthen this assumption.[84–86]

SUMMARY

Chronic widespread musculoskeletal pain, as defined by the ACR 1990 criteria, occurs in approximately 10% of the general population, women being significantly more often affected than men. The mechanisms responsible for the skewed gender ratio remain unknown. Although all ages are affected, the peak prevalence appears to be among those in the age group 50–74 years. The prevalence and incidence of such complaints among children and adolescents are insufficiently studied. Population studies of FM indicate that about 3–5% of the general population is affected, again with a significantly higher frequency among females.

Both chronic widespread musculoskeletal pain and FM occur rather frequently in both rheumatic and non-rheumatic disorders. Common to such disorders are a chronic and unpredictable course of disease and, rather often, unknown aetiopathogenesis and lack of available remittive therapy. These findings, and studies aimed at investigating possible risk factors for contracting chronic musculoskeletal pain, strongly indicate that both psychological and sociocultural factors are important for the development of such conditions.

REFERENCES

1. Forseth KØ. *Musculoskeletal Pain and Fibromyalgia: Prevalence, Incidence, Natural History and Predictors*. Thesis, University of Oslo, 2000.

2. Wolfe F, Smythe H, Yunus MB et al. The American College of Rheumatology 1990 criteria for the classification of fibromyalgia: report of the Multicenter Criteria Committee. *Arthritis Rheum* 1990; **33**: 160–172.

3. MacFarlane GJ, Croft PR, Schollum J et al. Widespread pain: is an improved classification possible? *J Rheumatol* 1996; **23**: 1628–1632.

4. Yunus MB. Gender differences in fibromyalgia and other related syndromes. *J Gender-Specific Med* 2002; **5**: 42–47.

5. Russell IJ. Is fibromyalgia a distinct clinical entity? The clinical investigator's evidence. *Baillière's Clin Rheumatol* 1999; **13**: 445–454.

6. Forseth KØ, Gran JT. The occurrence of fibromyalgia-like syndromes in a general female population. *Clin Rheumatol* 1993; **12**: 23–27.

7. Forseth KØ, Førre Ø, Gran JT. A 5.5 year prospective study of self-reported musculo-skeletal pain and of fibromyalgia in a female population: significance and natural history. *Clin Rheumatol* 1999; **18**:114–121.

8. Bergman S, Herrström P, Jacobsson LT et al. Chronic widespread pain: a three year follow up of pain distribution and risk factors. *J Rheumatol* 2002; **29**: 818–825.

9. Brattberg G, Thorslund M, Wikman A. The prevalence of pain in a general population. The results of a postal study in a county of Sweden. *Pain* 1989; **37**: 215–222.

10. Crook J, Rideout E, Browne G. The prevalence of pain complaints in a general population. *Pain* 1984; **18**: 299–314.

11. Jacobsson L, Lindgarde F, Manthorpe R. The commonest rheumatic complaints of over six weeks' duration in a twelve-month period in a defined Swedish population: prevalence and relationships. *Scand J Rheumatol* 1989; **18**: 353–360.

12. Andersson HI, Ejlertsson G, Leden I et al. Characteristics of subjects with chronic pain, in relation to local and widespread pain report. A prospective study of symptoms, clinical findings and blood tests in subgroups of a geographically defined population. *Scand J Rheumatol* 1996; **25**: 146–154.

13. Andersson HI. The epidemiology of chronic pain in a Swedish rural area. *Qual Life Res* 1994; **3**(Suppl 1): S19–S26.

14. Hunt IM, Silman AJ, Benjamin S et al. The prevalence and associated features of chronic widespread pain in the community using the 'Manchester' definition of chronic widespread pain. *Rheumatology* 1999; **38**: 275–279.

15. Jacobsson LT, Nagi DK, Pillemer SR et al. Low prevalence of chronic widespread pain and shoulder disorders among the Pima Indians. *J Rheumatol* 1996; **23**: 907–909.

16. Macfarlane TV, Blinkhorn A, Worthington HV et al. Sex hormonal factors and chronic widespread pain: a population study among women. *Rheumatology* 2002; **41**: 454–457.

17. Bergman S, Herrstöm P, Högstrøm K et al. Chronic musculoskeletal pain, prevalence rates, and sociodemographic associations in a Swedish population study. *J Rheumatol* 2001; **28**: 369–377.

18. Small E. Chronic musculoskeletal pain in young athletes. *Pediatr Clin North Am* 2002; **49**: 655–662.

19. Mikkelsson M, Salminen JJ, Kautiainen H. Non-specific musculoskeletal pain in preadolescents. Prevalence and 1-year persistence. *Pain* 1997; **73**: 29–35.

20. Campbell S, Clark S, Tindall E et al. Clinical characteristics of fibrositis 1. A 'blinded', controlled study of symptoms and tender points. *Arthritis Rheum* 1983; **26**: 817–824.

21. Hartz A, Kirchdoerfer E. Undetected fibrositis in primary care practice. *J Family Pract* 1987; **25**: 365–369.

22. Bazelmans E, Vercoulen JH, Galama JM et al. Prevalence of chronic fatigue syndrome and primary fibromyalgia syndrome in the Netherlands. *Ned Tijdschr Geneeskd* 1997; **141**: 1520–1523.

23. Marder WD, Meenan RF, Felson DT. The present and future adequacy of rheumatology manpower. *Arthritis Rheum* 1991; **34**: 1209–1217.

24. Alarcon-Segovia D, Ramos-Niembro F, Gonzales-Amaro RF. One thousand private rheumatology patients in Mexico city. *Arthritis Rheum* 1983; **26**: 688–689.

25. Calabozo-Raluy M, Llamazares-Gonzales AI, Munoz-Gallo MT et al. Sindrome de fibromialgia (fibrositis); tan frequente como disconcido. *Med Clin Barcelona* 1990; **94**: 173–175.

26. Reilly PA, Littlejohn OG. Peripheral arthralgic presentation of fibrositis/fibromyalgia syndrome. *J Rheumatol* 1992; **19**: 281–283.

27. Gran JT, Nordvaag BY. Referrals from general practitioners to an outpatient rheumatology clinic: disease spectrum and analysis of referral letters. *Clin Rheumatol* 2000; **19**: 450–454.

28. Wolfe F, Cathey M. Prevalence of primary and secondary fibrositis. *J Rheumatol* 1983; **10**: 965–968.

29. Buskila D, Neumann L, Odes LR et al. The prevalence of musculoskeletal pain and fibromyalgia in patients hospitalized on internal medicine wards. *Semin Arthritis Rheum* 2001; **30**: 411–417.

30. White KP, Speechley M, Harth M et al. Fibromyalgia in rheumatology practice: a survey of Canadian rheumatologists. *J Rheumatol* 1995; **22**: 722–726.

31. Yunus M, Masi A, Aldag J. Preliminary criteria for primary fibromyalgia syndrome (PFS): multivariate analysis of a consecutive series of PFS, other pain patients, and normal subjects. *Clin Exp Rheumatol* 1989; **7**: 63–69.

32. Makela M, Heliovaara M. Prevalence of primary fibromyalgia in the Finnish population. *BMJ* 1991; **303**: 216–219.

33. Raspe H, Baumgartner CH. The epidemiology of the fibromyalgia syndrome (FMS) in a German town. *Scand J Rheumatol* 1992; **94**(Suppl 8): abstract 038.

34. Farooqi A, Gibson T. Prevalence of the major rheumatic disorders in the adult population of North Pakistan. *Br J Rheumatol* 1998; **37**: 491–495.

35. Clark P, Burgos-Vargas R, Medina-Palma C et al. Prevalence of fibromyalgia in children: a clinical study of Mexican children. *J Rheumatol* 1998; **25**: 2009–2014.

36. Forseth KØ, Gran JT. The prevalence of fibromyalgia among women aged 20–49 years in Arendal, Norway. *Scand J Rheumatol* 1992; **21**: 74–78.

37. White KP, Speechley M, Harth M et al. The London fibromyalgia epidemiology study: the prevalence of fibromyalgia syndrome in London, Ontario. *J Rheumatol* 1999; **26**: 1570–1576.

38. White KP, Speechley M, Harth M et al. The London Fibromyalgia Epidemiologic Study: comparing the demographic and clinical characteristics in 100 random community cases of fibromyalgia versus controls. *J Rheumatol* 1999; **26**: 1577–1585.

39. Wolfe F, Ross K, Anderson J et al. The prevalence and characteristics of fibromyalgia in the general population. *Arthritis Rheum* 1995; **38**: 19–28.

40. Buskila D, Press J, Gedalia A et al. Assessment of nonarticular tenderness and prevalence of fibromyalgia in children. *J Rheumatol* 1993; **20**: 368–370.

41. Bowyer S, Roettcher P. Pediatric rheumatology database research group. Pediatric rheumatology clinic populations in the United States. Results of a 3-year survey. *J Rheumatol* 1996; **23**: 1968–1974.

42. Symmons DPM, Jones M, Osborne J. Pediatric rheumatology in the United Kingdom: data from the British Pediatric Rheumatology Group National Diagnostic Register. *J Rheumatol* 1996; **23**: 1975–1980.

43. Malleson PN, Fung MY, Rosenberg AM et al. The incidence of pediatric rheumatic diseases. *J Rheumatol* 1996; **23**: 1981–1987.

44. Hawley DJ. Fibromyalgia in the Danish population. *Scand J Rheumatol* 1994; **23**: 55–56.

45. Prescott E, Jacobsen S, Kjoller M et al. Fibromyalgia in the adult Danish population: II. A study of clinical features. *Scand J Rheumatol* 1993; **22**: 238–242.

46. Prescott E, Kjoller M, Jacobsen S et al. Fibromyalgia in the adult Danish population. I. A prevalence study. *Scand J Rheumatol* 1993; **22**: 233–237.

47. Andersson HI, Ejlertsson G, Leden I et al. Musculoskeletal chronic pain in general practice. Studies of health care utilisation in comparison with pain prevalence. *Scand J Primary Health Care* 1999; **17**: 87–92.

48. Forseth KØ, Gran JT, Førre Ø. A population study of the incidence of fibromyalgia among women aged 26–55 years. *Br J Rheumatol* 1997; **36**: 1318–1323.

49. Macfarlane GJ, McBeth J, Silman AJ. Widespread body pain and mortality: prospective population based study. *BMJ* 2001; **323**: 662–665.

50. Romano T. Fibrositis in men. *West Virginia Med J* 1988; **84**: 235–237.

51. Felson D. Epidemiologic research in fibromyalgia. *J Rheumatol* 1989; **16**(Suppl 19): 7–11.

52. Mikkelsson M, Kaprio J, Salminen JJ et al. Widespread pain among 11-year-old Finnish twin pairs. *Arthritis Rheum* 2001; **44**: 481–485.

53. Hagen KB, Bjørndal A, Uhlig T et al. A population study of factors associated with general practitioner consultation for non-inflammatory musculoskeletal pain. *Ann Rheum Dis* 2000; **59**: 788–793.

54. Pincus T, Callahan L, Burkhauser R. Most chronic diseases are reported more frequently by individuals with fewer than 12 years of formal education in the age 18–64 United States population. *J Chronic Dis* 1987; **40**: 984–985.

55. Andersson H, Ejlertsson G, Leden I. Widespread musculoskeletal chronic pain associated with smoking. An epidemiological study in a general rural population. *Scand J Rehab Med* 1998; **30**: 185–191.

56. McBeth J, MacFarlane GJ, Benjamin S et al. Features of somatization predict the onset of chronic widespread pain: results of a large population-based study. *Arthritis Rheum* 2001; **44**: 940–946.

57. Benjamin S, Morris S, McBeth J et al. The association between chronic widespread pain and mental disorder: a population-based study. *Arthritis Rheum* 2000; **43**: 561–567.

58. MacFarlane GJ, Morris S, Hunt IM et al. Chronic widespread pain in the community: the influence of psychological symptoms and mental disorder on healthcare seeking behaviour. *J Rheumatol* 1999; **26**: 413–419.

59. Brekke M, Hjortdahl P, Kvien TK. Severity of musculoskeletal pain: relations to socioeconomic inequality. *Social Sci Med* 2002; **54**: 221–228.

60. Hudson JI, Goldenberg DL, Pope Jr HG et al. Comorbidity of fibromyalgia with medical and psychiatric disorders. *Am J Med* 1992; **92**: 363–367.

61. White KP, Nielson WR, Harth M et al. Chronic widespread musculoskeletal pain with or without fibromyalgia: psychological distress in a representative community adult sample. *J Rheumatol* 2002; **29**: 588–594.

62. Magni G, Moreschi C, Luchini S et al. Prospective study on the relationship between depressive symptoms and chronic musculoskeletal pain. *Pain* 1994; **56**: 289–297.

63. Middleton GD, McFarlin JE, Lipsky PE. The prevalence and clinical impact of fibromyalgia in systemic lupus erythematosus. *Arthritis Rheum* 1994; **37**: 1181–1188.

64. Handa R, Aggarwall P, Wali JP et al. Fibromyalgia in Indian patients with SLE. *Lupus* 1998; **7**: 475–478.

65. Grafe A, Wollina U, Tebbe B et al. Fibromyalgia in lupus erythematosus. *Acta Dermato-Venereol* 1999; **79**: 62–64.

66. Ostuni P, Botsios C, Sfriso P et al. Prevalence and clinical features of fibromyalgia in systemic lupus erythematosus, systemic sclerosis and Sjøgren's syndrome. *Minerva Med* 2002; **93**: 203–209.

67. Ostuni P, Botsios C, Sfriso P et al. Fibromyalgia in Italian patients with primary Sjøgren's syndrome. *Joint Bone Spine* 2002; **69**: 51–57.

68. Bonafede RP, Downey DC, Bennett RM. An association of fibromyalgia with primary Sjøgren's syndrome: a prospective study of 72 patients. *J Rheumatol* 1995; **22**: 133–136.

69. Pendarvis WT, Pillemer SR. Widespread pain and Sjøgren's syndrome. *J Rheumatol* 2001; **28**: 2657–2659.

70. Vitali C, Tavoni A, Neri R et al. Fibromyalgia features inpatients with primary Sjøgren's syndrome. Evidence of a relationship with psychological depression. *Scand J Rheumatol* 1989; **18**: 21–27.

71. Buskila D, Gladman DD, Langevitz P et al. Fibromyalgia in human immunodeficiency virus infection. *J Rheumatol* 1990; **17**: 1202–1206.

72. Buskila D, Odes LR, Neumann L et al. Fibromyalgia in inflammatory bowel disease. *J Rheumatol* 1999; **26**: 1167–1171.

73. Palm Ø, Moum B, Jahnsen J et al. Fibromyalgia and chronic widespread pain in patients with inflammatory bowel disease: a cross-sectional population study. *J Rheumatol* 2001; **28**: 590–594.

74. Buskila D, Shnaider A, Neumann L et al. Musculoskeletal manifestations and autoantibody profile in 90 hepatitis C virus infected Israeli patients. *Semin Arthritis Rheum* 1998; **28**: 107–113.

75. Goulding C, O'Connell P, Murray FE. Prevalence of fibromyalgia, anxiety and depression in chronic hepatitis C virus infection: relationship to RT-PCR status and mode of acquisition. *Eur J Gastroenterol Hepatol* 2001; **13**: 507–511.

76. Simms RW, Zerbini CA, Ferrante N et al. Fibromyalgia syndrome in patients infected with human immunodeficiency virus. The Boston City Hospital Clinical AIDS Team. *Am J Med* 1992; **92**: 368–374.

77. Rea T, Russo J, Katon W et al. A prospective study of tender points and fibromyalgia during and after an acute viral infection. *Arch Intern Med* 1999; **159**: 865–870.

78. Dinerman H, Steere AC. Lyme disease associated with fibromyalgia. *Ann Intern Med* 1992; **117**: 281–285.

79. Barton A, Pal B, Whorwell PJ et al. Increased prevalence of sicca complex and fibromyalgia in patients with irritable bowel syndrome. *Am J Gastroenterol* 1999; **94**: 1898–1901.

80. Sperber AD, Atzmon Y, Neumann L et al. Fibromyalgia in the irritable bowel syndrome: studies of prevalence and clinical implications. *Am J Gastroenterol* 1999; **12**: 3541–3546.

81. Lubrano E, Iovino P, Tremolaterra F et al. Fibromyalgia in patients with irritable bowel syndrome. An association with the severity of the intestinal disorder. *Intl J Colorect Dis* 2001; **16**: 211–215.

82. Whitehead WE, Palsson O, Jones KR. Systematic review of the comorbidity of irritable colon syndrome with other disorders: what are the causes and implications? *Gastroenterology* 2002; **122**: 1140–1156.

83. Wolak T, Weitzman S, Harman-Boehm I et al. Prevalence of fibromyalgia in type 2 diabetes mellitus. *Harefuah* 2001; **140**: 1006–1009.

84. Bourdette DN, McCauley LA, Barkhuizen A et al. Symptom factor analysis, clinical findings, and functional status in a population-based case control study of Gulf War unexplained illness. *J Occupat Environ Med* 2001; **43**: 1026–1040.

85. Escalante A, Fischbach M. Musculoskeletal manifestations, pain, and quality of life in Persian Gulf War veterans referred for rheumatologic evaluation. *J Rheumatol* 1998; **25**: 2059–2061.

86. Grady EP, Carpenter MT, Koenig CD et al. Rheumatic findings in Gulf War veterans. *Arch Intern Med* 1998; **158**: 367–371.

87. Croft PR, Schollum J, Rigby AS et al. Chronic widespread pain in the general population. *Scand J Rheumatol* 1992; **94**(Suppl 8): abstract 084.

88. Croft P, Rigby AS, Boswell R et al. The prevalence of chronic widespread pain in the general population. *J Rheumatol* 1993; **20**: 710–713.

89. Abusdal UG, Hagen KB, Bjørndal A. Self-reported chronic muscle pain among women in Oslo. *Tidsskr Nor Lægeforen* 1997; **117**: 1606–1610.

90. Buskila D, Abramov G, Biton A et al. The prevalence of pain complaints in a general population in Israel and its implications for utilization of health services. *J Rheumatol* 2000; **27**: 1521–1525.

91. Lindell L, Bergman S, Petersson IF et al. Prevalence of fibromyalgia and chronic widespread pain. *Scand J Primary Health Care* 2000; **18**: 149–153.

92. Lydell C, Meyers OL. The prevalence of fibromyalgia in a South African community [abstract]. *Scand J Rheumatol* 1992; **94**(Suppl 8): S143.

93. Carmona L, Ballina J, Gabriel R et al. The burden of musculoskeletal diseases in the general population of Spain: results from a national study. *Ann Rheum Dis* 2001; **60**: 1040–1045.

The epidemiology of chronic generalized musculoskeletal pain in light of recent publications

Karin Ø. Forseth and Michael Shipley

Chronic generalized pain is widely present in the general population and its aetiology remains an enigma. The American College of Rheumatology (ACR) 1990 criteria[1] are international classification criteria for the fibromyalgia syndrome (FM), which is consequently a well-defined chronic pain condition, and therefore often addressed in epidemiological studies. When creating these criteria, associated non-specific symptoms were omitted in order to increase the specificity and sensitivity of the criteria. Nevertheless, such symptoms are an important part of FM and may contribute to the development of chronic pain[2] and often precede self-reported pain.[3] In the last few years a few more population studies have been done, and these have reported prevalences in the range 1.5–7.3%.[4, 5] These results confirm previously reported prevalences of 2–7% in different general populations. The wide range of prevalence values probably reflects a combination of real differences, and differences in methodology and the application of the ACR criteria.

The interesting discussion as to whether FM is a distinct entity or the end of a continuum has been ongoing for some years. Traditionally, like FM, some regional pain syndromes have also been considered as distinct entities. However, several studies have found a correlation between the number of painful sites (representing the spectrum from localized pain conditions to generalized pain), the number of tender points and the number of associated symptoms.[6, 7] This supports the view that chronic pain conditions may constitute a continuum of pain distribution from localized to widespread, rather than different entities.

In practice, in 70–80% of patients who later develop FM the disease starts with localized and intermittent pain. The number of painful sites usually increases slowly over many years, before the patient finally develops the full-blown picture of FM.[8, 9] This indicates strongly that those with localized pain have a higher risk of developing chronic pain than do others. The duration of pain may also play a role as a risk factor.[10] However, a large proportion of people with self-reported localized or regional pain do not report worsening, and may even improve.[11] It is important, therefore, to identify risk factors for the development of chronic widespread pain. Studies performed recently indicate that depression, perceived stress, substance abuse, coping resources, poor social support, current symptoms and perceptions on health may be risk factors.[2, 10] More prospective studies in this field are awaited and might provide more knowledge that may lead to successful preventative intervention in those with localized or regional pain.

Although the aetiology of chronic pain still remains an enigma, it is generally agreed that central sensitization and dysfunction of pain-modulating pathways are contributing factors in its pathogenesis. It is also agreed that chronic pain is often due to multiple causes, including a genetic predisposition. Recent evidence suggests that serotonin- and dopamine-related genes may play a role in the pathogenesis of chronic pain.[12] Hopefully the aetiology and pathogenesis will be further elucidated in the years to come.

REFERENCES

1. Wolfe F, Smythe H, Yunus MB et al. The American College of Rheumatology 1990 criteria for the classification of fibromyalgia: report of the Multicenter Criteria Committee. *Arthritis Rheum* 1990; **33**: 160–172.
2. Turk DC. The role of demographic psychosocial factors in transition from acute to chronic pain. Prog Pain Res Manage 1997; **8**: 185–213.
3. Forseth KØ. Risk factors for self-reported chronic pain among females; a prospective population study. *J Musculoskelet Pain* 1998; **6**(Suppl 2): 165.
4. Senna ER, De Barros AL, Silva EO et al. Prevalence of rheumatic diseases in Brazil: a study using the COPCORD approach. *J Rheumatol* 2004; **31**: 594–597.
5. White KP, Thompson J. Fibromyalgia syndrome in an Amish community: a controlled study to determine disease and symptom prevalence. *J Rheumatol* 2003; **30**(8):1835–1840.
6. Croft P, Burt J, Schollum J et al. More pain, more tender points: is fibromyalgia just one end of a continuous spectrum? *Ann Rheum Dis* 1996; **55**: 482–485.

7. Wolfe F. The relation between tender points and symptom variables: evidence that fibromyalgia is not a discrete disorder in the clinic. *Ann Rheum Dis* 1997; **56**: 268–271.

8. Egli R. *der Verlauf der generalisierten Tendomyopathie und seine Beeinflussung durch exogene und endogene Faktoren*. Insuguraldissertion, Basel University, 1987.

9. Brückle W, Lautenschläger J, Müller W. The course and topography of pain in fibromyalgia. *EULAR Bull* 1992; **1**: 12–18.

10. Forseth KØ, Husby G, Gran JT et al. Prognostic factors for the development of fibromyalgia in women with self-reported musculoskeletal pain. A prospective study. *J Rheumatol* 1999; **26**: 11.

11. MacFarlane G, Thomas E, Papageorgiou A et al. The natural history of chronic pain in the community: a better prognosis than in the clinic? *J Rheumatol* 1996; **23**: 1617–1620.

12. Buskila D, Neumann L, Press J. Genetic factors in neuromuscular pain. *CNS Spectr* 2005; **10**: 281–284.

Chapter 22

Chronic widespread pain and fibromyalgia

Richard E. Harris and Daniel J. Clauw

MISCONCEPTIONS ABOUT CHRONIC WIDESPREAD PAIN

Population-based studies of chronic widespread pain (CWP) suggest that approximately 10–12% of the population has this symptom at any given time.[1, 2] Chronic regional pain is found in 20–25% of the population.[3] Both these prevalence figures are remarkably similar in many different countries and cultures, and both regional and widespread pain occur about one and a half times as commonly in women as in men.

Some individuals with CWP meet the criteria for fibromyalgia syndrome (FM). The 1990 American College of Rheumatology (ACR) criteria for FM require that an individual has *both* a history of CWP and the finding of 11 of 18 possible tender points on examination.[4] The ACR criteria tender points are located in nine paired regions of the body, and if an individual reports pain when any of these regions is palpated with 4 kg of pressure, this is considered a positive tender point. Using the ACR criteria, the prevalence of FM in industrialized countries has been reported to range from 0.5% to 4% in the population.[1]

Although women are only one and a half times as likely to experience CWP as men, they are about ten times as likely to meet the criteria for FM. This disparity between the gender differential for CWP and FM is due solely to the ACR criteria requiring 11 of 18 tender points; this latter finding occurs 11 times more commonly in women than in men in population-based samples.[1, 5]

The tender point requirement in the ACR criteria not only causes FM to become an almost exclusively female disorder, it also skews FM patients towards displaying high levels of distress. Distress is typically operationalized as some combination of somatic symptoms and symptoms of anxiety and/or depression. Wolfe said it best when he commented that because of the association between tender points and distress in population-based studies, tender points are a 'sedimentation rate for distress'.[6] Until recently, it had been assumed that, because tender points were associated with distress, tenderness (an individual's innate sensitivity to mechanical pressure) was associated with distress.[7, 8] However, recent studies have suggested that this is not so.[9] Tender points do not accurately assess the tenderness of individuals, in large part because individuals may anticipate when and how much pressure will be applied; individuals who are anxious or 'expectant' have a tendency to 'bail out' as pressure is applied, because they do not want to experience even brief pain. More sophisticated measures of tenderness that present stimuli in a random, unpredictable fashion yield results that are totally independent of psychological status, but this method of experimental pain testing still shows that FM patients are more tender than controls. Thus, tender points are associated with distress, but tenderness (as measured by sophisticated pressure pain-threshold testing) is not. Therefore, modifying the ACR FM criteria to eliminate the requirement for 11 of 18 tender points would lead to a totally different disorder: one affecting far more men, with the group displaying considerably lower levels of distress.

However, the relationship between FM and distress is not solely due to tender points. CWP alone is somewhat associated with distress.[7, 10] Individuals with CWP are somewhat more likely to have high levels of distress, and individuals with high levels of distress are more likely to have CWP.[11] Recent longitudinal studies have even shown that this may be a bidirectional causal relationship rather than just an association, because individuals identified as having only CWP or distress at one point in time are more likely to develop the other symptom if followed longitudinally. However, these associations are modest. There are far more psychologically 'normal' individuals who develop CWP than distressed/depressed people who do, and there are far more CWP patients who do not develop distress/depression than those who do.[11]

In addition to CWP being somewhat associated with tender points and distress, many individuals with CWP also have other somatic symptoms, such as fatigue or memory difficulties. This clustering of somatic symptoms in the population gives rise to overlapping syndromes such as FM, chronic fatigue syndrome, multiple chemical sensitivity and somatoform disorders.[12] Population-based studies have been performed using factor analytic techniques to identify the seminal features of these conditions. In such studies the key symptoms that co-aggregate are multifocal pain, fatigue, memory difficulties and mood disturbances.[13] The term 'chronic multisymptom illnesses' has been coined by investigators from the Centers for Disease Control and Prevention in the USA to describe this symptom complex.[14] Population-based studies of individual symptoms (e.g. pain or fatigue) suggest that the greater the number of co-aggregated symptoms, the more likely that the syndrome will be permanent and the greater likelihood that the individuals will seek healthcare.[10] Other factors that predict the development or persistence of either widespread or regional pain include greater age, a family history of chronic pain, low social support, being an immigrant, being in a lower socio-economic class, and performing manual labour.[15, 16]

It is important to note that all the above-noted relationships between CWP and other somatic symptoms, as well as distress, also hold true for regional pain syndromes. Chronic low-back pain has been the best studied in this regard, and it is known that distress can lead to low-back pain, low-back pain can lead to distress, and low-back pain plus other somatic symptoms is less likely to resolve.[17] Other relationships have been demonstrated with other regional pain syndromes, with the strongest relationships occurring in other axial (i.e. shoulder and neck) structures.[15, 18, 19]

In addition to examining the predictors and comorbidities of CWP and FM, population-based studies have also examined the potential contribution of 'peripheral' or 'mechanical' factors in these and other chronic pain states. Although FM and CWP are generally acknowledged to be primarily 'central' in origin, there may also be prominent central mechanisms that are operative in regional pain syndromes. For example, population-based studies comparing the results of knee radiographs and/or magnetic resonance imaging (MRI) to pain have suggested a poor relationship between peripheral structure and pain in osteoarthritis of the knee.[20] Similarly, there is a poor relationship between radiographic, computed tomography or MRI images of the low back and symptoms.[21-24] In fact, there is a whole host of regional pain syndromes in which the peripheral or mechanical factors explain either no role, or a minor role, in generating a chronic pain state.

Thus, although many clinicians associate FM with women who display high levels of distress, much of this is an artefact of: (1) the ACR criteria that require 11 tender points, and (2) the fact that most studies of FM have originated from tertiary care centres, where healthcare-seeking behaviours lead to the fact that psychological and psychiatric comorbidities are much higher.[25] When all these biases are stripped away by examining CWP in population-based studies, a clearer picture of FM can be gleaned, and CWP becomes much like any other chronic pain syndrome.

FM: ONE OF A NUMBER OF OVERLAPPING DISORDERS

FM is one of many systemic and regional disorders that share common clinical features, including chronic fatigue syndrome, multiple chemical sensitivity and Gulf War illness, which may present with similar symptomatology.[26, 27] These conditions share as their common features: widespread or regional pain, involving either peripheral structures or viscera; a high frequency of symptoms, such as fatigue and cognitive difficulties; and dysfunction of visceral organs. The most common 'systemic' conditions in this spectrum are FM, chronic fatigue syndrome, and Gulf War illness, whereas the most common regional syndromes are irritable bowel syndrome, temporomandibular disorders, and migraine and tension headaches. Several studies have demonstrated that these conditions commonly present simultaneously in the same patient, and that individuals with one of these conditions are much more likely to have or develop another of these conditions.[27] Entities such as Gulf War illness and sick-building syndrome are referred to as 'exposure syndromes', because these illnesses can be diagnosed only if the individual has a given exposure, rather than by its symptoms.

Chronic fatigue syndrome, sometimes also called myalgic encephalomyelitis in the UK, is presently defined as severe fatigue accompanied by four of eight 'minor' symptoms: sore throat, tender nodes, myalgias, arthralgias, headaches, cognitive problems, sleep disorders and post-exertional malaise.[28] While the full syndrome is seen in only about 1% of the population, the primary symptom of chronic fatigue is reported by 10–20%. Multiple chemical sensitivity has no widely accepted definition but is broadly viewed as the presence of symptoms in multiple organ systems in response to multiple environmental stimuli. Somatoform disorders may affect up to 4% of the population (if subsyndromal somatization is included) and are defined as multiple unexplained physical symptoms.

It should be noted that, just as for FM, the criteria for all these disorders are arbitrary. In most cases, a group of experts took a symptom or finding that was continuously distributed across a wide range in the population (e.g. pain, fatigue or tenderness) and decided 'where to draw a line', such that on one side of the line, individuals had the syndrome, and on the other side they did not. Due to this, these criteria should not be used as rigid diagnostic factors, but instead should be used to help define the syndrome under consideration, enhance patient education and aid in forming effective treatment plans.

GENETIC, NEUROBIOLOGICAL, BEHAVIOURAL AND PSYCHOLOGICAL FACTORS IN FM AND RELATED CONDITIONS

Research has indicated a familial component to the development of FM because family members of patients already diagnosed display a higher risk for FM – as well as common overlapping conditions – than is seen in the general population.[27, 29] Arnold et al.[30] provide recent evidence in support of this hypothesis. The incidence of FM in relatives of patients with FM is greater than the incidence of rheumatoid arthritis in relatives of patients with rheumatoid arthritis. A similar strong family history of these related conditions has been noted in most conditions that fall within this spectrum. These data point to a genetic risk factor for these conditions.

Recent studies have begun to identify specific genetic polymorphisms that are associated with a higher risk of developing FM. To date, the serotonin 5-HT$_{2A}$ receptor polymorphism T/T phenotype, serotonin transporter, dopamine 4 receptor and COMT (catecholamine o-methyl transferase) polymorphisms have all been noted to be seen in higher frequency in FM.[31-33] It is of note that all these polymorphisms involve the metabolism or transport of monoamines, compounds that play a critical role in activity of the human stress response.

Perhaps the most informative recent study in this spectrum of illness is that by Diatchenko et al.,[34] which showed that certain COMT haplotypes are associated both with pain threshold and the subsequent development of temporomandibular disorders.[34]

As with most illnesses that may have a genetic underpinning, environmental factors may also play a prominent role in triggering the development of FM and related conditions. Environmental 'stressors' temporally associated with the development of FM or chronic fatigue syndrome include physical (and particularly skeletal) trauma, certain infections (e.g. hepatitis C, Epstein–Barr virus, parvovirus and Lyme disease), emotional stress and other regional pain conditions or autoimmune disorders.[29, 35-37] An excellent recent example of how illnesses such as FM might be triggered occurred in the setting of the deployment of troops to liberate Kuwait during the Gulf War in 1990 and 1991. The term 'Gulf War illnesses' is now commonly used to refer to a constellation of symptoms developed by some 5–15% of the 700,000 US troops deployed to the Persian Gulf in the early 1990s. The symptoms, which include headaches, muscle and joint pain, fatigue, memory disorders and gastrointestinal distress,[14, 38] were also seen in troops deployed from the UK.[39] The panels of experts who examined potential causes for these symptoms and syndromes found that the sickness could not be traced to any single environmental trigger, and noted the similarities between these individuals and those diagnosed with FM and chronic fatigue syndrome.

The above-noted relationship between autoimmune disorders and FM deserves special attention because of the relevance to practising clinicians. As many as 25% of patients correctly diagnosed with generalized inflammatory disorders, such as systemic lupus erythematosus, rheumatoid arthritis and ankylosing spondylitis, will also fulfil the ACR criteria for FM.[40] However, in clinical practice, this co-expression may go unrecognized, especially when the FM develops after the autoimmune disorder or regional pain syndrome. Although this causes clinical confusion when FM and autoimmune disorders are co-expressed, an equally vexing problem occurs when FM is misdiagnosed as an autoimmune disorder. This rarely occurs if an individual presents only with common somatic symptoms, such as fatigue, arthralgia and myalgia. More commonly, misclassification occurs if these symptoms are accompanied by

common FM features, such as morning stiffness, the subjective report of swelling of the hands and feet, or dermatological features that simulate autoimmune conditions such as malar flushing, livedo reticularis and Raynaud's-like paling or reddening of the hand. Another problem in this regard is that diagnostic testing in individuals may not clarify the picture. Laboratory tests used to detect the presence of autoimmunity (e.g. antinuclear antibody and circulating immune complexes) are frequently positive in healthy individuals, and may be more frequently positive in this spectrum of illness.[41, 42]

Once FM develops, the mechanisms responsible for ongoing symptom expression are probably complex and multifactorial. Due to the fact that disparate 'stressors' can trigger the development of these conditions, the human stress response has been closely examined for a causative role. The systems involved in this response are mediated primarily by the activity of the corticotropin-releasing hormone (CRH) nervous system, which is located in the hypothalamus, and the locus coeruleus (noradrenaline)–norepinephrine/autonomic (sympathetic) (LC–NE) nervous system, which is located in the brainstem. Recent research suggests that, although this system in humans has been highly adaptive throughout history, the stress response may be inappropriately triggered by a wide assortment of everyday occurrences that do not pose a real threat to survival, thus initiating the cascade of physiological responses more frequently than can be tolerated.[43]

The type of stress and the environment in which it occurs also have an impact on how the stress response is expressed. It has been noted that victims of accidents experience a higher frequency of FM and myofascial pain than do those who cause them, which is congruent with animal studies showing that the strongest physiological responses are triggered by events that are accompanied by a lack of control or support, and thus viewed or perceived as inescapable or unavoidable.[43, 44] In humans, daily 'hassles' and personally relevant stressors seem to be more capable of causing symptoms than do major catastrophic events that do not personally affect the individual.[45, 46]

Genetic differences also play a role in the expression of the biological response to stress, as well as in the systems that process sensory information. Data collected from animal studies show that there are inter- and intraspecies differences for the 'set points' for these systems. Set points may then be permanently altered by repeated exposure to environmental stressors. Certain studies in animals have indicated that early-life traumas are particularly likely to have a permanent effect on the animal's biological response to stress.[47] This notion is further supported by data indicating that patients with many of these conditions may be more likely than unaffected individuals to have experienced physical or sexual abuse in childhood, although these retrospective studies are methodologically problematic.

These theoretical links between neural stress systems and symptom expression have generally been supported by studies demonstrating changes in the hypothalamic–pituitary–adrenal (HPA) axis and the sympathetic nervous system.[48-52] HPA axis dysfunction in FM patients has been associated with clinical pain severity, and may be dramatically affected by a history of abuse in early life.[53] A recent study by McBeth et al.[54] suggests that HPA abnormalities predict the subsequent development of CWP. Previous studies have suggested that HPA abnormalities may predict the development of pain and fatigue in individuals deprived of regular exercise.[55] Thus, these most recent data suggest that HPA dysfunction, like COMT gene mutations, may represent risk factors for developing these conditions.

The most consistently detected objective abnormalities in FM have been those involving pain-processing systems. As FM is defined in part by tenderness, considerable work has been performed exploring the potential reason for this phenomenon. One of the earliest findings in this regard was that the tenderness in FM is not confined to tender points but, instead, extends throughout the entire body.[56] Theoretically, such diffuse tenderness could be either primarily due to psychological factors (e.g. hypervigilance, in which individuals are too attentive to their surroundings) or neurobiological factors (e.g. the plethora of factors that can lead to temporary or permanent amplification of sensory input). Two decades of experimental pain studies have shown that: (1) FM patients cannot detect electrical, pressure or thermal stimuli at lower levels than normal, but the point at which these stimuli cause pain or unpleasantness is lower;[57] and (2) these findings are noted even when stimuli are presented in a random, unpredictable fashion, suggesting that psychological factors such as hypervigilance are playing a minor role in modulating tenderness.[58] Experimental pain testing has also been used to look for evidence of possible mechanisms of the widespread allodynia (pain in response to normally non-painful stimuli) seen in FM. Such studies have suggested that there may be evidence of a decrease in neural signals that descend from the brainstem and normally inhibit the upward transmission of pain.[44, 59] Other studies, which have used different techniques, demonstrate that patients with FM exhibit altered temporal summation of pain stimuli administered as a thermal stimulus to skin or as a mechanical stimulus to muscle.[60, 61] These latter studies suggest a parallel between the human condition of FM and the 'wind-up' phenomenon that leads to hyperalgesia and allodynia, which has been studied extensively in animal models.[62]

Other data corroborating the veracity of FM patients' pain complaints have been collected using paradigms that are not dependent on subjective reports of patients. For example, Lorenz et al.[63] demonstrated altered laser-evoked potentials as an objective representation of the central nervous system response to cutaneous stimulation.

Functional imaging has also been very instructive in pain syndromes in general, and in FM in particular. Mountz et al.[64] were the first to demonstrate reduced thalamic blood flow under resting conditions (a finding noted in other chronic pain states). These findings have recently been replicated by a different group. A more recent study by Gracely et al.,[65] using functional MRI, demonstrated that the amount of pressure stimuli required to cause cerebral activation in pain-processing regions of the brain (e.g. the primary and secondary somatosensory cortices) was much lower in FM patients than in healthy controls. Interestingly, these differences seen in FM

patients are located in both sensory and affective pain-processing regions of the brain. Depressive symptoms are associated with evoked pain activity in affective regions of the brain, such as the amygdala and insula but not in classical sensory-encoding regions such as the primary and secondary somatosensory cortices.[66] It appears that two independent neural networks may function to code for differing aspects of pain: one for sensory and one for affective qualities.

Biochemical studies performed on samples from FM patients have supported the notion that there are central changes in pain processing that may be due to either high levels of pro-nociceptive peptides or low levels of anti-nociceptive peptides. For example, several studies have shown that patients with FM have approximately three-fold higher concentrations of substance P in cerebrospinal fluid when compared with normal controls.[67–69] Other chronic pain syndromes, such as osteoarthritis of the hip and chronic low-back pain, are also associated with elevated levels of substance P, although chronic fatigue syndrome (which is not defined on the basis of pain) is not.[70] Interestingly, once elevated, substance P levels do not appear to change dramatically, and also do not become elevated in response to acute painful stimuli. Thus, high levels of substance P appear to be a biological marker for the presence of chronic pain.

Other studies have shown that the principal metabolite of noradrenaline (norepinephrine), 3-methoxy-4-hydroxyphenethylene (MPHG), is lowered in the cerebrospinal fluid of FM patients.[71] This finding is important for two reasons: (1) a reduction in noradrenaline (norepinephrine)-mediated descending, pain-inhibitory pathways that descend to the spinal cord may be a potential mechanism for causing the allodynia and hyperalgesia associated with FM; and (2) some of the most effective drug therapies for FM provide augmentation of central adrenergic activity.

Serotonin levels may also be diminished in patients with this spectrum of disorders. Studies by Russell et al.[71] and Yunus et al.[72] have demonstrated reduced levels of serotonin and its precursor, L-tryphtophan, in the blood serum of patients with FM, as well as reduced levels of the principal metabolite 5-hydroxyindoleacetic acid (5-HIAA) in the cerebrospinal fluid, all of which suggest that defective synthesis or metabolism of serotonin could be a feature, at least in a subset of FM patients.

In addition to neurobiological mechanisms, behavioural and psychological factors also play a role in symptom expression in many FM patients. The rate of current psychiatric comorbidity in patients with FM may be as high as 30–60% in tertiary-care settings, and the rate of lifetime psychiatric disorders is even higher.[73, 74] Depression and anxiety disorders are the most commonly seen. However, recent data suggest that this high rate of comorbid mood disorders is partly an artefact of studying these conditions in tertiary-care samples. Individuals who meet the ACR criteria for FM who are identified in the general population do not have nearly this high a rate of identifiable psychiatric conditions.[25]

As already noted, population-based studies have demonstrated that distress can lead to pain, and pain to distress. In this latter instance, a typical pattern is that, as a result of pain and other symptoms of FM, individuals begin to function less well in their various roles. They may have difficulties with spouses, children and work inside or outside the home, which exacerbate symptoms and lead to maladaptive illness behaviours. These include isolation, cessation of pleasurable activities and reductions in activity and exercise. In the worst cases, patients become involved with disability and compensation systems that almost ensure that they will not improve.[75]

The complex interaction of biological, behavioural, and psychological mechanisms is not, however, unique to FM. Non-biological factors play a prominent role in symptom expression in all rheumatic diseases. In fact, in conditions such as rheumatoid arthritis and osteoarthritis, non-biological factors such as level of formal education, coping strategies and socio-economic variables account for more of the variance in pain report and disability than do biological factors, such as the joint-space width or sedimentation rate.[76, 77]

TREATMENT STRATEGIES: PHARMACOLOGICAL AND NON-PHARMACOLOGICAL THERAPY

FM, as yet incurable, must be managed as a chronic illness. Treatment approaches should include both pharmacological and non-pharmacological management of symptoms and, most importantly, patient education about the nature and course of the illness. Pharmacotherapy for FM is largely symptomatic as there is not yet adequate understanding of the pathogenesis of the disease.

Once this diagnosis (or a similar one) is considered, the practitioner should schedule a prolonged visit, or series of visits. This 'front-loading' of time pays tremendous long-term dividends for both the practitioner and patient. This is necessary for the physician to understand precisely what is bothering the patient, and for the patient to understand the goals of, and rationale for, treatment. In these visits, it is important to explore the symptoms that the individual is experiencing, the impact the condition is having on his or her life, the patient's perception of what is causing the symptoms, and the stressors that may be exacerbating the illness. Once this has been accomplished, the patient should be educated on the non-destructive nature of this condition, as well as the fact that meaningful improvement rarely occurs without active participation on his or her part (i.e. there is no 'magic bullet'). The savvy practitioner will soon realize that sometimes 'labels' such as FM may be helpful to accomplish these goals, whereas in other instances such labels are unnecessary and could even be harmful, although there are no data to support this.[78, 79]

For patients with mild symptoms, such counselling, along with intermittent analgesic therapy, is often enough. For patients whose symptoms are pronounced enough to limit daily function more aggressive therapy is typically necessary, in many cases using combinations of pharmacological and non-pharmacological approaches. Patients with FM should also be given reputable sources of information.

The pain of FM must be managed differently from the pain that occurs in most other rheumatic diseases, because FM pain is not due to inflammation or tissue damage. The best-supported pharmacological therapy for FM, for a number of reasons, is low doses of tricyclic antidepressants, such as amitriptyline and cyclobenzaprine.[80] These drugs have been effective in treating the pain associated with FM, especially when tolerance-promoting strategies are utilized (see below). This class of compounds also has demonstrated efficacy for comorbid conditions, including tension and migraine headaches, irritable bowel syndrome and non-cardiac chest pain. Tricyclic antidepressants provide the added benefit of improved sleep patterns in patients with disrupted sleep.

Cyclobenzaprine and amitriptyline are the two tricyclic agents most studied in the treatment of FM, and no difference has been found in effectiveness between these two. However, the clinical trials performed to date demonstrate only short-term benefits, as neither agent has been shown to be superior to placebo at 6 months of study. This could represent tachyphylaxis to these drugs, but is more likely to be due to these studies being underpowered and not designed to administer the optimal dose of the drug.

One of the big issues in the use of tricyclic antidepressants has been determining the optimal dosage for each individual. As tolerance to these drugs is problematic, it is recommended that treatment be initiated at low doses (10 mg or less) taken several hours before bedtime, with slow (10 mg) increases every week or two until an optimal dose is achieved (up to 40 mg of cyclobenzaprine, or 70–80 mg of amitriptyline).

Due to a better side-effect profile, newer antidepressants are frequently used in FM. The selective serotonin reuptake inhibitors (SSRIs) have been extensively studied, with conflicting results.[81–83] Although there are only anecdotal data to support this, many in the chronic-pain field feel that agents with greater adrenergic and/or dopaminergic activity, such as venlafaxine or nefazadone, may be of more benefit than pure serotinergic drugs. Pain management may also be achieved in FM patients with the use of tramadol.

Dual serotonin–norepinephrine reuptake inhibitors have demonstrated effectiveness in reducing FM pain levels. Both duloxetine[84] and milnacipran[85] have reduced FM pain in randomized, placebo-controlled trials. Interestingly, these effects seem to be independent of antidepressant effects, because as with most studies of antidepressants as analgesics, the presence or absence of comorbid depression did not influence the analgesic effect of either of these compounds.

A recent randomized controlled trial of pregabalin, a compound that binds to a subunit of voltage-gated calcium channels, suggested that pregabalin has analgesic effects in FM.[86] Although the precise mechanism of action of pregabalin in FM is unknown, it is thought that it reduces calcium influx into nerve terminals and thereby reduces neurotransmitter release. Analgesic, anticonvulsant and anxiolytic-like activity has been observed with this compound in animal models.[87]

Other symptoms may respond to other classes of medication. For example, fatigue is a significant problem in this spectrum of illnesses. In a review of the various pharmacological treatments used for fatigue across medical conditions, Guymer and Clauw[88] concluded that classes of compounds that raise central levels of noradrenaline (norepinephrine) or dopamine appear to be the most specific for the management of fatigue. Cognitive dysfunction is also a significant problem in some individuals with FM,[89] and may respond to similar classes of drugs. For insomnia, individuals who do not tolerate tricyclic drugs may benefit from alternatives, such as trazadone, zolpidem or clonazepam. A subset of FM patients with features of autonomic dysfunction, including those who may have neural-mediated hypotension, may benefit from the use of low-dose beta blockers and/or increased fluid and sodium/potassium intake. Finally, although both non-steroidal anti-inflammatory drugs (NSAIDs) and opioids are frequently used in FM, there are no randomized controlled trials supporting their efficacy.

The two best studied non-pharmacological therapies in FM in particular, and chronic pain in general, are cognitive–behavioural therapy and exercise. Both of these therapies have been shown to be efficacious in the treatment of FM, as well as a plethora of other medical conditions.[90–93] Both these treatments can lead to sustained (e.g. longer than 1 year) improvements and are very effective when an individual complies with therapy. The challenge for new studies examining these treatments is to improve long-term adherence and compliance and to move towards using modalities (e.g. the Internet and telemedicine) that will allow a larger number of patients access to these therapies.

Until these studies are performed, giving formal guidance, there are some general recommendations that have been made with respect to exercise. For example, high-impact exercise may be poorly tolerated in these patients, so only low-impact aerobic activities (e.g. walking, swimming, water aerobics or stationary cycling) should be considered initially. The occurrence of post-exertional worsening of symptoms may be reduced by utilizing low-impact conditioning programmes, initiated at a slow pace (sometimes beginning at only 5 minutes/day) that is gradually increased over time.

Other non-pharmacological therapies, many of which are considered complementary or alternative therapies in western medicine, may have some utility in FM.[94, 95] As with other diseases, there are few controlled trials to advocate their general use. Trigger-point injections, chiropractic manipulation, acupuncture and myofascial release therapy are among the more commonly used modalities that achieve varying levels of success. Two trials of acupuncture in FM have shown consistent findings that acupuncture is no better than sham treatments.[96, 97] However, the sham interventions themselves have been shown to be non-inert.[98] This suggests that the trials may not have been sufficiently powered to detect differences above the non-inert sham group. There is some evidence that the use of alternative therapies gives patients a greater sense of control over their illness, and in instances where this is accompanied by an improved clinical state, the decision to use these therapies is between physicians and patients themselves.

FUTURE RESEARCH DIRECTIONS

What is FM and how should it be defined?

Population-based studies have conclusively demonstrated that: (1) CWP is very common; (2) it is sometimes accompanied by tenderness, distress and other somatic symptoms; and (3) when this does occur, CWP is more likely to be permanent than transient and to lead individuals to seek healthcare.

The current definition of FM, which requires 11 of 18 tender points in addition to CWP, captures only about 20% of those individuals with CWP. We now know that, because of the tender point requirement, the definition selectively captures females and individuals with high levels of distress. What do we do when the other 80% of individuals with CWP present for medical care? What should we call them (if anything), what should we tell them is causing their symptoms and, most importantly, what can we do for them?

An equally important consideration with respect to including tender points in the ACR criteria is that they lack 'validity'. In spite of irrefutable data that the disturbance in pain processing in FM is widespread, it will be difficult to erase the notion that there is something wrong in those magical 18 locations in the body as long as we keep publishing those pictures of a woman with dots superimposed.

There are also potential problems with eliminating tender points from the FM definition. One problem is that the 'new' syndrome we define will probably affect a larger proportion of the population than FM currently does; the societal implications of this need to be considered. Also, the tender point requirement ensures that FM patients have not just pain but also hyperalgesia/allodynia, a finding that has been useful in elucidating the mechanisms of aberrant pain processing in FM. All these issues need to be considered as the research community re-thinks the ACR criteria.

It appears that our options in this regard are:

- Leave the definition as it is, but educate practitioners about the problems of rigidly adhering to these criteria in routine clinical practice.
- Consider adopting different research and clinical criteria. Research criteria could theoretically use more sophisticated measures of pain sensitivity that do not have the problems inherent to tender points, or researchers could study CWP, and examine how hyperalgesia/allodynia interact with other factors to lead to symptom expression.
- Eliminate the requirement for tender points entirely (at least for the definition used in clinical practice). Possibilities would include:
  – CWP (without evidence of an identifiable cause). This would affect 5–10% of the population, and all these individuals could be assumed to have a 'central' pain syndrome, and be treated as such.
  – CWP plus other somatic symptoms (e.g. fatigue, memory/cognitive and/or mood disturbances would be the best candidates based upon epidemiological factor analytical studies). This definition would be more restrictive than the one above, affecting 5% of the population.

- Move towards definitions that are more data derived than historical, and are based on the mechanisms of symptom expression in individual patients. Those of us who are self-confessed 'lumpers' vis-à-vis this spectrum of illness only do so because any previous attempt to 'split' has not been helpful, either in understanding these conditions or in treating patients more effectively. We are at the point, however, where we could consider definitions that would divide groups of individuals with CWP into subsets based on the presence or absence of hyperalgesia/allodynia (based on evoked-pain paradigms that are not confounded by distress, or on a yet to be identified simple laboratory measure), and/or of behavioural or psychological factors.

What causes CWP and FM?

In a given individual with FM, virtually the only thing that will be found on testing is that he or she has the defining features of the illness: CWP and tender points. As the definition of FM is based on a combination of clinical (i.e. self-report) and evoked (i.e. tenderness) pain, nearly all individuals with this spectrum of illness will have some identifiable central disturbance in pain processing, whether this is identified using functional imaging or by measuring cerebrospinal fluid substance P. The issues most germane are: (1) how do genetics and the environment interact to initiate these conditions, and (2) what mechanisms are operative in maintaining symptom expression?

There are numerous methodologies that can be used to answer these questions. Genetic studies of individuals with established FM and CWP that are now underway will give some clues as to the genetic underpinnings of these illnesses. With the rapid advances in genomics, the phenotypical characterization of subjects will soon become much more problematic than the assays examining differential DNA or gene expression. To answer most of the remaining questions regarding causation, we will need to shift our current paradigms and move towards:

- Longitudinal studies that:
  - follow individuals with FM serially as their symptoms wax and wane, either naturally or with interventions
  - identify populations enriched for individuals likely to develop these conditions, and follow neurobiological, behavioural and psychological factors serially as symptoms develop.
- Neurobiological studies that carefully examine psychological and behavioural factors as covariates, rather than exclude these individuals from study.
- Where possible, the use of population-based sampling for mechanistic studies. When this is not possible (well individuals randomly identified in the population will not consent to be involved in many of the types of testing paradigms that are required), careful consideration of control groups (e.g. examining the entire population of 'normals' rather than just the hyperhealthy who are totally asymptomatic, controlling for healthcare-seeking behaviour) is necessary.

WHO SHOULD BE TREATING FM? WHAT ARE THE MOST EFFECTIVE TREATMENTS?

Many rheumatologists express enormous frustration aimed specifically at FM patients, or the FM 'construct'. The most simplistic reason for this may be psychological distress on the part of patients, physicians or both. Patients with FM, especially those who meet the current criteria and present for secondary or tertiary care, display higher average levels of distress than do individuals with other rheumatic disorders. Previous unsatisfactory interactions with the healthcare system may increase the likelihood of an adversarial relationship between patient and physician. Distress on the part of physicians is probably due to the fact that mechanisms underlying FM symptoms are poorly understood and are outside the realm of mechanisms traditionally studied by rheumatologists (e.g. immunology, inflammation and connective-tissue biology). In addition, current pharmacological therapies are often ineffective, while non-pharmacological therapies require time to implement; moreover, dealing with contentious issues surrounding FM (e.g. disability compensation or litigation) is particularly frustrating and counterproductive.

Most of these issues are not the fault of the patient. Even in the worst settings, where patients present seeking disability compensation or litigation to relieve their predicament, there is a general acknowledgement that these symptoms are very real and that intentional amplification or malingering is extremely unusual. The logical approach to this conundrum is that we

---

PRACTICE POINTS

- Epidemiological studies suggest that the ACR criteria for FM, particularly the requirement for tender points, have led to some misconceptions about CWP; this symptom is only slightly more common in women than in men, and only modestly associated with distress.

- FM falls within a spectrum of overlapping systemic conditions (e.g. chronic fatigue syndrome and Gulf War illnesses) and regional conditions (e.g. irritable bowel syndrome, temporomandibular syndrome, and migraine and tension headaches) that share common mechanisms and effective treatments.

- The hallmark of this spectrum of illnesses is that individuals experience pain because of some disturbance in how the central nervous system processes sensory information, not because of damage or inflammation in peripheral tissues.

- Because of this, the most effective pharmacological treatments of FM are neuroactive compounds, especially those that raise central levels of noradrenaline (norepinephrine) or serotonin.

- Non-pharmacological therapies, such as aerobic exercise and cognitive–behavioural therapy, are underutilized in routine clinical practice and may be especially effective if combined with symptom-based pharmacological therapy.

RESEARCH AGENDA

- The current definition of FM needs to be reconsidered. Ideally, a new definition would be data derived and would classify patients into subgroups based on the underlying pathogenic mechanisms.

- Mechanistic studies of this spectrum of illnesses need to expand beyond comparing groups of FM patients with controls. Only longitudinal studies that examine individuals from when they are asymptomatic to symptomatic will be able to dissect which factors lead to symptom expression, and which may be epiphenomena or predisposing factors.

- New pharmacological therapies that target mediators of chronic 'central' pain need to be tested in FM, and strategies to increase compliance and adherence to non-pharmacological therapies such as exercise and cognitive–behavioural therapy must be addressed.

determine healthcare strategies that identify these individuals earlier, and intervene effectively before distress, psychiatric comorbidities, maladaptive illness behaviours and disability/compensation create therapeutic inertia. Examples of strategies that may help to improve our treatment of FM include:

- Use what we know works. Many treatments of proven efficacy, especially non-pharmacological interventions such as cognitive–behavioural therapy and exercise, are grossly underutilized in clinical practice. Even well-studied pharmacological therapies such as low doses of tricyclic antidepressant drugs are frequently ignored in lieu of classes of compounds (e.g. NSAIDs or SSRIs) that practitioners are more familiar with but which are less effective.

- Intervene earlier. Although there are no data to support this, nearly everyone in this field believes that we would be more likely to treat these conditions effectively if these individuals were identified and managed in primary care. The need for earlier intervention is a primary reason for considering a new definition of FM (or whatever we want to call it) that would be more inclusive. Given the frequency of visits required, and the attention to many aspects of the patient, primary care physicians may be better suited than rheumatologists to caring for these individuals.

- Develop new pharmacological treatments. There has been an explosion of knowledge regarding the neurobiology of chronic pain, and there is a parallel effort to develop drugs that target some of these mechanisms. FM is the prototypical 'central pain syndrome', and should be among the first conditions in which these new compounds are tested.

REFERENCES

1. Wolfe F, Ross K, Anderson J et al. The prevalence and characteristics of fibromyalgia in the general population. *Arthritis Rheum* 1995; **38**: 19–28.
2. Croft P, Rigby AS, Boswell R et al. The prevalence of chronic widespread pain in the general population. *J Rheumatol* 1993; **20**: 710–713.
3. Wolfe F, Ross K, Anderson J et al. Aspects of fibromyalgia in the general population: sex, pain threshold, and fibromyalgia symptoms. *J Rheumatol* 1995; **22**: 151–156.
4. Wolfe F, Smythe HA, Yunus MB et al. The American College of Rheumatology 1990 Criteria for the Classification of Fibromyalgia. Report of the Multicenter Criteria Committee. *Arthritis Rheum* 1990; **33**: 160–172.
5. White KP, Speechley M, Harth M et al. The London Fibromyalgia Epidemiology Study: the prevalence of fibromyalgia syndrome in London, Ontario. *J Rheumatol* 1999; **26**: 1570–1576.
6. Wolfe F. The relation between tender points and fibromyalgia symptom variables: evidence that fibromyalgia is not a discrete disorder in the clinic. *Ann Rheum Dis* 1997; **56**: 268–271.
7. White KP, Nielson WR, Harth M et al. Chronic widespread musculoskeletal pain with or without fibromyalgia: psychological distress in a representative community adult sample. *J Rheumatol* 2002; **29**: 588–594.
8. Croft P, Schollum J, Silman A. Population study of tender point counts and pain as evidence of fibromyalgia. *BMJ* 1994; **309**: 696–699.
9. Gracely RH, Grant MA, Giesecke T. Evoked pain measures in fibromyalgia. *Best Pract Res Clin Rheumatol* 2003; **17**: 593–609.
10. McBeth J, Macfarlane GJ, Hunt IM et al. Risk factors for persistent chronic widespread pain: a community-based study. *Rheumatology (Oxford)* 2001; **40**: 95–101.
11. McBeth J, Macfarlane GJ, Silman AJ. Does chronic pain predict future psychological distress? *Pain* 2002; **96**: 239–245.
12. Nisenbaum R, Reyes M, Mawle AC et al. Factor analysis of unexplained severe fatigue and interrelated symptoms: overlap with criteria for chronic fatigue syndrome. *Am J Epidemiol* 1998; **148**: 72–77.
13. Doebbeling BN, Clarke WR, Watson D et al. Is there a Persian Gulf War syndrome? Evidence from a large population-based survey of veterans and nondeployed controls. *Am J Med* 2000; **108**: 695–704.
14. Fukuda K, Nisenbaum R, Stewart G et al. Chronic multisymptom illness affecting Air Force veterans of the Gulf War. *JAMA* 1998; **280**: 981–988.
15. Bergman S, Herrstrom P, Jacobsson LT et al. Chronic widespread pain: a three year followup of pain distribution and risk factors. *J Rheumatol* 2002; **29**: 818–825.
16. White KP, Harth M, Speechley M et al. A general population study of fibromyalgia tender points in noninstitutionalized adults with chronic widespread pain. *J Rheumatol* 2000; **27**: 2677–2682.
17. Croft PR, Papageorgiou AC, Ferry S et al. Psychologic distress and low back pain. Evidence from a prospective study in the general population. *Spine* 1995; **20**: 2731–2737.
18. Nahit ES, Pritchard CM, Cherry NM et al. The influence of work related psychosocial factors and psychological distress on regional musculoskeletal pain: a study of newly employed workers. *J Rheumatol* 2001; **28**: 1378–1384.
19. Papageorgiou AC, Silman AJ, Macfarlane GJ. Chronic widespread pain in the population: a seven year follow up study. *Ann Rheum Dis* 2002; **61**: 1071–1074.
20. Felson DT, Zhang Y. An update on the epidemiology of knee and hip osteoarthritis with a view to prevention. *Arthritis Rheum* 1998; **41**: 1343–1355.
21. Frymoyer JW, Newberg A, Pope MH et al. Spine radiographs in patients with low-back pain. An epidemiological study in men. *J Bone Joint Surg Am* 1984; **66**: 1048–1055.
22. Boden SD, Davis DO, Dina TS et al. Abnormal magnetic-resonance scans of the lumbar spine in asymptomatic subjects. A prospective investigation. *J Bone Joint Surg Am* 1990; **72**: 403–408.
23. Jensen MC, Brant-Zawadzki MN, Obuchowski N et al. Magnetic resonance imaging of the lumbar spine in people without back pain. *N Engl J Med* 1994; **331**: 69–73.
24. Clauw DJ, Lauerman W, Dahlman M et al. Tenderness as a determinant of outcome in individuals with chronic low back pain (CLBP) [abstract]. *Arthritis Rheum* 1997; **40**(9 Suppl): S279.
25. Aaron LA, Bradley LA, Alarcon GS et al. Psychiatric diagnoses in patients with fibromyalgia are related to health care-seeking behavior rather than to illness [see comments]. *Arthritis Rheum* 1996; **39**: 436–445.
26. Aaron LA, Burke MM, Buchwald D. Overlapping conditions among patients with chronic fatigue syndrome, fibromyalgia, and temporomandibular disorder. *Arch Intern Med* 2000; **160**: 221–227.
27. Clauw DJ, Chrousos GP. Chronic pain and fatigue syndromes: overlapping clinical and neuroendocrine features and potential pathogenic mechanisms. *Neuroimmunomodulation* 1997; **4**: 134–153.
28. Fukuda K, Straus SE, Hickie I et al. The chronic fatigue syndrome: a comprehensive approach to its definition and study. International Chronic Fatigue Syndrome Study Group. *Ann Intern Med* 1994; **121**: 953–959.
29. Hudson JI, Goldenberg DL, Pope HGJ et al. Comorbidity of fibromyalgia with medical and psychiatric disorders. *Am J Med* 1993; **92**: 363–367.

30. Arnold LM, Hudson JI, Hess EV et al. Family study of fibromyalgia. *Arthritis Rheum* 2004; **50**: 944–952.

31. Bondy B, Spaeth M, Offenbaecher M et al. The T102C polymorphism of the 5-HT2A-receptor gene in fibromyalgia. *Neurobiol Dis* 1999; **6**: 433–439.

32. Offenbaecher M, Bondy B, de Jonge S et al. Possible association of fibromyalgia with a polymorphism in the serotonin transporter gene regulatory region. *Arthritis Rheum* 1999; **42**: 2482–2488.

33. Buskila D, Cohen H, Neumann L et al. An association between fibromyalgia and the dopamine D4 receptor exon III repeat polymorphism and relationship to novelty seeking personality traits. *Mol Psychiatry* 2004; **9**: 730–731.

34. Diatchenko L, Slade GD, Nackley AG et al. Genetic basis for individual variations in pain perception and the development of a chronic pain condition. *Hum Mol Genet* 2005; **14**: 135–143.

35. Buskila D, Neumann L, Vaisberg G et al. Increased rates of fibromyalgia following cervical spine injury. A controlled study of 161 cases of traumatic injury [see comments]. *Arthritis Rheum* 1997; **40**: 446–452.

36. Buskila D, Shnaider A, Neumann L et al. Fibromyalgia in hepatitis C virus infection. Another infectious disease relationship. *Arch Intern Med* 1997; **157**: 2497–2500.

37. White PD, Thomas JM, Amess J et al. The existence of a fatigue syndrome after glandular fever. *Psychol Med* 1995; **25**: 907–916.

38. Bourdette DN, McCauley LA, Barkhuizen A et al. Symptom factor analysis, clinical findings, and functional status in a population-based case control study of Gulf War unexplained illness. *J Occup Environ Med* 2001; **43**: 1026–1040.

39. Unwin C, Blatchley N, Coker W et al. Health of UK servicemen who served in Persian Gulf War. *Lancet* 1999; **353**: 169–178.

40. Clauw DJ, Katz P. The overlap between fibromyalgia and inflammatory rheumatic diseases: When and why does it occur? *J Clin Rheumatol* 1995; **1**: 335–341.

41. Bates DW, Buchwald D, Lee J et al. Clinical laboratory test findings in patients with chronic fatigue syndrome. *Arch Intern Med* 1995; **155**: 97–103.

42. Pincus T. A pragmatic approach to cost-effective use of laboratory tests and imaging procedures in patients with musculoskeletal symptoms. *Primary Care* 1993; **20**: 795–814.

43. Romero LM, Plotsky PM, Sapolsky RM. Patterns of adrenocorticotropin secretagog release with hypoglycemia, novelty, and restraint after colchicine blockade of axonal transport. *Endocrinology* 1993; **132**: 199–204.

44. Lautenbacher S, Rollman GB. Possible deficiencies of pain modulation in fibromyalgia. *Clin J Pain* 1997; **13**: 189–196.

45. Raphael KG, Natelson BH, Janal MN et al. A community-based survey of fibromyalgia-like pain complaints following the World Trade Center terrorist attacks. *Pain* 2002; **100**: 131–139.

46. Pillow DR, Zautra AJ, Sandler I. Major life events and minor stressors: identifying mediational links in the stress process. *J Pers Soc Psychol* 1996; **70**: 381–394.

47. Sapolsky RM. Why stress is bad for your brain. *Science* 1996; **273**: 749–750.

48. Crofford LJ, Pillemer SR, Kalogeras KT et al. Hypothalamic–pituitary–adrenal axis perturbations in patients with fibromyalgia. *Arthritis Rheum* 1994; **37**: 1583–1592.

49. Crofford LJ. The hypothalamic–pituitary–adrenal stress axis in fibromyalgia and chronic fatigue syndrome. *Z Rheumatol* 1998; **57**(Suppl 2): 67–71.

50. Adler GK, Kinsley BT, Hurwitz S et al. Reduced hypothalamic–pituitary and sympathoadrenal responses to hypoglycemia in women with fibromyalgia syndrome. *Am J Med* 1999; **106**: 534–543.

51. Petzke F, Clauw DJ. Sympathetic nervous system function in fibromyalgia. *Curr Rheumatol Rep* 2000; **2**: 116–123.

52. Martinez–Lavin M, Hermosillo AG, Rosas M et al. Circadian studies of autonomic nervous balance in patients with fibromyalgia: a heart rate variability analysis. *Arthritis Rheum* 1998; **41**: 1966–1971.

53. McLean SA, Williams DA, Harris RE et al. Momentary relationship between cortisol secretion and symptoms in patients with fibromyalgia. *Arthritis Rheum* 2005; **52**: 3660–3669.

54. McBeth J, Silman AJ, Gupta A et al. Altered hypothalamic pituitary adrenal (HPA) stress axis function influences the risk of new onset chronic widespread body pain (CWP): a population based prospective study. *IASP Abstracts* 2005; 1247-P117.

55. Glass JM, Lyden AK, Petzke F et al. The effect of brief exercise cessation on pain, fatigue, and mood symptom development in healthy, fit individuals. *J Psychosom Res* 2004; **57**: 391–398.

56. Granges G, Littlejohn GO. A comparative study of clinical signs in fibromyalgia/fibrositis syndrome, healthy and exercising subjects. *J Rheumatol* 1993; **20**: 344–351.

57. Lautenbacher S, Rollman GB, McCain GA. Multi-method assessment of experimental and clinical pain in patients with fibromyalgia. *Pain* 1994; **59**: 45–53.

58. Petzke F, Gracely RH, Khine A et al. *Pain* sensitivity in patients with fibromyalgia (FM): expectancy effects on pain measurements. *Arthritis Rheum* 1999; **42**(9 Suppl): S342.

59. Kosek E, Ekholm J. Modulation of pressure pain thresholds during and following isometric contraction. *Pain* 1995; **61**: 481–486.

60. Price DD, Staud R, Robinson ME et al. Enhanced temporal summation of second pain and its central modulation in fibromyalgia patients. *Pain* 2002; **99**: 49–59.

61. Staud R, Vierck CJ, Cannon RL et al. Abnormal sensitization and temporal summation of second pain (wind-up) in patients with fibromyalgia syndrome. *Pain* 2001; **91**: 165–175.

62. Price DD. Psychological and neural mechanism of the affective dimension of pain. *Science* 2000; **288**: 1769–1772.

63. Lorenz J, Grasedyck K, Bromm B. Middle and long latency somatosensory evoked potentials after painful laser stimulation in patients with fibromyalgia syndrome. *Electroencephalogr Clin Neurophysiol* 1996; **100**: 165–168.

64. Mountz JM, Bradley LA, Modell JG et al. Fibromyalgia in women. Abnormalities of regional cerebral blood flow in the thalamus and the caudate nucleus are associated with low pain threshold levels. *Arthritis Rheum* 1995; **38**: 926–938.

65. Gracely RH, Petzke F, Wolf JM et al. Functional magnetic resonance imaging evidence of augmented pain processing in fibromyalgia. *Arthritis Rheum* 2002; **46**: 1333–1343.

66. Giesecke T, Gracely RH, Williams DA et al. The relationship between depression, clinical pain, and experimental pain in a chronic pain cohort. *Arthritis Rheum* 2005; **52**: 1577–1584.

67. Welin M, Bragee B, Nyberg F et al. Elevated substance P levels are contrasted by a decrease in met-enkephalin-arg-phe levels in CSF from fibromyalgia patients. *J Musculoskelet Pain* 1995; **3**: 4.

68. Russell IJ, Orr MD, Littman B et al. Elevated cerebrospinal fluid levels of substance P in patients with the fibromyalgia syndrome. *Arthritis Rheum* 1994; **37**: 1593–1601.

69. Vaeroy H, Helle R, Forre O et al. Elevated CSF levels of substance P and high incidence of Raynaud phenomenon in patients with fibromyalgia: new features for diagnosis. *Pain* 1988; **32**: 21–26.

70. Evengard B, Nilsson CG, Lindh G et al. Chronic fatigue syndrome differs from fibromyalgia. No evidence for elevated substance P levels in cerebrospinal fluid of patients with chronic fatigue syndrome. *Pain* 1998; **78**: 153–155.

71. Russell IJ, Vaeroy H, Javors M et al. Cerebrospinal fluid biogenic amine metabolites in fibromyalgia/fibrositis syndrome and rheumatoid arthritis. *Arthritis Rheum* 1992; **35**: 550–556.

72. Yunus MB, Dailey JW, Aldag JC et al. Plasma tryptophan and other amino acids in primary fibromyalgia: A controlled study. *J Rheumatol* 1992; **19**: 90–94.

73. Boissevain MD, McCain GA. Toward an integrated understanding of fibromyalgia syndrome. I. Medical and pathophysiological aspects. *Pain* 1991; **45**: 227–238.

74. Hudson JI, Hudson MS, Pliner LF et al. Fibromyalgia and major affective disorder: a controlled phenomenology and family history study. *Am J Psychiatry* 1985; **142**: 441–446.

75. Hadler NM. If you have to prove you are ill, you can't get well. The object lesson of fibromyalgia. *Spine* 1996; **21**: 2397–2400.

76. Hawley DJ, Wolfe F. *Pain*, disability, and pain/disability relationships in seven rheumatic disorders: A study of 1,522 patients. *J Rheumatol* 1991; **18**: 1552–1557.

77. Callahan LF, Smith WJ, Pincus T. Self-report questionnaires in five rheumatic diseases: comparisons of health status constructs and associations with formal education level. *Arthritis Care Res* 1989; **2**: 122–131.

78. Hadler NM. Fibromyalgia, chronic fatigue, and other iatrogenic diagnostic algorithms. Do some labels escalate illness in vulnerable patients? *Postgrad Med* 1997; **102**: 161–166, comment 171.

79. White KP, Harth M. Classification, epidemiology, and natural history of fibromyalgia. *Curr Pain Headache Rep* 2001; **5**: 320–329.

80. O'Malley PG, Balden E, Tomkins G et al. Treatment of fibromyalgia with antidepressants. A meta-analysis. *J Gen Intern Med* 2000; **15**: 659–666.

81. Goldenberg D, Mayskiy M, Mossey C et al. A randomized, double-blind crossover trial of fluoxetine and amitriptyline in the treatment of fibromyalgia. *Arthritis Rheum* 1996; **39**: 1852–1859.

82. Wolfe F, Cathey MA, Hawley DJ. A double-blind placebo controlled trial of fluoxetine in fibromyalgia. *Scand J Rheumatol* 1994; **23**: 255–259.

83. Arnold LM, Hess EV, Hudson JI et al. A randomized, placebo-controlled, double-blind, flexible-dose study of fluoxetine in the treatment of women with fibromyalgia. *Am J Med* 2002; **112**: 191–197.

84. Arnold LM, Rosen A, Pritchett YL et al. A randomized, double-blind, placebo-controlled trial of duloxetine in the treatment of women with fibromyalgia with or without major depressive disorder. *Pain* 2005; **119**: 5–15.

85. Vitton O, Gendreau M, Gendreau J et al. A double-blind placebo-controlled trial of milnacipran in the treatment of fibromyalgia. *Hum Psychopharmacol* 2004; **19**(Suppl 1): S27–S35.

86. Crofford LJ, Rowbotham MC, Mease PJ et al. Pregabalin for the treatment of fibromyalgia syndrome: results of a randomized, double-blind, placebo-controlled trial. *Arthritis Rheum* 2005; **52**: 1264–1273.

87. Taylor CP. The biology and pharmacology of calcium channel alpha2-delta proteins Pfizer Satellite Symposium to the 2003 Society for Neuroscience Meeting. New Orleans, LA, 10 November 2003. *CNS Drug Rev* 2004; **10**: 183–188.

88. Guymer EK, Clauw DJ. Treatment of fatigue in fibromyalgia. *Rheum Dis Clin North Am* 2002; **28**: 367–378.

89. Park DC, Glass JM, Minear M et al. Cognitive function in fibromyalgia patients. *Arthritis Rheum* 2001; **44**: 2125–2133.

90. Williams DA, Cary MA, Glazer LJ et al. Randomized controlled trial of CBT to improve functional status in fibromyalgia. *Am Coll Rheumatol* 2000; **43**: S210.

91. National Institutes of Health. Integration of behavioral and relaxation approaches into the treatment of chronic pain and insomnia. NIH Technology Assessment Panel on Integration of Behavioral and Relaxation Approaches into the Treatment of Chronic Pain and Insomnia. *JAMA* 1996; **276**: 313–318.

92. Keefe FJ, Gil KM, Rose SC. Behavioral approaches in the multidisciplinary management of chronic pain: programs and issues. *Clin Psychol Rev* 1986; **6**: 87–113.

93. Janal MN. Pain sensitivity, exercise and stoicism. *J R Soc Med* 1996; **89**: 376–381.

94. Crofford LJ, Appleton BE. Complementary and alternative therapies for fibromyalgia. *Curr Rheumatol Rep* 2001; **3**: 147–156.

95. Harris RE, Clauw DJ. The use of complementary medical therapies in the management of myofascial pain disorders. *Curr Pain Headache Rep* 2002; **6**: 370–374.

96. Harris RE, Tian X, Williams DA et al. Treatment of fibromyalgia with formula acupuncture: investigation of needle placement, needle stimulation, and treatment frequency. *J Altern Complement Med* 2005; **11**: 663–671.

97. Assefi NP, Sherman KJ, Jacobsen C et al. A randomized clinical trial of acupuncture compared with sham acupuncture in fibromyalgia. *Ann Intern Med* 2005; **143**: 10–19.

98. Fargas-Babjak A. Acupuncture, transcutaneous electrical nerve stimulation, and laser therapy in chronic pain. *Clin J Pain* 2001; **17**(4 Suppl): S105–S113.

Chapter 23

Pharmacological therapies in fibromyalgia (chronic widespread pain)

Srinivas G. Rao and Robert M. Bennett

INTRODUCTION

As detailed elsewhere in this volume, the fibromyalgia syndrome (FM) is a common, chronic, widespread pain syndrome predominantly affecting middle-aged women. The management of FM patients involves a complex interplay between pharmacological management of pain and associated symptoms, and the use of non-pharmacological modalities. As the elimination of all FM symptoms (i.e. a cure) is not currently possible, the philosophy of management is symptom palliation and functional restoration. The presentation of FM symptomatology is highly variable, and each patient must have an individualized evaluation before deciding on an initial treatment plan.[1] Regular follow-up and modification of the initial management strategy is usually required, depending on the response pattern. As in other chronic pain states, there is often an existential crisis that goes through distinct phases, from denial, searching for 'the cure,' to eventual acceptance. The early phases of management (usually the first 2 years) require more 'hand-holding', until the patient has come to terms with their new existence.

SYMPTOMS AND COMORBID SYNDROMES OF FIBROMYALGIA

Chronic, widespread pain is the defining feature of FM, as reflected in the FM classification criteria adopted by the American College of Rheumatology in 1990.[2] FM patients display quantitative abnormalities in pain perception under experimental conditions, in the form of both allodynia (pain with innocuous stimulation) and hyperalgesia (increased sensitivity to painful stimuli).[3] Taken together, these data are suggestive of a state of sensitized pain perception in FM.[3-5]

FM patients typically have a number of complaints beyond pain; a list of commonly associated symptoms is presented in Table 23.1.[6,7] Fatigue is cited as a significant cause of morbidity for the vast majority of FM patients,[8,9] and it represents a significant problem in a variety of other chronic pain states.[10] The potential causes of fatigue in FM patients are manifold, but recent evidence suggests that sleep disturbances may play a particularly important role.[8] Sleep disturbances, particularly non-restorative sleep, are reported to occur in over three-quarters of FM patients.[11] Sleep electroencephalography has demonstrated a number of abnormalities in the sleep architecture of FM patients, especially during non-rapid eye movement (particularly slow-wave) sleep.[11,12] Other associated sleep syndromes seen commonly in FM patients include periodic limb movements of sleep/restless leg syndrome and sleep apnoea.[13]

As shown in Table 23.2,[14,15] patients with FM also frequently meet the diagnostic criteria for a number of other syndromes, particularly the class of conditions loosely referred to as the 'functional somatic syndromes'.[16] Such syndromes include irritable bowel syndrome, subsets of chronic low-back pain, temporomandibular disorder, chronic fatigue syndrome, interstitial cystitis, certain headache syndromes and multiple

Table 23.1. Frequency of symptoms in patients with FM

Symptom	% of patients affected
Musculoskeletal pain	100
Fatigue	96–100
Disturbed sleep	86–98
Restless legs	56

Table 23.2. Syndromes frequently comorbid with FM

Syndrome	Point prevalence (%)
Chronic low-back pain	67
Irritable bowel syndrome	59
Mood disorder	29
Temporomandibular joint disorder	24
Chronic tension-type headaches	23
Chronic fatigue syndrome	18
Multiple chemical sensitivities	18
Chronic pelvic pain	18
Interstitial cystitis	8

chemical sensitivity. These conditions are fundamentally characterized by a discrepancy between the degree of patient suffering and objective clinical findings. As a group, the functional somatic syndromes are typically more common in women than men, and they share a number of clinical features, including pain, psychological distress/affective disorders, sleep abnormalities, and fatigue.

Low-back pain represents one of the most common problems seen in primary care, with up to 70% of adults having at least one episode of such pain during the course of their lifetimes.[17] Most episodes are acute and self-limiting in nature. However, chronic low back pain, defined as pain persisting beyond 3 months, results in a great deal of morbidity and significant socio-economic costs.

Irritable bowel syndrome is a common disorder characterized by abdominal pain, bloating, and disturbed defaecation.[18] The prevalence of irritable bowel syndrome is estimated to be between 3% and 15% in the general population, depending on the diagnostic criteria employed; 60–70% of these patients are women.[19] Three subtypes of irritable bowel syndrome are recognized – diarrhoea, constipation and discomfort/pain predominant – and classification significantly impacts on therapy (see below).

Increased levels of psychological distress resulting in psychiatric syndromes are a common accompaniment of many painful chronic illnesses.[20, 21] Estimates of concurrent major depressive episode and FM range from 28.6% to 70%,[22] and about 60% of FM patients have a history of depressive illness.[23] Finally, recent work suggests that post-traumatic stress disorder and other anxiety disorders may also represent an important cause of psychological distress in FM.[24, 25]

Temporomandibular joint disorders are a cluster of common chronic orofacial pain syndromes of unknown aetiology. Patients are most often classified into one of three groups: myofascial, joint disorders and combined.[26] Patients in the latter two groups are similar to those with other functional somatic syndromes, as they are more typically women and report greater pain and distress than patients with purely anatomical abnormalities (for a review see Plesh et al.[26]). Temporomandibular joint disorders

are extremely common, with an overall estimated prevalence of 3.7% and 12% in men and women, respectively.[27]

Chronic tension-type headaches represent one of the most common forms of chronic headaches. As reviewed by Redillas et al.,[28] chronic tension-type headaches are defined by the presence of bilateral headaches that are mild to moderate in intensity, occurring more than 15 days per month for more than 6 months. The pain has a tightening or pressing quality that is not aggravated by physical activity. Associated symptoms include nausea, photophobia and phonophobia. The prevalence of chronic daily headache is estimated to be 2–3% in the general population.

Finally, other syndromes that are somewhat less frequently comorbid with FM include chronic fatigue syndrome, interstitial cystitis, chronic pelvic pain and multiple chemical sensitivity syndromes. Multiple definitions of chronic fatigue syndrome exist.[29] However, the widely employed CDC-1994 criteria[30] define chronic fatigue syndrome by the presence of severe fatigue in the context of four or more of the following symptoms: myalgia, arthralgia, sore throat, tender neck, cognitive difficulty, headache, post-exertional malaise and/or sleep disturbance. The overall prevalence of this syndrome is estimated to be 0.2–2.6% of the population, with the majority of those affected being women.[29] Interstitial cystitis, also referred to as irritable bladder or female urethral syndrome, is a chronic, debilitating disease characterized by bladder and pelvic pain, irritative voiding symptoms (i.e. urgency, frequency, nocturia and dysuria) and sterile urine. Prevalence is estimated at 0.3% in the general population in the USA, with 90% of the patients being women.[31] Unexplained chronic pelvic pain is a common (15–20% of women aged 18–50 years have chronic pelvic pain of ≥ 1 year duration), if poorly characterized, condition that results in significant disability and distress.[32] The pathogenesis of such pain is not well understood and is likely multifactorial in origin. Finally, multiple chemical sensitivity is characterized by sensitivity to numerous environmental exposures, with resultant unexplained symptoms in multiple organ systems. Women appear to be more commonly affected, although overall prevalence data have not been compiled.[33]

FIBROMYALGIA: TREATMENT STRATEGIES

A number of recent publications have reviewed the current state of FM therapy.[34–37] A summary of the results of randomized controlled trials performed in FM is given in Table 23.3; more recent results are given in italics. It should be noted that no therapeutic procedure currently holds an approval specifically for FM, although several compounds are in late-stage development. Furthermore, the number of randomized controlled trials published to date is relatively small compared to other chronic pain conditions such as neuropathic pain or even irritable bowel syndrome, although this situation is changing with increasing interest in and awareness of FM. This chapter focuses on the major classes of drugs used in the management of FM and its associated problems.

Antidepressants

The majority of clinical trials on FM have involved antidepressants of one class or another, as is evident from Table 23.3. Trials studying the oldest class of agents, tricyclic antidepressants, are most abundant, although several recent studies have focused on selective serotonin reuptake inhibitors (SSRIs) and 'atypical antidepressants', including dual reuptake inhibitors (DRIs) and monoamine oxidase inhibitors (MAOIs). Despite the multiplicity of antidepressant classes, practically all the agents that are currently in clinical use in the USA either directly or indirectly increase neurotransmission mediated by the monoamine neurotransmitters, particularly serotonin (5-HT) and/or norepinephrine (NE; also called noradrenaline) (see Table 23.3).[38] These activities are thought to underlie the antidepressant activity of these compounds, and such activities also appear to be an important mechanism by which these compounds effect centrally mediated analgesia.[38, 39]

Tricyclic antidepressants

Most tricyclic antidepressants (TCAs) increase the concentrations of 5-HT and/or NE by directly blocking their respective reuptake.[38] However, TCAs typically possess myriad other pharmacological activities, including the abilities to block certain cation channels as well as histamine-, acetylcholine-, and N-methyl-D-aspartate (NMDA)-mediated glutamatergic neurotransmission. Cation channel blockade can result in analgesia by generally decreasing neuronal excitability; indeed, this activity may underlie the analgesic efficacy of certain antiepileptic drugs. Increased NMDA-receptor-mediated glutamatergic neurotransmission has been implicated in the pathogenesis of chronic pain, and blocking this activity has been efficacious in relieving such pain in a variety of models and clinical states.

Unfortunately, the anticholinergic and antihistaminergic activities of TCAs contribute to the relatively poor side-effect profile of these agents. This point may be particularly relevant to the FM patient population, due to the relatively high prevalence of comorbid multiple chemical sensitivity (see Table 23.2). Despite these tolerability issues, the use of TCAs (particularly amitriptyline) to treat the symptoms of pain, poor sleep and fatigue associated with FM is supported by several randomized controlled trials.[40] Surprisingly, the story is less clear regarding the mood-elevating effects of these agents in the context of FM, perhaps as a result of the fact that most trials have evaluated sub-antidepressant doses of TCAs.[40] In most forms of major depressive disorder, however, the efficacy and remission rates of TCAs are equal or superior to those of other classes of agents, perhaps as a result of their effects on both serotonergic and noradrenergic systems.[41] TCAs also have an established track record in treating various forms of chronic pain, including the pain associated with other functional somatic syndromes. Double-blind, randomized controlled trials support the use of TCAs in irritable bowel syndrome,[42] temporomandibular joint disorders[26] and chronic low-back pain,[17] although the effect size in the latter appears to be small. Finally, while TCAs are not as efficacious as acute treatment for chronic tension-type headaches, they are an effective form of prophylaxis.[28]

Selective serotonin reuptake inhibitors

SSRIs have revolutionized the field of psychiatry, providing safe and effective treatment for common psychiatric conditions, including major depressive disorder, anxiety and social phobia. Much of their success is attributable to the fact that SSRIs display a much improved side-effect profile compared to TCAs, which, in turn, is a result of their much higher degree of pharmacological specificity. As implied by their name, SSRIs primarily inhibit the reuptake of 5-HT, and they typically lack the extra-monoaminergic activities that characterize TCAs. The SSRIs fluoxetine, citalopram, sertraline and paroxetine have each been evaluated in randomized, placebo-controlled trials in FM.[40, 43, 44] The results of these trials have been somewhat inconsistent, leaving some debate regarding the efficacy of the SSRIs, especially in comparison to TCAs. Two studies have demonstrated positive efficacy for fluoxetine, compared to either placebo or amitriptyline, in treating sleep, pain, fatigue and depression.[45, 46] However, a third study failed to demonstrate any significant improvement in pain, although mild improvements were noted in sleep and depression.[47] Two placebo-controlled trials of citalopram have been published. One was convincingly negative, with citalopram failing to demonstrate any improvements in pain, fatigue, sleep or mood.[48] The second study demonstrated that citalopram significantly improved mood, although other outcome measures did not improve.[49] One study comparing sertraline to amitriptyline demonstrated that the two compounds were equivalent in producing significant improvements in pain, sleep and fatigue.[50] Finally, a recent, large (116 patient), double blind, placebo-controlled trial of paroxetine in FM demonstrated that, while paroxetine did improve aspects of FM associated functional impairments, no difference in pain or sleep scores was noted between drug and placebo.[44] Taken together, SSRIs appear to be effective for treating certain FM symptoms, particularly mood. However, their effect sizes on pain, sleep and fatigue appear to be less robust in comparison to TCAs and other classes of agents.

Despite the wide use of SSRIs in the general population, surprisingly few randomized controlled trials assessing the efficacy of these agents in the functional somatic syndromes have been published. Two recently published randomized, placebo-controlled studies demonstrated that paroxetine[51] and fluoxetine[52] may be of some benefit in the treatment of irritable bowel syndrome. SSRIs do appear to be effective in prophylaxis for chronic tension-type headaches;[28] on the other hand, the use of SSRIs in chronic low-back pain is controversial.[17] Finally, in chronic pelvic pain, sertraline was found to be effective in improving mood, although no improvements in pain were noted.[53]

Dual reuptake inhibitors

DRIs are pharmacologically similar to some TCAs in their ability to inhibit the reuptake of both 5-HT and NE, a feature that may improve their analgesic efficacy.[38, 39, 54] Importantly, DRIs differ from TCAs in being generally devoid of significant activity at other receptor systems, and this selectivity results in diminished side-effects and enhanced tolerability.[38] Venlafaxine

Table 23.3. Pharmacotherapy for FM: summary of randomized controlled trials

Class[a]	Compound(s)	Pharmacology[b]	Treating FM symptoms[c]				Treating other functional somatic syndromes[d]
			Pain	Sleep	Fatigue	Mood	
Tricyclic antidepressants	Amitriptyline Clomipramine Doxepin	5-HT/NE reuptake blocker, cation channel blocker, NMDA antagonist, anticholinergic, antihistaminergic	+	+	+	−	IBS, TMJD, CLBP?; CTTH prophylaxis
SSRI antidepressants	Fluoxetine	5-HT reuptake blocker	+/−	+	+/−	+	CTTH prophylaxis
	Citalopram	5-HT reuptake blocker	−	−	−	+	CTTH prophylaxis
	Sertaline	5-HT reuptake blocker	+	+	+		CTTH prophylaxis
	Paroxetine	*5-HT reuptake blocker*	−	−			*CTTH prophylaxis*
SNRI antidepressants	Venlafaxine	5-HT > NE reuptake blocker	−	−	−	−	CTTH prophylaxis
	Duloxetine	*5-HT > NE reuptake blocker*	+	+	−	−	*CLBP? IC?*
	Milnacipran	*NE > 5-HT reuptake blocker*	+	+	+	+	
MAOI antidepressants	Moclobemide	Reversible inhibitor of MAO-A	−	−	−	−	CTTH prophylaxis, CFS
	Pirlindole	Reversible inhibitor of MAO-A	+	+	+	+	CTTH prophylaxis
NSAIDs	Ibuprofen Naproxen	Non-specific Cox inhibitor	−	−	−	−	CLBP, TMJD (short term)
Antiepileptics	*Pregabalin*	*Calcium channel blocker*	+	+	+	−	
Sedative–hypnotics	Zopiclone Zolpidem	BZ receptor agonist	−	+	−	−	
	γ-Hydroxybutyrate	(Unknown)	+	+	+		

Muscle relaxants	Cyclobenzaprine	5-HT, anticholinergic, antihistaminergic	+	+	+/−	+/−	IBS + FMS
Opiates	Morphine (intravenous)	Mu opiate receptor agonist					
	Tramadol	Mu agonist, 5-HT/NE reuptake blocker	+				CTTH, CLBP
	Tramadol + APAP	*Mu agonist, 5-HT/NE reuptake blocker, analgesic*	+	−			*CTTH, CLBP*
Other	Tropisetron	5-HT$_3$ antagonist	+	+		+	IBS?
	Pramipexole	*Dopamine$_{2,3}$ agonist*	+	+			
	Ketamine Dextromethorphan	NMDA antagonist	+				
	Growth hormone	Growth hormone	+	+			
	Prednisone	Corticosteroid	−	−			

[a]MAOI, monoamine oxidase inhibitor; NSAID, non-steroidal anti-inflammatory drug; SNRI, selective norepinephrine reuptake inhibitor; SSRI, selective serotonin reuptake inhibitor.

[b]BZ, benzodiazepine; 5-HT, serotonin; NE, norepinephrine (noradrenaline); NMDA, N-methyl-D-aspartate.

[c]+, beneficial; −, no benefit or detrimental; blank, not tested.

[d]CFS, chronic fatigue syndrome; CLBP, chronic low-back pain; CTTH, chronic tension-type headache; IBS, irritable bowel syndrome; IC, interstitial cystitis; TMJD, temporomandibular joint disorders.

and duloxetine are the two DRIs currently available within the USA. Venlafaxine is specifically indicated for depression and anxiety, while duloxetine is currently approved for depression and painful diabetic neuropathy.

Significant data support the use of venlafaxine in the management of neuropathic pain,[55–57] and data also indicate that this compound is effective in the prophylaxis of migraine and tension headaches.[58–60] Two open-label studies suggest that venlafaxine is useful in treating multiple symptoms of FM.[61, 62] However, these results were not replicated in a randomized, placebo-controlled trial.[63] Two reasons likely underlie the lack of efficacy seen in the latter trial: drug dosage and duration of treatment. The study by Dwight et al.[62] pushed each patient to their maximally tolerated dose or to a cap of 375 mg/day over the course of the 8-week trial; the overall mean dose taken by patients was 167 mg/day. The 6-week study by Zijlstra et al.,[63] on the other hand, had a single drug arm with a dose of 75 mg/day. The data suggest that venlafaxine is primarily an SSRI at lower doses (i.e. < 150 mg), with NE effects apparent only at higher doses.[13] Sayar et al.,[61] on the other hand, evaluated 75 mg/day in 15 patients over a 12-week period. Importantly, the authors did not detect any improvements in pain at the 6 week time point.

Pharmacologically, duloxetine is similar to venlafaxine in its preferential block of 5-HT reuptake over that of NE, although duloxetine is significantly more potent.[64] This agent is being developed for the FM indication, and the results of two randomized controlled trials of duloxetine in FM have recently been published.[65, 66] Generally, statistically significant improvements in pain and quality of life were seen with duloxetine 60 mg administered either once or twice daily. Curiously, while mood improved as well, the magnitude of the changes did not reach statistical significance, likely due to similar improvements in the placebo groups. Beyond FM, duloxetine has been shown in large, high-quality, randomized controlled trials to be effective in treating neuropathic pain[67, 68] and somatic complaints of patients with major depressive disorder.[69] The latter study did include a group of patients with low-back pain, although whether these patients were presenting predominantly with the acute or chronic conditions is not clear. Additionally, duloxetine had a small benefit in the management of stress urinary incontinence;[70] however, whether or not this may translate into a benefit in interstitial cystitis or chronic pelvic pain is also unclear.

Milnacipran is a DRI that is presently available in parts of Europe and in Japan for the treatment of depression. Milnacipran is unique among clinically available DRIs in its preferential blockade of NE reuptake over that of 5-HT.[64] Milnacipran is presently in Phase III clinical development for FM in the USA, and the results of a Phase II clinical trial were recently published.[71, 72] In a randomized, double-blind, placebo-controlled study, treatment with milnacipran resulted in statistically significant improvements in the pain, sleep, fatigue and mood of patients with FM. Assessments of milnacipran in other pain states, including other functional somatic syndromes, have not been published.

Monoamine oxidase inhibitors

Unlike TCAs and SSRIs, MAOIs increase monoamine levels by blocking their breakdown after release from the neuron. Non-enzyme-specific, irreversible MAOIs, such as phenelzine and tranylcypromine, have been on the market in the USA for many years as antidepressants, although concerns about potentially fatal interactions with certain foods and medications have limited their widespread use.[13] (Note, however, that transdermal delivery of such agents may reduce the risk of such adverse events.[73]) Moclobemide and pirlindole represent second-generation agents that show improved specificity and reversible receptor binding. Both these agents have been approved in Europe as antidepressants, although they are not presently available in the USA. Preliminary studies with moclobemide in FM failed to demonstrate significant analgesic activity when compared to amitriptyline.[13] However, a more recent study has demonstrated the efficacy of this compound in chronic fatigue syndrome, although effects were primarily limited to fatigue.[74] The results of a randomized, double-blind, placebo-controlled trial of pirlindole were more promising, with beneficial effects upon sleep, pain, fatigue and mood.[13] It is of interest to note that MAOIs show greater efficacy than TCAs in treating atypical depression, a particular depression subtype that is relatively common in patients with chronic pain conditions.[75] Finally, while MAOIs have not been tested extensively in other functional somatic syndromes, they do appear to be effective in prophylaxis against chronic tension-type headaches.[28]

Norepinephrine reuptake inhibitors

Reboxetine is a non-tricyclic norepinephrine reuptake inhibitor (NRI) antidepressant that is available in a number of European countries; it is currently unavailable in the USA. Both an open-label trial of reboxetine in 25 FM patients and a case report involving a patient with FM suggest that this compound may be useful for treating pain and fatigue.[76, 77] although more extensive follow-up studies are needed. Another NRI, atomoxetine, has recently been introduced to the US market for the treatment of attention-deficit hyperactivity disorder. While no formal trials of the use of this agent in the treatment of chronic pain have been reported, a letter outlining the beneficial effects of adjunctive therapy involving atomoxetine in two patients with FM was recently published.[78]

Non-steroidal anti-inflammatory drugs

Non-steroidal anti-inflammatory drugs (NSAIDs; including Cox-2-selective agents) and paracetamol (acetaminophen) are used by a large number of FM patients.[79] However, numerous studies have failed to confirm their effectiveness as analgesics in FM, although there is limited evidence that patients may experience enhanced analgesia when treated with combinations of NSAIDs and other agents.[80] This phenomenon may be a result of the fact that painful, inflammatory conditions – including osteoarthritis, rheumatoid arthritis and lupus – are frequently comorbid with FM. NSAIDs have been found to be moderately effective in the treatment of chronic low-back pain.[81] Well-controlled studies do not support the use of NSAIDS in temporomandibular joint disorder, although some patients do obtain short-term relief.[27] Finally, it should be noted that NSAID overuse may actually cause chronic daily headaches.[28]

Antiepileptic drugs

The majority of the antiepileptic drugs increase the seizure threshold through sodium- and/or calcium-channel blockade or by increasing inhibitory neurotransmission; this mechanism of action appears to underlie their analgesic activity as well.[13] Indeed, these compounds are widely used in the treatment of various chronic pain conditions, including postherpetic neuralgia and painful diabetic neuropathy.[82] Pregabalin is currently available in the USA as a scheduled drug for the treatment of epilepsy and diabetic and postherpetic neuralgia. The agent is also in development for FM, and the results of a large Phase II trial were recently published, demonstrating the efficacy of pregabalin in treating pain, sleep disturbances and fatigue in FM patients.[83] Several large studies support the use of this agent in neuropathic pain states,[84, 85] although no specific trials in other functional somatic syndromes have been reported. The precise mechanism of action of pregabalin is unknown, although its analgesic activities may result from the agent's ability to block certain calcium channels.[83] Gabapentin, a compound with similar pharmacology to pregabalin, is presently being tested in a double-blind, randomized controlled trial in FM, and the results are expected by the end of 2006.[86] Gabapentin is specifically indicated for the treatment of postherpetic neuralgia, and studies support its use in the symptomatic treatment of a variety of pain states as well as headache prophylaxis.[28, 82] Another antiepileptic drug, clonazepam, has demonstrated efficacy in treating jaw pain associated with temporomandibular joint disorder,[82] and is also a useful medication in the treatment of restless leg syndrome.[87] However, the widely used antiepileptic drug phenytoin was found to have no effect in irritable bowel syndrome.[82]

Sedative–hypnotic agents

Sedative–hypnotic drugs are widely used by FM patients.[79] A handful of studies have been published on the use of certain non-benzodiazepine hypnotics in FM, such as zopiclone and zolpidem. These reports have suggested that these agents can improve the sleep and, perhaps, fatigue of FM patients, although their effects on pain were not significant.[80]

γ-Hydroxybutyrate (GHB), a precursor of GABA with powerful sedative properties, is currently available in the USA for the treatment of cataplexy and excessive daytime sleepiness associated with narcolepsy. This agent is also being developed for the treatment of FM, and the results of a double-blind, placebo-controlled crossover study were recently published, demonstrating the agent's benefits in the pain, fatigue and sleep domains of FM.[88] However, GHB has significant abuse potential, and this fact may limit its availability for a common condition such as FM.

Several other agents typically classified as sedative–hypnotics have shown promise in the symptomatic treatment of FM in open-label studies. Melatonin, a dietary supplement, was shown to improve sleep and reduce tender-point counts.[13] Finally, patients with significant anxiety symptoms, including post-traumatic stress disorder or panic attacks, may benefit from the use of benzodiazepines, particularly in the early stages of management while waiting for the effects of antidepressant medications to optimize.[89]

Muscle relaxants
Cyclobenzaprine

Cyclobenzaprine is a muscle relaxant that was originally shown to be of some benefit in the management of FM in the mid-1980s.[80] Although typically classified as a muscle relaxant, cyclobenzaprine shares structural and pharmacological similarities with the TCAs.[38] The mechanism of action underlying the muscle-relaxing action of cyclobenzaprine is unclear, although it may be mediated by blockade of 5-HT$_2$ receptors.[38] Data generally support its use in FM, particularly in treating sleep and pain, and there are some data suggesting a synergistic effect when used with fluoxetine.[80, 90] The major problems that patients report with cyclobenzaprine are morning 'hangover' and dry mouth. In this respect, a recent report by Moldofsky et al.[91] on the efficacy of low-dose (1–4 mg) cyclobenzaprine is of special note. Finally, while one study suggests that cyclobenzaprine is effective in treating irritable bowel syndrome symptoms in the context of FM,[92] no randomized controlled trials specifically targeting other functional somatic syndromes have yet been performed.

Tizanidine

Tizanidine is a centrally acting alpha-2 adrenergic agonist that has been approved by the US Food and Drug Administration (FDA) for the treatment of muscle spasticity associated with multiple sclerosis and stroke. The literature suggests that this agent is a useful adjunct in treating several chronic pain conditions, including chronic daily headaches and low-back pain.[23] In a recent open-label trial, patients receiving tizanidine 4–24 mg/day reported significant improvements in several parameters, including sleep, pain and measures of quality of life.[93] Of particular interest was the demonstration that treatment with tizanidine resulted in a reduction in substance P levels within the cerebrospinal fluid of patients with FM. Substance P is an excitatory neurotransmitter that is thought to play a role in pain perception,[38] and multiple studies have confirmed elevated levels of substance P in the cerebrospinal fluid of patients with FM.

Opioids

Typical opioid receptor agonists such as morphine act at some combination of the μ, δ and κ opioid receptors. These receptors are located throughout the central nervous system, and all three receptors appear to play a role in analgesia.[38] Morphine and morphine-like compounds are widely used in many chronic pain states, including temporomandibular joint disorder[27] and subsets of chronic low-back pain.[81] Despite continuing lip service against the use of opioids in FM, a survey of academic medical centres in the USA reported that opioids were used in about 14% of patients.[79] The main problems related to long-term use of opioids are the effects on cognition, reduced motivation to pursue non-pharmacological treatment modalities, aggravation of depression and negative stigmatization by the medical profession and society in general.[23] The usually cited concerns regarding addiction are now known to be unfounded, addiction only occurring in about 0.5% of opioid-treated chronic pain patients.[23] However, problematic opioid use is reported in at least 5% of patients with chronic non-cancer pain on long-term opioid treatment.[94] All patients taking opioids can be expected to develop dependency; this however is not the same as addiction, but implies that this class of medications cannot be stopped abruptly without the patient experiencing withdrawal symptoms.

There have been only a few controlled clinical trials of the use of opioids in FM. Interestingly, acutely administered intravenous morphine was not found to be effective in treating FM pain.[95] Tramadol is another widely used analgesic that has a unique mechanism of action: weak μ agonist activity combined with 5-HT/NE reuptake inhibition.[23] Tramadol has been shown to be an effective treatment for several chronic pain conditions, including chronic daily headaches and low-back pain.[23] Three double-blind studies have demonstrated the efficacy and tolerability of tramadol in the management of FM pain and overall function, both as an isolated compound[23, 96] and in fixed combination with paracetamol.[97]

Other compounds

Finally, a few classes of agents that are not widely used clinically but that have shown promise in controlled trials bear mentioning: dopamine agonists, 5-HT$_3$ antagonists, NMDA antagonists, growth hormone and corticosteroids.

Dopamine agonists

Pramipexole is a dopamine agonist that is currently indicated for parkinsonism, and it is also widely used for the treatment of periodic limb movements during sleep. The results of a double-blind, placebo-controlled trial testing the efficacy of this agent in FM were recently published.[98] Statistically significant improvements in pain, fatigue, function and global well-being were noted, although only at the maximally recommended daily dose (4.5 mg) of pramipexole. Furthermore, while prescribing guidelines for this drug stipulate that this dose be given in a divided fashion (1.5 mg orally three times daily), in this study the full dose was administered all at once at night. That said, tolerability appeared to be similar overall to placebo, although increased anxiety and weight loss were noted in the treatment group. A high percentage of patients in both the drug and placebo groups experienced nausea. Follow-up studies to confirm the efficacy and tolerability of pramipexole are clearly warranted based on this finding.

5-HT$_3$ antagonists

Antiemetics that pharmacologically block 5-HT$_3$ receptors (e.g. ondansetron) have been approved for use in the USA for several years. Tropisetron, another 5-HT$_3$ antagonist, has been tested extensively in European FM patients and has been found to be modestly effective for the treatment of pain and sleep disturbances, although only within certain dose ranges.[99] As recently reviewed,[100] the 5-HT$_3$ antagonist alosetron (Lotronex) has been shown to be of use in managing the pain and diarrhoea in women with irritable bowel syndrome. Unfortunately, due to indiscriminate prescribing, some patients developed severe ileus, and there were several deaths; alosetron, was therefore withdrawn from the market in the USA in November 2000. The drug was reintroduced by the FDA in June 2002, although its use is now strictly limited. Physicians wishing to prescribe alosetron must now register with GlaxoSmithKline's 'Prescribing Program for Lotronex'.

NMDA antagonists

As mentioned above, certain TCAs are known to be NMDA receptor antagonists, although their activity in this regard is relatively weak (i.e. they are low-affinity agents).[38] Three studies have demonstrated that high-level NMDA receptor blockade (effected by the use of high-affinity agents or high doses of low-affinity compounds) can improve pain symptoms in FM patients.[13] However, such high-level blockade is associated with significant cognitive side-effects, thus potentially limiting the utility of this approach.

Growth hormone

Finally, it has been shown in numerous studies that FM patients display a variety of neuroendocrine abnormalities, including low levels of insulin-like growth factor-1 (IGF-1; also known as somatomedin-C) (for a review see Adler et al.[101]). IGF-1 is a factor produced in the liver, primarily in response to growth-hormone secretion. Bennett et al.[102] conducted a randomized, placebo-controlled, double-blind study of the clinical effects of growth-hormone therapy in 50 women with FM and predetermined low IGF-1 levels. The growth-hormone-treated group achieved a significant improvement in Fibromyalgia Impact Questionnaire (FIQ) scores and tender-point counts at 9 months compared to baseline, whereas no significant improvement was observed in the placebo group. Unfortunately, while growth-hormone therapy would appear to offer this subgroup of patients some symptomatic improvement, financial considerations limit the viability of growth hormone as a long-term therapy in this population.

Corticosteroids

Clinicians familiar with treating FM patients sometimes observe that moderate doses of corticosteroids (e.g. prednisone 30–100 mg), given for a concomitant condition such as asthma, result in a short-term improvement in pain and fatigue. There is only one study that has evaluated the effectiveness of corticosteroid therapy in FM.[103] In this double-blind, placebo, randomly assigned crossover trial, 14 days of prednisone (15 mg/day) was no more effective than placebo. However, FM is a common accompaniment of conditions such as rheumatoid arthritis and systemic lupus erythematosus, in which chronic corticosteroid therapy may be indicated. Furthermore, the withdrawal of corticosteroids in such patients may result in a syndrome that

PRACTICE POINTS

Tricyclic antidepressants (TCAs)

- TCAs, such as amitriptyline, are well suited for FM patients with comorbid chronic pain syndromes – including irritable bowel syndrome, temporomandibular joint syndrome and chronic low back pain – although patients with significant mood disorders may benefit from the addition of an SSRI (see below).

- Amitriptyline, in particular, should be started at a dose of 10 mg taken 1–2 hours before bedtime. The dose can then be gradually increased to a maximum of 50 mg/day, as required.

- Morning 'hangover', sicca symptoms and weight gain are problematic for some patients and may necessitate a lower dosage of TCAs. Patients with cardiac disorders predisposing to arrhythmias should not use TCAs.

Selective serotonin reuptake inhibitors (SSRIs)

- SSRIs are well suited for patients presenting with significant mood disorders and/or chronic tension-type headaches, particularly those not tolerant to the side-effects of TCA. The data suggest that combining SSRIs with low-dose TCAs can be synergistic. In general, standard antidepressant doses of SSRIs are utilized, although dose titration is a good idea to avoid side-effects.

Dual reuptake inhibitors (DRIs)

- Data from large, controlled trials support the use of duloxetine in treating the pain and improving overall quality of life in FM patients.

- Open-label data support the use of high-dose (i.e. > 150 mg/day) venlafaxine in FM, although a recent controlled trial of low-dose venlafaxine does not.

- Milnacipran appears promising, with unique pharmacology that bears resemblance to that of amitriptyline. However, it is presently available only in parts of Europe and in Japan and only for the treatment of depression.

Monoamine oxidase inhibitors (MAOIs)

- Based on their putative effects on monoaminergic neurotransmission, MAOIs may be reasonable agents for the treatment of FM symptoms. Second-generation drugs, such as pirlindole, or the use of delivery systems that bypass the gut and liver have both been shown to minimize the drug and food interactions of MAOIs.

Non-steroidal anti-inflammatory drugs (NSAIDs)

- Despite their poor showing in several randomized, controlled trials, NSAIDs likely have utility in suppressing peripheral pain generators resulting from concomitant osteoarthritis, rheumatoid arthritis, etc. Their use in chronic low-back pain is also supported by clinical trials. Care must be taken in using such medications in patients suffering from frequent headaches, due to rebound phenomena.

Antiepileptic drugs

- Pregabalin appears promising for the treatment of many FM symptoms, particularly pain and sleep disturbances.

PRACTICE POINTS – *continued*

Antiepileptic drugs – *continued*

- Gabapentin may represent an alternative to pregabalin, and results of a large, multicentre trial are expected by the end of 2006.

- Clonazepam may be a useful agent in FM patients with concomitant restless leg syndrome and/or anxiety disorders.

Sedative–hypnotic agents

- Zopiclone and zolpidem at standard doses have been shown to improve sleep in FMS patients. The importance of improving sleep in fibromyalgia should not be underrated, as a poor night's sleep has been shown to result in more pain and fatigue the next day.

- GHB may be beneficial in FMS; however, the significant abuse potential of this agent may limit its general availability.

- Patients with significant anxiety symptoms may benefit from the use of benzodiazepines, preferably in combination with psychotherapy.

Muscle relaxants

- Cyclobenzaprine 10–50 mg taken before bedtime appears to improve sleep and pain in FM patients, although side-effects (i.e. 'drug hangover') are common. Recent data suggest that very low doses of cyclobenzaprine may maintain the pain and sleep efficacy, while reducing side-effects of this drug.

- Trials support the use of tizanidine in a variety of chronic pain conditions, and open-label data suggest that it may be useful in FM. Care must be taken in using this compound, as tizanidine can cause transaminitis; liver function tests should be monitored monthly at first and every 3 months thereafter.

Opioids

- The usual dosage regimen is to start tramadol at 50 mg twice daily and increase the dose where indicated to a total maximum of 100 mg four times daily. The use of tramadol at a dose of > 100 mg every 6 hours is contraindicated due to an increased risk of seizures.

- Ultracet is a fixed-dose tablet consisting of tramadol 37.5 mg and paracetamol 325 mg. It is better tolerated than tramadol alone, has a faster onset of action and a longer duration of action. The dose range is 1 to 2 tablets two to four times daily.

Polypharmacy and drug–drug interactions

- Polypharmacy to tackle the symptoms and associated problems of FM may itself aggravate FM.

- The development of the 5-HT syndrome is of particular concern in patients taking multiple 5-HT modulating drugs. In particular, it is a risk in patients receiving tramadol combined with antidepressant drugs. The syndrome should be considered in any FM patient who is experiencing new symptoms such as hyperexcitability, muscle twitching, confusion, euphoria, diarrhoea, increased sweating, shivering or high body temperature.

Continued

mimics FM.[104] Current evidence suggests that the steroid-withdrawal syndrome is a result of increased circulating levels of interleukin-6 resulting from an impaired cortisol stress response.[105] Some elderly patients with a diagnosis of polymyalgia rheumatica may develop a secondary FM syndrome and require continued use of corticosteroids; in such cases the distinction between steroid-responsive polymyalgia rheumatica symptoms and FM symptoms is a difficult clinical challenge.

SUMMARY

As shown in Table 23.3, antidepressant agents represent the most thoroughly tested group of compounds in the FM armamentarium. TCAs, including amitriptyline and doxepin, are versatile and effective in treating the multiple symptoms associated with FM, irritable bowel syndrome, temporomandibular joint disorder and chronic low-back pain, as well as being useful in prophylaxis against chronic tension-type headaches. Unfortunately, tolerability remains a problem. Conversely, SSRIs show improved tolerability and have demonstrated much clearer activity against depressed mood in the context of FM compared with TCAs. However, their activity against other symptoms appears less robust. DRIs are a promising class of compounds, as they potentially combine the benefits of both TCAs and SSRIs. Duloxetine, in particular, has a significant amount of data supporting its use in treating the pain and overall quality-of-life issues in FM; the data supporting the use of venlafaxine is presently much more limited. A third DRI, milnacipran, was found to be effective against multiple domains of FM symptomatology, although this agent is not presently available in the USA. Finally, MAOIs show promise, particularly the newer compounds and formulations that lack food–drug interactions.

The antiepileptic agent pregabalin shows a great deal of promise in treating FM symptomatology, based on Phase II trial results. The related drug, gabapentin, is also in the midst of trials to test its efficacy in FM. Both agents are currently available in the USA. Sedative–hypnotic compounds such as zolpidem and zopiclone appear to be useful adjuncts for the treatment of disturbed sleep, and the use of tramadol to treat FM pain is supported by the results from three trials. NSAIDs, on the other hand, have not been shown to be particularly effective in FM, although they may still play a role in overall patient well-being by reducing the input from peripheral pain generators, including chronic low-back pain and temporomandibular joint disorders.

Some caveats regarding polypharmacy are warranted. As discussed above, the limitations of current therapy necessitate that many FM patients be treated with multiple drugs targeted at specific symptoms (pain, sleep and mood disorders) or associated problems, such as restless leg or irritable bowel syndrome. Indeed, the effective management of central sensitization often necessitates the use of medications that target different locations in pain pathways. For instance, the combined use of medications that target glutamatergic neurotransmission (e.g. gabapentin or pregabalin), μ opioid receptors (e.g. tramadol) and descending inhibitory pathways (e.g. TCAs or DRIs) may be employed in patients with pain that is difficult to treat. However, the resulting polypharmacy may itself aggravate FM. For instance, antiepileptic drugs, opioids, TCAs and muscle relaxants are common causes of increased fatigue. More critically, the use of multiple medications increases the risks of drug–drug interactions. For example, the development of the 5-HT syndrome is of particular concern in patients taking multiple 5-HT modulating drugs, particularly when those agents are predominantly metabolized by the CYP2D6 pathway.[106] This enzyme system catalyses the metabolism of a large number of drugs used in the management of FM, such as tramadol, opioids, TCAs, SSRIs, dextromethorphan and neuroleptic agents.[5] The CYP2D6 gene is highly polymorphic, with more than 70 allelic variants. A deficiency of the CYP2D6 enzyme is inherited as an autosomal-recessive trait in about 7% of caucasians and 1% of East Asians. Patients who inherit low CYP2D6 activity are at particular risk of developing the 5-HT syndrome. This problem should be considered in any FM patient who is experiencing new symptoms such as hyperexcitability, muscle twitching, confusion,

---

RESEARCH AGENDA

Dual reuptake inhibitors (DRIs)

- Definitive answers regarding the efficacy of venlafaxine are needed from the appropriate testing of high doses of this drug.

Monoamine oxidase inhibitors (MAOIs)

- The efficacy of second-generation MAOIs, such as pirlindole, and the use of MAOI delivery systems that bypass the gut and liver should be investigated more thoroughly in chronic pain states such as FM.

Norepinephrine reuptake inhibitors (NRIs)

- More robust studies are needed to support the use of NRIs in FM, although open-label data are promising. Hopefully, the availability of atomoxetine in the USA will encourage clinical testing of this compound in FM and other pain states.

5-HT$_3$ antagonists

- Tropisetron is not available in the USA, although it has been shown to be effective in treating pain, sleep and fatigue, and improving mood in FM, although only within a limited range of doses. Several 5-HT$_3$ antagonists are available in the USA, including alosetron, which is specifically indicated for the treatment of symptoms in women with severe diarrhoea predominant irritable bowel syndrome. It is presently unclear if alosetron improves FM symptoms, particularly at the doses used for irritable bowel syndrome therapy.

NMDA antagonists

- Newer NMDA receptor antagonists that bind to different sites on the NMDA receptor appear to significantly improve on the side-effect profile of older agents. However, the relative efficacy of these newer compounds in the treatment of pain is as yet unclear and needs to be elucidated.

euphoria, diarrhoea, increased sweating, shivering or high body temperature. If unrecognized, a 5-HT syndrome may progress to loss of consciousness and even death.[107]

It is worth re-emphasizing that, as present treatments target specific symptoms, individualized patient therapy is necessary, based on specific symptomatology, tolerance to side-effects, etc. Future research focusing on how the various manifestations of the functional somatic syndromes relate to one another will undoubtedly lead to a more rational targeting of drugs in these complex disorders.

REFERENCES

1. Bennett RM. The rational management of fibromyalgia patients. *Rheum Dis Clin North Am* 2002; **28**: 181–199.

2. Wolfe F, Smythe HA, Yunus MB et al. The American College of Rheumatology 1990 Criteria for the classification of fibromyalgia. Report of the Multicenter Criteria Committee. *Arthritis Rheum* 1990; **33**: 160–172.

3. Staud R, Smitherman ML. Peripheral and central sensitization in fibromyalgia: pathogenetic role. *Curr Pain Headache Rep* 2002; **6**: 259–266.

4. Price DD, Staud R. Neurobiology of fibromyalgia syndrome. *J Rheumatol* 2005; **75**(Suppl): 22–28.

5. Staud R. New evidence for central sensitization in patients with fibromyalgia. *Curr Rheumatol Rep* 2004; **6**: 259.

6. McCain GA. Fibromyalgia and myofascial pain. In: Wall PD, Melzack R (eds), *Textbook of Pain*, 3rd edn. Churchill Livingstone, Edinburgh, 1994, pp. 475–493.

7. Zachrisson O, Regland B, Jahreskog M et al. A rating scale for fibromyalgia and chronic fatigue syndrome (the FibroFatigue Scale). *J Psychosom Res* 2002; **52**: 501–509.

8. Nicassio PM, Moxham EG, Schuman CE et al. The contribution of pain, reported sleep quality, and depressive symptoms to fatigue in fibromyalgia. *Pain* 2002; **100**: 271–9.

9. Mease PJ, Clauw DJ, Arnold LM et al. Fibromyalgia syndrome. *J Rheumatol* 2005; **32**: 2270–2277.

10. Fishbain DA, Lewis J, Cole B et al. Multidisciplinary pain facility treatment outcome for pain-associated fatigue. *Pain Med* 2005; **6**: 299–304.

11. Moldofsky H. Management of sleep disorders in fibromyalgia. *Rheum Dis Clin North Am* 2002; **28**: 353–365.

12. Landis CA, Lentz MJ, Rothermel J et al. Decreased sleep spindles and spindle activity in midlife women with fibromyalgia and pain. *Sleep* 2004; **27**: 741–750.

13. Kranzler J, Gendreau J, Rao S. The psychopharmacology of fibromyalgia: a drug development perspective. *Psychopharmacol Bull* 2002; **36**: 165–213.

14. Aaron LA, Burke MM, Buchwald D. Overlapping conditions among patients with chronic fatigue syndrome, fibromyalgia, and temporomandibular disorder. *Arch Intern Med* 2000; **160**: 221–227.

15. Epstein SA, Kay G, Clauw D et al. Psychiatric disorders in patients with fibromyalgia. A multicenter investigation. *Psychosomatics* 1999; **40**: 57–63.

16. Manu P (ed.). *Functional Somatic Syndromes: Etiology, Diagnosis, and Treatment*. Cambridge University Press, New York, 1999.

17. Salerno SM, Browning R, Jackson JL. The effect of antidepressant treatment on chronic back pain: a meta-analysis. *Arch Intern Med* 2002; **162**: 19–24.

18. Ringel Y, Sperber AD, Drossman DA. Irritable bowel syndrome. *Annu Rev Med* 2001; **52**: 319–338.

19. Cremonini F, Talley NJ. Irritable bowel syndrome: epidemiology, natural history, health care seeking and emerging risk factors. *Gastroenterol Clin North Am* 2005; **34**: 189–204.

20. Katon W, Sullivan M, Walker E. Medical symptoms without identified pathology: relationship to psychiatric disorders, childhood and adult trauma, and personality traits. *Ann Intern Med* 2001; **134**: 917–925.

21. Giesecke T, Gracely RH, Williams DA et al. The relationship between depression, clinical pain, and experimental pain in a chronic pain cohort. *Arthritis Rheum* 2005; **52**: 1577–1584.

22. Thieme K, Turk DC, Flor H. Comorbid depression and anxiety in fibromyalgia syndrome: relationship to somatic and psychosocial variables. *Psychosom Med* 2004; **66**: 837–844.

23. Bennett RM. Pharmacological treatment of fibromyalgia. *J Function Synd* 2001; **1**: 79–92.

24. Sherman JJ, Turk DC, Okifuji A. Prevalence and impact of posttraumatic stress disorder-like symptoms on patients with fibromyalgia syndrome. *Clin J Pain* 2000; **16**: 127–134.

25. Cohen H, Neumann L, Haiman Y et al. Prevalence of post-traumatic stress disorder in fibromyalgia patients: overlapping syndromes or post-traumatic fibromyalgia syndrome? *Semin Arthritis Rheum* 2002; **32**: 38–50.

26. Plesh O, Curtis D, Levine J et al. Amitriptyline treatment of chronic pain in patients with temporomandibular disorders. *J Oral Rehab* 2000; **27**: 834–841.

27. Marbach JJ. Medically unexplained chronic orofacial pain. Temporomandibular pain and dysfunction syndrome, orofacial phantom pain, burning mouth syndrome, and trigeminal neuralgia. *Med Clin North Am* 1999; **83**: 691–710, vi–vii.

28. Redillas C, Solomon S. Prophylactic pharmacological treatment of chronic daily headache. *Headache* 2000; **40**: 83–102.

29. Ranjith G. Epidemiology of chronic fatigue syndrome. *Occup Med (London)* 2005; **55**: 13–19.

30. Fukuda K, Straus SE, Hickie I et al. The chronic fatigue syndrome: a comprehensive approach to its definition and study. International Chronic Fatigue Syndrome Study Group. *Ann Intern Med* 1994; **121**: 953–959.

31. Bouchelouche K, Nordling J. Recent developments in the management of interstitial cystitis. *Curr Opin Urol* 2003; **13**: 309–313.

32. American College of Obstetritians and Gynecologists. ACOG Practice Bulletin No. 51. Chronic pelvic pain. *Obstet Gynecol* 2004; **103**: 589–605.

33. Clauw DJ, Chrousos GP. Chronic pain and fatigue syndromes: overlapping clinical and neuroendocrine features and potential pathogenic mechanisms. *Neuroimmunomodulation* 1997; **4**: 134–153.

34. Yousefi P, Coffey J. For fibromyalgia, which treatments are the most effective? *J Fam Pract* 2005; **54**: 1094–1095.

35. Baker K, Barkhuizen A. Pharmacologic treatment of fibromyalgia. *Curr Pain Headache Rep* 2005; **9**: 301–306.

36. Mease P. Fibromyalgia syndrome: review of clinical presentation, pathogenesis, outcome measures, and treatment. *J Rheumatol Suppl* 2005; **75**: 6–21.

37. Offenbaecher M, Ackenheil M. Current trends in neuropathic pain treatments with special reference to fibromyalgia. *CNS Spectr* 2005; **10**: 285–297.

38. Rao SG. The neuropharmacology of centrally–acting analgesic medications in fibromyalgia. *Rheum Dis Clin North Am* 2002; **28**: 235–259.

39. Fishbain D. Evidence-based data on pain relief with antidepressants. *Ann Med* 2000; **32**: 305–316.

40. Miller LJ, Kubes KL. Serotonergic agents in the treatment of fibromyalgia syndrome. *Ann Pharmacother* 2002; **36**: 707–712.

41. Schatzberg AF. Noradrenergic versus serotonergic antidepressants: predictors of treatment response. *J Clin Psychiatry* 1998; **59**(Suppl 14): 15–18.

42. Ringel Y, Drossman DA. Irritable bowel syndrome: classification and conceptualization. *J Clin Gastroenterol* 2002; **35**(1 Suppl): S7–S10.

43. Arnold LM, Hess EV, Hudson JI et al. A randomized, placebo-controlled, double-blind, flexible-dose study of fluoxetine in the treatment of women with fibromyalgia. *Am J Med* 2002; **112**: 191–197.

44. Purcell C, Patkar A, Jiang W et al. A randomized, double-blind, placebo-controlled trial of paroxetine CR in fibromyalgia. IN: American Psychiatric Association Annual Meeting, New York, 2004.

45. Arnold LM, Hess EV, Hudson JI et al. A randomized, placebo-controlled, double-blind, flexible-dose study of fluoxetine in the treatment of women with fibromyalgia. *Am J Med* 2002; **112**: 191–197.

46. Goldenberg D, Mayskiy M, Mossey C et al. A randomized, double-blind crossover trial of fluoxetine and amitriptyline in the treatment of fibromyalgia. *Arthritis Rheum* 1996; **39**: 1852–1859.

47. Wolfe F, Cathey MA, Hawley DJ. A double-blind placebo controlled trial of fluoxetine in fibromyalgia. *Scand J Rheumatol* 1994; **23**: 255–259.

48. Anderberg UM, Marteinsdottir I, von Knorring L. Citalopram in patients with fibromyalgia – a randomized, double-blind, placebo-controlled study. *Eur J Pain* 2000; **4**: 27–35.

49. Norregaard J, Volkmann H, Danneskiold-Samsoe B. A randomized controlled trial of citalopram in the treatment of fibromyalgia. *Pain* 1995; **61**: 445–449.

50. Celiker R, Cagavi Z. Comparison of Amitriptyline and Sertraline in the treatment of fibromyalgia syndrome. American College of Rheumatology, 64th Annual Scientific Meeting, Philadelphia, PA, USA, Poster presentation, 1 November 2000.

51. Tabas G, Beaves M, Wang J et al. Paroxetine to treat irritable bowel syndrome not responding to high-fiber diet: a double-blind, placebo-controlled trial. *Am J Gastroenterol* 2004; **99**: 914–920.

52. Vahedi H, Merat S, Rashidioon A et al. The effect of fluoxetine in patients with pain and constipation-predominant irritable bowel syndrome: a double-blind randomized-controlled study. *Aliment Pharmacol Ther* 2005; **22**: 381–385.

53. Engel CC Jr, Walker EA, Engel AL et al. A randomized, double-blind crossover trial of sertraline in women with chronic pelvic pain. *J Psychosom Res* 1998; **44**: 203–207.

54. Mochizucki D. Serotonin and noradrenaline reuptake inhibitors in animal models of pain. *Hum Psychopharmacol* 2004; **19**(Suppl 1): S15–S19.

55. Sindrup SH, Bach FW, Madsen C et al. Venlafaxine versus imipramine in painful polyneuropathy: a randomized, controlled trial. *Neurology* 2003; **60**: 1284–1289.

56. Yucel A, Ozyalcin S, Koknel Talu G et al. The effect of venlafaxine on ongoing and experimentally induced pain in neuropathic pain patients: a double blind, placebo controlled study. *Eur J Pain* 2005; **9**: 407–416.

57. Mattia C, Paoletti F, Coluzzi F et al. New antidepressants in the treatment of neuropathic pain. A review. *Minerva Anesthesiol* 2002; **68**: 105–114.

58. Bulut S, Berilgen MS, Baran A et al. Venlafaxine versus amitriptyline in the prophylactic treatment of migraine: randomized, double-blind, crossover study. *Clin Neurol Neurosurg* 2004; **107**: 44–8.

59. Ozyalcin SN, Talu GK, Kiziltan E et al. The efficacy and safety of venlafaxine in the prophylaxis of migraine. *Headache* 2005; **45**: 144–152.

60. Adelman LC, Adelman JU, Von Seggern R et al. Venlafaxine extended release (XR) for the prophylaxis of migraine and tension-type headache: a retrospective study in a clinical setting. *Headache* 2000; **40**: 572–580.

61. Sayar K, Aksu G, Ak I et al. Venlafaxine treatment of fibromyalgia. *Ann Pharmacother* 2003; **37**: 1561–1565.

62. Dwight MM, Arnold LM, O'Brien H et al. An open clinical trial of venlafaxine treatment of fibromyalgia. *Psychosomatics* 1998; **39**: 14–17.

63. Zijlstra TR, Barendregt PJ, van de Laar MA. Venlafaxine in fibromyalgia: results of a randomized, placebo-controlled, double-blind trial. *Arthritis Rheum* 2002; **46**(9 Suppl): S105.

64. Stahl SM, Grady MM, Moret C et al. SNRIs: their pharmacology, clinical efficacy, and tolerability in comparison with other classes of antidepressants. *CNS Spectr* 2005; **10**: 732–747.

65. Arnold LM, Lu Y, Crofford LJ et al. A double-blind, multicenter trial comparing duloxetine with placebo in the treatment of fibromyalgia patients with or without major depressive disorder. *Arthritis Rheum* 2004; **50**: 2974–2984.

66. Arnold LM, Rosen A, Pritchett YL et al. A randomized, double-blind, placebo-controlled trial of duloxetine in the treatment of women with fibromyalgia with or without major depressive disorder. *Pain* 2005; **119**: 5–15.

67. Goldstein DJ, Lu Y, Detke MJ et al. Duloxetine vs. placebo in patients with painful diabetic neuropathy. *Pain* 2005; **116**: 109–118.

68. Raskin J, Pritchett YL, Wang F et al. A double-blind, randomized multicenter trial comparing duloxetine with placebo in the management of diabetic peripheral neuropathic pain. *Pain Med* 2005; **6**: 346–356.

69. Goldstein DJ. Duloxetine: a potential new treatment for depressed patients with comorbid pain. 10th World Congress on Pain, San Diego, CA, 2002.

70. Guay DR. Duloxetine for management of stress urinary incontinence. *Am J Geriatr Pharmacother* 2005; **3**: 25–38.

71. Gendreau RM, Thorn MD, Gendreau JF et al. Efficacy of milnacipran in patients with fibromyalgia. *J Rheumatol* 2005; **32**: 1975–1985.

72. Vitton O, Gendreau M, Gendreau J et al. A double-blind placebo-controlled trial of milnacipran in the treatment of fibromyalgia. *Hum Psychopharmacol* 2004; **19**(Suppl 1): S27–S35.

73. Robinson DS. Monoamine oxidase inhibitors: a new generation. *Psychopharmacol Bull* 2002; **36**: 124–138.

74. Hickie IB, Wilson AJ, Wright JM et al. A randomized, double-blind placebo-controlled trial of moclobemide in patients with chronic fatigue syndrome. *J Clin Psychiatry* 2000; **61**: 643–648.

75. Davidson J, Krishnan R, France R et al. Neurovegetative symptoms in chronic pain and depression. *J Affect Disord* 1985; **9**: 213–218.

76. Krell HV, Leuchter AF, Cook IA et al. Evaluation of reboxetine, a noradrenergic antidepressant, for the treatment of fibromyalgia and chronic low back pain. *Psychosomatics* 2005; **46**: 379–384.

77. Browne JJ, Chong S. The use of reboxetine in fibromyalgia and neuropathic pain; an open, non-randomised, prospective study. In: 10th World Congress of Pain, San Diego, CA, 2002.

78. Berigan T. The use of atomoxetine adjunctively in fibromyalgia syndrome. *Can J Psychiatry* 2004; **49**: 499–500.

79. Wolfe F, Anderson J, Harkness D et al. A prospective, longitudinal, multicenter study of service utilization and costs in fibromyalgia. *Arthritis Rheum* 1997; **40**: 1560–1570.

80. Lautenschlager J. Present state of medication therapy in fibromyalgia syndrome. *Scand J Rheumatol* 2000; **113**(Suppl): 32–36.

81. Deyo RA. Drug therapy for back pain. Which drugs help which patients? *Spine* 1996; **21**: 2840–2849; discussion 2849–2850.

82. Wiffen P, Collins S, McQuay H et al. Anticonvulsant drugs for acute and chronic pain. Cochrane Database Systematic Review, 2000(3): CD001133.

83. Crofford LJ, Rowbotham MC, Mease PJ et al. Pregabalin for the treatment of fibromyalgia syndrome: results of a randomized, double-blind, placebo-controlled trial. *Arthritis Rheum* 2005; **52**: 1264–1273.

84. Lesser H, Sharma U, LaMoreaux L et al. Pregabalin relieves symptoms of painful diabetic neuropathy: a randomized controlled trial. *Neurology* 2004; **63**: 2104–2110.

85. Rosenstock J, Tuchman M, LaMoreaux L et al. Pregabalin for the treatment of painful diabetic peripheral neuropathy: a double-blind, placebo-controlled trial. *Pain* 2004; **110**: 628–638.

86. Available at: http://www.clinicaltrials.gov (accessed 27 August 2006).

87. Hening W, Allen R, Earley C et al. The treatment of restless legs syndrome and periodic limb movement disorder. An American Academy of Sleep Medicine Review. *Sleep* 1999; **22**: 970–999.

88. Scharf MB, Baumann M, Berkowitz DV. The effects of sodium oxybate on clinical symptoms and sleep patterns in patients with fibromyalgia. *J Rheumatol* 2003; **30**: 1070–1074.

89. Kasper S, Resinger E. Panic disorder: the place of benzodiazepines and selective serotonin reuptake inhibitors. *Eur Neuropsychopharmacol* 2001; **11**: 307–321.

90. Tofferi JK, Jackson JL, O'Malley PG. Treatment of fibromyalgia with cyclobenzaprine: a meta-analysis. *Arthritis Rheum* 2004; **51**: 9–13.

91. Moldofsky H, Cesta A, Reynolds WJ et al. A double-blind, randomized, parallel study of the safety, efficacy and tolerability of very low-dosage cyclobenzaprine compared to placebo in subjects with fibromyalgia. *Arthritis Rheum* 2002; **46**(9 Suppl): S614.

92. Santandrea S, Montrone F, Sarzi-Puttini P et al. A double-blind crossover study of two cyclobenzaprine regimens in primary fibromyalgia syndrome. *J Int Med Res* 1993; **21**: 74–80.

93. Russell IJ, Michalek JE, Xiao Y et al. Therapy with a central alpha-2-adrenergic agonist [tizanidine] decreases cerebrospinal fluid substance P, and may reduce serum hyaluronic acid as it improves the clinical symptoms of the fibromyalgia syndrome. *Arthritis Rheum* 2002; **46**(9 Suppl): S614.

94. Portenoy RK, Foley KM. Chronic use of opioid analgesics in non-malignant pain: report of 38 cases. *Pain* 1986; **25**: 171–186.

95. Sorensen J, Bengtsson A, Backman E et al. Pain analysis in patients with fibromyalgia. Effects of intravenous morphine, lidocaine, and ketamine. *Scand J Rheumatol* 1995; **24**: 360–365.

96. Russell IJ, Kamin M, Bennett R et al. Efficacy of tramadol in treatment of pain in fibromyalgia. *J Clin Rheumatol* 2000; **6**: 250–257.

97. Bennett RM, Kamin M, Karim R et al. Tramadol and acetaminophen combination tablets in the treatment of fibromyalgia pain: a double-blind, randomized, placebo-controlled study. *Am J Med* 2003; **114**: 537–545.

98. Holman AJ, Myers RR. A randomized, double-blind, placebo-controlled trial of pramipexole, a dopamine agonist, in patients with fibromyalgia receiving concomitant medications. *Arthritis Rheum* 2005; **52**: 2495–2505.

99. Spath M, Stratz T, Farber L et al. Treatment of fibromyalgia with tropisetron – dose and efficacy correlations. *Scand J Rheumatol* 2004; **119**(Suppl): 63–66.

100. Moynihan R. Alosetron: a case study in regulatory capture, or a victory for patients' rights? *BMJ* 2002; **325**: 592–595.

101. Adler GK, Manfredsdottir VF, Creskoff KW. Neuroendocrine abnormalities in fibromyalgia. *Curr Pain Headache Rep* 2002; **6**: 289–298.

102. Bennett RM, Clark SC, Walczyk J. A randomized, double-blind, placebo-controlled study of growth hormone in the treatment of fibromyalgia. *Am J Med* 1998; **104**: 227–231.

103. Clark S, Tindall E, Bennett RM. A double blind crossover trial of prednisone versus placebo in the treatment of fibrositis. *J Rheumatol* 1985; **12**: 980–983.

104. Dixon RB, Christy NP. On the various forms of corticosteroid withdrawal syndrome. *Am J Med* 1980; **68**: 224–230.

105. Papanicolaou DA, Tsigos C, Oldfield EH et al. Acute glucocorticoid deficiency is associated with plasma elevations of interleukin-6: does the latter participate in the symptomatology of the steroid withdrawal syndrome and adrenal insufficiency? *J Clin Endocrinol Metab* 1996; **81**: 2303–2306.

106. Gnanadesigan N, Espinoza RT, Smith R et al. Interaction of serotonergic antidepressants and opioid analgesics: Is serotonin syndrome going undetected? *J Am Med Dir Assoc* 2005; **6**: 265–269.

107. Boyer EW, Shannon M. The serotonin syndrome. *N Engl J Med* 2005; **352**: 1112–1120.

Acute and postoperative pain

Chapter 24

How to implement an acute postoperative pain service: an update

Harald Breivik, Michele Curatolo, Geir Niemi, Håkon Haugtomt, Gunnvald Kvarstein, Luis Romundstad and Audun Stubhaug

WHY A WELL-ORGANIZED ACUTE PAIN SERVICE IS NEEDED

With the renaissance of epidural anaesthesia about 30 years ago, it soon became common practice to prolong epidural anaesthesia into the postoperative period. This made it possible to control dynamic pain, even after major surgery. It was documented that epidural analgesia reduces postoperative thromboembolism,[1] ileus and negative nitrogen balance.[2] However, hypotension, pronounced motor blockade, weak legs and inability to empty the urinary bladder were all frequent adverse effects of epidural bolus injections or continuous infusions of the high concentrations of local anaesthetics needed for prolonged epidural analgesia with local anaesthetics alone.

When morphine was added to local anaesthetics in the early 1980s, epidural analgesia improved, but respiratory depression, nausea and pruritus were common and potentially dangerous adverse effects.[3] This effective technique was therefore reserved for use in recovery rooms or intensive care units. It was not possible to keep many patients in the recovery ward or the intensive care unit solely for the purpose of giving epidural analgesia. Attempts to move patients with ongoing epidural infusions to the surgical wards were aborted when such complications occurred.

Consequently, surgeons and ward nurses lacked confidence in the safety of epidural analgesia. When we started to plan improvements in postoperative pain management, it was obvious that we first had to overcome these obstacles to wider use of the most effective pain-relieving methods available.

Similar experiences and obstacles impeded the introduction of intravenous opioid patient-controlled analgesia (PCA).[4]

Clearly, the many potential benefits from optimal and prolonged epidural analgesia and the increased comfort of patients receiving PCA could not be obtained without an organization that would make ward nurses confident in the care of patients with epidural analgesia and intravenous PCA. Our early experience led to the conclusion that a dedicated acute pain service was needed.[4, 5]

An important part of these early attempts to improve postoperative pain management was the development of a satisfactory balance between analgesic effects and adverse effects in low concentrations and slow infusion of bupivacaine, fentanyl and adrenalin (epinephrine) through an epidural catheter sited at an optimal segmental level (Figure 24.1). This easily convinced everybody concerned that it is possible to improve postoperative pain management dramatically, and that this can be achieved safely.[5, 6]

An acute pain service organization is needed for effective and safe postoperative pain management. The requirements for and aims of organizing such a service are summarized in Box 24.1.

IMPLEMENTING AN ACUTE PAIN SERVICE

The following is a summary of the lessons learned in Oslo and Berne over 15 years of setting up and implementing an acute pain service. Important factors for successfully implementing an effective acute postoperative pain service are listed in Box 24.2.

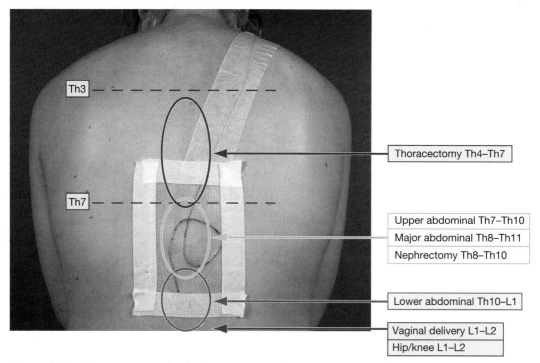

Figure 24.1. The standard triple component epidural solution containing bupivacaine 1 mg/mL, fentanyl 2 μg/mL and adrenalin 2 μg/mL causes segmental epidural analgesia when the drugs reach the spinal cord dorsal horn at the appropriate segmental level. Placement of the epidural catheter at an optimal segmental site, appropriate for the type and site of surgery, is therefore decisive for the quality of the analgesia produced. (See also Plate I of colour section, page xiii.)

Epidural analgesia on surgical wards

Initially, an anaesthetist and a pain nurse followed every patient closely, spending most of the working weekdays on patient care and intensive bedside training of the ward nurses, and on educational classes for ward nurses, surgeons and anaesthetists.

Box 24.1. The requirements for and aims of organizing an acute pain service for management of postoperative pain

A team of trained anaesthetists and nurses are needed to spend time and dedication to:

- fine tune an effective and safe thoracic epidural analgesia regimen on surgical wards
- establish safe intravenous opioid PCA on surgical wards
- make ward nurses confident in monitoring and handling pain pumps and epidural catheters, in monitoring effects, and in observing and treating any adverse effects
- teach anaesthetists in the operating room to place epidural catheters at optimal (thoracic) segmental levels
- teach and motivate on-call anaesthetists to help solve epidural-catheter and pain-pump problems during nights and at weekends
- focus on optimal pharmacological pain relief with non-opioid and opioid analgesics in order to improve postoperative pain relief for all surgical patients

---

Gradually ward nurses could take responsibility for monitoring and titrating epidural analgesia. Soon, nurses on the surgical wards as well as surgeons and physiotherapists realized that well-tailored epidural analgesia can make patients much more comfortable and satisfied with postoperative pain relief, and facilitates nursing care and mobilization of the patients. The patients could breathe deeply and cough effectively even after major thoracic or upper abdominal surgery. When we tried to discontinue epidural analgesia before the third day, the patients became very unhappy with the transition from only mild pain when coughing to strong pain, even at rest. A practice therefore developed of prolonging the epidural analgesia for 4–5 and even up to 7 days when needed after major thoracic or abdominal surgery.[4–6]

Intravenous opioid PCA

Reliable equipment for PCA by intravenous bolus injections of opioids became affordable about 15 years ago. Safe practice of PCA requires good knowledge of the pharmacokinetics of intravenous opioids. As with epidural analgesia, PCA also requires a major effort in the teaching and bedside training of ward nurses to make them confident in administering it. This is the only way to reduce user errors of PCA pumps and intravenous tubing to a minimum. Initially, several near accidents happened involving the use of the wrong intravenous-tubing connections and programming errors by insufficiently trained personnel. Complications caused by patients and relatives tampering with the PCA pumps also occurred. Training of nurses, investment in tamper-

Box 24.2. Important factors for successfully implementing an effective acute postoperative pain service

- Anaesthetist(s) should be able to spend most of their working days on the acute pain service
- Pain nurses must be trained, supervised and supported by an anaesthetist
- There must be continuous working day cover
- An ongoing educational programme for all health personnel involved in the care of surgical patients is essential
- Optimal epidural analgesia for severe dynamic pain should be prolonged for 3–7 days after major surgery
- Selected peripheral nerve blocks should be offered
- There should be standing orders for optimal pharmacological pain relief in all patients using paracetamol plus a NSAID (when tolerated), one dose of a glucocorticoid, and intramuscular, intravenous or oral opioid when needed
- A robust routine is essential to monitor pain-relieving effects, adverse effects, early symptoms of severe sedation and respiratory depression, infection or bleeding in the spinal canal
- There should be high preparedness for handling potentially dangerous complications: bleeding or infection in the spinal canal, severe sedation and respiratory depression

proof, reliable and fail-safe pumps, pharmacy-produced standard drug containers and standing orders for nurses eventually resulted in an effective and very safe PCA service.[4–6]

Improving traditional pharmacological analgesia

During our early attempts to implement epidural analgesia and intravenous opioid PCA it became obvious that most patients have to rely on traditional pharmacological pain relief. It was obvious also that analgesic medications were far from optimally prescribed and administered. By focusing attention on choice of drugs, positive drug interactions, route of administration, timing and dosing, it was possible to improve pharmacological pain relief markedly (see below). This then became an important part of the activities and responsibilities of our acute pain service.[6]

Organizing our model of the acute pain service

An organization with dedicated personnel and resources was obviously needed to enable more patients to benefit from these major advances in effective management of severe pain after major surgery. The first report of anaesthetist-based acute pain service teams was by Ready et al. in 1988.[7] We developed a nurse-based, anaesthesiologist-backed acute pain service organization in Norway and Switzerland,[4–6] as did Rawal in Sweden.[8] In most European countries this is achievable, provided the department of anaesthetics is able to dedicate enough anaesthetist back-up for the pain nurses. Understanding and support from the heads of the surgical departments are mandatory. Pain nurses without sufficient support from motivated and knowledgeable doctors

soon become frustrated by the lack of impact and appreciation of their efforts to improve pain management.

THE COST OF AN ACUTE POSTOPERATIVE PAIN SERVICE

The costs of a well-organized and effective postoperative pain service can be kept low by organizing the acute pain service with pain nurses trained by and with sufficient back-up and support from dedicated anaesthetists. A prerequisite for the success of this low-cost model is that everybody involved in the care of surgical patients understands the need for and is motivated to take part in upgrading postoperative pain management. In our experience this required a considerable effort in informing, convincing and motivating the 'opinion-makers' and people in administrative power in the hospital.[4–6]

A minimum personnel requirement is continuous pain-nurse cover during working days and a back-up of on-call anaesthetists for emergencies during nights and at weekends. Otherwise, small problems rapidly develop, frustrations accumulate and complications increase as the effectiveness of pain management decreases.[9, 10] More than 30% of epidural catheters malfunction during the first postoperative days.[11] Since implementing our acute pain service we have managed to maintain this problem at about 10%, even in our teaching hospitals where there are many trainees and a significant turnover of nurses on surgical wards.[6, 10]

We estimated that our acute pain service costs about US $5 per day, per surgical patient, based on the fact that about 10% of our patients receive epidural or intravenous PCA and the remaining surgical patients benefit from optimized pharmacological postoperative pain relief.[10]

We firmly believe that optimal postoperative pain relief not only increases patients' comfort but also reduces the incidence and severity of adverse effects and complications after surgery (Box 24.3).[2, 12, 13] Preventing only a few patients from developing atelectases and pulmonary infections saves considerable sums of money that would otherwise be spent on antibiotics and intensive care. Therefore, the costs of maintaining an effective acute pain service are easily saved many times over.[10] In addition patients' satisfaction with treatment is markedly increased.[6]

OPTIMIZING PHARMACOLOGICAL ANALGESIA WITH NON-OPIOID AND OPIOID ANALGESICS

Improving dosing, timing and route of administration of paracetamol

Any attempt to improve postoperative pain management should include the optimal use of paracetamol (acetaminophen). Paracetamol is safe in young and old patients, is effective and safe in correct doses, and can be given intravenously, by mouth or rectally.

Clinicians tend to use doses of paracetamol that are too low, especially in children.[14–16] If paracetamol is used as the only non-opioid analgesic, a dose of 1 g every 4 hours (i.e. 6 g per

24 hours) is needed to exploit fully its analgesic effects.[15] This dose of paracetamol is safe for the liver of otherwise healthy patients who require relief of acute pain for about a week after surgery.[15] For more prolonged pain relief, for patients with hepatic dysfunction and in patients on enzyme-P450-inducing agents (e.g. anticonvulsants and ethanol), the dose should not exceed 4 g/day.[9] Severely malnourished patients may have low glutathion, which is needed for neutralization of the reactive intermediary metabolite of paracetamol. If paracetamol is combined with a traditional non-steroidal anti-inflammatory drug (NSAID), 4 g/day will suffice for adult patients (see below about synergy between non-opioid analgesics).

Rectal administration of paracetamol is widely used in many countries, but absorption is slow and variable. Even 1.5 g of paracetamol given rectally can be ineffective.[17] Therefore, the initial rectal dose of paracetamol to adult patients should be 2 g followed by 1 g every 6 hours.

Intravenous administration of paracetamol is preferable when the patient is not able to take paracetamol orally and when gastric emptying is delayed. Paracetamol is usually completely absorbed from the small intestines when taken orally. Therefore the intravenous dose is equal to the oral dose. Juhl et al.[18] documented that there is a higher peak effect and longer duration of effect when an initial dose of 2 g is administered intravenously, compared with 1 g, and, importantly, they did not find hepatotoxic effects at this dose. The median time to rescue analgesic was more than 5 hours after the 2 g dose.[18] These results demonstrate that, provided a study has enough sensitivity by including patients with moderate to severe pain, a 'ceiling effect' of paracetamol at 1 g is not present. However, potential hepatotoxicity dictates that the subsequent doses should be 1 g.

Therefore, we now recommend that adult patients (above 50 kg) with normal nutritional status and not on liver-enzyme-inducing drugs, should be given a 2 g initial dose by mouth, intravenously (or rectally), followed by 1 g every 6 hours. It is important to remember that paracetamol is absorbed from the small intestine. When gastric emptying is slowed after surgery, due to pain or opioids, paracetamol absorption may be less rapid and complete.

Paracetamol dosing in children

After surgery, children tend to be given doses of paracetamol that are much too low. Korpela et al.[16] gave paracetamol rectally as a single dose up to 60 mg/kg body weight to children and documented that the need for rescue analgesia decreased as the dose of paracetamol increased. The dose–effect curve showed a median effective dose of paracetamol (ED_{50}) of 35 mg/kg. More than one-third of patients not receiving paracetamol had nausea after surgery, whereas none of the patients receiving paracetamol 60 mg/kg rectally had nausea.[16]

If the ED_{50} is 35 mg/kg rectally and the maximum safe dose of paracetamol for children is 120 mg/kg per 24 hours,[19] we should give at least 40 mg/kg as the initial rectal dose, followed by 20 mg/kg every 6 hours. This dosing regimen will not exceed the maximum safe dose of 120 mg/kg on the day of surgery and 80 mg/kg per 24 hours thereafter. For postoperative pain lasting around 3 days this dose is safe for otherwise healthy children.[19–23] For paracetamol treatment lasting more than 3 days a dose of 60 mg/kg of paracetamol probably should not be exceeded in 24 hours.[23]

Neonates (especially preterm) and infants below 3 months of age metabolize paracetamol more slowly than older children. In preterm (32–36 weeks) neonates and infants (younger than 3 months) the initial dose should be 20 mg/kg orally or 30 mg/kg rectally, and subsequent doses should be 20 mg/kg every 8 hours (every 6 hours for infants older than 3 months).[23]

Doses of intravenous paracetamol for children above 10 kg are 20 mg/kg, followed by 15 mg/kg every 6 hours.[24] For children below 1 year of age, the dose is 7.5 mg/kg every 6 hours.

Synergy between paracetamol and traditional NSAIDs

Whenever analgesic drugs that act via different mechanisms are administered at the same time, there is likely to be an additive

---

Box 24.3. Harmful effects of unrelieved postoperative pain that can be reduced by an effective acute postoperative pain service

- Respiratory functions:
  - decreased cough, forced vital capacity
  - atelectases, pneumonia, sepsis
- Cardiovascular functions:
  - tachycardia, hypertension, increased systemic vascular resistance
  - increased myocardial oxygen demand
  - ischaemic events, dysrhythmias, infarction
- Gastrointestinal functions:
  - nausea and vomiting
  - paralytic ileus
  - delayed oral nutrition
- Renal and urinary tract functions:
  - oliguria
  - urinary retention
- Endocrine and metabolic functions:
  - increased catabolism
  - impaired immune functions
- Psychological and mental functions:
  - disturbed sleep
  - anxiety
  - decreased cognitive capacity
- Pain modulation in the central nervous system:
  - chronic, intractable, neuropathic pain after surgery
- Hindering of nursing care and delaying and prolonging rehabilitation
- Increases hospital cost

or even supra-additive (synergistic) effect.[9] Paracetamol and NSAIDs relieve pain through different analgesic mechanisms.[25–30] NSAIDs inhibit both cyclo-oxygenase isoenzymes (Cox-1 and Cox-2) in the peripheral and central nervous systems. Paracetamol inhibits the release of prostaglandin E_2 in the spinal cord and has effects on serotonin (5-HT) mechanisms for spinal-pain inhibition. Both NSAIDs and paracetamol seem to reduce nitric oxide production in the central nervous system. At low, but not at high, concentrations of arachidonic acid, paracetamol inhibits Cox-2.[30] This explains why in animal studies supra-additive effects between paracetamol and traditional NSAIDs have been well documented. Peak effect, duration of analgesia and anti-inflammatory effects were all increased and prolonged when paracetamol and NSAIDs were coadministered to arthritic animals.[31, 32]

A controlled, double-blind trial on pain relief after surgical removal of impacted third molars provided evidence that it makes sense to coadminister paracetamol and diclofenac.[33] When paracetamol 1 g and diclofenac 100 mg were coadministered, pain relief was more pronounced and lasted much longer than when either paracetamol or diclofenac was given alone. Of particular clinical importance are the findings that coadministration of paracetamol and diclofenac caused superior and longer lasting pain relief with fewer side-effects than did paracetamol plus codeine (Figure 24.2).[33] These additive effects between paracetamol and other NSAIDs (e.g. ibuprofen) have been confirmed in other trials.[34–37] The side-effects of opioids, such as sedation, nausea and dizziness, can be reduced if paracetamol and an NSAID are coadministered.[33–36]

Single oral dose

- ● Paracetamol 1000 mg
- ○ Diclofenac 100 mg
- ▽ Paracetamol 1000 mg + codeine 60 mg
- ▼ Paracetamol 1000 mg + diclofenac 100 mg
- ■ Paracetamol 1000 mg + codeine 60 mg + diclofenac 100 mg

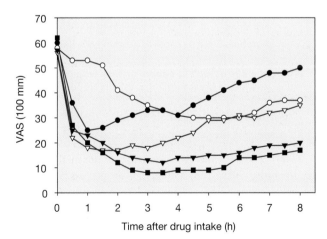

Figure 24.2. Combining paracetamol 1000 mg with diclofenac 100 mg relieves pain better and for much longer compared with either drug alone and with paracetamol 1000 mg plus codeine 60 mg. Modified from Breivik et al.[33]

There is now sufficient evidence available to recommend that a NSAID be added to paracetamol for short-term postoperative pain relief, unless there are any known contraindications to NSAIDs, such as allergy, gastrointestinal ulcer disease, potential bleeding problems, renal functional impairment or bronchospastic asthma.[37] When a NSAID is added, the dose of paracetamol can be kept well within a safe range (see above).

Several alternatives to diclofenac and ibuprofen are available in various countries for oral, rectal or intravenous administration: indomethacin, ketoprofen, tenoxicam and ketorolac. Methamizol is another non-opioid analgesic that is widely used in many parts of the world, but its use is prohibited in the Nordic countries because of its serious effects on bone marrow.

When using NSAIDs, either alone or in combination with paracetamol, the many contraindications and relative contraindications must always be kept in mind.

NSAIDs are contraindicated when patients have:

- actual or potential bleeding problems
- a history of gastrointestinal ulceration
- aspirin-sensitive asthma
- renal impairment
- hypovolaemia
- hyperkalaemia
- severe liver dysfunction
- congestive heart failure
- circulatory failure
- hypertension
- pre-eclampsia
- been on diuretics.

NSAIDs should be used with caution in:

- elderly patients, who often have significant renal impairment
- diabetic patients (renal impairment is likely)
- patients with widespread vascular disease
- patients on ACE inhibitors, beta blockers, cyclosporin or methotrexate.

The selective Cox-2 inhibitors should also be used with caution in most of the above-mentioned conditions, except for patients with bleeding problems. Actual gastrointestinal ulcerative problems may be exacerbated by Cox-2 inhibitors. These agents are certainly contraindicated in patients with coronary artery disease, cardiac failure, renal impairment, in patients with widespread vascular disease and in patients on diuretics or ACE inhibitors.[38]

Single-dose glucocorticoid for postoperative pain and nausea

The postoperative-pain-relieving effects of glucocorticoid drugs were studied in the early 1980s in several elegant RCTs conducted by Løkken and Skjelbred and their collaborators.[39] Recent studies have confirmed the analgesic effects of these drugs and the added benefit of antiemetic effects.[40, 41] When administered as a single dose after surgery glucocorticoids have no adverse effects on the gastrointestinal tract, kidney or liver, do not increase bleeding or postoperative infections, and do not impede wound healing. They seem to reduce postoperative fatigue and sensory changes and, possibly, the risk of chronic pain after surgery.[42]

No dose–effect studies have been done on these drugs, but intravenous dexamethasone at a dose of 4–8 mg for moderately extensive surgery and up to 16 mg for major and traumatic surgery (or methylprednisolone 40–125 mg) given at the end of the procedure appear to be effective in most cases. For children we administer dexamethasone 0.4 mg/kg (up to 4 mg). A much higher dose will cause transient hyperglycaemia, but no other adverse effects have been observed.[43]

Potent opioids for more severe postoperative pain

When epidural analgesia or neural blocks are not possible, patients with severe pain will require a potent opioid in addition to paracetamol and a NSAID. Opioid analgesics can be given by mouth or rectally, but a high first-pass metabolism makes them more effective by injection.

Oral, controlled-release opioid for postoperative analgesia after outpatient surgery

More extensive and painful surgery is now performed on an outpatient basis. These patients will often require potent opioids by mouth, in addition to paracetamol and NSAIDs. Immediate and controlled-release oxycodone have been documented to improve pain relief, quality of sleep, and nausea and vomiting after outpatient surgery of the knee.[44]

Nurse-controlled intramuscular administration of opioid

Harmer and Davies[45] found that, when nurses observe pain regularly, using a simple verbal categorical pain-intensity scale, and have standing orders to give morphine by intramuscular injection, most patients will get satisfactory pain relief at rest.

Standing orders for ward nurses to administer intramuscular morphine (or ketobemidone in Scandinavia) on surgical wards (prescribed jointly by the heads of the acute pain service and the surgical departments) should be in place as detailed in Box 24.4.

Nurse-controlled intravenous administration of opioid

Ward nurses trained to give morphine (or ketobemidone in Scandinavia) intravenously for severe postoperative pain according to standing orders use smaller doses and only 10 minutes between injections (see below). The pain-relieving effect comes on more rapidly and titration can be tailored quicker and better for both patients and nurses.[46]

Standing orders for nurse-administered intravenous morphine (or ketobemidone in Scandinavian countries) (prescribed jointly by the heads of the acute pain service and the surgical departments) should be in place as detailed in Box 24.5.

Box 24.4. Standing orders for intramuscular morphine (or ketobemidone in Scandinavia) on surgical wards (prescribed jointly by the heads of the acute pain service and the surgical departments)

If the patient has severe pain *despite taking* paracetamol plus a NSAID:

- *and* the patient is awake or only dozing intermittently
- *and* the respiratory rate is above 8 breaths/minute
- *and* the systolic blood pressure is above 100 mmHg
- *and* if more than 60 minutes have elapsed since the last intramuscular dose of morphine

   When all these conditions are present, the nurse has standing orders to give an intramuscular injection of:
   - morphine 5 mg to patients weighing 40–65 kg
   - morphine 10 mg to patients weighing 66–100 kg

If the patient is difficult to awaken and the respiratory rate slows to less than 8 breaths/minute, call the responsible doctor and

- give naloxone 0.1 mg intravenously
- repeat until the patient can easily be awakened and respiratory rate is 12 breaths/minute

---

Box 24.5. Standing orders for intravenous morphine (or ketobemidone in Scandinavia) on surgical wards (prescribed jointly by the heads of the acute pain service and the surgical departments)

If the patient has severe pain *despite taking* paracetamol plus a NSAID:

- *and* the patient is awake or only dozing intermittently
- *and* the respiratory rate is above 8 breaths/minute
- *and* the systolic blood pressure is above 100 mmHg
- *and* if more than 10 minutes have elapsed since the last intravenous dose of morphine

   When all these conditions are present, the nurse has standing orders to give an intravenous bolus injection of:
   - morphine 1 mg to patients weighing 40–65 kg
   - morphine 2 mg to patients weighing 66–100 kg

If the patient is difficult to awaken and the respiratory rate is less than 8 breaths/minute, call the responsible doctor and

- give naloxone 0.1 mg intravenously
- repeat until the patient can easily be awakened and the respiratory rate is 12 breaths/minute

---

ASPECTS OF A SUCCESSFUL PCA REGIMEN

Allow patients to take control of their pain relief

PCA was developed more than 30 years ago as a means of improving the effectiveness of opioid analgesia. The patient is the one best able to evaluate the need for analgesia and can find the best balance between the pain-relieving effect and the adverse effects of opioids, especially nausea, unpleasant sedation and cognitive dysfunctions. However, respiratory depression, nausea, hallucinations and nightmares are not less with opioid PCA than with nurse-controlled opioid administration.[47] PCA is now a widely used approach for the management of postoperative pain. Some important details from our experience during the last 15 years are described below.[6, 9]

Exploiting the morphine-sparing effect of paracetamol or NSAIDs

The morphine-sparing effect of paracetamol or NSAIDs can be exploited in order to reduce adverse effects of morphine PCA.

Oral paracetamol at 6 g per 24 hours reduces PCA morphine consumption and improves analgesia, reduces adverse effects and increases overall patient satisfaction.[15] Intravenous paracetamol 1 g every 6 hours similarly reduced PCA morphine consumption by almost 40% after orthopaedic surgery.[48]

NSAIDs also provide morphine-sparing effects and improve analgesia when coadministered with PCA morphine.[49] This may involve pharmacokinetic as much as pharmacodynamic interactions: NSAIDs transiently decrease renal function, impeding renal excretion of active morphine metabolites.[50–52] This may explain why a reduced consumption of PCA morphine is not always followed by reduced opioid side-effects.[53] Although the patient receives less morphine, the slower renal excretion causes accumulation of active morphine metabolites. These metabolites cause opioid analgesia as well as opioid side-effects.

Paracetamol plus NSAID with intravenous opioid PCA

The additive analgesic effects of paracetamol and diclofenac reduced morphine consumption with PCA more than when either agent was used alone.[17] Fletcher et al.[54] documented additive analgesic and morphine-sparing effects of paracetamol 1 g and ketoprofen 50 mg every 6 hours on pain relief at rest and during movement.

Non-opioid analgesic regimens with PCA intravenous opioid for adults

These regimens are summarized in Box 24.6.

NEURAXIAL AND PERIPHERAL NERVE BLOCKS FOR DYNAMIC PAIN AND REDUCED RISK OF COMPLICATIONS

Intense pain is experienced when the patient breathes deeply and coughs after thoracic or upper abdominal surgery. This dynamic pain can be relieved most effectively with neuraxial analgesia containing local anaesthetic agents, reinforced by an opioid and an α_2 agonist. This will enable the patient to breathe deeply, cough effectively and bring up impacted bronchial secretions, preventing atelectases, pneumonia, sepsis, hypoxaemia and ischaemic cardiac events, including postoperative myocardial infarction.

Box 24.6.   Non-opioid analgesic regimens with PCA intravenous opioid for adults

Basic analgesia with paracetamol and a glucocorticoid

- Paracetamol 2 g initial dose, followed by 1 g every 6 hours – administered intravenously, orally (or rectally)
- Dexamethasone 8–16 mg as a single dose intravenously at the end of surgery – alternative: methylprednisolone 40–125 mg

When there are no contraindications to NSAIDs

Reinforce and prolong paracetamol analgesia by adding one of these NSAIDs:

- diclofenac 50 mg every 8 hours – for intravenous, oral or rectal administration
- ketoprofen 100 mg every 8 hours – for intravenous, oral or rectal administration
- ketorolac 10–30 mg every 8 hours – for intravenous or oral administration
- ibuprofen 400 mg every 8 hours – for oral or rectal administration

---

Effective relief of dynamic pain after major orthopaedic surgery with peripheral blocks enables patients to move limbs, hastening rehabilitation of normal functions and reducing thromboembolic complications.

Continuous peripheral nerve blocks

Continuous cervical and brachial plexus blockade with catheter infusion of a local anaesthetic provides excellent analgesia and improves circulation and mobility of the upper extremity after shoulder, arm or hand surgery.[55] Patients recovering from major knee surgery, who received either femoral nerve block or epidural block for 72 hours, were able to move their knee joints more during the early days after surgery and had a shorter stay in the rehabilitation unit compared with patients having PCA intravenous morphine.[56] Intercostal nerve blocks and paravertebral blocks improve pulmonary function and reduce pulmonary complications.[12, 57]

Robust evidence for beneficial effects of optimal epidural analgesia

A number of studies and reviews form a substantial evidence base for the fact that prolonged and *optimal* epidural analgesia, as a most important part of a comprehensive rehabilitation programme, can reduce postoperative morbidity.[1–3, 12, 13, 58–70] Epidural local anaesthetics, with or without opioids, decrease the risk of postoperative pulmonary complications (atelectases and pneumonia) by 50–70% compared with systemic opioids.[12] Epidural opioids alone do not reduce significantly the risk of postoperative pulmonary complications.[12] This is also true for gastrointestinal motility after abdominal surgery: an epidural local anaesthetic shortens the time of intestinal paralysis after surgery compared with systemic or epidural morphine.[58–60]

Thus a local anaesthetic in epidural analgesia not only provides excellent pain relief, but also benefits cardiopulmonary and gastrointestinal functions. A Cochrane Review from 2006 of 13 randomized studies on 1224 patients having abdominal aortic surgery clearly shows that epidural analgesia provides better dynamic pain relief for 3 days, reduces the duration of tracheal intubation and postoperative mechanical ventilation, and reduces cardiac complications, including myocardial infarction, and gastric and renal complications.[70]

Less than optimal epidural analgesia: poor pain relief and increased risk of complications

Two negative studies illustrate that less than optimal epidural analgesia may not be beneficial to the patient.[71, 72] When almost 50% lost their epidural catheter, or never received an epidural catheter, but still were analysed as if they had received an epidural (intention-to-treat analyses), when various opioids and local anaesthetics were used in unknown doses, and no account is given in a multicentre study monitoring regime, this is likely to be far from an optimal epidural regimen.[72] When a high dose of fentanyl and a very low concentration of a local anaesthetic are administered epidurally and the effect on dynamic pain is no better than that of intravenous fentanyl, the epidural procedure cannot be optimal.[71]

Thoracic or lumbar epidural catheter?

It is now well established that, compared with a lumbar epidural, a thoracic epidural is more beneficial for patients who are at high risk of cardiopulmonary complications after thoracic or major abdominal surgery.[61, 63, 64, 73, 74]

Thoracic epidural analgesia has the following beneficial effects (with local anaesthetic with or without an opioid):[61–64]

- it dilates the stenotic coronary arteries and increases myocardial oxygen supply
- it decreases myocardial oxygen consumption
- it decreases myocardial ischaemic events and postoperative myocardial infarction
- it improves lung function and oxygenation
- it improves gastrointestinal motility.

Lumbar epidural (with local anaesthetic with or without an opioid) may be harmful to high-risk cardiac patients:[63, 73, 74]

- it dilates the arteries of the lower part of the body, with compensatory constriction in the upper part
- it constricts the coronary arteries
- it decreases myocardial oxygen supply
- it causes leg weakness and urinary retention
- it does not improve gastrointestinal motility
- it does not improve lung function.

Thus, *a lumbar epidural may even increase the cardiac risk* and does not improve pulmonary function or gastrointestinal motility. Lack of awareness of these important differences between thoracic and lumbar epidural analgesia is one of the important reasons for the confusion and conflicting opinions on the effects of epidural analgesia on outcome after surgery.[13]

Clearly, epidural catheters that are placed too low or too high, in a lateral root sleeve, and catheters that after correct positioning are dislocated out of the epidural space, will all give poor-quality pain relief. High concentrations and bolus doses of lipophilic opioids are rapidly absorbed and produce well-known systemic opioid adverse effects (nausea, vomiting, respiratory depression, sedation, dizziness, pruritus and urinary retention). These adverse effects ruin the quality of epidural pain relief. Several negative outcome studies clearly had poor control of, or did not document, these confounding factors. Only a well-tailored and optimally conducted epidural analgesia can be of benefit to the patient. Conducting an optimal epidural analgesia regimen requires knowledge and experience, and is definitely labour intensive.

INTRATHECAL ANALGESIA

Excellent dynamic pain relief can be achieved by subarachnoid infusion of a local anaesthetic, an opioid and an adrenergic drug. The dose needed is approximately 10% of the epidural dose. The fear of subarachnoid infection via the catheter canal is the reason why this technique is not more widely used. However, when an epidural catheter occasionally migrates through the meninges, or when an epidural catheter is accidentally placed in the subdural or subarachnoid space, we continue the infusion with 1/10 of the infusion rate, using the same analgesic mixture (see below).[6]

RISKS OF SERIOUS COMPLICATIONS FROM EPIDURAL AND INTRATHECAL ANALGESIA

Hypotension, sedation and respiratory depression

If a high dose of local anaesthetic is administered epidurally, hypotension, muscle weakness and urinary retention often result, even if the epidural catheter is in a low thoracic or thoracolumbar area. A high dose of any potent opioid will cause immediate and sometimes (especially after morphine) late respiratory depression and sedation. These are supra-spinal effects initially due to systemic absorption and later to cephalad migration of cerebrospinal fluid.

Epidural bleeding and epidural infection

These are rare, but potentially serious, complications that may cause permanent neurological damage if not diagnosed and treated early.

Infections are due to skin bacteria entering the epidural catheter insertion site, causing catheter tract infection in about 1 in 1000 epidurals for postoperative pain lasting more than about 3 days, and epidural abscess formation in about 1 in 10,000 postoperative epidurals.[75–77] There is increased *risk of infectious complications* in patients with diabetes, cancer, renal failure, in malnourished patients, patients on steroids and immunosuppressed patients. The risk of infection increases

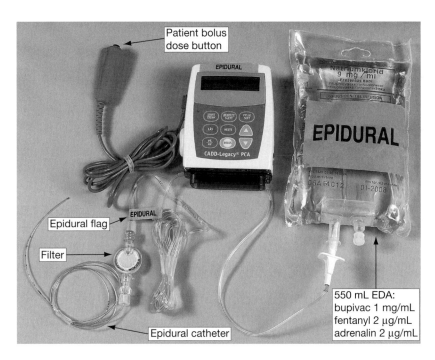

Figure 24.3. Our system for delivering continuous or patient-controlled epidural analgesia. The closed system reduces the risk of bacterial contamination. (See also Plate II of colour section, page xiii.)

when hygienic aspects of catheter care are suboptimal. Our system for delivering epidural analgesia is shown in Figure 24.3, and the hygiene precautions for affixing catheters are detailed in Figure 24.4.

Epidural haematomas are less frequent (1 in 4000 to 1 in 200,000) but progress more rapidly to irreversible ischaemic spinal cord damage.[75–77]

Risk factors for intraspinal bleeding are a history of clinical bleeding abnormalities, renal impairment, thrombocytes below 100,000, potent antiplatelet drugs (clopidogrel, triclopidin), warfarin with an International Normalized Ratio (INR) above 1.8, high-dose thromboprophylaxis with low-molecular-weight heparins or antithrombin drugs and thrombolytic drugs. Acetylsalicylic acid and NSAIDs increase the risk of bleeding slightly, but in combination with any other risk factor they may increase the likelihood of intraspinal bleeding significantly. Spinal deformities, spinal stenosis, ankylosing spondylitis and any 'difficult' epidural catheterization with a 'bloody tap' increase the risk of spinal bleeding. Elderly female patients with osteoporotic spinal vertebrae are especially high-risk patients with one intraspinal haematoma per 3600 patients after combined spinal epidural for knee arthroplasty.[77]

Early warning symptoms

These are increasing *leg weakness* and new *back pain*. These are easily missed if excessive doses of local anaesthetics are used, especially if lumbar epidural catheters are employed (leg weakness will already be a result of the epidural local anaesthetic motor block). When patients are heavily sedated or communication with patients is not possible, spinal cord functions cannot be followed easily (e.g. an intubated and ventilated patient). Monitoring routines must be robust enough to detect increasing leg weakness and new backache.[6, 76]

Treatment and prognosis

Early diagnosis, verified by magnetic resonance imaging (MRI) (a computed tomography (CT) scan is less sensitive), antibiotics and drainage of an abscess within 3 days of onset of leg weakness, lead to recovery in most cases. If delayed beyond 10 days from the onset of symptoms, prognosis is very poor.[75] The 'time of grace' is brief if intraspinal bleeding causes leg weakness. Verification of diagnosis with MRI and laminectomy within 10 hours of the onset of symptoms will recover spinal cord function in about 80% of cases. A delay of 24 hours will result in recovery of normal functions in less than 5% of cases.[76]

Unfortunately, because of a low index of suspicion for such rare complications and low awareness of the significance of early symptoms and lack of monitoring routines, diagnosis is far too often delayed beyond the time when recovery of spinal cord function is possible.[77]

OPTIMIZING THE EFFICACY AND SAFETY OF EPIDURAL ANALGESIA

The efficacy and safety of epidural analgesia improve when drugs with different mechanisms of analgesia are combined. The actions of each drug will reinforce each other and only small doses of each drug are needed for adequate pain relief. If these drugs have different and dose-related side-effects, adverse effects may decrease in frequency and severity as doses of each drug can be reduced.

During the last 15 years[4] we have used a mixture of:

- a local anaesthetic (bupivacaine 1 mg/mL)
- a lipophilic opioid (fentanyl 2 μg/mL)
- and an adrenergic drug (α_2-agonist) (adrenalin 2 μg/mL).

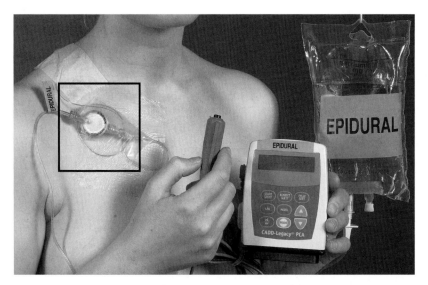

Figure 24.4. Strict hygienic precautions are necessary. Fix the epidural catheter with transparent adhesive covers. Do not change the tubing or filter unless they are contaminated. Inspect for signs of local inflammation (redness) and examine for local tenderness at the insertion site at least once daily. If there are signs of catheter site or catheter track infection, remove the catheter, culture the tip of the catheter and start antibiotics early. (See also Plate III of colour section, page xiv.)

Fix epi-catheter with Tegaderm/Opsite, and tape edges carefully

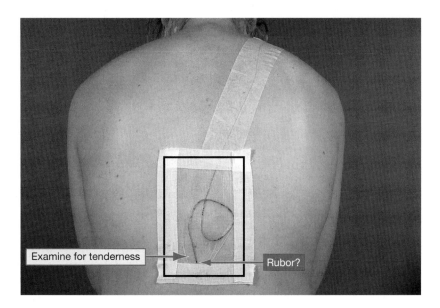

These three drugs produce spinal-cord analgesia by three different mechanisms that act on pain-impulse transmission in the spinal cord. Subanaesthetic doses of bupivacaine inhibit excitatory synaptic mechanisms in the spinal cord. Fentanyl and adrenalin increase inhibition of pain-impulse transmission from primary afferent nociceptive neurons to transmission neurons in the dorsal horn of the spinal cord:

- fentanyl acts on pre- and postsynaptic opioid receptors
- adrenalin (epinephrine) acts on pre- and postsynaptic α_2-receptors[78]
- subanaesthetic concentrations of bupivacaine inhibit Ca^{2+} flow and synaptic excitation.

Synergistic reinforcement between the different pain-inhibiting mechanisms[79] of these drugs allows for dose reduction (Figure 24.5).[80–84] These three drugs have different side-effect profiles, and when only small doses are needed of each of

the three drugs, dose-related respiratory depression, nausea, itching, gastrointestinal immobility, sedation, hypotension, urinary retention and leg weakness are observed infrequently and at low severity.[4–6, 85]

Nurses on the surgical wards are trained to titrate the infusion rate of the epidural analgesic mixture. When patients are awake and have stable vital signs, they are allowed to use the dose-release button to give themselves boluses when needed from the same epidural analgesic mixture (patient-controlled epidural analgesia) (see Figures 24.3 and 24.2).[80–85]

Adrenalin increases the effectiveness of epidural analgesia

In randomized, double-blind, crossover studies we documented the powerful effects of adrenalin in epidural infusions: pain intensity was practically zero at rest after major abdominal or thoracic surgery with an epidural mixture of bupivacaine (or

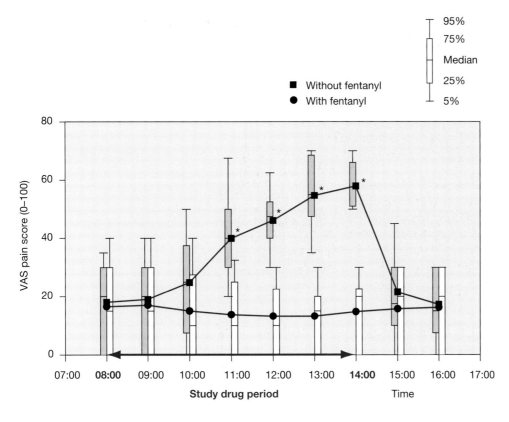

Figure 24.5. Epidural analgesia with bupivacaine 1 mg/mL and adrenalin 2 μg/mL is markedly improved by adding fentanyl 2 μg/mL. Modified from Niemi and Breivik.[81] Data from a double-blind, crossover study comparing bupivacaine and adrenalin with and without fentanyl.

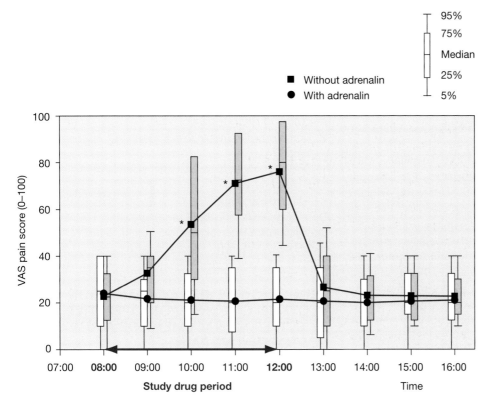

Figure 24.6. Epidural analgesia with bupivacaine 1 mg/mL and fentanyl 2 μg/mL is markedly improved by adding adrenalin 2 μg/mL. Modified from Niemi and Breivik.[83] Data from a double-blind, crossover study comparing bupivacaine and fentanyl with and without adrenalin.

ropivacaine) 1 mg/mL, fentanyl 2 μg/mL and adrenalin 2 μg/mL. When the adrenalin dose was reduced below 1.5 μg/mL, or removed from the mixture, pain increased at rest, and dramatically so during coughing, in spite of an increasing infusion rate, extra epidural bolus injections and morphine intravenous boluses for rescue analgesia. When the standard mixture with adrenalin 2 μg/mL was reintroduced, pain relief again became optimal (see Figure 24.6).[80–85]

Two positive interactions are possible between adrenalin and the two other analgesic drugs: pharmacokinetic interactions and pharmacodynamic interactions.

- *Pharmacokinetic interactions.* Adrenalin, a vasoconstrictor in the epidural space, slows and reduces the systemic absorption and systemic side-effects of fentanyl and bupivacaine.[80, 82, 83] Thus more of these two drugs can diffuse through the meninges and into the cerebrospinal fluid and spinal cord, where they exert their analgesic effects by different mechanisms.
- *Pharmacodynamic interactions.* Adrenalin, an α_2-receptor agonist, has an analgesic effect of its own in the spinal cord dorsal horn that is different from those of fentanyl and bupivacaine and therefore may interact in a supra-additive manner with these two drugs.[78–80]

Low-dose epidural infusion of adrenalin does not impair spinal cord blood flow. Adrenergic drugs do not cause vasoconstriction in central nervous system vessels. More than a century of experience using adrenalin with local anaesthetic drugs for subarachnoid anaesthesia and analgesia has documented that even very high doses of adrenalin (200–1000 µg) directly into the cerebrospinal fluid does not impair blood flow to the spinal cord. Experimental studies in dogs and cats have not shown any deleterious effects on the spinal cord blood flow from large doses of adrenalin directly into the subarachnoid space or into the epidural space. For references, see Niemi and Breivik,[80] Curatolo[84] and Niemi.[85]

Adrenalin increases the safety of epidural analgesia

In addition to its potentiating effect on analgesia produced by epidural infusion of small doses of bupivacaine and fentanyl, adrenalin also improves safety because it slows and reduces the absorption of fentanyl into the systemic circulation. The serum concentration of fentanyl was almost not measurable when adrenalin was added to the epidural infusion.[80] When adrenalin was removed from the epidural infusion, serum fentanyl concentrations increased and the patients experienced adverse effects (sedation, nausea and pruritus).[80] One patient illustrated this safety aspect of adrenalin in our standard epidural mixture. Due to an error in programming of the infusion pump, this patient received 80 mL/hour (instead of 8 mL/hour) for about 2 hours: except for excellent analgesia and leg weakness, there were no indications of toxic symptoms.

Adrenalin, by causing vasoconstriction in epidural vessels (as opposed to subarachnoid vessels, see above) and by increasing platelet adhesiveness, may reduce the risk of epidural haematoma when epidural catheterization has caused vessel injury.

During the last decade, annually more than 20,000 bags with this epidural analgesic mixture, sterile and with a documented shelf-life of at least 6 months[86] (125 mL for obstetric epidurals, 275 mL and 550 mL for postoperative epidural analgesia) have been supplied via our hospital pharmacy in Oslo to other hospitals in Norway, Iceland and Sweden. No complications have been reported to be caused by the epidural analgesic mixture per se.

A robust monitoring routine for effective and safe epidural analgesia

Observe and document every 4 hours (twice per nursing shift):
- pain intensity at rest and when moving, deep breathing, coughing
- upper and lower sensory level (using an ice cube in a glove)
- any leg weakness (or increasing leg weakness)
- any new backache
- any tenderness at the epidural catheter insertion site.

High index of suspicion for early symptoms of spinal haematoma or abscess, and high preparedness for verifying the diagnosis and evacuation of haematoma or abscess. If there is a suspicion of intraspinal bleeding or abscess (leg weakness, back pain):
- high preparedness for urgent MRI (or CT scan/myelography)
- and evacuation of a haematoma (within about 10 hours of the onset of increasing leg weakness)
- or antibiotics and drainage of an abscess (the time of grace is somewhat longer with an abscess, compared with bleeding, due to the more slowly developing compression of spinal cord blood supply).

Minimum requirements for monitoring when nursing time is limited (e.g. at night):
- Can the patient be easily awakened?
- Is the patient pain free at rest?
- Does the patient have only mild pain when coughing/ moving?
- Can the patient move legs as before?

If the answer is 'yes' to these four questions, the epidural is working as it should be and there is no serious complication.

Consider the following if communication with the patient becomes difficult (e.g. patient is intubated and ventilated):
- Does the patient respond with autonomic reflexes to painful stimuli?
- Does the patient move legs when stimulated?
- Signs of infection?
- Increased bleeding?

Does the patient really need the epidural? Is it safe to remove the epidural catheter (is the patient anticoagulated or having thrombolytic therapy)?

REDUCING THE RISK OF TRANSITION FROM ACUTE TO CHRONIC POSTOPERATIVE PAIN BY BETTER MANAGEMENT OF ACUTE POSTOPERATIVE PAIN

The incidence of chronic pain after surgery is high: up to two-thirds of patients have discomfort, and pain in and around the scar area 12 months after breast surgery, thoracotomy and sternotomy. Even after relatively minor surgery, such as inguinal hernia repair, hand surgery and hysterectomy, around 10% suffer long-lasting neuropathic pain that is often difficult to treat. Clearly, this is a major healthcare problem.[87, 88]

Unrelieved acute postoperative pain is associated with chronic postoperative pain. Acute pain impulses induce hypersensitivity of pain neurons in the spinal cord. This central hypersensitivity causes hyperalgesia and mechanical allodynia around the injured tissue and wound area. Normally, this gradually disappears within a few months after surgery. These hyperphenomena are in part caused by activity in excitatory synapses with glutamatergic transmissions via N-methyl-D-aspartate (NMDA) receptors. When the phenomena are aggravated and prolonged and do not regress normally, they may be the basis for chronic neuropathic pain after surgery.

Is 'acute neuropathic pain' after surgery a link to chronic postoperative pain?

Most patients have nerve damage and hyperalgesic, allodynic-type pain or discomfort after surgery. Touching the wound and the area around the wound causes painful sensations that are often quite severe during the first few days after surgery or trauma. Glutamate receptors in the spinal cord are involved in this normal central sensitization and secondary hyperalgesia, which responds poorly to traditional non-opioid and even potent opioid analgesics. However, the NMDA-glutamate-receptor antagonist ketamine, in small, subanaesthetic doses, has marked synergistic antihyperalgesic effects when coadministered with morphine: continuous small-dose intravenous infusion of ketamine (1–2 µg/kg/minute) for 72 hours during and after surgery removed the hypersensitive allodynic pain around the surgical wound.[89]

There is some evidence that perioperative neuraxial blockade and low-dose ketamine, systemic lidocaine and other antihyperalgesic drugs, such as gabapentin, pregabalin, amitryptiline and glucocorticoids, can abort or reduce the severity of acute neuropathic pain in the postoperative period. Although promising, it remains to be verified that such antihyperalgesic drugs reduce the risk of chronic neuropathic pain after surgery.[89, 90] Thus, combining a small dose of ketamine with morphine for intravenous PCA has been proven to be safe in large prospective studies for postoperative pain, but for the routine patients there did not seem to be advantages.[91, 92] A possible application for ketamine, with its narrow therapeutic range, may be continuous infusion for patients known to have risk factors for chronic neuropathic pain after surgery.

SUMMARY

Important factors for implementing a successful acute postoperative pain service are: well-trained pain nurses backed up by highly qualified and dedicated anaesthetists, an ongoing educational programme for all health personnel involved in the care of surgical patients, and the patients themselves. This service raises the standards of acute pain management throughout the hospital. The benefits in terms of increased patient satisfaction and improved outcome after surgery outweigh the costs of running an acute pain service.

Optimal dosing of paracetamol, exploiting its synergy with NSAIDs (when tolerated) and opioids (when needed), improves

PRACTICE POINTS

A successful postoperative pain management programme requires the following:

- All patients should, at least, be offered optimal pharmacological pain relief with:
  - appropriate combinations of paracetamol, a NSAID (when tolerated) and a glucocorticoid
  - and potent opioids administered by ward nurses with standing orders for intramuscular or intravenous administration (when needed).
- PCA with opioid bolus doses administered intravenously by the patient increases satisfaction with pain management but does not decrease side-effects. PCA with transcutaneous iontophoretic administration of fentanyl is an interesting new approach.[93]
- Patients at risk of developing postoperative respiratory and cardiac complications after major thoracic or abdominal surgery should be offered optimal epidural analgesia: a thoracic epidural infusion of small doses of local anaesthetic, a lipophilic opioid and adrenalin.
- An acute pain service team should be organized in all hospitals with specially trained and dedicated personnel for continuous daytime coverage with anaesthetist-backed pain nurses, as a minimum.
- An ongoing educational programme in which nurses on the surgical wards learn how to monitor pain, pain management, its effects and any side-effects, at least every 4 hours. This will help to 'make pain visible', focus attention on inadequate pain relief, and is a powerful tool in improving the quality of pain relief.
- To prevent permanent neurological damage from the rare, but potentially catastrophic complications of intraspinal bleeding or infection, the following are needed:
  - a high index of suspicion for detecting early signs of intraspinal bleeding or infection
  - vigilant monitoring of increasing leg weakness and any new backache
  - high preparedness for verifying the diagnosis with MRI (or CT scan)
  - high preparedness for rapid removal of intraspinal haematoma or abscess.
- Chronic neuropathic pain is common after surgery and a major healthcare problem. Unrelieved acute pain is a risk factor. Clinical research is needed to show whether perioperative administration of antihyperalgesic drugs, such as ketamine, antiepileptic, tricyclic or glucocorticoid drugs can reduce the risk.

pain relief at rest for most surgical patients. A single dose of a glucocorticoid reduces acute pain and has antiemetic effects. Well-tailored, optimal thoracic epidural analgesia relieves severe dynamic pain when coughing after thoracotomy or upper abdominal surgery. Peripheral nerve blocks reduce dynamic pain when moving limbs after major orthopaedic surgery. Neuraxial analgesia and some peripheral nerve blocks may facilitate

RESEARCH AGENDA

- It needs to be determined whether the risk of chronic postoperative neuropathic pain can be reduced by:
  - optimal perioperative epidural analgesia
  - NMDA-antagonist drugs, antiepileptic drugs, tricyclics or glucocorticoid drugs.

- A cost–benefit analysis is needed of optimal effective and safe postoperative pain management, with regard to:
  - morbidity
  - quality of life, short-term and long-term
  - economic costs and gains, direct and indirect

- It needs to be investigated whether **optimally conducted, well-tailored and monitored perioperative epidural analgesia** will facilitate rehabilitation and decrease the risk of pulmonary and cardiac morbidity after major surgery.

rehabilitation and reduce morbidity in patients at high risk of developing postoperative pulmonary infections and cardiac ischaemic events.

The highly effective high-tech methods (epidural and intravenous PCA) for postoperative pain management need robust monitoring routines to detect early symptoms of potentially serious complications. High preparedness is mandatory for diagnosing and treating rare but potentially serious respiratory depression, bleeding or infection in the spinal canal.

Chronic pain is common after surgery. Better acute pain relief is likely to reduce this distressing complication of surgery. Clinical studies involving optimal neuraxial analgesia, nerve blocks and antihyperalgesic drugs (NMDA antagonists, glucocorticoids, antiepileptics) will hopefully confirm that such approaches can reduce the risk of intractable chronic postoperative pain.

REFERENCES

1. Modig J, Hjelmstedt A, Sahlstedt B et al. Comparative influences of epidural and general anaesthesia on deep venous thrombosis and pulmonary embolism after total hip replacement. *Acta Chir Scand* 1981; **147**: 125–130.
2. Kehlet H. Modification of responses to surgery by neural blockade: clinical implications. In Cousins MJ, Bridenbough PO (eds), *Neural Blockade in Clincial Anesthesia and Management of Pain*, 3rd edn. Lippincott-Raven, Philadelphia, PA, 1998, pp. 129–175.
3. Stenseth R, Sellevold O, Breivik H. Epidural morphine for postoperative pain: experience with 1085 patients. *Acta Anaesthesiol Scand* 1985; **29**: 146–156.
4. Breivk H. Recommendations for foundation of a hospital-wide postoperative pain service – a European view. *Pain Digest* 1993; **3**: 27–30.
5. Breivik H. Pain management. *Baillière's Clin Anaesthesiol* 1994; **8**: 775–795.
6. Breivik H, Högström H, Niemi G et al. Safe and effective post-operative pain-relief: introduction and continuous quality-improvement of comprehensive post-operative pain management programmes. *Baillière's Clin Anaesthesiol* 1995; **9**: 423–460.
7. Ready LB, Oden R, Chadwick HS et al Development of an anaesthesiology-based postoperative pain management service. *Anesthesiolgy* 1988; **68**: 100–106.
8. Rawal N, Berggren L. Organization of acute pain service: a low cost model. *Pain* 1994; **57**: 117–123.
9. Breivik H. High-tech versus low-tech approaches to postoperative pain management. *Prog Pain Res Manage* 2000; **16**: 787–807.
10. Breivik H. Benefits, risks and economics of post-operative pain management programmes. *Baillière's Clin Anaesthesiol* 1995; **9**: 403–422.
11. Wheatley RG, Schug SA, Watson D. Safety and efficacy of postoperative epidural analgesia. *Br J Anaesth* 2001; **87**: 47–61.
12. Ballantyne JC, Carr DB, deFerranti S et al. The comparative effects of postoperative analgesic therapies on pulmonary outcome: cumulative meta-analyses of randomized, controlled trials. *Anaesth Analg* 1998; **86**: 598–612.
13. Breivik H. Postoperative pain management: why is it difficult to show that it improves outcome? *Eur J Anaesthesiol* 1998; **15**: 748–751.
14. Korpela R, Olkkola KT. Paracetamol – misused good old drug? *Acta Anaesthesiol Scand* 1999; **43**: 245–247.
15. Schug SA, Sidebotham DA, McGuinnety M et al. Acetaminophen as an adjunct to morphine by patient-controlled analgesia in the management of acute postoperative pain. *Anesth Analg* 1998; **87**: 368–372.
16. Korpela R, Korvenoja P, Meretoja OA. Morphine-sparing effect of acetaminophen in pediatric day-case surgery. *Anesthesiology* 1999; **91**: 442–447.
17. Montgomery JE, Sutherland CJ, Kestin IG et al. Morphine consumption in patients receiving rectal paracetamol and diclofenac alone and in combination. *Br J Anaesth* 1996; **77**: 445–447.
18. Juhl G, Norholt SE, Tonnesen E et al. Analgesic efficacy and safety intravenous paracetamol (acetaminophen) administered as 2 g starting dose following 3rd molar surgery. *Eur J Pain* 2006; **10**: 371–377.
19. Gaukroger PB. Paediatric analgesia: Which drug? Which dose? *Drugs* 1991; **41**: 52–59.
20. Birmingham PK, Tobin MJ, Henthorn TK et al. Twenty-four-hour pharmacokinetics of rectal acetaminophen in children. An old drug with new recommendations. *Anesthesiology* 1997; **87**: 244–252.
21. Birmingham PK, Tobin MJ, Fisher DM, Henthorn TK, Hall SC, Coté CJ. Initial and subsequent dosing of rectal acetaminophen in children. *Anesthesiology* 2001; **94**: 385–389.
22. Hansen TG, O'Brien K, Morton NS et al. Plasma paracetamol concentrations and pharmacokinetics following rectal administration in neonates and young infants. *Acta Anaesthesiol Scand* 1999; **43**: 855–859.
23. Arana A, Morton NS, Hansen TG. Treatment with paracetamol in infants. *Acta Anaesthesiol Scand* 2001; **45**: 20–29.
24. Murrat I, Baujard C, Foussat C et al. Tolerance and analgesic efficacy of a new i.v. paracetamol solution in children after inguinal hernia repair. *Pediatr Anesth* 2005; **15**: 663–670.
25. Malmberg AB, Yaksh TL Antinociceptive actions of spinal nonsteroidal anti-inflammatory agents on the formalin test in the rat. *J Pharm Exp Ther* 1992; **263**: 136–146.
26. Tjølsen A, Lund A, Hole K. Antinociceptive effect of paracetamol in rats is partly dependent on spinal serotonergic systems. *Eur J Pharmacol* 1991; **193**: 193–201.
27. Björkman R, Hallman KM, Hedner T et al. M. Acetaminophen blocks spinal hyperalgesia induced by NMDA and substance P. *Pain* 1994; **57**: 259–264.
28. Björkman R. Central antinociceptive effects of non-steroidal anti-inflammatory drugs and paracetamol. Experimental studies in the rat. *Acta Anaesthesiol Scand* 1995; **39**: 103S.
29. Muth-Selbach US, Tegeder I, Brune K et al. Acetaminophen inhibits spinal prostaglandin E_2 release after peripheral noxious stimulation. *Anesthesiology* 1999; **91**: 231–239.
30. Graham GG, Scott KF. Mechanisms of action of paracetamol. *Am J Therapeut* 2005; **12**: 46–55.
31. Wong S, Gardocki JF. Anti-inflammatory and antiarthritic evaluation of acetaminophen and its potentiation of tolmetin. *J Pharmacol Exp Therapeut* 1983; **226**: 625–632.
32. Fletcher D, Benoist JM, Gautron M et al. Isobolographic analysis of interactions between intravenous morphine, propacetamol, and diclofenac in carrageenin-injected rats. *Anesthesiology* 1997; **87**: 317–326.
33. Breivik EK, Barkvoll P, Skovlund E. Combining diclofenac with acetaminophen or acetaminophen–codeine after oral surgery: a randomized, double-blind single-dose study. *Clin Pharmacol Ther* 1999; **66**: 625–635.
34. Legeby M, Sandelin K, Wickman M et al. Analgesic efficacy of diclofenac in combination with morphine and paracetamol after mastectomy and immediate breast reconstruction. *Acta Anaesthesiol Scand* 2005; **49**: 1360–1366.
35. Pickering AE, Bridge HS, Nolan J et al. Double-blind, placebo-controlled analgesic study of ibuprofen or rofecoxib in combination with paracetamol for tonsillectomy in children. *Br J Anaesth* 2002; **88**: 72–77.
36. Menhinick KA, Gutman JL, Regan JD et al. The efficacy of pain control following nonsurgical root canal treatment using ibuprofen or a combination of ibuprofen and acetaminophen in a randomized, double-blind, placebo-controlled study. *Int Endodontol J* 2004; **37**: 531–541.

37. Hyllestad M, Jones S, Pedersen JL et al. Comparative effect of paracetamol, NSAIDs or their combination in postoperative pain management: a qualitative review. Br J Anaesth 2002; 88: 199–214.

38. Jones SF, Power I. Postoperative NSAIDs and COX-2 inhibitors: cardiovascular risks and benefits. Br J Anaesth 2005; 95: 281–284.

39. Skjelbred P, Løkken P. Post-operative pain and inflammatory reaction reduced by injection of a corticosteroid. A controlled trial in bilateral oral surgery. Eur J Clin Pharmacol 1982; 21: 391–396.

40. Romundstad L, Breivik H, Niemi G et al. Methylprednisolone intravenously 1 day after surgery has sustained analgesic and opioid-sparing effects. Acta Anaesthesiol Scand 2004; 48: 1223–1231.

41. Romundstad L, Breivik H, Roald H et al. Methylprednisolone reduces pain, emesis, and fatigue after breast augmentation surgery: a single-dose, randomized, parallel-group study with methylprednisolone 125 mg, parecoxib 40 mg, and placebo. Anesth Analg 2006; 102: 418–425.

42. Romundstad L, Stubhaug A, Skolleborg K et al. Chronic pain and sensory changes after cosmetic augmentation–mammoplasty: long term effects of pre-incisional administration of methylprednisolone. Pain 2006; 124: 92–99.

43. Sauerland S, Nagelschmidt M, Mallmann P et al. Risks and benefits of pre-operative high dose methylprednisolone in surgical patients: a systematic review. Drug Safety 2000; 23: 449–461.

44. Reuben SS, Connelly NR, Maciolek H. Postoperative analgesia with controlled-release oxycodone for outpatient anterior cruciate ligament surgery. Anesth Analg 1999; 88: 1286–1291.

45. Harmer M, Davies KA. The effect of education, assessment and a standardised prescription on postoperative pain management. Anaesthesia 1998; 53: 424–430.

46. Borchgrevink P, Hval B, Jystad Å et al. Changing from i.m. to nurse controlled i.v. morphine on ward – is it dangerous? 9th World Congress on Pain, Vienna, 22–27 August 1999, Abstract No. 230.

47. Walder B, Schafer M, Henzi I et al. Efficacy and safety of patient-controlled opioid analgesia for acute postoperative pain. A quantitative systematic review. Acta Anaesthesiol Scand 2001; 45: 795–804.

48. Delbos A, Boccard E. The morphine-sparing effect of propacetamol in orthopedic postoperative pain. J Pain Symptom Manage 1995; 10: 279–286.

49. Etches RC, Warriner CB, Badner N et al. Continuous intravenous administration of ketorolac reduces pain and morphine consumption after total hip or knee arthroplasty. Anesth Analg 1995; 81: 1175–1180.

50. Irwin MG, Roulseon CJ, Jones RDM. Peri-operative administration of rectal diclofenac sodium. The effect on renal function in patients undergoing minor orthopedic surgery. Eur J Anaesthesiol 1995; 12: 403–405.

51. Hobbs GJ. Ketorolac alters the kinetics of morphine metabolites. Br J Anaesth 1997; 78: 95.

52. Tighe KE, Webb AM, Hobbs GI. Persistently high plasma morphine-6-glucuronide levels despite decreased hourly patient-controlled analgesia morphine use after single-dose diclofenac: potential for opioid related toxicity. Anesth Analg 1999; 88: 1137–1142.

53. Marret E, Kurdi O, Zufferey P et al. Effects of nonsteroidal antiinflammatory drugs on patient-controlled analgesia morphine side effects: meta-analysis of randomized controlled trials. Anesthesiology 2005; 102: 1249–1260.

54. Fletcher D, Nègre I, Barbin C et al. Postoperative analgesia with iv propacetamol and ketoprofen combination after disc surgery. Can J Anaesth 1997; 44: 479–485.

55. Niv D, Raj PP, Erdine S. Efficacy of permanent indwelling catheters used for regional analgesia. Prog Pain Res Manage 2000; 16: 935–949.

56. Capdevila X, Barthelet Y, Biboulet P et al. Effects of perioperative analgesic technique on the surgical outcome and duration of rehabilitation after major knee surgery. Anesthesiology 1999; 91: 8–15.

57. Richardson J, Lonnquist PA Thoracic paravertebral block. Br J Anaesth 1998; 81: 230–238.

58. Wattwil M, Thoren T, Hennerdal S et al. Epidural analgesia with bupivacaine reduces postoperative paralytic ileus after hysterectomy. Anesth Analg 1989; 68: 353–358.

59. Liu SS, Carpenter RL, Meal JM. Epidural anesthesia and analgesia. Their role in postoperative outcome. Anesthesiology 1995; 82: 1474–1506.

60. Steinbrook RA. Epidural anesthesia and gastrointestinal motility. Anesth Analg 1998; 86: 837–844.

61. Blomberg S, Emanuelsson H, Kvist H. Effects of thoracic epidural anesthesia on coronary arteries and arterioles in patients with coronary artery disease. Anesthesiology 1990; 73: 840–847.

62. Stenseth R, Bjella L, Berg EM et al. Effects of thoracic epidural analgesia on pulmonary function after coronary artery bypass surgery. Eur J Cardiothorac Surg 1996; 10: 859–865.

63. Van Aken H, Gogarten W, Rolf N. Epidural anesthesia in cardiac risk patients Anesth Analg 1999; 89(Rev Course Suppl): 104–110.

64. Van Aken H, Rolf N. Thoracic epidural anaesthesia. Clin Anaesthesiol 1999; 13: 1–109.

65. Scheinin H, Virtanen T, Kentala E et al. Epidural infusion of bupivacaine and fentanyl reduces perioperative myocardial ischaemia in elderly patients with hip fracture – a randomized controlled trial. Acta Anaesthsiol Scand 2000; 44: 1061–1070.

66. Tenling A, Joachimsson PO, Tydén H et al. Thoracic epidural analgesia as an adjunct to general anaesthesia for cardiac surgery. Effects on pulmonary mechanics. Acta Anaesthesiol Scand 2000; 44: 1071–1076.

67. O'Connor CJ, Tuman KJ. Epidural anesthesia and analgesia for coronary artery bypass graft surgery: still forbidden territory? Anesth Analg 2001; 93: 523–525.

68. Park WY, Thompson JS, Lee KK et al. Effect of epidural anesthesia and analgesia on perioperative outcome. A randomized, controlled veterans affairs cooperative study. Ann Surg 2001; 234: 560–571.

69. Scott NB, Turfrey DJ, Ray DAA et al. A prospective randomized study of the potential benefits of thoracic epidural anesthesia and analgesia in patients undergoing coronary artery bypass grafting. Anesth Analg 2001; 93: 528–535.

70. Nishimori M, Ballantyne JC, Low JHS. Epidural pain relief versus systemic opioid-based pain relief for abdominal aortic surgery. Cochrane Database of Systematic Reviews 2006, Issue 3 (19 July 2006).

71. Norris EJ, Beattie C, Perler BA et al. A double-masked randomized trial comparing alternative combinations of intraoperative anesthesia and postoperative analgesia in abdominal aortic surgery. Anesthesiology 2001; 95: 1054–1067.

72. Rigg JRA, Jamrozik K, Myles PS et al. Epidural anaesthesia and analgesia and outcome of major surgery: a randomised trial. Lancet 2002; 359: 1276–1282.

73. Rodgers A, Walker N, Schug S et al. Reduction of postoperative mortality and morbidity with epidural or spinal anaesthesia: results from overview of randomized trials. BMJ 2000; 321: 1493–1497.

74. Beattie WS, Badner NH, Choi P. Epidural analgesia reduces postoperative myocardial infarction: a meta-analysis. Anesth Analg 2001; 93: 853–858.

75. Breivik H. Infectious complications of epidural anaesthesia and analgesia. Curr Opinion Anaesthesiol 1999; 12: 573–577.

76. Breivik H. Neurological complications in association with spinal and epidural analgesia – again. Acta Anaesthesiol Scand 1998; 42: 609–613.

77. Moen V, Dahlgren N, Irestedt L. Severe neurological complications after central neuraxial blockades in Sweden 1990–1999. Anesthesiology 2004; 101: 950–959.

78. Collins JG, Kitahata LM, Suzukawa M. Spinally administered epinephrine suppresses noxiously evoked activity of WDR neurons in the dorsal horn of the spinal cord. Anesthesiology 1984; 60: 269–275.

79. Solomon RE, Gebhart GF. Synergistic antinociceptive interaction among drugs administered to the spinal cord. Anesth Analg 1994; 78: 1164–1172.

80. Niemi G, Breivik H. Adrenaline markedly improves thoracic epidural analgesia produced by a low-dose infusion of bupivacaine, fentanyl and adrenaline after major surgery. Acta Anaesthesiol Scand 1998; 42: 897–909.

81. Niemi, G. Breivik, H. Epidural fentanyl markedly improves thoracic epidural analgesia in a low-dose infusion of bupivacaine, adrenaline and fentanyl. A randomized, double-blind crossover study with and without fentanyl. Acta Anaesthesiol Scand 2001; 45: 221–232.

82. Niemi G, Breivik H. The minimally effective concentration of adrenaline in a low-concentration thoracic epidural analgesic infusion of bupivacaine and fentanyl after major surgery. A randomized, double blind, dose-finding study. Acta Anaesthesiol Scand 2003; 47: 439–450.

83. Niemi G, Breivik H. Epinephrine markedly improves thoracic epidural analgesia produced by a small-dose infusion of ropivacaine, fentanyl and epinephrine after major thoracic or abdominal surgery: a randomized, double-blind, cross-over study with and without epinephrine. Anesth Analg 2002; 94: 1598–1605.

84. Curatolo M. Is epinephrine unfairly neglected for postoperative epidural mixtures? Anesth Analg 2002; 94: 1381–1383.

85. Niemi G. Optimizing epidural analgesia. Medical Thesis for Doctor of Medical Sciences, Faculty of Medicine, University of Oslo, Norway, 2004.

86. Kjønniksen I, Brustugun J, Niemi G et al. Stability of an epidural analgesic solution containing adrenaline, bupivacaine and fentanyl. Acta Anaesthesiol Scand 2000; 44: 864–867.

87. ANZCA. Acute Pain Management: Scientific Evidence. Australian and New Zealand College of Anaesthetists and Faculty of Medicine, Melbourne, 2005.

88. Power I. Recent advances in postoperative pain therapy. Br J Anaesth 2005; 95: 43–51.

89. Stubhaug A, Breivik H, Eide PK et al. Mapping of punctate hyperalgesia surrounding a surgical incision demonstrates that ketamine is a powerful suppressr of central sensitisation to pain following surgery. Acta Anaesthesiol Scand 1997; 41: 1124–1132.

90. Rowbotham DJ. Gabapentin: a new drug for postoperative pain?. Bt J Anaesth 2006; 96: 152–155.

91. Sveticic G, Gentilini A, Eichenberger U et al. Combinations of morphine with ketamine for patient controlled analgesia. A new optimization method. *Anesthesiology* 2003; **98**: 1195–1205.

92. Sveticic G, Eichenberger U, Curatolo M. Safety of mixture of morphine with ketamine for postoperative patient-controlled analgesia: An audit with 1026 patients. *Acta Anaesthesiol Scand* 2005; **49**: 870–875.

93. Viscusi ER, Reynolds L, Tait S et al. An iontophoretic fentanyl patient-activated analgesic delivery system for postoperative pain: A double-blind, placebo-controlled trial. *Anesth Analg* 2006; **102**: 188–194.

Chapter 25

The effect of postoperative epidural analgesia on perioperative morbidity and mortality

Christopher L. Wu and Matthew D. Caldwell

INTRODUCTION

Surgery is associated with a series of potentially detrimental physiological effects. The disturbances in physiology following surgery may result in postoperative mortality and morbidity. Much of the perioperative pathophysiology is centred on the surgical or neuroendocrine stress response, which may result in a wide range of physiological responses and adversely affect many organ systems. In general, many of these physiological responses begin in the intraoperative period and will extend well into the postoperative period; however, the precise pathophysiology and aetiology of some of these responses have not been completely elucidated.

Both systemic opioid analgesics and regional analgesic techniques are commonly used by anaesthesiologists for control of postoperative pain, and although systemic use of opioids is effective in the treatment of postoperative pain, use of regional analgesic techniques provides physiological benefits in attenuation of perioperative surgical pathophysiology, which may not be conferred by use of systemic opioids. It is unlikely that pain control per se will decrease perioperative morbidity.[1] Here the discussion is focused on the effect of regional neuraxial (epidural) analgesic techniques, as the data suggest that this type of postoperative analgesic technique may influence patient morbidity to a greater extent than systemic opioids. Nevertheless, no matter which type of postoperative analgesic technique or agent is used, it is important, as part of the concept of multimodal analgesia,[2] effectively to control the patient's postoperative pain in order to facilitate patient participation in their own convalescence.

PERIOPERATIVE PATHOPHYSIOLOGY

General pathophysiology

Surgical trauma typically results in the neuroendocrine stress response, a combination of local inflammatory (e.g. cytokines, prostaglandins and leukotrienes) and systemic neuroendocrine metabolic elements, which in effect produces a hypermetabolic, catabolic state resembling semi-starvation.[3] Transmission of afferent neural and nociceptive stimuli from the periphery to the central nervous system, particularly the hypothalamus, results in an efferent stress response that includes increases in catabolic hormones, such as catecholamines, cortisol, renin, aldosterone and glucagon. In turn, this results in hyperglycaemia, muscle protein catabolism (negative nitrogen balance) and increased lipolysis. The extent of the contribution of individual local inflammatory mediators to the stress response is uncertain.

The extent of the stress response is influenced by many factors, including the type of anaesthesia (regional versus general anaesthesia) and intensity of surgical injury, with the extent of the stress response being proportional to the degree of surgical trauma.[4, 5] Unlike the response seen with regional anaesthesia, use of general anaesthesia, with the possible exception of a high-dose opioid regimen,[6] does not significantly attenuate the perioperative stress response. The specific factors that initiate and potentiate the stress response are not completely known.

The detrimental physiological effects of the stress response may affect other organ systems, including the coagulation, immune and cardiovascular systems. The hypercoagulable state that occurs in the postoperative period is associated with enhancement of coagulation (e.g. decreased levels of natural anticoagulants, such as protein C), increased platelet reactivity, plasma viscosity and levels of procoagulants (such as von

Willebrand factor), and inhibition of fibrinolysis.[7] Although the precise aetiology of the postoperative hypercoagulability is not clear, potentiation of coagulation by the stress response may be an important factor.[8]

The stress response may also potentiate postoperative immunosuppression. Like that of postoperative hypercoagulability, the exact aetiology of postoperative immunosuppression is uncertain; however, the surgical stress response results in elevated levels of cortisol and epinephrine, which may be important in mediating some aspects of postoperative immunosuppression.[9, 10] Similar to that seen with the surgical stress response, the degree of immunosuppression is related to the severity of surgical injury.[11]

Finally, the hormones released as a result of the neuroendocrine stress response may affect other systems. Increased levels of catecholamines released as part of the stress response may cause increases in heart rate, which may result in postoperative myocardial ischaemia or infarction in higher risk cardiac patients. Hyperglycaemia may contribute to poor wound healing and depression of immune function.[12] In addition, negative nitrogen balance and protein catabolism may hinder overall patient convalescence. Thus, the neuroendocrine stress response resulting from surgical injury may cause a wide range of potentially adverse physiological responses and may potentiate the hypercoagulable and immunosuppressive states in the postoperative period.

Pathophysiology of specific organ systems
Cardiovascular system
Sympathetic nervous system activation, either through the stress response or inadequate analgesia, may increase heart rate, contractility and blood pressure, and may be important in the development of myocardial ischaemia and infarction in the postoperative period. Although increases in myocardial oxygen demand may not necessarily correlate with the occurrence of myocardial ischaemia,[13] any increase in myocardial oxygen consumption may increase myocardial oxygen demand and result in myocardial ischaemia and even increases in the size of myocardial infarction.[14]

Sympathetic activation may also decrease myocardial oxygen supply through coronary vasoconstriction, and may override local metabolic coronary vasodilatation.[15] This may result in myocardial ischaemia or infarction, the incidence of which typically peaks in the postoperative period.[16] Furthermore, the postoperative hypercoagulable state may contribute to the development of myocardial ischaemia and infarction.[17]

Pulmonary system
Unlike that following lower abdominal, peripheral or laparoscopic surgery, there is a pronounced decrease in postoperative respiratory function after upper abdominal and thoracic surgery. This decrease in pulmonary function occurs within 24 hours postoperatively, with a return to preoperative levels over the next 2 weeks and may be significant (e.g. vital capacity at 40% of preoperative levels after upper abdominal surgery).[18] Postoperative decreases in respiratory function may be due, in part, to inadequate analgesia, diaphragmatic dysfunction and increase in upper abdominal and intercostal muscle tone.[8] Patients with poor pain control may breathe less deeply, have an inadequate cough and be unable to fully cooperate with physical therapy, and therefore may be more likely to develop postoperative pulmonary complications.[18, 19] Complete control of pain alone will not completely prevent a decrease in postoperative pulmonary function,[20] as diaphragmatic dysfunction, independent of the extent of analgesia, occurs as a result of spinal reflex inhibition of phrenic nerve activity.[21] In addition, increased lower intercostal and abdominal muscle tone during exhalation further decreases lung volumes as a result of cephalad displacement of the diaphragm.[22]

Postoperative decreases in pulmonary function may be caused by abnormalities in gas exchange as a result of alveolar hypoventilation, ventilation–perfusion mismatches or right-to-left shunting, which in turn may lead to pulmonary complications, including hypoxaemia, atelectasis, pneumonia and respiratory failure. Certain patient populations, such as those with advanced age, pre-existing pulmonary disease (including smoking), obesity, severe pain, and undergoing thoracic or upper abdominal surgery, may be at higher risk for development of postoperative pulmonary complications.

Gastrointestinal system
Gastrointestinal ileus generally occurs following abdominal surgery. Complete return of gastrointestinal motility returns typically within 2–3 days in uncomplicated cases but may develop into a more severe, protracted form of paralytic ileus. Postoperative ileus is the combination of inhibitory inputs from central and systemic sources, spinal reflexes and local factors.[23] Similar to that seen in spinal reflex inhibition of the phrenic nerve and diaphragmatic function, there is spinal reflex inhibition of gastrointestinal tract function.[8, 24] In addition, any factors that increase sympathetic efferent stimulation (e.g. neuroendocrine stress response and excessive pain) will diminish organized gastrointestinal activity and inhibit return of gastrointestinal function. Likewise, any factors that diminish sympathetic efferent and increase parasympathetic efferent activity will facilitate return of gastrointestinal function. Finally, use of opioids for postoperative analgesia may also inhibit return of gastrointestinal motility.

EFFECT OF POSTOPERATIVE REGIONAL ANALGESIA ON MORBIDITY AND MORTALITY

Use of both intraoperative regional anaesthesia and postoperative epidural analgesia can attenuate the pathophysiology that occurs following surgery, and is associated with a reduction in mortality and morbidity when compared to general anaesthesia. Some studies have incorporated a combination of intraoperative regional anaesthesia followed by postoperative epidural analgesia and demonstrated a decrease in patient morbidity; however, the great majority of the research has focused on the question of intraoperative regional (neuraxial) versus general anaesthesia.[25] A recent meta-analysis (CORTRA) of all randomized data (a total of 141 trials consisting of 9559 subjects) comparing intraoperative neuraxial versus general anaesthesia demonstrated that the use of intraoperative neuraxial anaesthesia reduced overall mortality by approximately 30% and was associated with one less death per 100 patients within 30 days of randomization.[25]

On the other hand, few studies have controlled for or specifically investigated the effect of postoperative epidural analgesia on postoperative mortality or morbidity. This is unfortunate, as some pathophysiological processes and complications, such as deep venous thrombosis formation, will begin in the intraoperative period,[26] while others, such as myocardial ischaemia and infarction, will peak in the postoperative period.[16] Analysis of the Medicare database suggests that the presence of postoperative epidural analgesia is associated with a significantly lower odds of death at 7 days (odds ratio (OR) 0.52; 95% confidence interval (CI) 0.38–0.73; $p = 0.0001$) and 30 days (OR 0.74; 95% CI 0.63–0.89; $p = 0.0005$) after various surgical procedures;[27] however, there are many limitations of this type of study design in examining this issue. Thus, it may be difficult to differentiate the extent of the contribution of intraoperative anaesthesia versus postoperative analgesia on improvements in patient outcomes, especially in light of the fact that the aetiologies of certain perioperative pathophysiologies (e.g. stress response, hypercoagulable state, immunosuppression and postoperative delirium) have not been completely elucidated.

Although the overall efficacy of perioperative epidural anaesthesia and analgesia on mortality is controversial, due in part to some of the methodological issues present (see below), there are some data that demonstrate the benefits of postoperative epidural analgesia, possibly as a result of the provision of superior analgesia and certain physiological benefits. During the discussion here of the effect of postoperative epidural analgesia on patient morbidity, it is important to keep in mind that the term 'epidural analgesia' is not used generically. Any benefits of postoperative epidural analgesia on improvement in patient morbidity are limited to an appropriate placement of catheter insertion in relation to the site of surgery (thoracic versus lumbar) and the use of an appropriate analgesic agent (local anaesthetic versus opioid). The role of postoperative epidural analgesia in facilitating patient recovery as part of a multimodal analgesic and recovery regimen is discussed.

Gastrointestinal system

Postoperative ileus is estimated to cost approximately US $750 million annually.[28] A delay in return of postoperative gastrointestinal function will prevent initiation of enteral feeding, enhance the stress response, increase the incidence of septic complications and decrease wound healing.[29–31]

Use of epidural analgesia with local anaesthetics can diminish some of the adverse physiological effects that contribute to postoperative ileus. Specifically, inhibition of sympathetic outflow (and increased influence of the parasympathetic system) resulting from the sympathectomy provided by local anaesthetics administered through the thoracic epidural catheter will facilitate gastrointestinal motility. The decrease in the amount of opioids used may also contribute to an accelerated return of gastrointestinal function. In addition, the local anaesthetic used in the epidural analgesic regimen may inhibit the spinal reflex inhibition of the gastrointestinal tract,[8, 32] and may also be absorbed systemically to facilitate return of gastrointestinal motility.[33] Finally, use of thoracic epidural analgesia with a local anaesthetic-based solution does not contribute to anastomatic dehiscence[34] and actually will increase gut mucosal blood flow and possibly mucosal tissue oxygenation.[35]

Randomized clinical trials investigating recovery of gastrointestinal function after abdominal and other types of surgery have consistently shown that use of postoperative thoracic epidural analgesia with a local anaesthetic-based regimen, compared with systemic opioid analgesia, will allow earlier return of gastrointestinal function and earlier fulfilment of discharge criteria (Table 25.1). No study has shown an advantage of systemic opioids over epidural analgesia with regard to recovery of gastrointestinal motility after abdominal surgery.[28] It appears that the duration of postoperative epidural analgesia, the location of catheter placement (thoracic versus lumbar) and the analgesic agent used (local anaesthetic versus opioid) will influence recovery of gastrointestinal function. Unlike other trials showing a benefit of epidural analgesia, the two randomized trials that did not demonstrate any difference in return of postoperative gastrointestinal motility between epidural and systemic opioid analgesia removed the epidural catheter within 24 hours of surgery, which may have been too brief a period to provide any significant physiological benefits of epidural analgesia.[37, 45] In addition, compared to patients who had a lumbar location for epidural catheter placement, those who had a thoracic placement for abdominal surgery had a significantly earlier return of bowel function and improved analgesia.[50] Finally, randomized trials have demonstrated that, when compared to those who received epidural opioids for postoperative analgesia, patients who received epidural local anaesthetics had an earlier return of gastrointestinal motility following abdominal surgery.[38, 44, 51, 52]

Pulmonary system

Use of thoracic epidural analgesia with a local anaesthetic-based regimen can preserve postoperative pulmonary function after upper abdominal and thoracic surgery, not only by providing superior analgesia, but also by attenuating the spinal reflex inhibition of diaphragmatic function.[8] Patients with thoracic epidural analgesia (versus systemic opioids) have lower pain scores and less sedation postoperatively,[53] which will allow the patients to participate actively in postoperative pulmonary physiotherapy and, in turn, decrease the incidence of postoperative pulmonary complications.[54, 55]

A recent meta-analysis investigating the effect of several postoperative analgesic therapies on postoperative pulmonary complications combined data from 48 randomized controlled trials.[53] Compared to those who received systemic opioids, patients who received postoperative epidural analgesia with local anaesthetics had a significantly increased P_aO_2 and a decreased

Table 25.1. Summary of randomized trials comparing the effect of regional anaesthesia–analgesia versus general anaesthesia–systemic opioids on gastrointestinal recovery in patients undergoing abdominal surgery

Study	Surgical procedure	No. of subjects	Gastrointestinal recovery*	
			Favours epidural	No difference
Rawal et al. (1984)[36]	Gastroplasty	30	X	
Wallin et al. (1986)[37]	Cholecystectomy	30		X
Scheinin et al. (1987)[38]	Colonic	60	X	
Ahn et al. (1988)[39]	Colonic	30	X	
Wattwil et al. (1989)[40]	Hysterectomy	40	X	
Bredtmann et al. (1990)[41]	Colectomy	116	X	
Seeling et al. (1990)[42]	Cholecystectomy	214	X	
Jayr et al. (1993)[43]	Major abdominal	153	X	
Liu et al. (1995)[44]	Colectomy	54	X	
Neudecker et al. (1999)[45]	Laparoscopic sigmoidectomy	20		X
Cassady et al. (2000)[46]	Spine fusion	33	X	
Mann et al. (2000)[47]	Major abdominal	70	X	

*Generally defined as passage of faeces, flatus or radio-opaque markers, or return of bowel sounds. See also Jorgensen et al.[48]

incidence of pulmonary infections and overall complications, despite there being no differences in surrogate measures of pulmonary function (e.g. forced expiratory volume in 1 second, functional vital capacity and peak expiratory flow rate) between groups. Compared to those who received systemic opioids, patients who received postoperative epidural opioids had a lower incidence of atelectasis, but did not have a significant decrease in the incidence of pulmonary complications. Use of intercostal blocks, wound infiltration or intrapleural analgesia was not associated with any significant decrease in the incidence of pulmonary complications.[53]

Other: cardiovascular, coagulation, cognitive and immune function

Although postoperative thoracic epidural analgesia with a local-anaesthetic-based solution appears to decrease postoperative pulmonary and gastrointestinal morbidity, the benefits are not as clear for other organ systems (e.g. cardiovascular, coagulation, cognitive and immune function). The data on the effect of regional anaesthesia and analgesia on these organ systems is equivocal at best, despite some physiological evidence that use of epidural analgesia may attenuate adverse physiological responses in these systems after surgery. Certainly there are methodological issues regarding the investigation of the effect of postoperative epidural analgesia on these and other organ systems, as has been described elsewhere.[56]

Cardiovascular system

The majority of cardiovascular events, including myocardial ischaemia, myocardial infarction, congestive heart failure, ventricular arrhythmias and sudden death, occur in the immediate postoperative period (within the first 72 hours following

surgery).[16] Postoperative myocardial ischaemia may be present in up to 40% of high-risk patients, silent in nature, and a predictor of patient outcome.[57, 58] Use of postoperative thoracic epidural analgesia could, theoretically, diminish cardiac-related morbidity by attenuating the stress response and hypercoagulability, improving postoperative analgesia and providing a favourable redistribution of coronary blood flow. There are physiological data to suggest that thoracic epidural analgesia with local anaesthetics can decrease the severity of myocardial ischaemia and the size of infarction, block sympathetically mediated coronary vasoconstriction and improve coronary flow to areas at risk for ischaemia.[59–62] The use of postoperative epidural analgesia has been shown to significantly decrease the incidence of myocardial ischaemia and infarction.[63] Another meta-analysis[64] demonstrated that use of thoracic, but not lumbar, epidural analgesia significantly decreases the incidence of postoperative myocardial infarction. The fact that thoracic but not lumbar epidural analgesia decreased the incidence of postoperative myocardial infarction nicely corroborates the experimental data on the physiological benefits of thoracic epidural analgesia.

Effects on coagulation

The postoperative hypercoagulable state may lead to vaso-occlusive (e.g. vascular graft failure) and thromboembolic events (e.g. deep venous thrombosis and pulmonary embolism) and, in part, contributes to the over 200,000 deaths annually in the USA.[8, 65] Use of regional anaesthetic techniques, especially with local anaesthetics, may lessen the effects of the postoperative hypercoagulable state by increasing peripheral blood flow, preserving fibrinolytic activity, attenuating increases in coagulation factors and decreasing blood viscosity.[7] Although there are a lot of randomized data that suggest the use of intraoperative regional anaesthesia will decrease the incidence of hypercoagulable-related events when compared to that from general anaesthesia,[25, 66–69] the effect of postoperative epidural analgesia on incidence of hypercoagulable-related events has not been studied as extensively. There is some evidence that continuation of postoperative regional analgesia with local anaesthetics may be associated with a lower incidence of deep venous thrombosis.[70, 71] It is unclear whether patients who receive postoperative epidural analgesia with local anaesthetics will continue to enjoy the physiological benefits that would result in a lower incidence of hypercoagulable-related events when compared to those who receive systemic opioids. An important confounding factor in many trials investigating the effect of either intraoperative or postoperative regional anaesthetic techniques on perioperative thromboembolic events is the lack of concurrently used systemic thromboembolic (anticoagulant) prophylaxis; however, some retrospective data suggest that regional anaesthesia will provide a benefit in diminishing the incidence of deep venous thrombosis regardless of the presence or absence of prophylaxis.[72]

Effects on cognition

Postoperative delirium may cost Medicare approximately US $2 billion per year.[73] Postoperative cognitive dysfunction may be present in approximately 26% of elderly patients 1 week after major non-cardiac surgery, with long-term cognitive dysfunction (3 months after surgery) present in about 10% of patients.[74] The decline in mental function reaches a nadir during the first postoperative week, with delays in recovery of mental function associated with poor patient outcomes.[75, 76] Delirium is associated with increased mortality and longer length of hospital stay, as cognitive functional measures have been shown to be strong predictors of long-term mortality after hospitalization.[77, 78]

The mechanisms of postoperative cognitive dysfunction and delirium are unclear; however, the perioperative use of psychoactive medications (anticholinergic drugs, meperidine and benzodiazepines) and higher levels of postoperative pain have been associated with the development of postoperative delirium and a decrease in postoperative mental status.[79–82] Despite the potential benefits of regional anaesthetic techniques in decreasing the incidence of cognitive dysfunction and delirium by the provision of superior analgesia[83] and avoidance of psychoactive medications, use of intraoperative regional anaesthesia has not been shown to improve postoperative cognitive function compared to those who received general anaesthesia.[84] However, the effect of postoperative regional analgesia on cognitive function has not been carefully examined. At this time, it is unclear whether use of postoperative epidural analgesia with a local anaesthetic-based regimen as part of a multimodal approach to patient convalescence can diminish the incidence of postoperative cognitive dysfunction.

Immunity

The immunodepression that occurs postoperatively following surgery under general anaesthesia may contribute to the development of infections, increase in cost of care, and enhance tumour growth and metastases.[85] Use of regional anaesthetic techniques may preserve perioperative immune function by attenuating the stress response, decreasing perioperative blood loss and the need for blood transfusions (which may be immunosuppressive), and decreasing the use of opioids, which may contribute to immunodepression.[9, 86, 87] Although some data suggest that intraoperative regional anaesthesia is associated with a lower risk of developing pneumonia or other infections,[25] the effect of postoperative epidural analgesia on immunodepressive-related outcomes has not been thoroughly investigated. Until the pathophysiology of perioperative immunodepression is elucidated, any benefits of postoperative epidural analgesia on the preservation of perioperative immune function may be difficult to determine.

Methodological issues

As previously mentioned, the overall effect of perioperative epidural anaesthesia–analgesia on mortality is unclear, despite the physiological and analgesic benefits provided by epidural analgesia, which may result in decreased cardiovascular, pulmonary, gastrointestinal and coagulation-related morbidity. No randomized controlled trial since 1997 (the last year for data inclusion into the CORTRA meta-analysis) has shown a reduction in mortality with use of neuraxial anaesthesia. The controversy of whether epidural anaesthesia–analgesia can reduce perioperative mortality persists, due in part to the presence of methodological issues (e.g. small sample sizes, study-design-related issues and inadequate evaluation of the postoperative period) in currently available studies. For instance, one of the most significant limitations in currently available studies is the inadequate sample size, such that all trials are underpowered to determine the efficacy of an intervention such as epidural anaesthesia for a rare outcome such as death. The actual number of subjects needed for such a trial is quite large: ~24,000 patients for a high-risk group (vascular patients)[88] or ~1.2 million subjects for a lower risk group (e.g. total hip replacement).[89] In addition, 'epidural analgesia' has been considered a single generic entity; however, the various factors that are incorporated in postoperative epidural analgesia (e.g. analgesic regimen, catheter placement and multimodal approach; see below) may influence patient outcomes. Other methodological issues examining the 'regional versus general' question have been discussed in greater detail elsewhere.[56]

Patient-orientated outcomes

Since epidural analgesia does provide superior postoperative pain control,[83] epidural analgesia may have a beneficial effect on patient-orientated outcomes, such as patient satisfaction, quality of life and quality of recovery, when compared to systemic opioids. When compared to intravenous patient-controlled analgesia with opioids, epidural analgesia provided superior postoperative pain control,[83] and it is associated with preservation of health-related quality of life (HRQL) after abdominal surgery.[90] Compared to systemic opioids for postoperative pain control, epidural (and peripheral nerve) analgesia results in higher patient satisfaction.[91] Patient-orientated outcomes such as

HRQL and satisfaction are widely accepted as valid endpoints, and may be adversely affected by higher levels of postoperative pain. Thus, postoperative epidural analgesia may improve patient-orientated outcomes, although there are many methodological issues in measuring these endpoints.

Importance of epidural catheter location

The benefits of postoperative epidural analgesia are maximized when the catheter is inserted in a location corresponding to the dermatomes covered by the surgical incision (Table 25.2). Since the catheter tip is located in relatively close proximity to the dermatome of surgical incision, appropriate insertion of an epidural catheter may allow for a lower dose of epidural analgesic agents and potentially reduce the amount of analgesic drug-induced side-effects, such as pruritus, nausea, vomiting and lower extremity motor block. For surgical procedures covered by the thoracic dermatomes, insertion of a thoracic rather than a lumbar epidural catheter may provide segmental analgesia, thus sparing the lumbar–sacral segments. This may result in a lower incidence of urinary retention and motor block, and possibly less hypotension due, in part, to a lower amount of local anaesthetic used and the limited extent of sympathetic block.[92–95] Finally, physiological benefits may not be seen with lumbar catheters.[50] Thus, placement of a thoracic epidural catheter for surgical procedures covered by the thoracic dermatomes optimizes postoperative analgesia by allowing for a more intense segmental analgesia, while minimizing side-effects (e.g. lower extremity motor block) that would interfere with the patient's ability to participate in their own convalescence.

Importance of analgesic agent

The ability of postoperative epidural analgesia potentially to diminish the pathophysiology that occurs following surgery is dependent on the type of agents used (opioids versus local anaesthetics) in the analgesic regimen. The physiological benefits and maximal attenuation of perioperative pathophysiology occurs primarily with use of a local-anaesthetic-based rather than an opioid-based epidural analgesic solution. Local anaesthetics have the capability to block afferent and efferent signals to and from the spinal cord, thus suppressing the surgical stress response[96] and spinal reflex inhibition of diaphragmatic and gastrointestinal function. Unlike local anaesthetics, opioids cannot completely block transmission of afferent input from the periphery into the spinal cord.[3] In addition, the local anaesthetic used in the epidural regimen may be absorbed systematically and exert various systemic effects, including facilitating return of gastrointestinal motility,[33] decreasing blood viscosity[7] and diminishing inflammation.[97]

Clinical trials have demonstrated the advantages of using a local-anaesthetic-based epidural analgesic solution. Four randomized trials have shown that, when compared to epidural opioids for postoperative analgesia, the use of a local-anaesthetic-based epidural solution resulted in an earlier recovery of gastrointestinal motility after abdominal surgery.[38, 44, 51, 52] Unlike those who received epidural opioids, patients who received epidural local anaesthetics had a lower incidence of

Table 25.2. Appropriate location of epidural catheter insertion for various types of surgery

Type of surgery	Epidural catheter placement
Thoracic	T4–8
Upper abdominal:	T6–7
gastrectomy	
hepatic resection	
Whipple resection	
Mid-abdominal:	T7–10
cystoprostatectomy	
nephrectomy	
Lower abdominal:	T9–12
abdominoperineal repair	
colectomy	
total abdominal hysterectomy	
Lower extremity:	L1–4
total hip or knee replacement	

pulmonary complications.[53] Thus, use of a local-anaesthetic-based regional technique appears to provide several advantages, compared to using opioid-based techniques, in diminishing perioperative morbidity in certain organ systems.

MULTIMODAL APPROACH TO PATIENT CONVALESCENCE

Although epidural analgesia does confer some physiological benefits by attenuating perioperative pathophysiology, it is unclear whether use of epidural analgesia in itself may be sufficient to decrease perioperative morbidity and mortality. However, use of epidural analgesia as part of a multimodal approach to perioperative management may facilitate patient recovery and improve patient-related outcomes. The multimodal approach to control perioperative pathophysiology and facilitate patient convalescence postoperatively emphasizes attenuation of the perioperative stress response, effective pain control, early patient mobilization, and early enteral feeding or return of gastrointestinal function.[2] Clearly, many of these goals can be achieved by using a local-anaesthetic-based analgesic solution administered through an appropriately located epidural catheter.

The multimodal approach (which may incorporate perioperative use of epidural analgesia) to control postoperative pathophysiology has been shown to facilitate patient recovery for a number of surgical procedures. In patients undergoing abdominothoracic oesophagectomy, patients who participated in a multimodal approach had a shorter time to extubation, superior analgesia, earlier return of bowel function and earlier fulfilment of intensive-care-unit discharge criteria.[98] In another trial, a multimodal approach implemented in patients undergoing colon resection reduced length of hospitalization from 6–10 days to a median of 2 days.[99] Finally, patients undergoing major urological procedures had a reduction in hormonal and

PRACTICE POINTS

- Postoperative epidural analgesia provides superior analgesia and physiological benefits. Although there are methodological issues in the interpretation of available studies, there are data suggesting that perioperative epidural analgesia may be associated with a decrease in postoperative pulmonary, cardiac, coagulation and gastrointestinal complications.

- Epidural analgesia is not a generic intervention. Specific management (i.e. analgesic drug (local anaesthetic versus opioid), catheter-incision congruency, duration of epidural analgesia and use as part of a multimodal regimen) of the postoperative epidural regimen may influence outcome.

metabolic stress and an improvement in convalescence with a multimodal approach using thoracic epidural analgesia.[100]

SUMMARY

The pathophysiology that occurs following surgery may cause many detrimental physiological effects, which in turn may result in postoperative morbidity and mortality. Use of perioperative regional anaesthetic techniques, including postoperative epidural analgesia, can attenuate these adverse physiological changes, which may result in an improvement in patient morbidity, especially in return of gastrointestinal function[36, 39, 40–47, 101] and preservation of postoperative pulmonary function. Although perioperative epidural analgesia may provide benefits in decreasing perioperative morbidity and mortality, use of epidural analgesia is not without risk,[101] as rare neurological complications, such as epidural haematoma (<1:10,000) or epidural abscess (<1:20,000), may occur.

There are many issues still to be resolved, including elucidating the pathophysiology of certain postoperative disorders, determining the extent of the contribution of intraoperative anaesthesia versus postoperative analgesia to any decreases in mortality and morbidity, and assessing the role of postoperative epidural analgesia in facilitating patient convalescence (multimodal analgesia). In addition, there are other potential benefits

RESEARCH AGENDA

- Further research is needed to elucidate the effect of epidural analgesia (versus other techniques such as intravenous patient-controlled analgesia) on patient-orientated outcomes such as quality of recovery, quality of life and patient satisfaction.

- Randomized controlled trials are needed to determine the optimal postoperative regimens for conditions such as obstructive sleep apnoea and postoperative cognitive dysfunction.

of postoperative epidural analgesia, including improvements in analgesia and patient satisfaction. Finally, although we have focused on epidural analgesia, other regional analgesic techniques, such as continuous peripheral catheter analgesia, may also potentially provide decreases in patient morbidity through similar physiological benefits as that discussed for epidural analgesia.

REFERENCES

1. Rosenberg J, Kehlet H. Does effective postoperative pain management influence surgical morbidity? *Eur Surg Res* 1999; **31**: 133–137.
2. Kehlet H. Multimodal approach to control postoperative pathophysiology and rehabilitation. *Br J Anaesth* 1997; **78**: 606–617.
3. Kehlet H. Modification of responses to surgery by neural blockade: clinical implications. In: Cousins MJ, Bridenbaugh PO (eds), *Neural Blockade in Clinical Anesthesia and Management of Pain*, 3rd edn. Lippincott-Raven, Philadelphia, PA, 1998, pp. 129–175.
4. Chernow B, Alexander HR, Smallridge RC et al. Hormonal responses to graded surgical stress. *Arch Intern Med* 1987; **147**: 1273–1278.
5. Glaser F, Sannwald GA, Buhr HJ et al. General stress response to conventional and laparoscopic cholecystectomy. *Ann Surg* 1995; **221**: 372–380.
6. Anand KJS, Hickey PR. Halothane–morphine compared with high-dose sufentanil for anesthesia and postoperative analgesia in neonatal cardiac surgery. *N Engl J Med* 1992; **326**: 1–9.
7. Rosenfeld BA. Benefits of regional anesthesia on thromboembolic complications following surgery. *Regional Anesth* 1996; **21**: S9–S12.
8. Liu S, Carpenter RL, Neal JM. Epidural anesthesia and analgesia: their role in postoperative outcome. *Anesthesiology* 1995; **82**: 1474–506.
9. Tonnesen E, Brinklov MM, Christensen NJ et al. Natural killer cell activity and lymphocyte function during and after coronary artery bypass grafting in relation to the endocrine stress response. *Anesthesiology* 1987; **67**: 526–533.
10. Davis JM, Albert JD, Tracy KJ et al. Increased neutrophil mobilization and decreased chemotaxis during cortisol and epinephrine infusions. *J Trauma* 1991; **31**: 725–732.
11. Salo M. Effects of anaesthesia and surgery on the immune response. *Acta Anaesthesiol Scand* 1992; **36**: 201–220.
12. Pomposelli JJ, Baxter JK 3rd, Babineau TJ et al. Early postoperative glucose control predicts nosocomial infection rate in diabetic patients. *J Parenteral Enteral Nutr* 1998; **22**: 77–81.
13. Leung JM, O'Kelly BF, Mangano DT. Relationship of regional wall motion abnormalities to hemodynamic indices of myocardial oxygen supply and demand in patients undergoing CABG surgery. *Anesthesiology* 1990; **73**: 802–814.
14. Flatley KA, DeFily DV, Thomas JX. Effects of cardiac sympathetic nerve stimulation during adrenergic blockade on infarct size in anesthetized dogs. *J Cardiovasc Pharmacol* 1985; 7: 673–679.
15. Johannsen UJ, Mark AL, Marcus ML. Responsiveness to cardiac sympathetic nerve stimulation during maximal coronary dilation produced by adenosine. *Circulation Res* 1982; **50**: 510–517.
16. Mangano DT, Hollenberg M, Fergert G et al. Perioperative myocardial ischemia in patients undergoing noncardiac surgery – I: incidence and severity during the 4 day perioperative period. *J Am Coll cardiol* 1991; **17**: 843–850.
17. Trip MD, Volkert MC, van Capelle FJL et al. Platelet hyperreactivity and prognosis in survivors of myocardial infarction. *N Engl J Med* 1990; **322**: 1549–1554.
18. Craig DB. Postoperative recovery of pulmonary function. *Anesth Analges* 1981; **60**: 46–52.
19. Kavanagh BP, Katz J, Sandler AN. Pain control after thoracic surgery: a review of current techniques. *Anesthesiology* 1994; **81**: 737–759.
20. Simonneau G, Vivien A, Sartene R et al. Diaphragmatic dysfunction induced by upper abdominal surgery. Role of postoperative pain. *Am Rev Respir Dis* 1983; **128**: 899–903.
21. Fratacci M-D, Kimball WR, Wain JC et al. Diaphragmatic shortening after thoracic surgery in humans: effects of mechanical ventilation and thoracic epidural anesthesia. *Anesthesiology* 1993; **79**: 654–665.
22. Duggan J, Drummond GB. Activity of lower intercostal and abdominal muscle after upper abdominal surgery. *Anesth Analges* 1987; **66**: 852–855.
23. Livingston EH, Passaro EP Jr. Postoperative ileus. *Digest Dis Sci* 1990; **35**: 121–132.

24. Glise H, Abrahamsson H. Reflex inhibition of gastric motility: patho-physiological aspects. *Scand J Gastroenterol* 1984; **89**(Suppl): 77–82.

25. Rodgers A, Walker N, Schug S et al. Reduction of postoperative mortality and morbidity with epidural or spinal anaesthesia: results from overview of randomised trials. *BMJ* 2000; *321*: 1493–1496.

26. Sharrock NE, Ranawat CS, Urquhart B et al. Factors influencing deep vein thrombosis following total hip arthroplasty under epidural anesthesia. *Anesth Analges* 1993; **76**: 756–771.

27. Wu CL, Hurley RW, Anderson GF et al. Effect of postoperative epidural analgesia on morbidity and mortality following surgery in Medicare patients. *Region Anesth Pain Med* 2004; **29**: 525–533.

28. Steinbrook RA. Epidural anesthesia and gastrointestinal motility. *Anesth Analges* 1998; **86**: 837–844.

29. Saito H, Trocki O, Alexander JW et al. The effect of route of nutrient administration on the nutritional state, catabolic hormone secretion, and gut mucosal integrity after burn injury. *J Parenteral Enteral Nutr* 1987; **11**: 1–7.

30. Moore FA, Feliciano DV, Andrassay RJ et al. Early enteral feeding, compared with parenteral, reduces postoperative septic complications. *Ann Surg* 1992; **216**: 172–183.

31. Shou J, Lappin J, Minnard EA et al. Total parenteral nutrition, bacterial trans-location, and host immune function. *Am J Surg* 1994; **167**: 145–150.

32. Rimback G, Cassuto J, Wallin G et al. Inhibition of peritonitis by amide local anesthetics. *Anesthesiology* 1988; **69**: 881–886.

33. Groudine SB, Fisher HA, Kaufman RP et al. Intravenous lidocaine speeds the return of bowel function, decreases postoperative pain, and shortens hospital stay in patients undergoing radical prostatectomy. *Anesth Analges* 1998; **86**: 235–239.

34. Worsley MH, Wishart HY, Peebles Brown DA et al. High spinal nerve block for large bowel anastomosis. *Br J Anaesth* 1988; **60**: 836–840.

35. Sielenkamper AW, Eicker K, Van Aken H. Thoracic epidural anesthesia increases mucosal perfusion in ileum of rats. *Anesthesiology* 2000; **93**: 844–851.

36. Rawal N, Sjostrand U, Christoffersson E et al. Comparison of intramuscular and epidural morphine for postoperative analgesia in the grossly obese: influence on postoperative ambulation and pulmonary function. *Anesth Analges* 1984; **63**: 583–592.

37. Wallin G, Cassuto J, Hogstrom S et al. Failure of epidural anesthesia to prevent postoperative paralytic ileus. *Anesthesiology* 1986; **65**: 292–297.

38. Scheinin B, Asantila R, Orko R. The effect of bupivacaine and morphine on pain and bowel function after colonic surgery. *Acta Anaesthesiol Scand* 1987; **31**: 161–164.

39. Ahn H, Bronge A, Johansson K et al. Effect of continuous postoperative epidural analgesia on intestinal motility. *Br J Surg* 1988; **75**: 1176–1178.

40. Wattwil M, Thoren T, Hennerdal S et al. Epidural analgesia with bupivacaine reduces postoperative paralytic ileus after hysterectomy. *Anesth Analges* 1989; **68**: 353–358.

41. Bredtmann RD, Herden HN, Teichmann W et al. Epidural analgesia in colonic surgery: results of a randomized prospective study. *Br J Surg* 1990; **77**: 638–642.

42. Seeling W, Bruckmooser KP, Hufner C et al. No reduction in postoperative complications by use of catheterized epidural analgesia following major abdominal surgery. *Anaesthesist* 1990; **39**: 33–40.

43. Jayr C, Thomas H, Rey A et al. Postoperative pulmonary complications. Epidural analgesia using bupivacaine and opioids versus parenteral opioids. *Anesthesiology* 1993; **78**: 666–676.

44. Liu SS, Carpenter RL, Mackey DC et al. Effects of perioperative analgesic technique on rate of recovery after colon surgery. *Anesthesiology* 1995; **83**: 757–765.

45. Neudecker J, Schwenk W, Junghans T et al. Randomized controlled trial to examine the influence of thoracic epidural analgesia on postoperative ileus after laparoscopic sigmoid resection. *Br J Surg* 1999; **86**: 1292–1295.

46. Cassady JF Jr, Lederhaas G, Cancel D et al. A randomized comparison of the effects of continuous thoracic epidural analgesia and intravenous patient-controlled analgesia after posterior spine fusion in adolescents. *Regional Anesth and Pain Medicine* 2000; **25**: 246–253.

47. Mann C, Pouzeraate Y, Boccara G et al. Comparison of intravenous or epidural patient-controlled analgesia in the elderly after major abdominal surgery. *Anesthesiology* 2000; **92**: 433–441.

48. Jorgensen H, Wetterslev J, Moiniche S et al. *Epidural Local Anaesthetics versus Opioid-based Analgesic Regimens on Postoperative Gastrointestinal Paralysis, PONV and Pain after Abdominal Surgery*. Cochrane Review. The Cochrane Library 2001; 3.

49. Hjortso NC, Neumann P, Frosig F et al. A controlled study on the effect of epidural analgesia with local anaesthetics and morphine on morbidity after abdominal surgery. *Acta Anaesthesiol Scand* 1985; **29**: 790–796.

50. Scott AM, Starling JR, Ruscher AE et al. Thoracic versus lumbar epidural anesthesia's effect on pain control and ileus resolution after restorative protocolectomy. *Surgery* 1996; **120**: 688–697.

51. Thoren T, Wattwil M. Effects on gastric emptying of thoracic epidural analgesia with morphine or bupivacaine. *Anesth Analges* 1988; **67**: 687–694.

52. Thorn SE, Wickborn G, Philipson L et al. Myoelectric activity in the stomach and duodenum after epidural administration of morphine or bupivacaine. *Acta Anaesthesiol Scand* 1996; **40**: 773–778.

53. Ballantyne JC, Carr DB, deFerranti S et al. The comparative effects of postoperative analgesic therapies on pulmonary outcome: cumulative meta-analyses of randomized, controlled trials. *Anesth Analges* 1998; **86**: 598–612.

54. Stiller KR, Munday RM. Chest physiotherapy for the surgical patient. *Br J Surg* 1992; **79**: 745–749.

55. Morran CG, Finlay IG, Mathieson M et al. Randomized controlled trial of physiotherapy for postoperative pulmonary complications. *Br J Anaesth* 1983; **55**: 1113–1117.

56. Wu CL, Fleisher LA. Outcomes research in regional anesthesia and analgesia. *Anesth Analges* 2000; **91**: 1232–1242.

57. Mangano DT, Browner WS, Hollenberg M et al. Association of perioperative myocardial ischemia with cardiac morbidity and mortality in men undergoing noncardiac surgery. *N Engl J Med* 1990; **323**: 1781–1788.

58. McCann RL, Clements FM. Silent myocardial ischemia in patients undergoing peripheral vascular surgery: incidence and association with perioperative cardiac morbidity and mortality. *J Vasc Surg* 1989; **9**: 583–587.

59. Davis RF, DeBoer LW, Maroko PR. Thoracic epidural anesthesia reduces myocardial infarct size after size after coronary artery occlusion in dogs. *Anesth Analg* 1986; **65**: 711–717.

60. Rolf N, Van de Velde M, Wouters PF et al. Thoracic epidural anesthesia improves functional recovery from myocardial stunning in conscious dogs. *Anesth Analges* 1996; **83**: 935–940.

61. Klassen GA, Bramwell RS, Bromage PR et al. Effect of acute sympathectomy by epidural anesthesia on the canine coronary circulation. *Anesthesiology* 1980; **52**: 8–15.

62. Kock M, Blomberg S, Emanuelsson H et al. Thoracic epidural anesthesia improves global and regional left ventricular function during stress-induced myocardial ischemia in patients with coronary artery disease. *Anesth Analges* 1990; **71**: 625–630.

63. Nishimori M, Ballantyne JC, Low JHS. Epidural pain relief versus systemic opioid-based pain relief for abdominal aortic surgery. Cochrane Database of Systematic Reviews 2006, Issue 3 (19 July 2006).

64. Beattie WS, Badner NH, Choi P. Epidural analgesia reduces postoperative myocardial infarction: a meta-analysis. *Anesth Analges* 2001; **93**: 853–858.

65. Clagett GP, Anderson FA, Heit J et al. Prevention of venous thrombo-embolism. *Chest* 1995; **108**: 312S–334S.

66. Sorenson RM, Pace NL. Anesthetic techniques during surgical repair of femoral neck fractures: a meta-analysis. *Anesthesiology* 1992; **77**: 1095–1104.

67. Christopherson R, Beattie C, Frank SM et al. Perioperative morbidity in patients randomized to epidural or general anesthesia for lower extremity vascular surgery. *Anesthesiology* 1993; **79**: 422–434.

68. Rosenfeld BA, Beattie C, Christopherson R et al. The effects of different anesthetic regimens on fibrinolysis and the development of postoperative arterial thrombosis. *Anesthesiology* 1993; **79**: 435–443.

69. Tuman KJ, McCarthy RJ, March RJ et al. Effects of epidural anesthesia and analgesia on coagulation and outcome after major vascular surgery. *Anesth Analges* 1991; **73**: 696–704.

70. Jorgensen LN, Rasmussen LS, Nielsen PT et al. Antithrombotic efficacy of continuous extradural analgesia after knee replacement. *Br J Anaesth* 1991; **66**: 8–12.

71. Dalldorf PG, Perkins FM, Totterman S et al. Deep venous thrombosis following total hip arthroplasty: effect of prolonged postoperative epidural anesthesia. *J Arthroplasty* 1994; **9**: 611–616.

72. Eriksson BI, Ekman S, Baur M et al. Regional block anaesthesia versus general anaesthesia. Are different antithrombotic drugs equally effective in patients undergoing hip replacement? Retrospective analysis of 2354 patients under-going hip replacement receiving either recombinant hirudin, unfractionated heparin or enoxaparin. [abstract]. *Thromb Haemostas* 1997; **77**: PS1992.

73. Levkoff SE, Besdine RW, Wetle T. Acute confusional states (delirium) in the hospitalized elderly. *Ann Rev Gerontol Geriatr* 1986; **6**: 1–26.

74. Moller JT, Cluitmans P, Rasmussen LS et al. Long-term postoperative cognitive dysfunction in the elderly: ISPOCD1 study. *Lancet* 1998; **351**: 857–861.

75. Riis J, Lomholt B, Haxholdt O et al. Immediate and long-term mental recovery from general versus epidural anesthesia in elderly patients. *Acta Anaesthesiol Scand* 1983; **27**: 44–49.

76. Edwards H, Rose EA, Schorow M et al. Postoperative deterioration in psychomotor function. *JAMA* 1981; **245**: 1342–1343.

77. Inouye SK, Peduzzi PN, Robison JT et al. Importance of functional measures in predicting mortality among older hospitalized patients. *JAMA* 1998; **279**: 1187–1193.

78. Francis J, Martin D, Kapoor WN. A prospective study of delirium in hospitalized elderly. *JAMA* 1990; **263**: 1097–1101.

79. Duggleby W, Lander J. Cognitive status and postoperative pain: older adults. *J Pain Sympt Manage* 1994; **9**: 19–27.

80. Marcantonio ER, Juarez G, Goldman L et al. The relationship of postoperative delirium with psychoactive medications. *JAMA* 1994; **272**: 1518–1522.

81. Dyer CB, Ashton CM, Teasdale TA. Postoperative delirium: a review of 80 primary data-collection studies. *Arch Intern Med* 1995; **155**: 461–465.

82. Lynch EP, Lazor MA, Gellis JE et al. The impact of postoperative pain on the development of postoperative delirium. *Anesth Analges* 1998; **86**: 781–785.

83. Block BM, Liu SS, Rowlingson AJ et al. Efficacy of postoperative epidural analgesia: a meta-analysis. *JAMA* 2003; **290**: 2455–2463.

84. Wu CL, Hsu W, Richman JM et al. Postoperative cognitive function as an outcome of regional anesthesia and analgesia. *Reg Anesth Pain Med* 2004; **29**: 257–268.

85. Ben-Eliyahu S, Yirmiya R, Liebeskind JC et al. Stress increases metastatic spread of a mammary tumor in rats: evidence for mediation by the immune system. *Brain, Behavior, and Immunity* 1991; 5: 193–205.

86. Amato AC, Pescatori M. Effect of perioperative blood transfusions on recurrence of colorectal cancer: meta-analysis stratified on risk factors. *Dis Colon Rectum* 1998; **41**: 570–585.

87. de Leon-Casasola OA. Immunomodulation and epidural anesthesia and analgesia. *Regional Anesth* 1996; **21**: S24–S25.

88. Bode RH Jr, Lewis KP, Zarich SW et al. Cardiac outcome after peripheral vascular surgery. Comparison of general and regional anesthesia. *Anesthesiology* 1996; **84**: 3–13.

89. Liu SS. Bank robbers and outcomes research. *Reg Anesth Pain Med* 2003; **28**: 262–264.

90. Carli F, Mayo N, Klubien K et al. Epidural analgesia enhances functional exercise capacity and health-related quality of life after colonic surgery: results of a randomized trial. *Anesthesiology* 2002; **97**: 540–549.

91. Wu CL, Naqibuddin M, Fleisher LA. Measurement of patient satisfaction as an outcome of regional anesthesia and analgesia: a systematic review. *Reg Anesth Pain Med* 2001; **26**: 196–208.

92. Liu SS, Allen HW, Olsson GL. Patient-controlled epidural analgesia with bupivacaine and fentanyl on hospital wards: prospective experience with 1.030 surgical patients. *Anesthesiology* 1998; **88**: 688–695.

93. Brennum J, Arendt-Nielsen L, Secher NH et al. Quantitative sensory examination in human epidural anaesthesia and analgesia: effects of lidocaine. *Pain* 1992; **51**: 27–34.

94. Chisakuta AM, George KA, Hawthorne CT. Postoperative epidural infusion of a mixture of bupivacaine 0.2% with fentanyl for upper abdominal surgery. A comparison of thoracic and lumbar routes. *Anaesthesia* 1995; **50**: 72–75.

95. Magnusdottir H, Kirno K, Riksten SE et al. High thoracic epidural anesthesia does not inhibit sympathetic nerve activity in the lower extremities. *Anesthesiology* 1999; **91**: 1299–1304.

96. Rutberg H, Hakanson E, Anderberg B et al. Effects of the extradural administration of morphine, or bupivacaine, on the endocrine response to upper abdominal surgery. *Br J Anaesth* 1984; **56**: 233–238.

97. Hollman MW, Durieux ME. Local anesthetics and the inflammatory response? A new therapeutic indication? *Anesthesiology* 2000; **93**: 858–875.

98. Brodner G, Pogatzki E, Van Aken H et al. A multimodal approach to control postoperative pathophysiology and rehabilitation in patients undergoing abdominothoracic esophagectomy. *Anesth Analges* 1998; **86**: 228–234.

99. Basse L, Jakobsen D, Billesbolle P et al. A clinical pathway to accelerate recovery after colonic resection. *Ann Surg* 2000; **232**: 51–57.

100. Brodner G, Van Aken H, Hertle L et al. Multimodal perioperative management – combining thoracic epidural analgesia, forced mobilization, and oral nutrition – reduces hormonal and metabolic stress and improves convalescence after major urologic surgery. *Anesth Analges* 2001; **92**: 1594–1600.

101. Horlocker TT, Wedel DJ. Neurologic complications of spinal and epidural anesthesia. *Reg Anesth Pain Med* 2000; **25**: 83–98.

Chapter 26

Prevention and treatment of hyperalgesia and persistent neuropathic pain after surgery

Audun Stubhaug and Harald Breivik

INTRODUCTION

All surgical procedures carry a risk of triggering persistent pain caused by tissue and nerve injury. The incidence varies from 5% to 80% (Table 26.1), and pain intensity and degree of functional impairment caused by chronic postsurgical pain varies from mild to intolerable and disabling.[1–8]

Thus chronic postoperative pain is common and an important health problem. Although only a small portion of those reporting persistent discomfort and pain after surgery

Table 26.1. Prevalence of chronic pain after various types of surgery

Type of surgery	Prevalence (%)
Breast[6, 7]	11–49
Thoracotomy[6, 7]	5–67
Cholecystectomy[6, 7]	3–56
Inguinal hernia[6, 7]	1–63
Vasectomy[7]	0–37
Sternotomy[1]	28
Hip arthroplasty[4]	28
Knee arthroplasty[10]	19
Dupuytren's surgery[43]	5–40
Wrist fracture[43]	7–37
Ankle surgery[43]	14
Arthroscopic knee surgery[43]	2–4
Carpal tunnel surgery[43]	2–5

have severe and disabling pain conditions, even after a simple operation such as an inguinal hernia repair 16.6% had impairment of daily activities 1 year after surgery.[8] Therefore, with the large number of patients undergoing surgery worldwide, many individuals will suffer ill-health because of this adverse effect of surgical trauma. In a recent large-scale survey of chronic pain in 16 countries, one in five adults reported chronic pain that had lasted for a median time of more than 7 years and was rated 5 or more on a 10-point numerical pain scale.[9] Of those reporting chronic pain, 15% had pain after surgery or trauma. Significant impact on working life, social and daily life and mental health was reported by a majority of the respondents with chronic pain.[9]

WHAT IS CHRONIC PAIN AFTER SURGERY?

Unfortunately, most publications simply report the presence, and sometimes the intensity, of spontaneous pain after surgery. Pain that persists for 3 months or more after surgery has been considered chronic postoperative pain. In order to characterize and classify chronic pain, as a minimum we need information about the quality of the pain experienced and the results of a clinical examination.

It is crucial to know whether the postsurgical pain was developed after surgery or was a continuation of similar pain present before surgery. Stanos et al.[10] assessed prospectively the incidence of criteria for complex regional pain syndrome type I (CRPS-I) in patients following knee-replacement surgery. They found that 42% met the International Association for the Study of Pain (IASP) criteria 4 weeks and 3 months after surgery, while 19% still met the criteria 6 months after the operation. However, 13.5% had significant pain also before surgery, including allodynia and oedema, as well as temperature, colour and sweating asymmetry. Similarly, preoperative pain can be an important indication for surgery in a number of surgical procedures, for example cholecystectomy and orthopaedic procedures.

A thorough examination and classification of the pain is necessary to rule out other causes of chronic pain, such as recurrent malignancy or infection. Chronic postoperative pain may present as several different syndromes.

Chronic postsurgical pain conditions can be characterized by documenting whether there is:

- spontaneous pain
- evoked pain, such as lancinating pain evoked from a trigger zone
- allodynia to gentle touch
- hypoaesthesia
- dysaesthesia.

It is obvious that simply to assess the intensity of spontaneous pain is not adequate if we want to study the efficacy of interventions. A call for uniform assessment of post-herniorrhaphy pain can be expanded to chronic postsurgical pain in general.[11] An example of how postoperative pain should be analysed is illustrated in Figure 26.1.

Patients with a postoperative continuation of presurgical pain should be treated as a separate group.

Since spontaneous resolution of pain seems to be frequent during the first few months, only pain that persists for more than 6 months should be evaluated as possible chronic postoperative pain.

FACTORS ASSOCIATED WITH INCREASED RISK OF CHRONIC PAIN AFTER SURGERY

Pain before surgery, severe and insufficiently relieved acute pain soon after surgery, immobilization (e.g. in a cast), reoperations, radiation and cytotoxic drug therapy for cancer, hypervigilant personality and genetic factors are all associated with a greater risk of developing chronic pain after surgery.[2–8, 11–14]

A strong association between poorly managed and severe pain during the first few days after surgery does not necessarily mean a causal relationship, but it raises an important question: Will effective relief of acute postoperative pain reduce the risk of chronic postoperative pain? If acute pain and chronic pain are separate consequences of injury, as indicated in Figure 26.2, relief of acute pain may not necessarily reduce the risk of chronic pain after surgery.[13] If less acute pain reduces the risk of chronic pain after surgery, this may be linked more to the type of pain management than to the reduction in intensity of acute pain. Thus, drugs that have antihyperalgesic effects, such as local anaesthetic drugs, antiepileptic drugs and tricyclic antidepressants, may have both analgesic and antihyperalgesic effects. Only the latter effect may be related to a reduced risk of chronic neuropathic pain after tissue injury.

Although most analgesics given at the start of a noxious stimulation seem to reduce the development of hyperalgesia, only the N-methyl-D-aspartate (NMDA) receptor antagonists (e.g. ketamine) have been shown to reduce hyperalgesia that is already established.[15] It is reasonable that patients with one or more known risk factors receive special attention and that the focus is on possible preventive measures for avoiding the development of chronic pain when surgery is unavoidable. Optimal management of dynamic pain after surgery, with analgesic and antihyperalgesic drugs, as well as early mobilization are essential (see below).

POSSIBLE MECHANISMS INVOLVED IN THE PATHOGENESIS OF CHRONIC PAIN AFTER SURGERY

In their search of mechanisms of post-injury pain and hypersensitivity, basic neuroscientists have focused on the

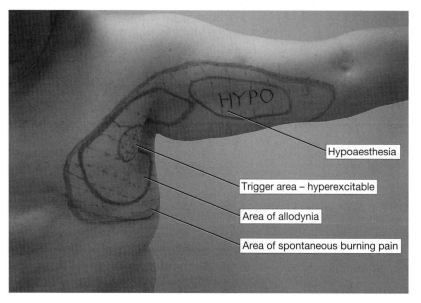

Figure 26.1. Analysis of components of chronic pain after mastectomy.

An area of *hypoaesthesia* is a result of section of the peripheral sensory nerves. This is a sign of nerve injury.

A *trigger area* where *hyperexcitable peripheral nerves* cause *ectopic discharges*, and pain occurring *spontaneously* or after *stimulation by pressure or movement*. This type of pain may be relieved by a sodium-channel blocker; lidocaine topically or intravenously.

An area of *allodynia* (i.e. pain provoked by light touch) indicates central nervous system sensitization. Lidocaine, NMDA blockers or opioids may reduce this pain component.

An area of *spontaneous, burning pain*, is most likely due to central maladaptation and dysfunction of pain-modulating neurons. Amitriptyline, gabapentin, pregabalin and opioids may reduce this pain component.

(See also Plate IV of colour section, page xiv.)

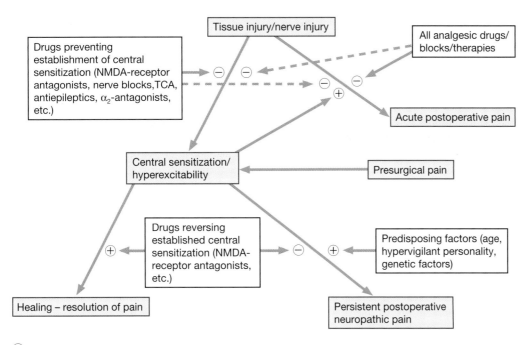

Figure 26.2. Model proposing relationships between surgical trauma and tissue and nerve injury, acute pain, central nervous system plasticity and development of chronic postoperative neuropathic pain. Possible augmenting or diminishing factors and treatments are also shown.

plasticity in the nervous system following tissue and nerve injury.[16–18] Tissue injury induces *peripheral sensitization* of nociceptors, and the subsequent afferent barrage induces a hyperexcitable state in the spinal cord dorsal horn, which is often referred to as *central sensitization*. Nerve injury can produce the same result. These changes explain the increased pain sensation to previously painful stimuli (*hyperalgesia*) and pain induced by previously non-painful stimuli (*allodynia*) that occur after acute injury, as well as in chronic pain conditions. Nerve injury also induces changes in ion-channel expression of neuronal cell membranes that lead to spontaneous depolarization in both injured and in neighbouring non-injured neurons.

Complex mechanisms act in the central nervous system, including glial cell activation.[19–24] Neuronal cell death, in part from excessive and prolonged excitation (e.g. excitotoxic effects from prolonged glutamate release from interneurons as well as activated glial cells) may contribute to persistent and irreversible changes in pain-modulating mechanisms. Several interacting receptor systems and intracellular messenger systems are involved. Molecular changes in neurons after tissue injury turn on genes, causing synthesis of new proteins and growth factors that cause abnormal growth of nerve fibres, maladaptive reconnections and hypersensitivity of nerve cells. Changes in sodium-channel expression are important aspects of these functional changes.

In summary, it seems unlikely that we can expect one simple drug treatment to prevent such neuroplastic changes and their sometimes detrimental adverse effects leading to prolonged and pronounced pain and misery after tissue injury. Rather, a combination of drugs may be needed (see below).

Lack of regression of the promoter of repair

Normal sensitization of peripheral nociceptors and central sensitization in the spinal cord dorsal horn neurons both create hyperalgesia and allodynia in the postoperative period in the area surrounding the surgical wound. This postoperative pain is a promoter of repair, by creating a region of increased sensitivity near the injured tissue. This minimizes movement and contact trauma of the injured part of the body until healing has occurred. Normally, this hypersensitivity regresses after a few weeks, diminishing to mild soreness that eventually disappears altogether. However, in some unfortunate patients this regression of the normal and useful hyperalgesia and allodynia does not occur. Hyperalgesia and allodynia persist and reduce function and the quality of life of the patient. Apart from the risk factors listed above that are associated with a higher incidence of chronic pain after surgery, we know little of why some patients end up with debilitating chronic pain, while most patients after the same type of surgery do not.

IS PREVENTION OF CHRONIC PAIN AFTER SURGERY POSSIBLE?

We can hope to be able to reduce the incidence and severity of chronic neuropathic pain after surgery by optimal management of acute postoperative pain. However, as indicated in Figure 26.2, perceived acute pain can be an epiphenomenon to the plastic changes taking place in the central nervous system after tissue and nerve injury.[25] Traditional analgesic drugs may have only a minor modifying effect on nervous system plasticity, and may not be effective in reversing already established central sensitization. This is especially important in patients with long-lasting presurgical neuropathic pain conditions.

On the other hand, drugs that are only weak analgesics for acute pain may be more effective in controlling central sensitization and the transition from acute to chronic pain. Agents such as α_2-agonists, glutamate NMDA receptor antagonists, sodium-channel blockers (local anaesthetics and others) and drugs that modify functions of calcium channels and release of excitatory transmitters are candidate co-analgesics for further clinical research in this area. Glucocorticoids reduce hypersensitivity after tissue trauma and surgery,[26, 27] possibly through a diminished activation of spinal glial cells.[23, 24]

LOCAL ANAESTHETICS AND OPIOID-RECEPTOR AGONISTS

In animal research it is well documented that pre-injury treatment with local anaesthetics or opioids can prevent post-injury hyperexcitability in the spinal cord. Woolf and Wall[28] showed that the amount of morphine required to prevent the development of spinal hyperexcitability was ten-fold less than the amount required to reverse it when it was well established. This discovery led to the idea of pre-emption of pain. Pre-emptive analgesia is still a controversial topic in humans. The idea is to prevent central sensitization. However, in major surgery in humans it is obvious that sensitization can occur both during surgery and postoperatively.[29] This explains why a single intervention during surgery has only a minor effect on postoperative pain and hyperalgesia. Obviously, in clinical practice, the sensitizing stimulus continues after surgery and must be treated both intra- and postoperatively.

Preventive or pre-emptive analgesia?

The above considerations have led to the introduction of *preventive analgesia* as a more pragmatic concept: we have to start inhibiting noxious input and central sensitization as soon as surgery starts and continue it during surgery and for as long after surgery as the pain impulses are strong.[29] The original definition of pre-emptive analgesia, in which pretreatment is expected to have a lasting effect after surgery, has been proven by numerous studies to be futile.[29]

Although no perfect study in humans has yet been published, a modest evidence base for the beneficial effect of opioids (with or without local anaesthetics) is available. A small dose (10 mg) of preoperative morphine did reduce postoperative pain, analgesic requirements and hypersensitivity in patients undergoing gynaecological laparatomies.[30] Human experimental research confirms that pre-injury morphine reduces secondary hyperalgesia, while the same dose post-injury does not.[31] Epidural opioids with a local anaesthetic seem to be more potent than intravenous opioids: pre-incisional treatment with epidural lidocaine and fentanyl 4 μg/kg in patients undergoing gynaecological laparatomies resulted in significantly lower pain scores, opioid requirements and less hyperalgesia compared with a placebo.[32]

In a prospective, randomized trial Sentürk et al.[33] compared the effects of three different analgesia techniques in 69 thoracotomy patients. Two groups received thoracic epidural analgesia, either with preoperative initiation (pre-TEA) or postoperative initiation (post-TEA). The third group had patient-controlled intravenous analgesia with morphine (iv-PCA). The patients receiving pre-TEA with bupivacaine and morphine had significantly less pain postoperatively than did those in the other groups, and a significantly lower incidence of pain after 6 months (45%) compared with the iv-PCA group (78%).

In a double-blind trial in 60 patients undergoing spinal fusion with bone graft from the iliac crest, Reuben et al.[34] examined the effect of local morphine 5 mg at the graft site compared with placebo and intramuscular morphine. Local morphine reduced postoperative pain, and after 1 year only 5% had persistent pain compared with 32% in the placebo group and 37% in the intramuscular morphine group. These two studies are small and have methodological shortcomings, and should be replicated before definite conclusions are drawn.

ANTIHYPERALGESIC DRUGS: THE NEED FOR GOOD CLINICAL TRIALS

A number of drugs and drug classes have been shown to reduce hyperphenomena after tissue injury in animal studies: glutamate-receptor antagonists (ketamine), α_2-adrenergics (clonidine and adrenalin), drugs that modify functions of calcium channels (e.g. gabapentin and pregabalin), serotonin inhibitors/antagonists (amitriptyline and ketanserine), glucocorticoids, paracetamol (acetaminophen), cyclo-oxygenase inhibitors and specific sodium-channel blockers. Clinical research in this field will require additional outcome variables that more directly measure the phenomena related to the development of chronic pain, such as central sensitization.[35, 36] Ketamine, the only clinically useable and available glutamate antagonist, reduces postoperative hyperalgesia and persistent pain.[35, 37] Glucocorticoids reduce acute pain after surgery[26] and persistent hyperaesthesia,[27] and may contribute to reduced long-term pain after surgery.[23, 24] Cyclo-oxygenase inhibitors and paracetamol have similar, but weaker, effects.[24]

The optimal timing and length of treatment are other open questions, especially in cases where presurgical pain is present. A combination of several treatment approaches may be necessary. The final test of the clinical usefulness of a treatment strategy aimed at preventing chronic postoperative neuropathic pain will be adequately sized, randomized, double-blind (whenever applicable), single- or multicentre trials.

SECONDARY PREVENTION: AGGRESSIVE TREATMENT OF ACUTE NEUROPATHIC PAIN EARLY AFTER SURGERY

Clearly it is important to identify early those at risk and those patients who show early signs and symptoms of acute neuropathic pain after surgery,[38] in the acute to subacute phase following surgery or an accidental injury. Those patients who have severe and abnormal sensory changes, hyperphenomena and pain 4–6 weeks after surgery, often have similar or worse pain 1 year later.[3, 27] Therefore, it must be important that patients having clear signs and symptoms of acute neuropathic pain during the first few weeks after surgery receive early and aggressive interventions. Since the same mechanism can give rise to different symptoms and one symptom may arise from different mechanisms, in these high-risk patients it seems prudent to treat pain aggressively with a sodium-channel blocker (lidocaine, topically and intravenously), a calcium-channel-modifying drug (gabapentin or pregabalin[39–42]), a glucocorticoid (effects on glial activation), as well as an opioid, a cyclo-oxygenase inhibitor, paracetamol, and possibly amitriptyline, clonidine and ketanserine.[32, 35]

TREATMENT OF ESTABLISHED CHRONIC POSTSURGICAL NEUROPATHIC PAIN

The treatment of established chronic postsurgical neuropathic pain is often difficult. While it is not the main focus of this chapter, the options are described here briefly.[43, 44] Antiepileptic drugs (e.g. carbamazepine, phenytoin, gabapentin and pregabalin) and tricyclic antidepressants (e.g. amitriptyline) will relieve some of the pain in some patients. Neuromodulation

with spinal cord (dorsal columns) stimulation via epidural electrodes helps some patients. Transcutaneous nerve stimulation sometimes helps. Opioids may reduce the intensity of pain and suffering in some patients, but these should be added to the treatment regimen only when non-drug modalities and optimal dosing of antiepileptic and antidepressant drugs have failed to relieve pain and to increase function and quality of life.

REFERENCES

1. Meyerson J, Thelin S, Gordh T et al. The incidence of chronic post-sternotomy pain after cardiac surgery – a prospective study. *Acta Anaesthesiol Scand* 2001; **45**: 940–944.
2. Kroner K, Krebs B, Skov J et al. Immediate and long-term phantom breast syndrome after mastectomy: incidence, clinical characteristics and relationship to premastectomy breast pain. *Pain* 1989; **39**: 327–334.
3. Callesen T, Bech K, Kehlet H. Prospective study of chronic pain after groin hernia repair. *Br J Surg* 1999; **86**: 1528–1531.

4. Nikolajsen L, Brandsborg B, Lucht U et al. Chronic pain following total hip arthroplasty: a nationwide questionnaire study. *Acta Anaesth Scand* 2006; **50**: 495–500.

5. Gehling M, Scheidt CE, Niebergall H et al. Persistent pain after elective trauma surgery. *Acute Pain* 1999; **2**: 110–114.

6. Perkins FM, Kehlet H. Chronic pain as an outcome of surgery. A review of predictive factors. *Anesthesiology* 2000; **93**: 1123–1133.

7. Macrae WA. Chronic pain after surgery. *Br J Anaesth* 2001; **87**: 88–98.

8. Bay-Nielsen M, Prkins FM, Kehlet H. Pain and functional impairment 1 year after inguinal herniorrhaphy – a nationwide questionnaire study. *Ann Surg* 2001; **233**: 1–7.

9. Breivik H, Collett B, Ventafridda V et al. Survey of chronic pain in Europe: prevalence, impact on daily life, and treatment. *Eur J Pain* 2006; **10**: 287–333.

10. Stanos SP, Harden RH, Wagner-Raphael R et al. A prospective clinical model for investigating the development of CRPS. In: Harden RN, Baron R, Jänig W (eds), *Complex Regional Pain Syndrome, Progress in Pain Research and Management.* IASP Press, Seattle, WA, 2001, pp. 151–164.

11. Kehlet H, Bay-Nielsen M, Kingsnorth A. Chronic postherniorrhaphy pain – a call for uniform assessment. *Hernia* 2002; **6**: 178–181.

12. Katz J, Jackson M, Kavanagh BP et al. Acute pain after thoracic surgery predicts long-term post-thoracotomy pain. *Clin J Pain* 1996; **12**: 50–55.

13. Tasmuth T, Kataja M, Blomqvist C et al. Treatment-related factors predisposing to chronic pain in patients with breast cancer – a multivariate approach. *Acta Oncol* 1997; **36**: 625–630.

14. Katz J, Poleshuck EL, Audrus CH et al. Risk factors for acute pain and its persistence following breast cancer surgery. *Pain* 2005; **119**: 16–25.

15. Woolf CJ, Thompson SW. The induction and maintenance of central sensitization is dependent on N-methyl-D-aspartic acid receptor activation; implications for the treatment of post-injury pain hypersensitivity states. *Pain.* 1991; **44**: 293–299.

16. Coderre TJ, Katz J, Vaccarino AL et al. Contribution of central neuroplasticity to pathological pain: review of clinical and experimental evidence. *Pain* 1993; **52**: 259–285.

17. Woolf CJ, Salter MW. Neuronal plasticity: increasing the gain in pain. *Science* 2000; **288**: 1765–1769.

18. Woolf CJ. Dissecting out mechanisms responsible for peripheral neuropathic pain: Implications for diagnosis and therapy. *Life Sci* 2004; **74**: 2605–2610.

19. Coward K. Aitken A. Powell A et al. Plasticity of TTX-sensitive sodium channels PN1 and brain III in injured human nerves. *Neuroreport* 2001; **12**: 495–500.

20. Lai J. Hunter JC. Porreca F. The role of voltage-gated sodium channels in neuropathic pain. *Curr Opin Neurobiol* 2003; 13: 291–297.

21. Waxman SG, Dib-Hajj S, Cummins TR et al. Sodium channels and their genes: dynamic expression in the normal nervous system, dysregulation in disease states. *Brain Res* 2000; **886**: 5–14.

22. Watkins LR, Maiers SF. Immune regulation of central nervous system functions: from sickness responses to pathological pain. *J Int Med* 2005; **257**: 139–155.

23. Takeda K, Sawamura S, Sekiyama H et al. Effect of methylprednisolone on neuropathic pain and spinal glial activation in rats. *Anesthesiology* 2004; **100**: 1249–1257.

24. Takeda K, Sawamura S, Tamai H et al. Role for cyclooxygenase 2 in the development and maintenance of neuropathic pain and spinal glial activation. *Anesthesiology* 2005; **103**: 837–844.

25. Stubhaug A. Can opioids prevent post-operative chronic pain? *Eur J Pain* 2005; **9**: 153–156.

26. Romundstad L, Breivik H, Roald H et al. Methylprednisolone reduces pain, emesis, and fatigue after breast augmentation surgery: a single dose, randomized, parallel-group study with methylprednisolone 125 mg, parecoxib 40 mg, and placebo. *Anesth Analges* 2006; **102**: 418–425.

27. Romundstad L, Breivik H, Roald H et al. Chronic pain and sensory changes after augmentation mammoplasty: long term effects of preincisional administration of methylprednisolone. *Pain* 2006; **124**: 92–99.

28. Woolf CJ, Wall PD. Morphine-sensitive and morphine-insensitive actions of C-fibre input on the rat spinal cord. *Neurosci Lett* 1986; **64**: 221–225.

29. Breivik H, Breivik EK, Stubhaug A. Clinical aspects of pre-emptive analgesia: prevention of post-operative pain by pretreatment and continued optimal treatment. *Pain Rev* 1996; **3**: 63–78.

30. Richmond CE, Bromley LM, Woolf CJ. Preoperative morphine pre-empts postoperative pain. *Lancet* 1993; **342**: 73–75.

31. Warncke T, Stubhaug A, Jorum E. Preinjury treatment with morphine or ketamine inhibits the development of experimentally induced secondary hyperalgesia in man. *Pain* 2000; **86**: 293–303.

32. Katz J, Cohen L, Schmid R et al. Postoperative morphine use and hyperalgesia are reduced by preoperative but not intraoperative epidural analgesia: implications for preemptive analgesia and the prevention of central sensitization. *Anesthesiology* 2003; **98**: 1449–1460.

33. Sentürk M, Ozcan PE, Talu GK et al. The effects of three different analgesia techniques on long-term postthoracotomy pain. *Anesth Analges* 2002; **94**: 11–15.

34. Reuben SS, Vieira P, Faruqi S et al. Local administration of morphine for analgesia after iliac bone graft harvest. *Anesthesiology* 2001; **95**: 390–394.

35. Stubhaug A, Breivik H, Eide PK et al. Mapping of punctuate hyperalgesia surrounding a surgical incision demonstrates that ketamine is a powerful suppressor of central sensitization to pain following surgery. *Acta Anaesthesiol Scand* 1997; **41**: 1124–1132.

36. Stubhaug A. Quantitative sensory testing in clinical trials: what does it get you? In: Giamberardino MA (ed.), *Pain 2002. An Updated Review.* IASP Press, Seattle, WA, 2002, pp. 131–136.

37. Lavand'homme P, De Kock M, Waterloos H. Intraoperative epidural analgesia combined with ketamine provides effective preventive analgesia in patients undergoing major digestive surgery. *Anesthesiology* 2005; **103**: 681–683.

38. Power I. Recent advances in postoperative pain therapy. *Br J Anaesth* 2005; **95**: 43–51.

39. Gilron I, Orr E, Tu D et al. A placebo-controlled randomized clinical trial of perioperative administration of gabapentin, rofecoxib and their combination for spontaneous and movement-evoked pain after abdominal hysterectomy. *Pain.* 2005; **113**: 191–200.

40. Fassoulaki A, Triga A, Melemeni A et al Multimodal analgesia with gabapentin and local anesthetics prevents acute and chronic pain after breast surgery for cancer. *Anesth Analg* 2005; **101**: 1427–1432.

41. Fassoulaki A, Stamatakis E, Petropoulos G et al. Gabapentin attenuates late but not acute pain after abdominal hysterectomy. *Eur J Anaesthesiol* 2006; **23**: 136–141.

42. Rowbotham DJ. Gabapentin: a new drug for postoperative pain? *Br J Anaseth* 2006; **96**: 152–155.

43. Finnerup NB, Otto M, McQuay HJ et al. Algorithm for neuropathic pain treatment: an evidence based proposal. *Pain* 2005; **118**: 289–305.

44. Kehlet H, Jensen ST, Woolf CJ. Persistent postsurgical pain: risk factors and prevention. *Lancet* 2006; **367**: 1618–1625.

SECTION 8

Management strategies

Chapter 27

Pain management and quality in healthcare

Lesley A. Colvin and Ian Power

INTRODUCTION

The alleviation of pain is central to the role of the anaesthetist, who is uniquely placed to deliver effective analgesia using a combination of appropriately directed pharmacological and interventional techniques. Before going on to consider how pain can best be managed in the perioperative setting, we need to be clear what exactly we are treating and why. The International Association for the Study of Pain (IASP) definition states 'Pain is an unpleasant sensory and emotional experience associated with actual or potential tissue damage or described in terms of such damage'.[1] This reflects the complex nature of pain perception, with many factors influencing the expression of pain and distress in the individual. The biopsychosocial model (Figure 27.1) outlines some of the factors involved. Although this chapter is limited mainly to the management of acute postoperative pain, many of the areas discussed can be applied to other pain settings.

A basic assumption is that it is beneficial to relieve pain. This is not only a humanitarian and ethical right, but also has a sound economic basis. Prompt and effective management of pain will allow early re-establishment of function, minimizing any associated disability. This will consequently decrease economic costs. It has been estimated that acute pain costs Australian society up to $10 billion per year. Strategies to maximize delivery of effective analgesia and to utilize the benefits from this can lead to a decrease in hospital stay, with benefits for both patients and society.[2]

CURRENT PAIN MANAGEMENT

Pain is one of the commonest symptoms for which a patient consults their general practitioner. Despite this, many studies have found that pain is not well managed by our profession. In one survey, more than 70% of adults believed pain to be

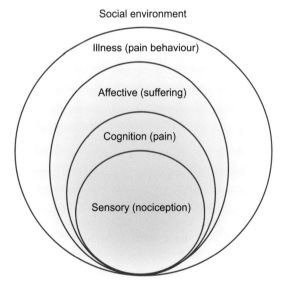

Social environment

Illness (pain behaviour)

Affective (suffering)

Cognition (pain)

Sensory (nociception)

Figure 27.1. The biopsychosocial model. This model indicates the multidimensional nature of pain and pain experience that must be considered in all patients in pain.

inevitable after surgery, with this being a significant cause of fear and anxiety prior to surgery. Unfortunately, Australian, British and American audits of pain management show that these fears may indeed be justified. About a decade ago, a report on pain after surgery highlighted significant deficiencies in this area.[3, 4] Some improvements have been made, but many aspects of acute pain management could still be improved (Box 27.1).

An audit of 3000 UK hospital patients found that up to 87% of patients reported severe or moderate pain.[5] Another study

Box 27.1. Challenging areas for acute pain management and possible influences contributing to make management difficult

Potentially difficult patient areas
- Neonates and infants
- Elderly
- Burns
- Trauma
- Cancer
- Head injury/impaired consciousness level
- Drug abuse

Possible influences: patient factors
- Assessment difficulties
- Fear of addiction
- Expectation of pain and disability
- Pharmacokinetic variability
- Social and cultural influences
- Opioid tolerance

Potentially difficult healthcare worker areas
- Cultural and attitudinal barriers
- Low priority on importance of pain relief
- Communication problems
- Inadequate assessment

Possible influences: system factors
- Inadequate funding and staffing
- Poor knowledge base and training
- Influences of legal prescribing requirements
- Ineffective or lack of evidence for treatment available

involving 3000 patients in 15 UK hospitals found that by introducing a programme of education for staff, formal assessment and use of simple algorithms for pain management, moderate to severe pain could be reduced from 37% to 13%.[6] A prospective audit carried out by the Picker Institute found that within a UK hospital setting around 58% of patients had moderate to severe pain.[7] In France, an audit of the effectiveness of introducing a quality assurance programme over 1 year found that pain control could be improved by education of all staff involved, systematic assessment and use of protocol-driven provision of modern analgesic techniques. This was without requiring specially qualified personnel in every ward area.[8] Another European study had similar results, with a significant improvement in acute pain management after surgery by the introduction of a nurse-led, anaesthetist-supervised acute pain service. Education and the provision of regular, simple analgesics were thought to be the main factors contributing to the improvement in analgesia.[9]

Pain management has been traditionally divided into acute and chronic, often with different strategies used in treatment. As more is understood about nociceptive transmission and rapid plasticity within the peripheral and central nervous systems, the rigid division between acute and chronic becomes unhelpful. If pain is viewed as a continuum, difficult pain problems presenting acutely should become easier to diagnose and treat. One important area that is not yet understood is the factors predisposing to developing persistent pain. The 'difficult patient' that anaesthetists are asked to assess, several days after surgery, could simply be more susceptible to rapid plastic changes, resulting in altered nociceptive processing. Alternatively, there may be more complex factors regulating pain perception and the expression of pain in particular individuals (see Figure 27.1).

The incidence of persistent pain after surgery is probably underestimated, with a minority of sufferers attending a chronic pain clinic. One study found that about 20% of patients attending pain clinics did so because of pain related to surgery.[10] Studies in this area are of mixed quality, often with a non-standard definition of chronic pain and variable assessment measures.[11] A recent review concluded that there is a need for research in this area to determine predisposing factors and causes.[12]

In developing strategies to improve management of acute pain, it is important to base these on the best evidence currently available, with careful assessment of both safety and efficacy for any intervention.[13] Regularly updated and high-quality websites can be used, such as the Oxford Pain Website[14] and the Cochrane Database.[15] Use of meta-analysis and systematic reviews should help to provide definitive management plans, although these must be flexible enough for individual patient variation. It is clear that current management of acute pain is far from ideal (see Box 27.1). Principles for optimizing treatment of post-operative pain need to be developed, providing pain relief that allows early mobilization and return to normal function.

This chapter covers each of the following areas:

- pain mechanisms
- assessment
- treatment
- approaches to achieving high-quality pain management.

PAIN MECHANISMS

A clear understanding of the pathways involved in nociceptive transmission and how these can be affected by tissue injury is essential for a logical approach to pain management. The following section gives a brief overview of the scientific basis of nociceptive transmission.

Nociceptive transmission

Figure 27.2 shows the neuraxis (the peripheral and central nervous system) involved in sensory processing and gives a framework for understanding the changes occurring as a result of tissue injury.[18–21] This is a dynamic system that responds to sensory input, tissue damage and other factors, with significant modifications occurring in the neuraxis even in the immediate postoperative period.

Non-specialized free nerve endings transduce high-intensity noxious stimuli in the periphery, resulting in action potential

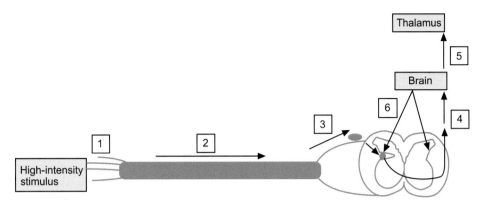

Figure 27.2. Basic pain pathway. (1) A high-intensity stimulus activates polymodal nociceptors in the periphery. (2) These unmodified bare nerve endings initiate action potential generation in small, myelinated A-δ fibres and unmyelinated C fibres, within a mixed peripheral nerve. (3) Impulses ascend and enter the spinal cord via the dorsal root, synapsing with second-order neurons in the superficial dorsal horn (the substantia gelatinosa) and Rexed's lamina V (mainly A-δ fibres). (4) From the first central synapse, onward transmission includes activation of neurons within the anterolateral spinothalamic tract. Larger myelinated A-δ fibres have also been shown to enter the dorsal horn, synapsing predominantly in laminae III and IV. A low-intensity stimulus, such as light touch, rather than a noxious stimulus would be required to activate these neurons.[16, 17] (5) The ascending pathways give off branches within the brainstem, then synapse in the thalamus, from where multiple areas within the brain are activated. (6) Descending systems, originating in the periaqueductal grey matter in the midbrain and the nucleus raphe magnus in the pons exert modulatory influences in the spinal cord.

generation in primary sensory neurons. Unmyelinated C fibres and small myelinated A-δ fibres are predominantly involved in nociceptive transmission. The cell bodies of all sensory fibres are situated in the dorsal root ganglia, close to the spinal cord. This is where the nucleus lies and where all neurotransmitters necessary for chemical transmission at the synapses are synthesized, before peripheral and central transport to axon terminals.[22]

Specific receptors and channels have been identified in nociceptors involved in transducing particular types of noxious stimuli, with the potential for developing targeted and peripherally acting analgesics. For example, noxious thermal stimuli may activate vanilloid receptors, which are members of the transient receptor potential (TRP) family of ion channels.[23] Primary sensory neurons synapse in the dorsal horn of the spinal cord in a precise somatotopic map of peripheral structures. The majority of C fibres and A-δ fibres synapse in laminae I and II of the superficial dorsal horn, in the substantia gelatinosa, with some A-δ fibres terminating in lamina V. Complex modulation of dorsal horn neurons can occur both via intrinsic spinal mechanisms and descending systems. The second-order projection neurons ascend to the brain in specific tracts.[22]

Within the spinal cord, the main neurotransmitter involved in fast synaptic transmission is glutamate, acting at the ionotropic receptor, the α-amino-3-hydroxyl-5-methyl-4-isoxazole propionic acid (AMPA) receptor. Neuropeptides, such as substance P are also released in response to noxious stimulation.[24, 25]

At the level of the thalamus, multiple areas of the brain can be activated, reflecting the complex nature of pain perception. This has been studied in the clinical setting, using brain imaging techniques such as functional magnetic resonance imaging (fMRI) to study the cortical response to nociceptive stimuli, with the most consistently activated areas including the insular and the anterior cingulated regions.[26–28] There is increasing evidence of the complex interaction between the brain and the spinal cord in pain processing.[29, 30] The descending brainstem systems modulate nociceptive input – this may either be inhibitory or excitatory.[31, 32]

Response to tissue injury

Acute pain has been described as 'physiological' pain, whereas 'pathological' pain can occur in the absence of ongoing tissue injury (Box 27.2).[33] In the perioperative period a variety of peripheral and central changes can contribute to an alteration in nociceptive processing. Why these responses can persist in some individuals is as yet poorly understood.

The immediate response to a noxious stimulus results in encoding for intensity, duration and location, resulting in perception of acute pain in that area. As a result of tissue injury, this direct relationship can alter, with subsequent changes in signs and symptoms (Table 27.1). The relative importance of

---

Box 27.2. Physiological versus pathological pain

Physiological pain
- Acute
- Initiates withdrawal response: removes from further injury
- Protective function
- Immobilizes to allow healing

Pathological pain
- Can be acute or develop over time
- Ongoing tissue damage not necessarily present
- Maladaptive
- Reduces level of function
- Disability and distress

Peripheral responses

As a result of tissue injury, peripheral changes can affect both action potential generation and chemical transmission. Peripheral sensitization can occur, with a resultant alteration in response. Specific animal models of tissue injury may contribute to our understanding of pain mechanisms and the way in which the neuraxis responds to peripheral injury.[35, 36] After surgery, the exact changes can depend on the nature of the tissue injury. For example, after thoracotomy, there may be a combination of an acute inflammatory response and peripheral nerve injury.

Inflammation

As a result of tissue damage a cascade of responses may be initiated that result in an inflammatory response with a decrease in activation threshold of peripheral nociceptors.[37] Several peripheral receptors may have a role in the inflammatory process. For example, there is a family of cation channels termed the acid-sensing ion channel (ASIC) family that responds specifi-cally to reduced pH, a dominant factor in inflammation.[38, 39] Another family of G-protein-coupled receptors, the proteinase-activated receptors (PARs), also appears to be involved in inflammatory processes.[40, 41]

Alterations in regional blood flow, recruitment of immune cells and release of inflammatory mediators are all involved in the inflammatory process (Figure 27.3) (for a review see Kidd and Urban[42]). Cytokines may act as inflammatory mediators via kinase-linked receptors to alter gene expression at a cellular level. For example, mitogen-activated protein kinases (MAPK), such as extracellular signal-regulated protein kinase (ERK) and p38, are activated by inflammatory mediators in both primary sensory and secondary order dorsal horn neurons.[43] The interaction between inflammatory mediators and receptors on sensory neurons is key to this process of peripheral sensitization (Table 27.2). There are also changes in neuropeptide synthesis within the dorsal root ganglia (Table 27.3).

Nerve injury

As a result of damage to peripheral nerves, the precise relationship between stimulus and coded input is lost. There are

Table 27.1. Altered symptoms and signs after tissue injury

Symptom/sign	Description	Possible mechanisms
Spontaneous pain	Pain arising without peripheral stimulus	Ectopic discharges
		Summation of subthreshold electrical activity initiating action potentials
Allodynia	Pain arising from innocuous stimulus	Lower nociceptors threshold (peripheral); rewiring (central)
Primary hyperalgesia	Exaggerated pain response in injured area	Increased neuronal activation; after-discharges of stimulated neurons
Secondary hyperalgesia	Exaggerated pain response outwith injured area	Altered receptive field size; recruitment of previously silent synapses

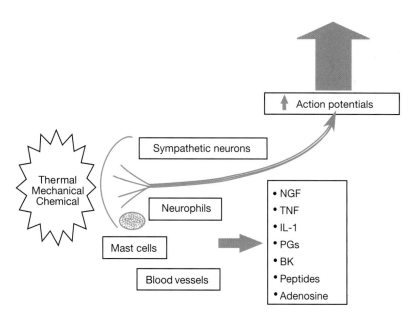

Figure 27.3. Peripheral inflammatory response. Tissue damage can initiate a series of responses that result in local alterations in blood flow, changes in autonomic activity and recruitment of immune cells into the area. A variety of substances is released into the damaged area, including nerve growth factor (NGF), cytokines such as tumour necrosis factor (TNF) and interleukin-1 (IL-1), prostaglandins (PG) and bradykinin (BK), as well as peptides such as substance P and purines such as adenosine. The pH in the area may also decrease. One result of these changes is an increase in responsiveness of sensory neurons, with a resultant increased input into the spinal cord.

Table 27.2. Peripheral receptors important in nociceptive processing after tissue damage

Receptor	Type	Putative ligands	References
Vanilloid	Several subtypes, non-selective cation channel	Capsaicin, thermal stimuli, protons, anandamide	Szallasi et al. (1999)[44]
Acid-sensing ion channels (ASIC)	Several subtypes throughout CNS; ion channel	Protons (low pH)	Waldmann et al. (1997[39]
Purinergic	Several subtypes; ionotropic	Adenosine and phosphorylated compounds	Burnstock et al. (1996)[45]
Proteinase-activated receptor	Several subtypes; G-protein-coupled	Proteinases, e.g. tryptase, trypsin	Vergnalle et al. (2001)[46]

Table 27.3. Neuropeptide changes in dorsal root ganglia after inflammation or peripheral nerve injury

Neuropeptide	Normal	Inflammation	Nerve injury
Substance P	Small cells	↑	
Calcitonin gene-related peptide	Small cells	↑	↓
Somatostatin	Small cells	→	↓
Neuropeptide Y	Little present	→	↑
Galanin	Little present	→	↑

changes in both action potential generation and neuronal transport (Figure 27.4).[47, 48] There are also major alterations in the synthesis of neurotransmitters within the dorsal root ganglia (see Table 27.3).[51, 52] During nerve regeneration, axonal sprouts generate neuronal activity, and ectopic activity can develop at the site of neuromas or at the dorsal root ganglia. The resultant barrage of activity to the spinal cord can contribute to central changes.[47]

Central responses
Spinal cord

A complex series of responses occur in the spinal cord as a result of peripheral injury. Some of these changes are similar in both inflammation and nerve injury, with amplification of sensory transmission.

- Acutely, the phenomenon known as 'wind up' occurs in response to repeated noxious stimulation.[53] The key neurotransmitters involved in this include glutamate, acting via the N-methyl-D-aspartate (NMDA) receptor, and substance P, acting via the neurokinin (NK-1) receptor[54]. During normal sensory transmission, the NMDA receptor is blocked by magnesium. As a result of repeated high-intensity stimulation the voltage-dependent magnesium block is lifted and NMDA receptors are activated by any subsequent release of glutamate.[55] Certain NMDA receptor subtypes may interact with a family of proteins known as the membrane-associated guanylate kinase family (MAGUK), including protein complexes such as PSD-95/SAP90, which may play a significant role in neuropathic pain.[56]
- Changes in gene transcription can occur rapidly, with early alterations in activity of immediate early genes (IEGs) within

dorsal horn neurons. Within minutes of intense noxious stimulation, an increase in IEG protein products, such as c-fos and c-jun, can be found.[57–59]

- There are major changes in neurotransmitter levels, both in the dorsal root ganglia and within the spinal cord itself, with several hundred genes being either up- or down-regulated, altering the character of subsets of primary sensory neurons.[60] The specific nature of these changes is dependent on the type and severity of tissue damage.[61]
- After nerve injury, central terminations of sensory neurons, mainly C fibres, degenerate in the spinal cord. This may be related to loss of retrogradely transported neurotrophins from the periphery, such as NGF and GDNF (glial derived neurotrophic factor). Trans-synaptic degeneration may also occur with loss of second-order neurons possibly related to factors at the time of nerve injury. Earlier studies have reported sprouting of A-β fibres into the superficial dorsal horn after nerve injury, but there is considerable debate as to whether or not this may be an artefact due to immunohistochemical techniques.[62–64] In addition, alterations in sympathetic neurons have been found, with sprouts forming around sensory cell bodies in the dorsal root ganglia.[65]
- There is increasing interest in the role of glial cells in some pathological pain states, with the possibility for new drug targets.[66, 67]

Brain

Using brain-imaging techniques such as positron emission tomography and scanning and fMRI, it has been possible to study neuronal responses to both acute and chronic pain in humans.[27] It is not yet known if these techniques can differentiate between excitatory and inhibitory neuronal activity, but they do provide a non-invasive way of assessing neuronal response within the brain.[68] Changes in cortical responses have been found in complex regional pain syndrome and phantom limb pain.[69] Studies of upper-limb amputees have revealed a strong positive correlation between cortical remapping and phantom limb pain.[70, 71] This could be due to alterations in cortical anatomy or unmasking of previously silent synapses.[72] There is some evidence from primate studies that cortical and subcortical neurons can sprout some distance in response to peripheral nerve injury.[73, 74]

PAIN ASSESSMENT

Firstly we need to consider why it is important to assess pain:

- Poor pain assessment is a barrier to good pain control.[75]
- Regular assessment of pain can improve pain management. The use of pain charts has been shown to increase the quality of analgesia. This may be related more to actually having a chart rather than to the details of the chart itself.[76, 77] There is, however, some evidence that pain assessment by both doctors and nurses may underestimate pain severity.[78]

- A reliable technique is needed to compare the efficacy of different treatments.[79, 80]
- From a clinical perspective, it is important to know not just how effective a treatment or intervention is, but also the level of risk associated with it. This can be assessed by calculating the number-needed-to-harm (NNH), as outlined in McQuay and Moore.[13]

For research and detailed audit, assessment of pain can include complex tools to study all aspects of pain perception, but for day-to-day ward-based practice, a quick and simple assessment is required. If it becomes too complex, then the likelihood is that due to staffing and time constraints, the assessment will not be carried out, and analgesia will not be delivered appropriately.[81]

In everyday clinical practice, we need a means of assessment that is simple and practical, yet will reliably predict difficult pain problems to allow early intervention. One example of this is in the Clinical Standards Advisory Board (CSAG) Report on Services for Patients with Back Pain,[82] where early intervention is guided by following detailed protocols that highlight 'red flags' (requiring specialist medical assessment) and 'yellow flags' (requiring psychological intervention).

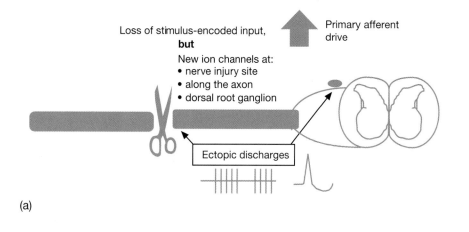

(a)

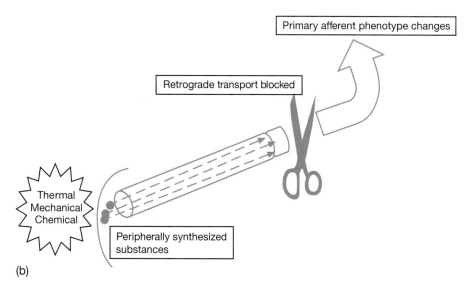

(b)

Figure 27.4. Peripheral nerve injury changes. (a) Spontaneous ectopic discharges develop at the nerve injury site and within the dorsal root ganglia after nerve injury. There is some evidence that these are related to the generation of spontaneous pain.[49] Mechanosensitive areas may also develop around the nerve injury site. (b) Alterations in neuronal transport as a result of nerve injury may contribute to the alterations in the characteristic neurotransmitters synthesized by primary sensory neurons in the dorsal root ganglia. There is some evidence that growth factor substances such as NGF may be important in this process.[50]

Assessment tools

As pain is a subjective experience, varying between individuals, it could be argued that to attempt to quantify and objectively assess pain is misleading.[83] Given that there is no definitive physiological variable that changes in a predictable fashion with pain experience, a reliable and sensitive way of interpreting patient reporting of pain must be used. These can be divided into measurements of pain intensity or relief and broader measures of pain experience.

Pain intensity measures

These can be (Figure 27.5):

- categorical
- visual–analogue
- numerical.

Simple rating scales can be used, either verbal or numerical. To be useful, a rating scale must be simple, with minimal reassessment variability and be sensitive enough to reflect response to treatment. A 100-mm visual–analogue scale (VAS) is often used, and has been shown to be reliable over time, with little to choose between this and an 11-point numerical rating scale. Both have been shown to be more robust in clinical use than a four-point verbal rating scale.[84, 85] The use of different pain-measurement techniques can make comparisons between different studies difficult. Comparing results from many randomized controlled trials, it was found that a score of > 30 mm on a VAS for pain intensity was equivalent to moderate or greater pain.[86] More recently, the use of simple global rating scales has received attention as a means of comparing treatment efficacy.[79]

Questionnaires

Many questionnaires have been designed to measure the overall pain experience; most are used in the research setting. Before using a particular questionnaire, it is important to assess that it has been validated for use in that setting. Factors such as ethnicity must be considered.[87] Another example is the widely used McGill Pain Questionnaire, which has been validated extensively, but may be more robust as a total score, rather than individual scores for each component of pain perception.[88]

A mechanistic approach

The use of quantitative sensory testing could be one way to try to link our improved understanding of sensory mechanisms of pain, with diagnosis and directed treatment in the clinic. This technique uses detailed and quantifiable ways in which to test for sensory response to specific stimuli, such as graded thermal or mechanical stimuli. Areas of allodynia, hyperalgesia and reduced sensation can be mapped. This technique has been used in the assessment of postherpetic neuralgia, where it is claimed that it is possible to differentiate between peripherally and centrally maintained pains.[89–91]

Accurate assessment of pain is essential to formulate a cohesive and effective management plan. Difficult pain problems can be a mixture of acute tissue injury, neuropathic or radicular pain, exacerbated by anxiety about the underlying disease. An example is outlined in the case history in Box 27.3.

TREATMENT

The scientific evidence for the safe and effective treatment of acute pain has recently been rigorously examined by a Working Party of the Faculty of Pain Medicine of the Australian and New Zealand College of Anaesthetists, and published as the document *Acute Pain Management: Scientific Evidence.*[92]

Paracetamol

Systematic reviews have found that paracetamol (acetaminophen) is effective when taken alone or in combination for mild to moderate pain, or as an adjunct to opioids.[13, 93, 94] In one study, 61 American Society of Anesthesiologists (ASA) physical status I and II patients were enrolled in a double-blind, randomized, placebo-controlled, parallel study to investigate the effect of a combination of paracetamol and morphine after open reduction and internal fixation of acute limb fractures. Patients were given either oral paracetamol (1 g every 4 hours) or placebo as an adjuvant to morphine by patient-controlled analgesia (PCA) postoperatively. The paracetamol group had lower pain scores on day 1 (2.1 versus 3.3; $p = 0.03$), a shorter average duration of PCA use (35.8 versus 45.5 hours; $p = 0.03$), and greater overall patient satisfaction.[94] Paracetamol is therefore an effective postoperative

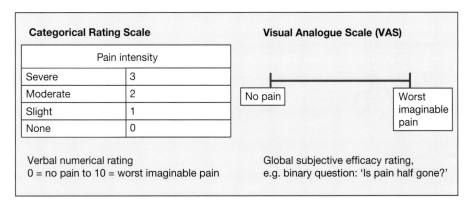

Figure 27.5. Pain measurement: these scales can be used to measure pain intensity or pain relief.

analgesic, with potency slightly less than a standard dose of morphine or the non-steroidal anti-inflammatory drugs (NSAIDs).[95, 96] The availability of intravenous paracetamol has enhanced and extended the use of paracetamol as a fundamental component of analgesia.[96–98] In one recent study performed after surgery for removal of impacted third molar teeth, the administration of one intravenous preparation, propacetamol, in repeated doses (2 g followed by 1 g) had a significant analgesic effect indistinguishable from that of intramuscular morphine (10 mg followed by 5 mg), but with improved tolerability.[99] More research is required as some studies have found either less impressive opioid sparing with intravenous paracetamol,[100, 101] or evidence of a ceiling to the analgesia at low doses.[16]

Nitroxyparacetamol (or nitroacetaminophen) is a promising new nitric oxide releasing version of paracetamol with analgesic and anti-inflammatory properties, which may be less hepatotoxic.[17] In the future nitroxyparacetamol may be a safer, while still effective, alternative to paracetamol.

Box 27.3. Case history: management of a difficult case

An 18-year-old boy had thoracic surgery for excision of a recurrent osteosarcoma. He had been treated for 4 years at the local children's hospital, but on this occasion the surgery was carried out in the regional neurosurgical unit. His pain was difficult to deal with postoperatively, with respiratory depression resulting from his use of patient-controlled analgesia (PCA) morphine, but without adequate analgesia. Nursing staff found him and his family difficult to deal with. Assessment revealed high levels of parental anxiety, significant pain both at rest and on movement, and allodynia in a radicular distribution.

Key points

- Social issues: parents unhappy about move from familiar environment of children's hospital; lower staffing levels with no specialist paediatric training
- Emotional: adolescence and patient wish for more independence; fear of underlying cancer and of the future; concern about addiction to morphine
- Sensory changes: neuropathic pain, with non-opioid responsive component

As a result of careful assessment several treatment strategies were used:

- Pharmacological: PCA ketamine, transfer onto oral long-acting opioids, regular paracetamol/NSAIDs, addition of adjuvant analgesia (amitriptyline and gabapentin) (number needed to treat noted)
- Discussion with nursing staff: involvement of Macmillan nurse from children's hospital
- Liaison with inpatient palliative care service, including psychology input

The patient was reassessed at regular intervals, and discharged home with good pain control and continued support organized in the community setting.

NSAIDs and Cox-2 inhibitors

Systematic reviews have found that NSAIDs are effective for mild to moderate pain, and are useful adjuncts for severe pain.[13, 93] However, NSAID use is restricted by side-effects (peptic ulceration, antiplatelet actions, aspirin-induced asthma and renal dysfunction), although in clinical practice the incidence of such adverse effects may be minimized by careful patient selection.[92] New drugs were developed that selectively inhibit the inducible cyclo-oxygenase enzyme Cox-2, and spare the constitutive Cox-1, and a review indicated that these Cox-2 inhibitors could represent a significant safety advance and permit their more widespread use for acute pain relief.[102] Unfortunately, this desired outcome has not been achieved because of associated cardiovascular thrombotic events that led to the voluntary withdrawal of rofecoxib, and remains the subject of considerable controversy.[103]

Opioids

Opioids are the basis of the management of moderate to severe pain, but they have significant side-effects (sedation, respiratory depression, nausea and vomiting, depression of gastrointestinal motility and disruption of sleep patterns). Possibly the most serious limitation of opioid use is inability to control movement-associated pain after surgery. In general, patients given systemic opioids after major surgery achieve adequate analgesia at rest but not during movement, when they may suffer severe discomfort. As a result, the patient minimizes any movement, but modern postoperative rehabilitation regimens following major surgery are dependent on analgesia that encourages mobilization.[92, 104]

Local anaesthetic techniques

Systematic reviews have found that the use of local anaesthetics for central neural blockade is effective for the relief of postoperative pain, is opioid sparing, and therefore facilitates early rehabilitation.[92] In addition, neural components of the stress response are blunted by epidural local anaesthesia, and this can be associated with a reduction in perioperative medical complications.[105, 106] A cumulative meta-analysis of randomized controlled trials on the comparative effects of postoperative analgesic therapies on pulmonary outcome confirmed that the use of epidural analgesia is associated with less postoperative respiratory morbidity.[105] Multimodal perioperative management after major urological surgery, employing thoracic epidural analgesia to enable mobilization and oral nutrition, reduces hormonal and metabolic stress and aids convalescence.[106]

Epidural local anaesthetics are often used in combination with low doses of epidural opioids, which are added to improve the analgesia.[92] Unfortunately, even small opioid doses given alone spinally may produce urinary retention, pruritus, nausea and a reduction in gut motility. For example, epidural morphine, but not bupivacaine, inhibits gastric motility on the day after cholecystectomy.[107]

The use of local anaesthetics for analgesia is not only restricted to the treatment of nociceptive pain by large nerve blockade; lidocaine given systemically is effective for the relief of neuropathic pain.[92] This antineuropathic or 'anti-allodynic' effect of lidocaine was confirmed in a rat model of neuropathic pain and the site of action was found to be predominantly peripheral.[108]

Tramadol

Tramadol is a synthetic analgesic with both opioid agonist and spinal and central nervous system effects through noradrenergic and serotonergic pathways, with minimal sedation, respiratory depression, gastrointestinal stasis or abuse potential. The two enantiomers of tramadol may be analgesic by complementary mechanisms.[109] In one study of patients having hysterectomy, the subjects were given tramadol 3 mg/kg or morphine 0.2 mg/kg at wound closure. The authors found that tramadol was as effective as morphine in providing postoperative analgesia, while permitting more rapid psychomotor recovery.[110] In a recent review the analgesic efficacy of tramadol was considered to be less than morphine, and the drug is listed by the World Health Organization as a weak opioid.[92]

Ketamine

The use and efficacy of low-dose ketamine in the management of acute postoperative pain was confirmed in a recent review; ketamine reduces postoperative morphine requirements.[111] Unfortunately, even low doses of ketamine can produce side-effects, such as hallucinations, and so alternative NMDA antagonists (e.g. dextromethorphan) are being assessed. In one study, dextromethorphan given by mouth before laparotomy significantly reduced intraoperative opioid requirements.[112] Low-dose ketamine therapy is also effective for the relief of neuropathic pain.[92]

Clonidine

Clonidine and other α_2 agonists can provide effective postoperative analgesia, although side-effects of sedation and hypotension limit general use.[113] Traditional use has concentrated on spinal or epidural administration of clonidine to take advantage of the known attenuating effect of stimulating spinal α_2 receptors on pain perception.[92]

Antidepressants and anticonvulsants

Systematic reviews confirm that tricyclic antidepressants and anticonvulsants are effective for the relief of neuropathic pain.[13, 92, 94] The anti-allodynic effects and the sites of action (peripheral, spinal or central) of amitriptyline, gabapentin and lidocaine were investigated using a rat model of neuropathic pain. All were effective; gabapentin acted centrally and lidocaine peripherally, whereas amitriptyline appeared to have multiple sites of action.[108] In addition to the effect on neuropathic pain, it is now evident that the preoperative administration of gabapentin can reduce postoperative pain and opioid requirements.[92]

Comparing different analgesics

McQuay and Moore[13] proposed a method of comparing different drugs: the number needed to treat (NNT). This is the number of patients who must be given active drug for one to achieve at least 50% relief of pain, compared with placebo. An NNT of 1 describes an event that occurs in every patient given treatment, but not with placebo. It would be exceptional in clinical studies for the treatment to be 100% effective and the placebo completely ineffective, and NNTs of 2 or 3 indicate effective analgesia (Table 27.4). The NNT for neuropathic pain for efficacy and adverse effects (NNH = number needed to harm; see above) are known for the anticonvulsants and tricyclic antidepressants (e.g. carbamazepine)[13] (Table 27.5).

APPROACHES TO ACHIEVING HIGH-QUALITY PAIN MANAGEMENT

Neuropathic pain in the postoperative period and the prevention of chronicity

Neuropathic pain is common after some surgical operations, and attempts must be made to prevent chronicity.[12, 114–116] The problem is dysfunction in the peripheral or central nervous system, as discussed previously. Possible causes can include nerve damage by surgical section, compression, stretching, ischaemia or infection. Changes in the neuraxis can take days to develop, and could explain the lack of efficacy of pre-emptive analgesia. Neuropathic pain is more likely in the postoperative period, when persistent central changes may be favoured (e.g. inadequate analgesia in the perioperative period, large operations or pre-existing pain).[114, 116]

It is essential to recognize and treat neuropathic pain after surgery, which may take a number of forms:[92]

- pain in the absence of ongoing tissue damage
- pain in an area of sensory loss
- paroxysmal, spontaneous pain
- allodynia, hyperalgesia, dysaesthesias

Table 27.4. The number needed to treat for various analgesics[13]

Drug	Number needed to treat
Codeine 60 mg	16.7
Paracetamol 1000 mg	4.6
Morphine 10 mg intramuscular	2.9
Ibuprofen 400 mg	2.7
Diclofenac 50 mg	2.3
Paracetamol 1000 mg + codeine 60 mg	1.9

Table 27.5. The number needed to treat: carbamazepine[13]

Condition	Efficacy	Adverse events	Severe events
Trigeminal neuralgia	2.6	3.4	24
Diabetic neuropathy	3.0	2.5	20

- burning, pulsing, stabbing pain
- poor response (not unresponsiveness) to opioids.

Perioperative neuropathic pain can be controlled initially with systemic lidocaine (1 mg/kg per hour) or ketamine (5–10 mg/hour), and later with an oral tricyclic antidepressant or anticonvulsant.

Pre-emptive and preventive analgesia

It has been proposed that effective analgesia given prior to an insult can act pre-emptively and reduce central sensitization and postoperative pain.[117] Evidence of this from animal experiments is convincing, but clinical studies are less impressive.[116] Clinical studies of pre-emptive analgesia can suffer from poor design, containing confounding factors such as the necessity of providing anaesthesia and analgesia to control groups.[118] Pre-emptive therapy with a single agent given before surgery is likely to fail, as afferent neuronal activity into the spinal cord continues for some time afterwards. To have any chance of producing a clinically significant effect, pre-emptive analgesia must include a strategy for modulating the sustained neuronal input into the spinal cord in the postoperative period. It appears that the timing of a single analgesic manoeuvre, as in pre-emptive analgesia, does not reduce postoperative pain significantly.[118] However, there is evidence that some analgesic interventions can reduce postoperative pain or analgesic use, exceeding the duration of action of the drug, which can be defined as preventive analgesia.[92]

Multimodal analgesia

There is evidence of the benefits of employing multimodal analgesia after surgery.[119] NSAIDs, paracetamol, local anaesthetics, other non-opioid analgesics and opioids are given in combination to improve analgesia and reduce side-effects.[92] Non-opioid analgesics contribute significantly to multimodal analgesia and recovery of the patient by minimizing opioid side-effects (e.g. opioid-induced gastrointestinal stasis). It is possible to eliminate pain after surgery using multimodal analgesia, with a significant reduction in total opioid consumption. Evidence from recent research has suggested that the use of multimodal analgesia after major surgery can hasten recovery and reduce costs.[106] Kehlet and Dahl[119] have proposed that the 'pain-free state' should be used to facilitate postoperative mobilization and oral feeding in a process of acute rehabilitation. Multimodal analgesia has the particular advantage over unimodal systemic opioid administration of providing excellent pain relief upon movement, thus allowing early mobilization, and is therefore a fundamental component of 'fast-track' surgery.[2]

SUMMARY

This chapter has addressed the question of pain management and quality in healthcare by considering pain mechanisms, assessment, treatment and approaches to achieving high-quality pain relief. The essential point about pain mechanisms is that injury can result in many changes, both peripherally and centrally, that can influence nociceptive transmission and pain perception. More information is required about these processes in the expectation that preventive strategies might be possible. The accurate assessment of pain is fundamental to the diagnosis of different pain states and also to the appraisal of treatment success or failure. Assessment of pain is particularly important in difficult pain problems that may have mixed nociceptive and neuropathic features. There is a continuing need to develop clinical assessments that may enlighten us about the predisposition of some individuals to develop chronic pain after acute injury. The scientific evidence for the use of different agents for the treatment of pain is increasing rapidly, and so the concepts of the number needed to treat (NNT) and the number needed to harm (NNH) should be expanded so that clinicians and patients have reliable information on the risk/benefit ratios of commonly used analgesics. With the rapid expansion in understanding of pain mechanisms, we need to know which analgesics can modify these changes. Pre-emptive analgesia should be reconsidered using strategies for modulating the

---

PRACTICE POINTS

There is a need to improve pain management in terms of:[3]

- Education:
  - of staff and patients[6, 120]
  - in the understanding of pain mechanisms.[112, 122]

- Assessment:
  - adequate and regular patient assessment improves pain control[123, 124]
  - difficult acute pain may be neuropathic.[125]

- Treatment:
  - implement a multidisciplinary approach[9]
  - utilize modern analgesic techniques when appropriate[126]
  - consider the risks versus benefits of available treatments.[13]

- Systems:
  - pain management should be made a priority[127, 128]
  - adequate staffing levels and motivation are important.[67, 129]

RESEARCH AGENDA

- Improve understanding of underlying mechanisms of pain.[130, 131]
- Link clinical presentation with underlying mechanisms.[122, 132, 133]
- Improve assessment, using validated measures.[134]
- To expand the evidence base for particular treatment modalities.[13, 135]
- Role of multimodal analgesia.[126]

sustained neuronal input into the spinal cord in the postoperative period. More outcome studies are required to explore the true value of multimodal analgesia, and the question of the prevention of chronic pain after surgery must be addressed.

REFERENCES

1. Merskey H, Bogduk N. *Classification of Chronic Pain: Descriptions of Chronic Pain Syndromes And Definitions of Pain Terms*. IASP Press, Seattle, WA, 1994.
2. Wilmore DW, Kehlet H. Management of patients in fast track surgery. *BMJ* 2001; **322**: 473–476.
3. The Royal College of Surgeons of England, The College of Anaesthetists. *Report of the Working Party on Pain After Surgery*. HMSO, London, 1990.
4. Justins DM. Postoperative pain: a continuing challenge. *Ann R Coll Surg England* 1992; **74**: 78–79.
5. Bruster S, Jarman B, Bosanquet N et al. National survey of hospital patients. *BMJ* 1994; **309**: 1542–1546.
6. Harmer M, Davies KA. The effect of education, assessment and a standardised prescription on postoperative pain management. The value of clinical audit in the establishment of acute pain services. *Anaesthesia* 1998; **53**: 424–430.
7. Straw P, Bruster S, Richards N et al. Sit up, take notice. *Health Serv J* 2000; **5704**: 24–26.
8. Mann C, Beziat C, Pouzeratte Y et al. [Quality assurance program for postoperative pain management: impact of the Consensus Conference of the French Society of Anesthesiology and Intensive Care]. *Ann Fr Anesth Reanim* 2001; **20**: 246–254.
9. Bardiau FM, Braeckman MM, Seidel L et al. Effectiveness of an acute pain service inception in a general hospital. *J Clin Anesth* 1999; **11**: 583–589.
10. Davies HTO, Crombie IK, Macrae WA et al. Pain clinic patients in northern Britain. *Pain Clin* 1992; **5**: 129–135.
11. Macrae WA, Davies HTO. Chronic postsurgical pain. In: Crombie IK (ed.), *Epidemiology of Pain*. IASP Press, Seattle, WA, 1999, pp. 125–142.
12. Macrae WA. Chronic pain after surgery. *Br J Anaesth* 2001; **87**: 88–98.
13. McQuay H, Moore A. *An Evidence-based Resource for Pain Relief*. Oxford University Press, Oxford, 1998.
14. Oxford Pain Website: http://www.jr2.ox.ac.uk/bandolier/index.html (accessed 29 August 2006).
15. Cochrane Database of Systematic Reviews: http://www.cochrane.org (accessed 27 August 2006).
16. Hahn TW, Mogensen T, Lund C et al. Analgesic effect of i.v. paracetamol: possible ceiling effect of paracetamol in postoperative pain. *Acta Anaesthesiol Scand* 2003; **47**: 138–145.
17. Futter LE, al-Swayeh OA, Moore PK. A comparison of the effect of nitroparacetamol and paracetamol on liver injury. *Br J Pharmacol* 2001; **132**: 10–12.
18. Swett JE, Woolf CJ. The somatotopic organization of primary afferent terminals in the superficial laminae of the dorsal horn of the rat spinal-cord. *J Comp Neurol* 1985; **231**: 66–77.
19. Stamford JA. Descending control of pain. *Br J Anaesth* 1995; **75**: 217–227.
20. Cervero F, Iggo A. The substantia gelatinosa of the spinal cord: a critical review. *Brain* 1980; **103**: 717–772.
21. Bouhassira D, Chitour D, Villaneuva L et al. The spinal transmission of nociceptive information: modulation by the caudal medulla. *Neuroscience* 1995; **69**: 931–938.
22. Willis WD, Coggeshall RE. *Sensory Mechanisms of the Spinal Cord*, 2nd edn. Plenum, New York, 1991.
23. Wang H, Woolf CJ. Pain TRPs. *Neuron* 2005; **46**: 9–12.
24. Duggan AW, Hendry IA, Morton CR et al. Cutaneous stimuli releasing immunoreactive substance P in the dorsal horn of the cat. *Brain Res* 1988; **451**: 261–273.
25. Allen BJ, Rogers SD, Ghilardi JR et al. Noxious cutaneous thermal stimuli induce a graded release of endogenous substance P in the spinal cord: imaging peptide action in vivo. *J Neurosci* 1997; **17**: 5921–5927.
26. Berman HH, Kim KHS, Talati A et al. Representation of nociceptive stimuli in primary sensory cortex. *Neuroreport* 1998; **9**: 4179–4187.
27. Davis KD. The neural circuitry of pain as explored with functional MRI. *Neurol Res* 2000; **22**: 313–317.
28. Peyron R, Laurent B, Garcia-Larrea L. Functional imaging of brain responses to pain. A review and meta-analysis (2000). *Clin Neurophysiol* 2000; **30**: 263–288.
29. Eccleston C, Crombez G. Attention and pain: merging behavioural and neuroscience investigations. *Pain* 2005; **113**: 7–8.
30. Tracey I, Ploghaus A, Gati JS et al. Imaging attentional modulation of pain in the periaqueductal grey in humans. *J Neurosci* 2002; **22**: 2748–2752.
31. Porreca F, Ossipov MH, Gebhart GF. Chronic pain and medullary descending facilitation. *Trends Neurosci* 2002; **25**: 319–325.
32. Dickenson AH. Gate control theory of pain stands the test of time. *Br J Anaesth* 2002; **88**: 755–757.
33. Woolf CJ. Recent advances in the pathophysiology of acute pain. *Br J Anaesthesia* 1989; **63**: 139–146.
34. Woolf CJ, Mannion RJ. Neuropathic pain: aetiology, symptoms, mechanisms, and management. *Lancet* 1999; **353**: 1959–1964.
35. Kim KJ, Yoon YW, Chung JM. Comparison of three rodent neuropathic pain models. *Exp Brain Res* 1997; **113**: 200–206.
36. Abram SE. Necessity for an animal model of postoperative pain. *Anesthesiology* 1997; **86**: 1015–1017.
37. Schaible H-G, Grubb BD. Afferent and spinal mechanisms of joint pain. *Pain* 1993; **55**: 5–54.
38. Voilley N. Acid-sensing ion channels (ASICs): new targets for the analgesic effects of non-steroid anti-inflammatory drugs (NSAIDs). *Curr Drug Target Inflamm Allergy* 2004; **3**: 71–79.
39. Waldmann R, Champigny G, Bassilana F et al. A proton-gated cation channel involved in acid-sensing. *Nature* 1997; **386**: 173–177.
40. Vergnolle N, Ferazzini M, D'Andrea MR et al. Proteinase-activated receptors: novel signals for peripheral nerves. *Trends Neurosci* 2003; **26**: 496–500.
41. Noorbakhsh F, Vergnolle N, Hollenberg MD et al. Proteinase-activated receptors in the nervous system. *Nature Rev Neurosci* 2003; **4**: 981–990.
42. Kidd BL, Urban LA. Mechanisms of inflammatory pain. *Br J Anaesth* 2001; **87**: 3–11.
43. Ji RR. Mitogen-activated protein kinases as potential targets for pain killers. *Curr Opin Investig Drug* 2004; **5**: 71–75.
44. Szallasi A, Blumberg PM. Vanilloid (capsaicin) receptors and mechanisms. *Pharmacol Rev* 999; **51**: 159–211.
45. Burnstock G, Wood JN. Purinergic receptors: their role in nociception and primary afferent neurotransmission. *Curr Opin Neurobiol* 1996; **6**: 526–532.
46. Vergnalle N, Bunnett NW, Sharkey KA et al. Proteinase-activated receptor-2 and hyperalgesia: a novel pain pathway. *Nature Med* 2001; **7**: 821–826.
47. Arnarson A, Michaelis M, Janig W. Development of ectopic spontaneous activity, mechano- and thermosensitivity in axotomized sural nerve fibres in rats. *Pflug Archiv Eur J Physiol* 1997; **433**: P201.
48. Tal M, Devor M. Ectopic discharge in injured nerves: comparison of trigeminal and somatic afferents. *Brain Res* 1992; **579**: 148–151.
49. Ossipov MH, Lai J, Malan P et al. Spinal and supraspinal mechanisms of neuropathic pain. *New Medicat Drug Abuse* 2000; **909**: 12–24.
50. Friedman B, Wong V, Lindsay RM. Axons, Schwann cells and neurotrophic factors. *Neuroscientist* 1995; **1**: 192–198.
51. Nahin RL, Ren K, De León M et al. Primary sensory neurons exhibit altered gene expression in a rat model of neuropathic pain. *Pain* 1994; **58**: 95–108.
52. Hokfelt T, Zhang X, Wiesenfeld-Hallin Z. Messenger plasticity in primary sensory neurons following axotomy and its functional implications. *Trends Neurosci* 1994; **17**: 22–29.
53. Davis SN, Lodge D. Evidence for involvement of *N*-methyl-D-aspartic acid receptors in 'wind up' of class 2 neurons in the dorsal horn of the rat. *Brain Res* 1987; **424**: 402–406.
54. Thompson SW, Dray A, Urban L. Injury-induced plasticity of spinal reflex activity: NK1 neurokinin receptor activation and enhanced A- and C-fiber mediated responses in the rat spinal cord in vitro. *J Neurosci* 1994; **14**: 3672–3687.
55. Woolf CJ, Thompson SWN. The induction and maintenance of central sensitization is dependent on *N*-methyl-D-aspartic acid receptor activation; Implications for the treatment of post-injury pain hypersensitivity states. *Pain* 1991; **44**: 293–299.
56. Garry EM, Fleetwood-Walker SM. Organizing pains. *Trends Neurosci* 2004; **27**: 292–294.
57. DeLander GE, Schott E, Brodin E et al. Spinal expression of mRNA for immediate early genes in a model of chronic pain. *Acta Physiol Scand* 1997; **161**: 517–525.
58. Leah JD, Sandkuhler J, Herdegen T et al. Potentiated expression of fos protein in the rat spinal cord following bilateral noxious cutaneous stimulation. *Neuroscience* 1992; **48**: 525–532.
59. Munglani R, Hunt SP. Molecular biology of pain. *BJA* 1995; 75: 186–192.
60. Costigan M, Woolf CJ. No DREAM, No pain. Closing the spinal gate. *Cell* 2002; **108**: 297–300.
61. Honore P, Rogers SD, Schwei MJ et al. Murine models of inflammatory, neuropathic and cancer pain each generates a unique set of neurochemical

changes in the spinal cord and sensory neurons. *Neuroscience* 2000; **98**: 585–598.

62. Coggeshall RE, Lekan HA, Doubell TP et al. Central changes in primary afferent fibers following peripheral nerve lesions. *Neuroscience* 1997; **77**: 1115–1122.

63. Doubell TP, Woolf CJ. Growth-associated protein 43 immunoreactivity in the superficial dorsal horn of the rat spinal cord is localized in atrophic c- fiber, and not in sprouted a-fiber, central terminals after peripheral nerve injury. *J Comp Neurol* 1997; **386**: 111–118.

64. Tong YG, Wang HF, Ju G et al. Increased uptake and transport of cholera toxin B-subunit in dorsal root ganglion neurons after peripheral axotomy: possible implications for sensory sprouting. *J Comp Neurol* 1999; **404**: 143–158.

65. McLachlan EM, Janig W, Devor M et al. Peripheral nerve injury triggers noradrenergic sprouting within dorsal root ganglia. *Nature* 1993; **363**: 543–545.

66. Wieseler-Frank J, Maier SF, Watkins LR. Glial activation and pathological pain. *Neurochem Intl* 2004; **45**: 389–395.

67. Watkins LR, Maier SF. Glia: a novel drug discovery target for clinical pain. *Nature Rev Drug Disc* 2003; **2**: 973–985.

68. Logothetis NK, Guggenberger H, Peled S et al.. Functional imaging of the monkey brain. *Nature Neurosci* 1999; **2**: 555–562.

69. Eisenberg E, Chistyakov AV, Yudashkin M et al. Evidence for cortical hyperexcitability of the affected limb representation area in CRPS: a psychophysical and transcranial magnetic stimulation study. *Pain* 2005; **113**: 99–105.

70. Flor H, Elbert T, Knecht S et al. Phantom-limb pain as a perceptual correlate of cortical reorganization following arm amputation. *Nature* 1995; **375**: 482–484.

71. Karl A, Birbaumer N, Lutzenberger W et al. Reorganization of motor and somatosensory cortex in upper extremity amputees with phantom limb pain. *J Neurosci* 2001; **21**: 3609–3618.

72. Birbaumer N, Lutzenberger W, Montoya P et al. Effects of regional anesthesia on phantom limb pain are mirrored in changes in cortical reorganization. *J Neurosci* 1997; **17**: 5503–5508.

73. Florence SL, Taub HB, Kaas JH. Large-scale sprouting of cortical connections after peripheral injury in adult macaque monkeys. *Science* 1998; **282**: 1117–1121.

74. Florence SL, Hackett TA, Strata F. Thalamic and cortical contributions to neural plasticity after limb amputation. *J Neurophys* 2000; **83**: 3154–3159.

75. Von Roenn JH, Cleeland CS, Gonin R et al. Physician attitudes and practice in cancer pain management. *Ann Intern Med* 1993; **119**: 121–126.

76. Rawal N, Berggren L. Organization of acute pain services: a low cost model. *Pain* 1994; **57**: 117–123.

77. Gould TH, Crosby DL, Harmer M et al. Policy for controlling pain after surgery: effect of sequential changes in management. *BMJ* 1992; **305**: 1187–1193.

78. Krivo S, Reidenberg MM. Assessment of patients' pain. *N Engl J Med* 1996; **334**: 59.

79. Collins SL, Edwards J, Moore RA et al. Seeking a simple measure of analgesia for mega-trials: is a single global assessment good enough? *Pain* 2001; **91**: 189–194.

80. Jenkinson C, Carroll D, Egerton M et al. Comparison of the sensitivity to change of long and short form pain measures. *Qual Life Res* 1995; **4**: 353–357.

81. McQuay H, Moore A, Justins DM. Treating acute pain in hospital. *BMJ* 1997; **314**: 1531–1535.

82. Rosen M et al. Back Pain. Report of a CSAG Committee on Back Pain. HMSO, London, 1994.

83. Cox P. The fallibility of pain scores. *Anaesthesia* 2001; **56**: 499–500.

84. DeLoach LJ, Higgins MS, Caplan AB et al. The visual analogue scale in the immediate postoperative period: intrasubject variability and correlation with a numeric scale. *Anesth Analges* 1998; **86**: 102–106.

85. Hartrick CT. A four-category verbal rating scale (VRS-4), an 11-point numeric rating scale (NRS-11), and a 100-mm visual analog scale (VAS) were compared in the assessment of acute pain after oral surgery. *Clin J Pain* 2001; **17**: 104–105.

86. Collins SL, Moore RA, McQuay HJ. The visual analogue pain intensity scale: what is moderate pain in millimetres? *Pain* 1997; **72**: 95–97.

87. Bergstrom G, Jensen IB, Bodin L et al. Reliability and factor structure of the Multidimensional Pain Inventory – Swedish Language Version (MPI-S). *Pain* 1998; **75**: 101–110.

88. Turk DC, Rudy TE, Salovey P. The McGill Pain Questionnaire reconsidered: confirming the factor structure and examining appropriate uses. *Pain* 1985; **21**: 385–397.

89. Attal N, Brasseur L, Parker F et al. Effects of gabapentin on the different components of peripheral and central neuropathic pain syndromes: a pilot study. *Eur Neurol* 1998; **40**: 191–200.

90. Attal N, Bouhassira D. Mechanisms of pain in peripheral neuropathy. *Acta Neurol Scand* 1999; **100**: 12–24.

91. Rowbotham M, Harden N, Stacey B et al. Gabapentin for the treatment of postherpetic neuralgia – a randomized controlled trial. *JAMA* 1998; **280**: 1837–1842.

92. Australian and New Zealand College of Anaesthestists. *Acute Pain Management: Scientific Evidence*, 2nd edn. Faculty of Pain Medicine, Australian and New Zealand College of Anaesthestists, 2005. Available at: http://www.anzca.edu.au/publications/acutepain.htm (accessed 27 August 2006).

93. McQuay H. Acute pain. In: Tramer MJ (ed.), *Evidence-based Resource in Anaesthesia & Analgesia*. BMJ Books, London,: 2000, pp. 87–103.

94. Schug SA, Sidebotham DA, McGuinnety M et al. Acetaminophen as an adjunct to morphine by patient-controlled analgesia in the management of acute postoperative pain. *Anesth Analges* 1998; **87**: 368–372.

95. Barden J, Edwards J, Moore A et al. *Single Dose Oral Paracetamol (Acetaminophen) for Postoperative Pain*. Cochrane Database of Systematic Reviews 2004; 1.

96. Kehlet H, Werner MU. Role of paracetamol in acute pain management. *Drugs* 2003; **63**: 15–22.

97. Prescott LF. Future perspectives with paracetamol. *Drugs* 2003; **63**: 51–56.

98. Burkle H, Gogarten W, Van Aken H. Intravenous non-opioid analgesics in anaesthesia – the role of paracetamol, metamizol, tenoxicam and parecoxib in the perioperative treatment of acute pain. *Anasthesiol Intensivmed* 2003; **44**: 311–320.

99. Van Aken H., Thys L, Veekman L et al. Assessing analgesia in single and repeated administrations of propacetamol for postoperative pain: comparison with morphine after dental surgery. *Anesth Analges* 2004; **98**: 159–165.

100. Lahtinen P, Kokki H, Hendolin H. Propacetamol as adjunctive treatment for postoperative pain after cardiac surgery. *Anesth Analges* 2002; **95**: 813–819.

101. Aubrun F, Kalfon F, Mottet P et al. Adjunctive analgesia with intravenous propacetamol does not reduce morphine-related adverse effects. *Br J Anaesth* 2003; **90**: 314–319.

102. Kam PCA, Power I. New selective COX-2 inhibitors. *Pain Rev* 2000; **7**: 3–13.

103. Jones SF, Power I. Editorial I: postoperative NSAIDs and COX-2 inhibitors: cardiovascular risks and benefits. *Br J Anaesth* 2005; **95**: 281–284.

104. Kehlet H. Organizing postoperative accelerated recovery programmes. *Regional Anesth* 1996; **21**: 149–151.

105. Ballantyne JC, Carr DB, Deferranti S et al. The comparative effects of postoperative analgesic therapies on pulmonary outcome: cumulative meta-analyses of randomized controlled trials. *Anesth Analges* 1998; **86**: 598–612.

106. Brodner G, Van Aken H., Hertle L et al. Multimodal perioperative management combining thoracic epidural analgesia, forced mobilization, and oral nutrition reduces hormonal and metabolic stress and improves convalescence after major urologic surgery. *Anesth Analges* 2001; **92**: 1594–1600.

107. Thorn SE, Wattwil M, Naslund I. Postoperative epidural morphine, but not epidural bupivacaine, delays gastric-emptying on the 1st day after cholecystectomy. *Regional Anesth* 1992; **17**: 91–94.

108. Abdi S, Lee DH, Chung JM. The anti-allodynic effects of amitriptyline, gabapentin, and lidocaine in a rat model of neuropathic pain. *Anesth Analges* 1998; **87**: 1360–1366.

109. Eggers KA, Power I. Tramadol [editorial]. *Br J Anaesth* 1995; **74**: 247–249.

110. Coetzee JF, Vanloggerenberg H. Tramadol or morphine administered during operation: a study of immediate postoperative effects after abdominal hysterectomy. *Br J Anaesth* 1998; **81**: 737–741.

111. Schmid RL, Sandler AN, Katz J. Use and efficacy of low-dose ketamine in the management of acute postoperative pain: a review of current techniques and outcomes. *Pain* 1999; **82**: 111–125.

112. Grace RF, Power I, Zammit A et al. Preoperative dextromethorphan reduces intraoperative but not postoperative morphine requirements after laparatomy. *Anesth Analges* 1998; **87**: 1135–1138.

113. Sandler AN. The role of clonidine and alpha(2)-agonists for postoperative analgesia. *Can J Anaesth* 1996; **43**: 1191–1194.

114. Perkins FM, Kehlet H. Chronic pain as an outcome of surgery. *Anesthesiology* 2000; **93**: 1123–1133.

115. Hayes C, Molloy AR. Neuropathic pain in the perioperative period. In: Molloy AR, Power I (eds), *Acute and Chronic Pain*. Lippincott-Raven, Philadelphia, PA, 1997, pp. 67–81.

116. Cousins MJ, Power I, Smith G. Pain – a persistent problem. *Regional Anesth Pain Med* 2000; **25**: 6–21.

117. Woolf CJ, Chong MS. Preemptive analgesia – treating postoperative pain by preventing the establishment of central sensitization. *Anesth Analg* 1993; **77**: 362–379.

118. Kissin I. Preemptive analgesia. *Anesthesiology* 2000; **93**: 1138–1143.

119. Kehlet H, Dahl JB. The value of 'multimodal' or 'balanced analgesia' in postoperative pain treatment. *Anesth Analges* 1993; **77**: 1048–1056.

120. Dalton JA, Blau W, Lindley C et al. Changing acute pain management to improve patient outcomes: an educational approach. *J Pain Symptom Manage* 1999; **17**: 277–287.

121. Woolf CJ, Salter MW. Neuronal plasticity-increasing the gain in pain. *Science* 2000; **288**:1765–1768.

122. Jensen TS, Baron R. Translation of symptoms and signs into mechanisms in neuropathic pain. *Pain* 2003; **102**: 1–8.

123. Chibnall JT, Tait RC. Pain assessment in cognitively impaired and unimpaired older adults: a comparison of four scales. *Pain* 2001; **92**: 173–186.

124. Willson H. Factors affecting the administration of analgesia to patients following repair of a fractured hip. *J Adv Nurs* 2000; **31**: 1145–1154.

125. Wilson JA, Colvin LA, Power I. Acute neuropathic pain after surgery. *R Coll Anaesth Bull* 2002; **15**:739–743.

126. Wilmore DW, Kehlet H. Management of patients in fast track surgery. *BMJ* 2001; **322**: 473–476.

127. Anderson KO, Mendoza TR, Valero V et al. Minority cancer patients and their providers: pain management attitudes and practice. *Cancer* 2000; **15**: 1929–1938.

128. Anderson KO, Richman SP, Hurley J et al. Cancer pain management among underserved minority outpatients: perceived needs and barriers to optimal control. *Cancer* 2002; **94**: 2295–2304.

129. Parsons G, Edwards P. Acute pain algorithm. *Prof Nurse* 1999; **15**: 136.

130. Ji RR. Peripheral and central mechanisms of inflammatory pain, with emphasis on MAP kinases. *Curr Drug Targets Inflamm Allergy* 2004; **3**: 299–303.

131. Julius D, Basbaum AI. Molecular mechanisms of nociception. *Nature* 2001; **413**: 203–210.

132. Rasmussen PV, Sindrup SH, Jensen TS et al. Symptoms and signs in patients with suspected neuropathic pain. *Pain* 2004; **110**: 461–469.

133. Dworkin RH, Backonja M, Rowbotham MC et al. Advances in neuropathic pain: diagnosis, mechanisms, and treatment recommendations. *Arch Neurol* 2003; **60**: 1524–1534.

134. Wallace K, Reed B, Pasero C et al. Staff nurses' perceptions of barriers to effective pain management. *J Pain Sympt Manage* 1995; **10**: 204–213.

135. Smith LA, Moore RA, McQuay HJ et al. Using evidence from different sources: an example using paracetamol 1000 mg plus codeine 60 mg. *BMC Med Res Methodol* 2001; **1**: 1.

Chapter 28

Drug combinations in pain management: a review of the published evidence and methods to find optimal combinations

Gorazd Svetičič and Michele Curatolo

INTRODUCTION

The rationale underlying the practice of combining drugs in pain management is based mainly on two considerations. First, single drugs do not always provide satisfactory pain relief: combining drugs that act at different receptors and pain mechanisms may enhance pain relief. Second, single drugs that provide satisfactory pain relief may cause, at the same time, unacceptable side-effects. Drug combinations may allow a reduction in the amount of the single components to achieve the same analgesic effect with a lower incidence of side-effects. Clearly, this is true if the drug interaction is in favour of the analgesic effect, rather than of toxicity.

Despite the above considerations, combining drugs is still not always supported by the published evidence. Moreover, the optimal doses of each drug in most combination regimens remain unknown.

This chapter is divided into two parts. In the first, an overview of the literature comparing drug combinations with single drugs is provided. In the second, the problem of optimizing therapeutic regimens is analysed and new optimization methods for clinical research are presented. This chapter is an update of a previously published work.[1]

DRUG COMBINATIONS IN PAIN MANAGEMENT

This section is not intended to cover all drug combinations that have been investigated or may be used in pain management. Rather, it focuses on selected combinations for the management of acute postoperative, chronic musculoskeletal, neuropathic and cancer pain. The aim is to evaluate the evidence that drug combinations are superior to single-drug regimens in clinical pain.

Medline and the authors' database were searched. Among the retrieved hits, only clinical investigations comparing a single drug with a combination of the same drug with one or more additional drugs were considered. Whenever systematic reviews were found, they were used for evaluating the literature. Otherwise, randomized controlled trials, selected by the authors based on a personal evaluation of their validity, were presented.

The main results of the review are summarized in Table 28.1.

Postoperative pain
Systemic analgesia

Opioids–NSAIDs A meta-analysis[2] of 22 prospective, randomized, double-blind studies including 2307 patients showed a 30–50% sparing effect on morphine consumption. NSAIDs significantly decreased postoperative nausea and vomiting by 30%, nausea alone by 12%, vomiting alone by 32% and sedation by 29%. Pruritus, urinary retention and respiratory depression were not significantly decreased.

A recent study[3] on 1003 patients confirmed the morphine-sparing effect and reduction of opioid-related side-effects in the early postoperative period.

The addition of a NSAID to paracetamol (acetaminophen) and opioid patient-controlled analgesia (PCA) following mastectomy and immediate breast reconstruction reduced opioid consumption and improved pain relief during the first 20 hours

Table 28.1. Summary results of the efficacy of drug combinations in pain management

Drug combination	Effect
Acute postoperative pain	
Adding NSAIDs to opioid	Mostly better analgesia and less side-effects
Adding paracetamol to opioid	Morphine sparing effect with unclear benefit
Paracetamol and a NSAID	Probably better than either component alone
Adding weak opioid to paracetamol	Questionable usefulness in minor surgery
Adding weak opioid to a NSAID	Questionable usefulness in minor surgery
Adding intravenous ketamine to opioid	Questionable usefulness
Adding epidural opioid to local anaesthetic	Useful
Adding epidural local anaesthetic to opioid	Useful
Adding clonidine to epidural mixtures	Unclear benefit
Adding adrenalin to epidural mixtures	Useful at least for thoracic epidural analgesia
Neuropathic pain (peripheral nerve injury, postherpetic neuralgia, diabetic polyneuropathy)	Very limited data on postherpetic neuralgia, no data on peripheral nerve injury or diabetic polyneuropathy
Chronic musculoskeletal pain (fibromyalgia, low back and neck pain)	Sparse inconsistent data on fibromyalgia, no data on low-back or neck pain
Cancer pain Various combinations of opioids, NSAIDs, paracetamol and ketamine	Very limited data, possible usefulness of adding NSAIDs, paracetamol or ketamine to opioids

NSAID, non-steroidal anti-inflammatory drug.

at rest but failed to do so during mobilization.[4] There was no difference regarding opioid related side-effects. Postoperative blood loss was higher with diclofenac.

One systematic review has analysed the effect of adding the weak opioid codeine to the NSAID ibuprofen for postoperative pain.[5] Included papers considered minor surgery, mostly dental pain. The analgesic effect of ibuprofen was increased by only 8% by codeine, and adverse effects were increased.

Opioids–paracetamol   The meta-analysis that compared intravenous morphine PCA alone with morphine PCA combined with acetaminophen administered orally or intravenously after major surgery showed a significant morphine-sparing effect but failed to demonstrate a reduction in the incidence of morphine-related adverse effects or an improvement in patient satisfaction in the postoperative period.[6]

In an investigation on paediatric patients, paracetamol improved pain relief, reduced morphine consumption and reduced opioid-induced nausea and vomiting in a dose-dependent fashion.[7] In a systematic review, the combination of tramadol with paracetamol was superior to either component alone.[8] Three systematic reviews found the addition of codeine to paracetamol to improve pain relief.[9–11] In two of these,[9, 10] the combination was associated with an increased incidence of side-effects. Another systematic review found little objective evidence to support prescribing a combination of paracetamol and dextropropoxyphene in preference to paracetamol alone in moderate pain:[12] the difference in pain intensity between the combination and paracetamol alone was only 7.3%.

Opioids–ketamine   A systematic review showed that, compared to morphine alone, intravenous PCA with ketamine and morphine did not improve analgesia.[13] A meta-analysis including the same randomized controlled trials did not clarify the role of ketamine as a component of postoperative analgesia.[14] The trials included were of limited size, groups rarely exceeding 30 patients, and there was a major problem of wide variability in clinical settings, ketamine regimens and outcome measures. A recently completed randomized controlled study performed on a larger patient population after major elective orthopaedic surgery using the morphine–ketamine combination suggested by the results of an optimizing study,[15] showed no benefit in adding ketamine to morphine for PCA in terms of the incidence of unsatisfactory treatment, adverse effects, pain scores or consumption of administered drugs (G. Sveticic, unpublished work, 2007).

Paracetamol–NSAIDs   One systematic review[16] found the concurrent use of paracetamol and a NSAID to be superior to paracetamol alone. However, no evidence was found of a superior analgesic effect of the combination compared with the NSAID alone. Another systematic review[17] also found that the addition of a NSAID to paracetamol may confer additional analgesic efficacy. Unlike the former review, it concluded from the limited data available that paracetamol may enhance analgesia when added to a NSAID.

In more recent studies, a combined treatment with propacetamol and diclofenac provided only a minor advantage over monotherapy with respect to postoperative analgesia or the incidence of side-effects in adult tonsillectomy patients.[18] Addition of ibuprofen (but not rofecoxib) to paracetamol following tonsillectomy in children reduced the need for early analgesia, but there were no differences in pain score, side-effects or blood loss between the combination and monotherapy 4 and 8 hours after operation.[19]

The combination of ibuprofen with paracetamol may be more effective than ibuprofen alone in the management of postoperative endodontic pain.[20] Following surgical removal of wisdom teeth, a combination of diclofenac and paracetamol for acute pain had a superior analgesic effect compared with diclofenac, paracetamol, or paracetamol with codeine after oral surgery, supporting the practice of adding a NSAID and not an opioid to paracetamol.[21]

Summary   The addition of a NSAID to an opioid is probably beneficial, either in terms of analgesia, side-effects or both. Adding paracetamol to morphine following major surgery showed a significant morphine-sparing effect but no reduction of side-effects or patient satisfaction, while the combination of paracetamol and an opioid might be beneficial following moderately painful procedures. The literature on the combination of paracetamol with a NSAID does not consistently show a clear superiority to either component alone. Different therapy regimens, types of operation and outcome measurements may account for the variability of the results. In addition, no study had enough power to analyse a possible increase in the incidence of rare serious adverse effects. For instance, it is unclear whether the paracetamol–NSAID combination carries a higher risk of renal failure than either component alone. Moreover, the impact of combinations as routine analgesic regimens on overall costs is unclear.

The evidence supporting the addition of a weak opioid to paracetamol or a NSAID is weak. Intuitively, moderate pain responding well to paracetamol or to NSAIDs is unlikely to benefit significantly from adding other analgesics. Combining ketamine with opioids after a major surgery showed no benefit compared to opioid monotherapy. The potential usefulness of combination regimens in patients in whom treatment with an opioid alone is unsatisfactory still needs to be investigated.

Epidural analgesia

Adding opioids to local anaesthetics   Opioids are currently employed for epidural or intrathecal use despite the fact that some studies appear to show that epidural or intrathecal administration of opiates may not produce analgesia with a selective spinal mechanism or that the analgesia produced is not superior to that produced by intravenous opiate monotherapy, according to Bernards.[22]

However, lumbar epidural local anaesthetics alone are associated with a higher incidence of motor block than their combination with an opioid.[23, 24] For thoracic epidural analgesia, adding an opioid to a local anaesthetic probably improves pain control.[25, 26] The incidence of side-effects is either decreased,[27] unchanged[26] or even increased.[25, 28] The effect of adding an opioid to a local anaesthetic probably depends on the type and dose of opioid used. In a crossover study,[26] the addition of low concentrations of fentanyl (i.e. 2 μg/mL) to a bupivacaine–epinephrine thoracic epidural infusion strongly improved analgesia without increasing side-effects.

Adding local anaesthetics to opioids   Studies have shown either a benefit[29] or no advantage[23, 30] of adding a local anaesthetic to pure opioid solutions. It is likely that local anaesthetics do not confer benefits when added to high-dose opioids, as high doses may provide adequate analgesia even when used alone. However, several dose-dependent side-effects may result from opioid administration.[31] Most studies were not sufficiently powered to analyse whether opioids alone are associated with more respiratory depression than are mixtures of low-dose opioids with local anaesthetics. Moreover, pathophysiological data support the superiority of local anaesthetics to opioids in reducing cardiovascular and respiratory morbidity, as well as the duration of postoperative paralytic ileus.[32] The authors believe that combinations of low doses of local anaesthetics with opioids should be preferred to opioids alone for postoperative pain relief.

Adding clonidine to epidural mixtures   The addition of clonidine to a bupivacaine–fentanyl infusion produced an improvement in analgesia,[33] but also a higher incidence of hypotension.[34, 35] However, better pain relief without an increase in side-effects was produced by the addition of a single injection of clonidine to caudal[36] or epidural[37] bupivacaine. Perhaps clonidine could have a role in lumbar epidural analgesia: the concentration of local anaesthetic may be reduced by the additional use of clonidine, with a possible decrease in the incidence of motor block. Studies on this issue are lacking.

Adding adrenalin to epidural mixtures   The addition of adrenalin to mixtures of opioids with local anaesthetics has proven beneficial for thoracic epidural analgesia in most reported studies.[38–41] Therefore, the limited use of adrenalin in current practice seems unjustified.[42] Results concerning lumbar epidural analgesia are less consistent and require further investigation.[29, 43–47]

Summary   Combinations of low doses of a local anaesthetic, an opioid and adrenalin are superior to single-drug regimens. The role of clonidine is still unclear.

Neuropathic pain

The literature was searched for all possible drug combinations used for neuropathic pain. The focus was set on peripheral nerve injury, postherpetic neuralgia and diabetic polyneuropathy.

Unfortunately, we were able to identify only two studies comparing a combination with a single-drug regimen. The addition of the neuroleptic fluphenazine to the antidepressant amitriptyline did not improve analgesia in patients with postherpetic neuralgia.[48] Gabapentin and morphine combined achieved better analgesia at lower doses of each drug than either agent singly, with constipation, sedation and dry mouth as the most frequent adverse effects in patients with diabetic neuropathy and postherpetic neuralgia.[49] At the maximal tolerated dose, the gabapentin–morphine combination resulted in a higher frequency of constipation than gabapentin alone and a higher frequency of dry mouth than morphine alone.

Summary   The literature on drug combinations in neuropathic pain is almost non-existent. Compared with our previous review,[1] we found only one additional study.[49] Although we can not rule out the possibility that our search may have missed some randomized controlled trials, there is certainly a need for research on drug combinations in this difficult pain condition.

Chronic musculoskeletal pain

The focus of the search was on unlimited combinations of analgesics in fibromyalgia, low-back pain and neck pain. In addition, specific searches were conducted on combinations of NSAIDs, paracetamol and opioids.

As in our previous review,[1] no study on drug combinations in neck or low-back pain was found. In the light of the enormous medical, social and economic implications of these pain syndromes, such absence of data is disconcerting.

In fibromyalgia, the addition of ibuprofen to the muscle relaxant cyclobenzaprine improved morning stiffness.[50] A combination of naproxen with amitriptyline was slightly, but not significantly, better than amitriptyline alone.[51] Combinations of NSAIDs with benzodiazepines were investigated in two studies. The combination of tenoxicam with bromazepam was only marginally more effective than tenoxicam alone, but not better than placebo.[52] The combination of ibuprofen with alprazolam produced a more pronounced clinical improvement than either drug alone.[53]

Summary   Because of the extreme paucity of evidence, the authors cannot draw any conclusion regarding the usefulness of combination regimens in chronic musculoskeletal pain.

Cancer pain

The search was conducted on the following drug combinations: opioids–NSAIDs, opioids–paracetamol, NSAIDs–paracetamol, opioids–anticonvulsants, opioids–antidepressants and opioids–ketamine. Very few studies were found.

The addition of diclofenac to intravenous PCA with morphine reduced morphine consumption.[54] There was a trend for reduced pain scores, which did not reach statistical significance. Two placebo-controlled studies found that adding ibuprofen to the oxycodone–paracetamol combination[55] or methadone[56] significantly decreased pain scores without increasing side-effects. Another randomized controlled study showed that adding ketorolac to morphine produced better analgesia, slowed the morphine escalation and reduced the maximum morphine dose.[57] Conversely, adding codeine to diclofenac did not affect pain scores.[58]

Adding paracetamol improved pain and well-being without major side-effects in patients with cancer and persistent pain despite a strong opioid regimen.[59]

The use of low doses of ketamine reduced morphine consumption and pain scores, but a dose-dependent increase in central side-effects was observed.[60, 61]

Summary   The limited published evidence suggests that adding NSAIDs, paracetamol or ketamine to opioids may be useful. Randomized controlled trials on other combinations are lacking.

FINDING THE OPTIMAL DRUG COMBINATION

The problem of identifying the optimal combination

In general, drug combinations are investigated by comparing two or more groups of patients, each of which receives a different combination. However, this approach is challenged by a serious problem: the number of possible combinations. If we combine two different drugs and analyse two doses for each drug, $2^2 = 4$ different combinations exist. However, if the therapeutic range of the drugs under investigation is wide, we may want to analyse a higher number of different doses, e.g. five. In this case, we have to analyse $5^2 = 25$ different combinations. If we want to add an additional variable, e.g. another drug or the time interval between the doses, the number of possible combinations increases to $5^3 = 125$. Therefore, only a small part of all possible combinations is investigated in a randomized controlled trial. Such a trial allows conclusions pertaining to the combinations analysed, and the optimal combination may not be tested.

Thus, there is a need for methods to identify optimal combinations of therapeutic regimens. Actually, optimization models have existed for a long time and are commonly applied to real economic problems.[62] Conversely, despite its great importance, the problem of optimizing therapeutic regimens has received very little formal attention in medicine.[63]

In this section an optimization method and a surface modelling method that can be applied to clinical research are presented. To our knowledge, only three human clinical studies using this method have been published, all by our research group.[15, 64, 65] The well-being model was applied to the combination of intravenous morphine with ketamine.

Direct search optimization method

The optimization method presented is called 'direct search'. The principle is simple. The optimum is searched stepwise. Initially, a few combinations are tested. On the basis of the results obtained, new combinations are identified and investigated in a stepwise manner, until the optimal one is reached. Basically, the information obtained from the analysis of the combinations at each step is used to move away from the 'bad' combinations in the direction of the 'good' ones, and thus towards the optimum. In this way, it is not necessary to explore all possible combinations.

In the following, three direct search methods are presented, from the basic one to the latest development in clinical research.

Simplex method   The 'simplex' method[62] has been applied mainly to mathematical and industrial problems. It is presented here because it illustrates well the principles of optimization models (Figure 28.1). The main disadvantage of this method for applications in clinical research is the excessive weight given to each combination. Measurements performed in a clinical setting are usually characterized by a large variability. Therefore, a certain combination can perform as the worst one merely as a result of chance. Since the step direction is given by the position of the worst combination (see Figure 28.1), an incorrect estimation would direct the procedure towards an incorrect point.

Partition method   In order to avoid the excessive weight given to the worst combination by the simplex method, Berenbaum developed the 'partition' optimization model (Figure 28.2), which he then applied to an animal chemotherapy study.[63]

We implemented this method in clinical studies to optimize a postoperative epidural regimen[64, 65] and intravenous PCA with morphine and ketamine.[15] For these studies we developed a new partition method that addresses some limitations of Berenbaum's original approach. For example, partitioning the complex by cutting the ranked list at its halfway point (see Figure 28.2) is arbitrary. Theoretically, the worst combination of the 'good' subgroup and the best combination of the 'bad'

subgroup could be characterized by very similar and clinically indistinguishable pain scores. In this case, it would be more productive for the optimization procedure if these two combinations belonged to the same subgroup, as this would result in a more reliable calculation of the centroids of the 'good' and 'bad' subgroups (see Figure 28.2). We achieved this by partitioning the complex using a probabilistic model. The effect of this amended approach is illustrated in Figure 28.3. The specific procedure has been described in detail elsewhere.[15, 65]

The method also provides a multiple regression model to deal with the occurrence of unacceptable side-effects. More details about the method can be found in the literature.[15, 63–66]

Role of optimization methods in clinical research

The results of optimization studies cannot be considered conclusive. Rather, they may identify the range of the optimal com-

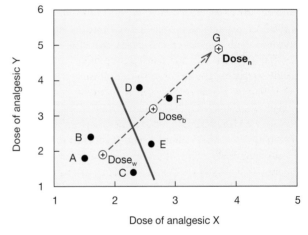

Figure 28.2. Berenbaum's partition method for direct search. The main rationale is to avoid the excessive weight given to the worst combination by the simplex method (see Figure 28.1). In the example illustrated, a complex of six combinations A–F of two analgesics X and Y is represented. These combinations are ranked from the best to the worst, according to their analgesic effect (e.g. the mean pain score). It is important to note that differences in pain scores do not need to be statistically significant, so it is not necessary to analyse large sample sizes. Once the combinations have been ranked, they are 'partitioned' into two equal subgroups: the worst (A–B–C) and the best (D–E–F) combinations. The continuous line divides the two subgroups. Then, the mean doses of the combinations of each subgroup are calculated, and two virtual combinations, i.e. the centroid of the worst three and the centroid of the best three combinations, are identified (Dose$_w$ and Dose$_b$, respectively). The new combination G of the optimization procedure is calculated as Dose$_n$ = Dose$_b$ + α(Dose$_b$ - Dose$_w$), where α is a positive number (in this case α = 1.3). In this way, the relative position of the three worst combinations in the ranking does not influence the direction of the next step, because the mean of the doses is considered when calculating the new combination G. Assuming that the worst of the six initial combinations in our example is A, this combination is discarded and the new combination G is tested on an additional group of patients. The above ranking and partition procedure is repeated on the new complex of six combinations (B–G), of which five (B–F) were tested in the previous phase.

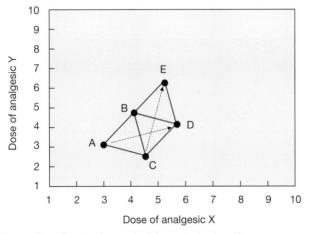

Figure 28.1. The simplex method for optimization. For a problem of *n* variables, an initial complex of *n* + 1 empirically chosen combinations is analysed. In the example illustrated, two analgesics X and Y are combined, i.e. *n* + 1 = 3 combinations are initially analysed (combinations A, B and C). These combinations must form the vertices of an equilateral triangle. After analysing these combinations, the one characterized by the worst analgesic effect (in this example combination A) is discarded. The basic principle of the method is to move away from the 'bad' combinations in the direction of the 'good' ones. A new combination D is determined by reflecting the triangle ABC on the axis BC of the initial complex (i.e. the axis of the two 'good' combinations). Combination D of the new complex BCD is analysed in an additional group of patients, without need of re-testing combinations B and C. The worst combination of the complex BCD (i.e. combination C) is discarded and the new combination E is determined. The procedure is stopped when no further improvement in the therapeutic effect is obtained.

ponents of a therapeutic regimen: the wide range of possibilities, giving rise to an enormous number of possible combinations, is 'narrowed' to a small range of potentially useful combinations, which can then be analysed in randomized controlled trials. Therefore, optimization studies complement randomized controlled trials, rather than being an alternative to them. Furthermore, prospective observational studies, investigating the best combinations on large sample sizes, should be carried out to assess the incidence of rare complications. We believe that optimization procedures are more scientifically based than the pure empirical selection criteria of drug combinations, and should therefore be preferred to them.

The well-being model: a new drug interaction model for positive and negative effects

When addressing the question of optimal drug combinations, one cannot avoid considering side-effects also. As an extension of a previously published interaction model,[67] we proposed a method for studying drug interactions that also takes into consideration their side-effects.[68] A general outcome parameter identified as 'patient's well-being' was defined by superposition of positive and negative (i.e. side-effects) effects. Response

surfaces for patient's well-being were constructed, their shape depending on the pharmacodynamic characteristics of the individual drugs and on their interaction type, by algebraically adding the sigmoid-shaped positive- and negative-effect curves. Simulations were performed to test the effect of the different parameters on the shape of the well-being surface (Figure 28.4). Finally, the model was applied to a clinical question, the combination of intravenous morphine and ketamine, to show its potential usefulness in identifying optimal drug infusion regimens (V. Sartori, unpublished work, 2005). The proposed approach allowed the response surface to be drawn for the combination of intravenous morphine and ketamine, and the optimal-effect compartment concentration ranges to be targeted during drug administration to be identified. The new framework could help in exploring the issue of optimal drug administration in clinical practice.

SUMMARY

In acute postoperative pain, various combinations of NSAIDs, paracetamol and opioids are superior to single drugs in terms of analgesic effect and/or side-effects. However, the combination of paracetamol and morphine after major surgery did not reduce the incidence of morphine-related adverse effects or increase patient satisfaction in the postoperative period. In addition, there is mostly no evidence that rare severe adverse

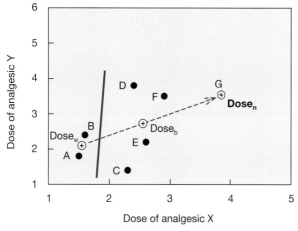

Figure 28.3. The model proposed by Berenbaum was improved by choosing a more rational approach to partitioning the complexes into 'good' and 'bad' subgroups. To allow direct comparison with the original model, the same initial six combinations (A–F) as in Figure 28.2 were used as the starting complex. Combinations A–F were ranked according to the pain scores allocated, and combinations C and B were placed in positions 4 and 5, respectively. According to Berenbaum's original method (see Figure 28.2) the complex would be partitioned into two equal halves, so that both combinations C and B would belong to the 'bad' subgroup. However, we assume that the mean pain score for combination C is very close to the one of combination E, so that the difference would be clinically indistinguishable. Conversely, the pain score for combination C is much lower than the pain score for combination B. The probabilistic model implemented here then allocates combination C to the 'good' rather than to the 'bad' subgroup, unlike in Berenbaum's method. This changes the direction of the search procedure, as indicated by the different position of the new combination G in this graph compared with its position in Figure 28.2.

PRACTICE POINTS

- In acute postoperative pain, various combinations of NSAIDs, paracetamol and opioids should be preferred to single-drug regimens after major surgery. In minor surgery, drug combinations should be used only when single drugs provide inadequate pain relief.

- There is conflicting evidence that adding ketamine to systemic opioids is beneficial in routine postoperative pain therapy.

- Combinations of low doses of local anaesthetics, opioids and adrenalin are superior to single-drug regimens in epidural postoperative analgesia.

- The rationale underlying the use of drug combinations applies also to neuropathic and chronic musculoskeletal pain, but there is an almost complete lack of published data for use of combination regimens in these cases.

- The very limited data on cancer pain suggest that adding NSAIDs, paracetamol or ketamine to opioids may be beneficial.

- Randomized controlled trials allow conclusions pertaining to the specific combinations to be analysed. Because of the high number of possible combinations of a therapeutic regimen, the optimal combination may not be tested.

- Optimization models exist and have been used in a few clinical trials.

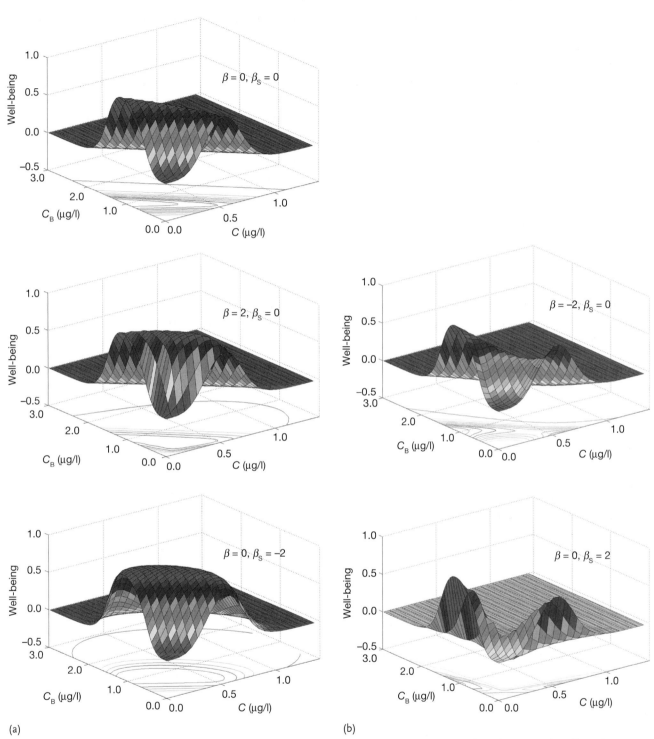

(a)   (b)

Figure 28.4. (a) Well-being surface for various values of the interaction parameter for positive effect (β) and negative (β_S) effect. The effect of the parameters on the shape of the well-being surface assessed by the sensitivity analysis is consistent with the interpretation in terms of synergy and antagonism and with common clinical knowledge. Considering the interaction parameter, a synergism in the positive effect ($\beta > 0$) or antagonism in negative effect ($\beta_S < 0$) results in the surface that reaches a higher well-being value than a zero interaction constellation, and forms a plateau. This means that the same effect can be reached by more than just one drug concentration combination of drugs A and B. (b) In the same way, the interactions between the negative effects can be interpreted in terms of synergy and antagonism: a positive value of β_S indicates synergy between the negative effects, while a negative value indicates antagonism. In the latter case, the surface reaches lower well-being values for a given combination of drugs, and forms a depression. This means that a single drug results in a better effect than a combination. C is the concentration of drug A and C_B is the concentration of drug B in the effect compartment. (See also Plate V of colour section, page xv.)

RESEARCH AGENDA

- Randomized, controlled trials performed on large patient populations are needed to assess the cost/benefit ratio of drug combinations and their safety in terms of rare adverse effects.
- Research on drug combinations may offer a perspective of better treatment for cancer, neuropathic and chronic musculoskeletal pain.
- Existing optimization methods should be used more widely in clinical research.
- The currently available optimization methods should be improved by methodological studies.

effects are not increased by drug combinations. Adding ketamine to intravenous morphine for postoperative pain therapy showed no benefit in routine use. The potential usefulness of this drug combination in opioid-resistant pain needs to be studied further. For epidural postoperative analgesia, combinations of low doses of a local anaesthetic, an opioid and adrenalin are superior to single-drug regimens. The role of epidural clonidine is still unclear. There is a disappointing lack of data on the advantages of drug combinations over single drugs in neuropathic and chronic musculoskeletal pain. Based on very limited data, adding NSAIDs, paracetamol or ketamine to opioids may be useful in cancer pain. Other combinations are unexplored.

The problem of how to find the optimal combination of therapeutic regimens has received very little attention in medicine. Because of the enormous number of possible combinations, randomized controlled trials may fail to test the optimal combination. The direct search method is a stepwise optimization procedure that has been used in three clinical investigations of postoperative analgesia. A drug-interaction model for studying drug interactions that also takes into consideration the drug side-effects is being investigated. A wider use of optimization methods in clinical research is desirable.

REFERENCES

1. Curatolo M, Sveticic G. Drug combinations in pain treatment: a review of the published evidence and a method for finding the optimal combination. *Best Pract Res Clin Anaesthesiol* 2002; 16: 507–519.
2. Marret E, Kurdi O, Zufferey P et al. Effects of nonsteroidal antiinflammatory drugs on patient-controlled analgesia morphine side effects: meta-analysis of randomized controlled trials. *Anesthesiology* 2005; 102: 1249–1260.
3. Cepeda MS, Carr DB, Miranda N et al. Comparison of morphine, ketorolac, and their combination for postoperative pain: results from a large, randomized, double-blind trial. *Anesthesiology* 2005; 103: 1225–1232.
4. Legeby M, Sandelin K, Wickman M et al. Analgesic efficacy of diclofenac in combination with morphine and paracetamol after mastectomy and immediate breast reconstruction. *Acta Anaesthesiol Scand* 2005; 49: 1360–1366.
5. Po AL, Zhang WY. Analgesic efficacy of ibuprofen alone and in combination with codeine or caffeine in post-surgical pain: a meta-analysis. *Eur J Clin Pharmacol* 1998; 53: 303–311.
6. Remy C, Marret E, Bonnet F. Effects of acetaminophen on morphine side-effects and consumption after major surgery: meta-analysis of randomized controlled trials. *Br J Anaesth* 2005; 94: 505–513.
7. Korpela R, Korvenoja P, Meretoja OA. Morphine-sparing effect of acetaminophen in pediatric day-case surgery. *Anesthesiology* 1999; 91: 442–447.
8. Edwards JE, McQuay HJ, Moore RA. Combination analgesic efficacy: individual patient data meta-analysis of single-dose oral tramadol plus acetaminophen in acute postoperative pain. *J Pain Symptom Manage* 2002; 23: 121–130.
9. de Craen AJ, Di Giulio G, Lampe-Schoenmaeckers JE et al. Analgesic efficacy and safety of paracetamol–codeine combinations versus paracetamol alone: a systematic review. *BMJ* 1996; 313: 321–325.
10. Moore A, Collins S, Carroll D et al. *Single Dose Paracetamol (Acetaminophen), With and Without Codeine, for Postoperative Pain.* Cochrane Database Systematic Review 2000: CD001547.
11. Zhang WY, Li Wan Po A. Analgesic efficacy of paracetamol and its combination with codeine and caffeine in surgical pain – a meta-analysis. *J Clin Pharm Ther* 1996; 21: 261–282.
12. Li Wan Po A, Zhang WY. Systematic overview of co-proxamol to assess analgesic effects of addition of dextropropoxyphene to paracetamol. *BMJ* 1997; 315: 1565–1571.
13. Subramaniam K, Subramaniam B, Steinbrook RA. Ketamine as adjuvant analgesic to opioids: a quantitative and qualitative systematic review. *Anesth Analg* 2004; 99: 482–495.
14. Elia N, Tramer MR. Ketamine and postoperative pain – a quantitative systematic review of randomised trials. *Pain* 2005; 113: 61–70.
15. Sveticic G, Gentilini A, Eichenberger U et al. Combinations of morphine with ketamine for patient-controlled analgesia: a new optimization method. *Anesthesiology* 2003; 98: 1195–1205.
16. Romsing J, Moiniche S, Dahl JB. Rectal and parenteral paracetamol, and paracetamol in combination with NSAIDs, for postoperative analgesia. *Br J Anaesth* 2002; 88: 215–226.
17. Hyllested M, Jones S, Pedersen JL et al. Comparative effect of paracetamol, NSAIDs or their combination in postoperative pain management: a qualitative review. *Br J Anaesth* 2002; 88: 199–214.
18. Hiller A, Silvanto M, Savolainen S et al. Propacetamol and diclofenac alone and in combination for analgesia after elective tonsillectomy. *Acta Anaesthesiol Scand* 2004; 48: 1185–1189.
19. Pickering AE, Bridge HS, Nolan J et al. Double-blind, placebo-controlled analgesic study of ibuprofen or rofecoxib in combination with paracetamol for tonsillectomy in children. *Br J Anaesth* 2002; 88: 72–77.
20. Menhinick KA, Gutmann JL, Regan JD et al. The efficacy of pain control following nonsurgical root canal treatment using ibuprofen or a combination of ibuprofen and acetaminophen in a randomized, double-blind, placebo-controlled study. *Int Endod J* 2004; 37: 531–541.
21. Breivik EK, Barkvoll P, Skovlund E. Combining diclofenac with acetaminophen or acetaminophen–codeine after oral surgery: a randomized, double-blind single-dose study. *Clin Pharmacol Ther* 1999; 66: 625–635.
22. Bernards CM. Understanding the physiology and pharmacology of epidural and intrathecal opioids. *Best Pract Res Clin Anaesthesiol* 2002; 16: 489–505.
23. Cooper DW, Ryall DM, McHardy FE et al. Patient–controlled extradural analgesia with bupivacaine, fentanyl, or a mixture of both, after Caesarean section. *Br J Anaesth* 1996; 76: 611–615.
24. Gogarten W, Van de Velde M, Soetens E et al. A multicentre trial comparing different concentrations of ropivacaine plus sufentanil with bupivacaine plus sufentanil for patient-controlled epidural analgesia in labour. *Eur J Anaesthesiol* 2004; 21: 38–45.
25. Finucane BT, Ganapathy S, Carli F et al. Prolonged epidural infusions of ropivacaine (2 mg/ml) after colonic surgery: the impact of adding fentanyl. *Anesth Analg* 2001; 92: 1276–1285.
26. Niemi G, Breivik H. Epidural fentanyl markedly improves thoracic epidural analgesia in a low-dose infusion of bupivacaine, adrenaline and fentanyl. A randomized, double-blind crossover study with and without fentanyl. *Acta Anaesthesiol Scand* 2001; 45: 221–232.
27. Torda TA, Hann P, Mills G et al. Comparison of extradural fentanyl, bupivacaine and two fentanyl–bupivacaine mixtures of pain relief after abdominal surgery. *Br J Anaesth* 1995; 74: 35–40.
28. Lorenzini C, Moreira LB, Ferreira MB. Efficacy of ropivacaine compared with ropivacaine plus sufentanil for postoperative analgesia after major knee surgery. *Anaesthesia* 2002; 57: 424–428.
29. Cohen S, Lowenwirt I, Pantuck CB et al. Bupivacaine 0.01% and/or epinephrine 0.5 microg/ml improve epidural fentanyl analgesia after cesarean section. *Anesthesiology* 1998; 89: 1354–1361.
30. Poopalalingam R, Chow MY, Wong LT. Patient-controlled epidural analgesia after thoracic and upper abdominal surgery using sufentanil with and without bupivacaine 0.125%. *Singapore Med J* 2003; 44: 126–130.
31. Chaney MA. Side effects of intrathecal and epidural opioids. *Can J Anaesth* 1995; 42: 891–903.

32. Liu S, Carpenter RL, Neal JM. Epidural anesthesia and analgesia. Their role in postoperative outcome. *Anesthesiology* 1995; **82**: 1474–1506.

33. Forster JG, Rosenberg PH. Small dose of clonidine mixed with low-dose ropivacaine and fentanyl for epidural analgesia after total knee arthroplasty. *Br J Anaesth* 2004; **93**: 670–677.

34. Mogensen T, Eliasen K, Ejlersen E et al. Epidural clonidine enhances postoperative analgesia from a combined low-dose epidural bupivacaine and morphine regimen. *Anesth Analg* 1992; **75**: 607–610.

35. Paech MJ, Westmore MD, Speirs HM. A double-blind comparison of epidural bupivacaine and bupivacaine–fentanyl for caesarean section. *Anaesth Intensive Care* 1990; **18**: 22–30.

36. Lee JJ, Rubin AP. Comparison of a bupivacaine–clonidine mixture with plain bupivacaine for caudal analgesia in children. *Br J Anaesth* 1994; **72**: 258–262.

37. Carabine UA, Milligan KR, Moore J. Extradural clonidine and bupivacaine for postoperative analgesia. *Br J Anaesth* 1992; **68**: 132–135.

38. Niemi G, Breivik H. Adrenaline markedly improves thoracic epidural analgesia produced by a low-dose infusion of bupivacaine, fentanyl and adrenaline after major surgery. A randomised, double-blind, cross-over study with and without adrenaline. *Acta Anaesthesiol Scand* 1998; **42**: 897–909.

39. Niemi G, Breivik H. Epinephrine markedly improves thoracic epidural analgesia produced by a small-dose infusion of ropivacaine, fentanyl, and epinephrine after major thoracic or abdominal surgery: a randomized, double-blinded crossover study with and without epinephrine. *Anesth Analg* 2002; **94**: 1598–1605.

40. Sakaguchi Y, Sakura S, Shinzawa M et al. Does adrenaline improve epidural bupivacaine and fentanyl analgesia after abdominal surgery? *Anaesth Intensive Care* 2000; **28**: 522–526.

41. Verborgh C, Van der Auwera D, Noorduin H et al. Epidural sufentanil for postoperative pain relief: effects of adrenaline. *Eur J Anaesthesiol* 1988; **5**: 183–191.

42. Curatolo M. Is epinephrine unfairly neglected for postoperative epidural mixtures? *Anesth Analg* 2002; **94**: 1381–1383.

43. Cohen S, Amar D, Pantuck CB et al. Epidural patient-controlled analgesia after cesarean section: buprenorphine–0.015% bupivacaine with epinephrine versus fentanyl–0.015% bupivacaine with and without epinephrine. *Anesth Analg* 1992; **74**: 226–230.

44. Forster JG, Niemi TT, Aromaa U et al. Epinephrine added to a lumbar epidural infusion of a small-dose ropivacaine–fentanyl mixture after arterial bypass surgery of the lower extremities. *Acta Anaesthesiol Scand* 2003; **47**: 1106–1113.

45. Huang KS, Tseng CH, Cheung KS et al. Influence of epinephrine as an adjuvant to epidural morphine for postoperative analgesia. *Ma Zui Xue Za Zhi* 1993; **31**: 245–248.

46. Ngan Kee WD, Khaw KS, Ma ML. The effect of the addition of adrenaline to pethidine for patient-controlled epidural analgesia after caesarean section. *Anaesthesia* 1998; **53**: 1012–1016.

47. Semple AJ, Macrae DJ, Munishankarappa S et al. Effect of the addition of adrenaline to extradural diamorphine analgesia after caesarean section. *Br J Anaesth* 1988; **60**: 632–638.

48. Graff–Radford SB, Shaw LR, Naliboff BN. Amitriptyline and fluphenazine in the treatment of postherpetic neuralgia. *Clin J Pain* 2000; **16**: 188–192.

49. Gilron I, Bailey JM, Tu D et al. Morphine, gabapentin, or their combination for neuropathic pain. *N Engl J Med* 2005; **352**: 1324–1334.

50. Fossaluzza V, De Vita S. Combined therapy with cyclobenzaprine and ibuprofen in primary fibromyalgia syndrome. *Int J Clin Pharmacol Res* 1992; **12**: 99–102.

51. Goldenberg DL, Felson DT, Dinerman H. A randomized, controlled trial of amitriptyline and naproxen in the treatment of patients with fibromyalgia. *Arthritis Rheum* 1986; **29**: 1371–1377.

52. Quijada-Carrera J, Valenzuela-Castano A, Povedano-Gomez J et al. Comparison of tenoxicam and bromazepan in the treatment of fibromyalgia: a randomized, double-blind, placebo-controlled trial. *Pain* 1996; **65**: 221–225.

53. Russell IJ, Fletcher EM, Michalek JE et al. Treatment of primary fibrositis/fibromyalgia syndrome with ibuprofen and alprazolam. A double-blind, placebo-controlled study. *Arthritis Rheum* 1991; **34**: 552–560.

54. Bjorkman R, Ullman A, Hedner J. Morphine-sparing effect of diclofenac in cancer pain. *Eur J Clin Pharmacol* 1993; **44**: 1–5.

55. Stambaugh JE Jr, Drew J. The combination of ibuprofen and oxycodone/acetaminophen in the management of chronic cancer pain. *Clin Pharmacol Ther* 1988; **44**: 665–669.

56. Ferrer-Brechner T, Ganz P. Combination therapy with ibuprofen and methadone for chronic cancer pain. *Am J Med* 1984; **77**: 78–83.

57. Mercadante S, Fulfaro F, Casuccio A. A randomised controlled study on the use of anti-inflammatory drugs in patients with cancer pain on morphine therapy: effects on dose-escalation and a pharmacoeconomic analysis. *Eur J Cancer* 2002; **38**: 1358–1363.

58. Minotti V, De Angelis V, Righetti E et al. Double-blind evaluation of short-term analgesic efficacy of orally administered diclofenac, diclofenac plus codeine, and diclofenac plus imipramine in chronic cancer pain. *Pain* 1998; **74**: 133–137.

59. Stockler M, Vardy J, Pillai A et al. Acetaminophen (paracetamol) improves pain and well-being in people with advanced cancer already receiving a strong opioid regimen: a randomized, double-blind, placebo-controlled cross-over trial. *J Clin Oncol* 2004; **22**: 3389–3394.

60. Lauretti GR, Lima IC, Reis MP et al. Oral ketamine and transdermal nitroglycerin as analgesic adjuvants to oral morphine therapy for cancer pain management. *Anesthesiology* 1999; **90**: 1528–1533.

61. Mercadante S, Arcuri E, Tirelli W et al. Analgesic effect of intravenous ketamine in cancer patients on morphine therapy: a randomized, controlled, double-blind, crossover, double-dose study. *J Pain Symptom Manage* 2000; **20**: 246–252.

62. Spendley W, Hext G, Himsworth F. Sequential applications of simplex designs in optimisation and evolutionary operation. *Technometrics* 1962: 441–461.

63. Berenbaum MC. Direct search methods in the optimisation of cancer chemotherapy regimens. *Br J Cancer* 1990; **61**: 101–109.

64. Curatolo M, Schnider T, Petersen-Felix S et al. A direct search procedure to optimize combinations of epidural bupivacaine, fentanyl, and clonidine for postoperative analgesia. *Anesthesiology* 2000; **92**: 325–337.

65. Sveticic G, Gentilini A, Eichenberger U et al. Combinations of bupivacaine, fentanyl, and clonidine for lumbar epidural postoperative analgesia: a novel optimization procedure. *Anesthesiology* 2004; **101**: 1381–1393.

66. Berenbaum MC. What is synergy? *Pharmacol Rev* 1989; **41**: 93–141.

67. Minto CF, Schnider TW, Short TG et al. Response surface model for anesthetic drug interactions. *Anesthesiology* 2000; **92**: 1603–1616.

68. Zanderigo E, Sartori V, Sveticic G et al. The well-being model: a new drug interaction model for positive and negative effects. *Anesthesiology* 2006; **104**: 742–753.

Chapter 29
How do we manage chronic pain?

Hans-Georg Schaible and Horacio Vanegas

INTRODUCTION

Pain is the sensation that usually arises when an external or internal agent, called a *noxious stimulus,* causes real or potential damage to a bodily tissue. The neural encoding and further processing elicited by such stimuli is called *nociception.* Pain researchers have classified pain into three categories according to the pathophysiological mechanisms involved, namely:

- *Nociceptive pain that is elicited by noxious stimulation of normal tissue.* Normally, pain arises only when the stimulus is sufficiently intense to potentially or actually damage the tissue (e.g. twisting a joint or burning the skin). This type of pain constitutes a warning signal that helps avoid damage to our body.
- *Nociceptive pain that is elicited when the tissue is in a pathological condition.* This type of pain typically arises when the tissue is inflamed or damaged. The patient may complain about *spontaneous pain,* previously painful stimuli can elicit an exaggerated pain sensation (*hyperalgesia*) and stimuli of intensities that are normally not painful (e.g. palpation or movement of a joint or brushing of the skin) now elicit pain (*allodynia*). Finally, the patient often feels pain in neighbouring body regions, although these are not inflamed or damaged. This is called *referred pain* or secondary hyperalgesia and allodynia. In short, as a result of tissue damage the nociceptive system becomes more sensitive. This type of pain can become chronic.
- *Neuropathic pain that is elicited when peripheral nerves or neurons in the central nervous system themselves are damaged.* This type of pain is often burning or shooting. In many cases it occurs spontaneously (continuously or episodically) and it is often not related to the application of stimuli. In addition, allodynia and hyperalgesia can be found. Neuropathic pain is usually considered abnormal, as it does not indicate the presence of damage in the innervated tissue. Neuropathic pain may be associated with other sensory abnormalities or sensory deficits, is often chronic, and is difficult to treat.

Each of these pain states is characterized by a set of neuronal mechanisms. The following sections briefly describe these mechanisms and thus the target sites for intervention, with emphasis on inflammatory and neuropathic pain. The various forms of pain therapy are then described within the framework of neuroanatomy, neurophysiology and neuropharmacology.

GENERAL PLAN OF THE PAIN (NOCICEPTIVE) SYSTEM

Figure 29.1 shows a scheme of the nociceptive system. Nociceptive messages are carried from the tissue into the central nervous system (CNS) by the primary afferent neurons, which are called nociceptors. These neurons have a small cell body in the dorsal root (spinal) ganglia or the trigeminal ganglion, and axons with little or no myelin (A-δ and C fibres, respectively). The axonal processes to the periphery reach the tissues, where they form sensory endings. The axonal processes to the spinal cord or the trigeminal nuclei branch into central terminations that form synapses on second-order neurons. In the case of nociceptive pain the action potentials arise at the peripheral sensory endings of nociceptors. In the case of neuropathic pain the action potentials may also arise proximally to the sensory ending, e.g. in the course of the damaged axon or in the dorsal root ganglion. By contrast, neurons with large-diameter cell bodies and large-diameter, thickly myelinated processes (A-β fibres) are excited by small mechanical forces and their activation elicits non-painful sensations such as touch and movement. In the case of neuropathic pain, however, stimulation of the sensory endings of A-β fibres may cause allodynia (e.g. brush-evoked pain).

Primary nociceptive afferents synthesize the excitatory neurotransmitter glutamate as well as pronociceptive neuropeptides such as substance P and the calcitonin gene-related peptide (CGRP). Substance P and CGRP are transported into both the peripheral and the central endings. At the peripheral sensory endings substance P and CGRP can be released, whereupon they induce a so-called 'neurogenic inflammation' and excite the nociceptive endings. When the so-elicited action potentials arrive at the central endings, substance P and CGRP are released together with glutamate, and excite spinal neurons.[1]

Many second-order neurons in the spinal cord have long axons which form tracts that ascend to the brainstem and the thalamus. Other second- and higher order neurons are involved in motor reflex circuits and in autonomic responses. Thus an afferent barrage in nociceptors sets in motion segmental motor reflexes, generalized autonomic reflexes and the flow of pain messages towards the brainstem, the thalamus and, finally, the cerebral cortex.[1] For transmission of nociceptive information to the cerebrum, the spinothalamic tracts are most important. Excitation of neurons in the cerebral cortex[2,3] gives rise to the experience of pain, with its psychophysical and affective components. Psychophysical components are the location, intensity, character (e.g. burning, pressing or tearing) and duration of the perceived damage. Affective components are the unpleasantness and rejection that are integral elements of the pain experience. The primary and secondary somatosensory cortices seem to be responsible for the psychophysical aspects of pain, whereas limbic cortices such as the cingulate gyrus and the insula are responsible for the affective aspects of pain. A clinical state of depression or dysphoria may additionally develop as a consequence of chronic pain.

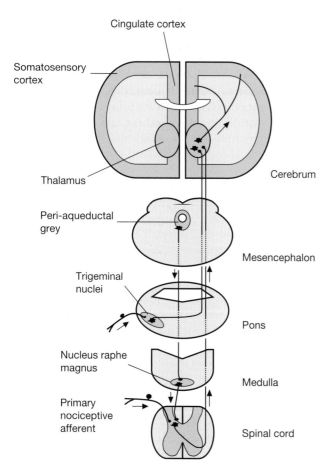

Figure 29.1. General plan of the nociceptive system.

Pain messages also arrive at various regions of the brainstem, notably the nucleus raphe magnus and adjacent structures in the medulla as well as the grey matter around the sylvian aqueduct. These structures are elements of the so-called descending pain-control system, which sends impulses to the trigeminal and spinal relay stations, and thus diminishes or enhances the pain elicited by chronic tissue or nerve lesions.[4,5]

PERIPHERAL MECHANISMS OF NOCICEPTION

The peripheral sensory endings of nociceptors are excited by large mechanical forces, as well as by a variety of chemical agents that are released as a consequence of trauma or inflammation.[6] Many such factors may also increase the sensitivity of (i.e. sensitize) the nociceptors. Some of these nociceptors, called 'silent nociceptors', become excitable only after sensitization.[7] Peripheral (i.e. nociceptor) sensitization underlies pathological nociceptive pain (e.g. chronic inflammatory pain).[1,7]

The chemical agents that excite and sensitize nociceptors may act directly on their membrane or may sensitize it to directly acting agents. Peptides such as substance P, CGRP and bradykinin, inflammatory mediators such as interleukins and tumour necrosis factor α (TNFα), autacoids such as prostaglandins (PGs) and prostacyclin, potassium ions released during trauma, and hydrogen ions released during inflammation, all contribute to the generation of pain signals.

In neuropathic pain the damaged and adjacent nerve fibres are subject to an inflammatory process.[1] In addition, the trophic changes induced by the damage include alterations in the expression, responsiveness and distribution of sodium, potassium and calcium membrane channels. Both the surrounding inflammation and the channel alterations lead to increased excitability and instability, spontaneous discharges at both the damaged site and the dorsal root ganglion, and long-lasting responses to stimulation. Finally, postganglionic sympathetic fibres invade the dorsal root ganglion, and the membrane of primary afferents becomes sensitive to adrenergic mediators. The contribution of the sympathetic system to neuropathic pain may thus be considerable.

CENTRAL MECHANISMS OF NOCICEPTION

Peripheral sensitization or nerve damage induces an exaggerated flow of impulses towards the spinal cord and the trigeminal nuclei. These messages excite spinal neurons and render them hyperexcitable (central sensitization).[8] Together with peripheral sensitization, central sensitization underlies nociceptive pain under pathological conditions such as inflammation and nerve damage.[7,9] It is not clear yet whether or for how long central sensitization can persist after peripheral sensitization has disappeared.

Presynaptic as well as postsynaptic events contribute to central sensitization.[1] Central terminals of primary afferents release increased amounts of transmitters. This process is dependent on the entrance of calcium ions into the presynaptic endings of the central terminals through voltage-gated N-type and P/Q-type calcium channels.[10] Glutamate, the most important excitatory transmitter, is released and binds to different receptor types. Of particular importance are the *N*-methyl-D-aspartate (NMDA)-type receptors, which allow calcium ions to flow into the neurons. Calcium activates intracellular molecular pathways that enhance neuronal excitability. Furthermore, substance P and CGRP are released in the spinal cord, where they activate neurokinin 1 and CGRP receptors, respectively, and thus contribute to central sensitization.[11] Also, phospholipase A_2 mediates the release of arachidonic acid from the cell membrane and the cyclo-oxygenases (Cox-1 and Cox-2) turn it into PGs at an increasing pace in both neurons and glial cells.[12, 13] PGs excite and sensitize nociceptive spinal neurons[14] and, together with substance P and CGRP, may further increase the release of glutamate and facilitate its effect on the relay neurons.[12] The spinal action of immunological mediators, such as interleukin-1β[15] and nuclear factor kappa B (NF-kB),[16] also contributes to neuronal hyperexcitability. Additional mechanisms contribute to central sensitization during peripheral nerve damage.[1] In the primary afferents involved there is an upregulation of the pronociceptive neuropeptides cholecystokinin (CCK) and vasoactive intestinal peptide (VIP), and these are probably released at their spinal cord terminals. The general increase in nociceptive activity in the spinal cord is probably also aided by an inactivation of GABAergic inhibitory neurons,[1] and PGs may induce an attenuation of glycinergic inhibition in the dorsal horn,[17] with the consequent increase in excitability.

Finally, intracellular mediators, such as calcium and protein kinases, triggered by activation of glutamatergic ionotropic and metabotropic receptors, lead to long-term changes in neuronal responsiveness.[18, 19] Particularly interesting for the transition into chronicity are the induction of immediate early genes and the slow and long-lasting phenotypical changes in spinal neurons.[20]

The highly increased flow of nociceptive messages during peripheral and central sensitization reaches brainstem structures, which are responsible for the descending control of nociceptive transmission.[4] During inflammation, descending inhibition predominates over facilitation in pain circuits with input from the inflamed tissue, and thus attenuates primary hyperalgesia, while descending facilitation predominates over inhibition in circuits with input from neighbouring tissues, and thus facilitates secondary hyperalgesia. The (primary) hyperalgesia and allodynia of the neuropathic syndrome are also facilitated by the descending system. Simultaneously there is an inhibition of secondary neuronal pools and thus hypoalgesia in regions outside the damaged nerve's territory.

MECHANISMS OF CHRONIC PAIN

Chronic pain in humans has been arbitrarily defined as pain lasting for more than 6 months.[21] The pathophysiological mechanisms that occur in prolonged acute, clinically relevant, pain states (see above) may also be at work in chronic pain states (Tables 29.1 and 29.2). In addition, further neuronal mechanisms may occur in chronic pain states that are not found under prolonged acute conditions. Studies on experimental models will have to reveal which players (ions, transmitters, receptors, cytokines, intracellular mediators, genes) are most important in different pain states and different painful diseases.

Chronic pain may result from the persistence of pathological conditions that activate the nociceptive system, such as in rheumatoid diseases, which are per se chronic. It is also theoretically possible that the peripheral pathology subsides but the changes induced in primary afferents and CNS structures

Table 29.1. Neuronal mechanisms of chronic pain

Mechanism	Example
Persistent activation of nociceptors	Abnormal mechanical conditions of the tissue
Persistent peripheral sensitization	Chronic inflammation or axonal damage
Persistent ectopic discharges in nociceptors	At a nerve lesion site or dorsal root ganglion
Persistent central sensitization	Due to persistent peripheral sensitization, peripheral ectopic discharges or long-lasting changes in spinal neurons
Increased descending facilitation	Secondary hyperalgesia during inflammation
Loss of segmental or descending inhibition	Reduced function of local GABAergic and glycinergic neurons
Structural changes of neurons and synaptic connections	Sprouting of sympathetic fibres on spinal ganglion neurons

Table 29.2. Molecular mechanisms of chronic pain

Mechanism	Example
Upregulation of transmitters and modulators	The pronociceptive substance P and CGRP in dorsal root ganglia during inflammation
Upregulation of receptors in nociceptors and in neurons of the CNS	Bradykinin receptors in nociceptors during chronic inflammation; adrenergic receptors in damaged nerve fibres
Changes in the expression of ion channels	Upregulation of peripheral TTX-resistant sodium channels in inflammation, and downregulation after nerve damage
Phenotypical changes in primary afferents	De novo expression of substance P by non-nociceptive afferents

persist. Furthermore, numerous psychological and social factors have an influence on the persistence of pain.[22, 23]

PRINCIPLES OF ANALGESIC DRUG THERAPY

Most of this section is a description of the rationale for drug treatment of inflammatory pain, but some attention is also paid to neuropathic pain. As outlined in previous sections, several levels of potential intervention are available (Table 29.3). At all levels the drug or procedure should reduce the excitability of the neurons involved in nociceptive processing.

Reduction of inflammation and reduction of activation and sensitization of nociceptive sensory endings

The reduction of peripheral sensitization is a key approach in the treatment of inflammatory pain. This implies both attenuating the inflammatory process and decreasing the hyperexcitability of primary afferents. The ideal approach would be one that antagonizes mediators that affect both neurons and tissue

cells and thus foster both inflammation and hyperexcitability. Among a variety of plausible targets, current therapy is mainly focused on PGs by using Cox inhibitors (Table 29.4), but there are new promising trends.[24]

Cox inhibitors

PGs are produced by Cox-1 and Cox-2, and PG synthesis can be blocked by the traditional non-steroidal anti-inflammatory drugs (NSAIDs), which inhibit both Cox-1 and Cox-2, and by selective Cox-2 inhibitors.[12, 25, 26] In most tissues Cox-1 is constitutively expressed, whereas the expression of Cox-2 is induced.[12] Induction of Cox during inflammation is responsible for a considerable elevation of PG levels. PGs, in particular PGE_2 and PGI_2, facilitate voltage-dependent sodium and calcium channels and thus increase the excitability of nociceptors. PGs also sensitize nociceptive afferents to algogenic mediators such as potassium ions, hydrogen ions and bradykinin. PGs thus play a key role in peripheral sensitization.[7, 12] Furthermore, PGs are also released in the spinal cord and also contribute to central sensitization.[12] NSAIDs and selective Cox-2 inhibitors thus relieve pain by acting both peripherally and centrally.

Table 29.3. Approaches in pain therapy and their site of action

Site	Current therapy	Potential therapy
Encephalon		
Cerebrum	Opioids Antidepressants Psychosocial therapy	
Brainstem	NSAIDs Opioids Antidepressants	Cannabinoids
Spinal cord	NSAIDs Selective Cox-2 inhibitors Opioids α_2-Agonists Antidepressants	Selective NMDA antagonists Neurokinin-1 antagonists CGRP antagonists Gabapentinoids Calcium channel blockers Adenosine agonists
Primary afferent		
Axon	Local anaesthetics Anticonvulsants Adrenergic blockers	Sodium channel blockers
Sensory endings	Local anaesthetics Opiods Capsaicin Anticonvulsants	Sodium channel blockers Vanilloid antagonists Bradykinin antagonists Opioids Cannabinoids
Tissue	NSAIDs Selective Cox-2 inhibitors Adrenal steroids Physical therapy	NO-NSAIDs Bradykinin antagonists PG receptor antagonists LOX-Cox inhibitors Cannabinoids Cytokine antagonists

CGRP, calcitonin gene related peptide; Cox, cyclooxygenase; NMDA, N-methyl-D-aspartate receptor; LOX, lipoxygenase; NSAID, non-steroidal anti-inflammatory drug; PG, prostaglandin.

Table 29.4. World Health Organization analgesic ladder for non-malignant and malignant chronic pain

First step	NSAID, selective Cox-2 inhibitor, paracetamol
	± adjuvant
If pain persists or increases: Second step	Opioid for mild-to-moderate pain
	± non-opioid
	± adjuvant
If pain persists or increases: Third step	Opioid for moderate-to-strong pain
	± non-opioid
	± adjuvant

Adjuvant: tricyclic antidepressants, anticonvulsants, local anaesthetics, antiarrhythmics

Inhibition of Cox-1 has the disadvantage that it also prevents the normal synthesis of PGs that protect the tissue (e.g. in the gastrointestinal system). The selective Cox-2 inhibitors offer the advantage of reducing the pathologically enhanced PG production that results from Cox-2 induction but not the 'physiological' PG production by Cox-1.[12, 26] However, some selective Cox-2 inhibitors have recently been suspected of inducing serious cardiovascular problems, and their therapeutic use is presently under consideration. An interesting alternative is offered by molecules of traditional NSAIDs sterified to a nitric oxide (NO) donor moiety (NO-NSAIDs or CINODs). Although high concentrations of NO in damaged tissues and spinal cord contribute to hyperalgesia, the slow and moderate release of NO by, for example, NO– naproxen or NO–paracetamol (acetaminophen) may protect the gastrointestinal mucosa by improving the microcirculation and other defence mechanisms.[27]

The analgesic effect of NSAIDs is limited ('ceiling' effect),[21] for several reasons. Firstly, although NSAIDs reduce PG production, other inflammatory mediators may also act on nociceptive sensory endings. Secondly, pain can also be produced by mechanisms independent of PG production. Ectopic discharges in damaged neurons, for example, depend on a host of other factors (see above).[28] Furthermore, in addition to PGs, through the action of 5-lipoxygenases pronociceptive leukotrienes are also derived from arachidonic acid. Therefore, compounds such as licofelone (ML 3000) have been developed that inhibit 5-lipoxygenase, Cox-1 and Cox-2 simultaneously, and which reportedly have an improved gastric tolerability.[27]

Other compounds that act on the sensory nerve terminal

Nociceptive afferents are excited by capsaicin, the active compound of hot peppers, by activating TRPV1 vanilloid receptors.[29] These ion channels are crucial for thermal hyperalgesia and inflammatory pain, and their sensitivity can be modulated by inflammatory mediators. Interestingly, capsaicin excites and then desensitizes the nociceptive neurons, and thus capsaicin creams are used for topical analgesia.[24] However, capsaicin may eventually kill the primary afferents and also abolish normal pain.

A high proportion of nociceptive afferents express receptors for bradykinin, a very powerful algesic neuropeptide that is released under inflammatory conditions. Bradykinin 2 receptors are expressed under normal conditions whereas bradykinin 1 receptors seem to be mainly expressed during inflammation and thus constitute analgesic targets.[30] While experimental compounds such as bradyzide have been shown to reduce inflammatory hyperalgesia, no antagonist has been successfully used in humans.[27]

Tissue acidosis is characteristic of inflammation. Pain afferents express ion channels that are activated by hydrogen ions, the so-called ASICs, with the consequent generation of action potentials. Locally applied NSAIDs reduce cutaneous and corneal acid induced pain, an action curiously independent of Cox inhibition. NSAIDs also prevent the inflammation-induced ASIC upregulation. These two effects probably contribute to the analgesic action of NSAIDs during inflammation.[31] Research into the relationships between NSAIDs and ASICs might yield therapeutically useful compounds.

A substantial proportion of primary afferents express opioid receptors, and the expression of these receptors increases during inflammation. Morphine and other opiates cause prolonged analgesia when applied locally after joint or dental surgery.[32] Ideally, opioids with only peripheral, not central, effects should be developed. Also, drugs should be developed that induce immunocompetent cells to release endogenous opioids upon primary afferents.[27]

Most dorsal root ganglion neurons express receptors for the neuropeptide somatostatin.[33] There is evidence that a tonic activation of somatostatin receptors stabilizes neuronal excitability.[34] Furthermore, somatostatin receptor agonists are antinociceptive and anti-inflammatory, because they reduce neurogenic inflammation.[35, 36] Somatostatin receptor agonists are therefore a possible target for the future.

The main cannabinoid of marijuana (Δ^9-tetrahydrocannabinol), the endogenous cannabinoids (anandamide, 2-arachidonylglycerol and others) and synthetic cannabinoid agonists produce analgesia by acting both at the peripheral tissues and at the CNS. The peripheral effects are exerted on primary afferents and involve a reduction in neurogenic inflammation thanks to an increase in the local release of endogenous opioids.[27] Ideally, cannabinoids should be developed with good analgesic action but devoid of their typical depressant effects on motricity and body temperature.

Activation of nuclear factor kappa B (NF-κB) seems to be involved in chronic inflammatory pain and inflammation-induced bone destruction. Drugs traditionally used for treating chronic arthritis, such as gold salts, glucocorticoids and flurbiprofen, in fact inhibit the activation of NF-κB.[27] Drugs with similar actions and fewer side-effects might offer some promise for the future.

Blockade of action potentials in peripheral nerves

An effective way to treat or prevent pain is the blockade of action potentials in peripheral nerves. Since conduction blockers such as local anaesthetics have a rather short action, this approach cannot be used for the persistent treatment of pain. Another problem with this approach is that sensations other than pain, as well as movement, can also be impaired or abolished. Furthermore, the aim of antinociceptive treatment is to eliminate pathophysiological pain, not pain as a warning signal. Nevertheless, because thin nociceptive fibres are more sensitive than thick (e.g. touch and motor) fibres to the effect of local anaesthetics, systemic administration of low doses of, for example, lidocaine has been experimentally tested for the treatment of pain.

Primary afferents express two types of sodium channel: tetrodotoxin (TTX)-sensitive and TTX-resistant channels. The TTX-resistant sodium channels are only expressed in nociceptive primary afferents and are upregulated during inflammation. They are probably important for the generation of the action potential in primary endings, because mice that lack them have hypoalgesia for mechanical stimuli. TTX-resistant sodium channels are also involved in the conduction of action potentials towards the CNS. Since they are upregulated during inflammation and facilitated by inflammatory mediators such as PGE_2 and CGRP, they may offer a target for analgesia during inflammation. During nerve damage, on the other hand, TTX-resistant sodium channels are downregulated and partly replaced by more sensitive and faster TTX-sensitive sodium channels. In this case, these fast channels would be the ideal target for analgesia.[28]

In cases of peripheral nerve damage the primary afferents become sensitive to adrenergic mediators, and there is evidence for an adrenergic component in inflammatory pain. Particularly for neuropathic pain, depletion of adrenergic mediators with drugs like guanetidine, and partial blockade of the sympathetic system, have shown to be successful analgesic manipulations.

Reduction of excitatory synaptic transmission and of hyperexcitability in the central nociceptive system

For effective pain treatment, central sensitization must also be reduced. Thus the exaggerated action of excitatory mediators plus the spinal neuronal hyperexcitability must be attenuated, and neuronal inhibition must be enhanced.

Reduction of the action of excitatory mediators

Since glutamate is the major excitatory transmitter in the CNS, NMDA receptor antagonists are considered for the treatment of pain.[7, 9] Ketamine at non-narcotic doses is a specific NMDA receptor antagonist, and it reduces pain.[37] However, the presently available NMDA antagonists are too general and cannot be used for the long-lasting treatment of pain, because they produce unwanted effects on many neuronal circuits in the CNS. Another option would be antagonists at neuropeptide receptors involved in central sensitization. Thus neurokinin 1 (substance P) receptor and CGRP receptor antagonists have been developed, although their use as analgesics remains to be evaluated.

The action of mediators can be reduced by blocking the calcium channels that are involved in their release. N- and P/Q-type calcium channel blockers reduce behavioural pain responses and nociceptive neuronal responses in animals, as well as subjective pain in humans.[10] Calcium channel blockers, either alone for neuropathic pain[10] or in combination with, for example, opiates for other types of pain, are a possibility for the future, provided that compounds with limited side-effects can be developed. The anticonvulsant gabapentin is likely to act on calcium channels, and has been successfully used against neuropathic pain.

Opioid agonists also inhibit release of mediators.

Opioids

Drugs that bind to opioid receptors are the most powerful analgesic compounds known to date.[21] Three different groups of opioid receptors are known, namely μ, δ and κ receptors. All clinically used opiates such as morphine have highest affinities for the μ receptor, which is the most abundant receptor in the spinal cord. Activation of opioid receptors on presynaptic endings causes a reduction in the release of glutamate and other excitatory mediators from nociceptive afferent fibres. Activation of opioid receptors on nociceptive postsynaptic neurons inhibits them by hyperpolarization. This dual pre- and postsynaptic action may be a key to their effectiveness.

For many years opioids have been mainly used for the treatment of severe cancer pain, in particular at the final stage, and for intense pain after surgery, etc. Use of opioids for severe non-malignant pain, such as in rheumatoid arthritis, has been under discussion since the views on tolerance and addiction have changed. It is claimed that opioids do not necessarily induce tolerance to their analgesic effects and addiction (psychological dependence) if they are given in a strict regimen. However, opioids should only be given if non-opioidergic drugs are insufficient for analgesia (see Table 29.4).[21]

Unfortunately, peripheral nerve damage induces a downregulation of opioid receptors in the spinal terminals of primary afferents and also an upregulation of the anti-opioid peptide cholecystokinin (CCK).[1] Opiates have, therefore, often a poor effect on neuropathic pain.

Other compounds that act in the CNS

As already mentioned, traditional NSAIDs and the selective Cox-2 inhibitors act not only in the periphery but also in the CNS.[12] In cases of peripheral inflammation there is an induction of spinal Cox-2 that leads to an increased synthesis of spinal PGs, and these contribute to making spinal nociceptive neurons hyperexcitable (central sensitization). Spinal application of a variety of traditional NSAIDs or selective Cox-2 inhibitors prevents neuronal hyperexcitability as well as behavioural hyperalgesia, and orally administered NSAIDs or Cox inhibitors[38, 39] reach sufficiently high concentrations in the spinal cord. Therefore part of the analgesic effect of Cox inhibitors is due to their spinal action. Also paracetamol, a potent analgesic compound, has a clear effect on the CNS.[21]

Finally, further hope is based on experiments that show an antinociceptive effect of adenosine agonists at the spinal cord level.[40]

Increase of inhibitory processes (descending inhibition)

The descending pain-control system normally functions in association with endogenous opioids such as endorphins, encephalins and endomorphin.[5] Endogenous opioids act on structures such as the periaqueductal grey matter and the rostral ventromedial medulla, and thus reduce the flow of pain messages at the spinal cord and supraspinal relay stations.

Although the descending pain-control system may facilitate certain nociceptive circuits (see above), exogenous opiates such as morphine activate generalized descending inhibition by acting on structures where endogenous opioids normally act.[5] This contributes to the strong analgesic action of opiates. Some NSAIDs[41] as well as cannabinoids[42] also activate the descending pain-control system, and a similar activation is probably the basis for the analgesic effect of antidepressants.[43] Indeed, antidepressants affect serotoninergic synapses,[43] and serotonin plays a key role at many levels of the descending pain control system. Another important neurotransmitter of descending inhibitory axons is norepinephrine,[5] and thus α_2-adrenergic agonists such as clonidine induce analgesia when applied to the spinal cord.

Finally, the analgesic effect of drug administration depends not only on the pharmacological action of the drug but also on its placebo effect, i.e. on the degree to which the patient (and even the doctor) hopes or expects a beneficial outcome.[44] The placebo effect may result from an unconscious activation of the endogenous opioid system. Plausibly much of the beneficial effect of several therapeutic manipulations (including acupuncture), physical therapy, psychosocial therapy and rituals, is due to a placebo-like activation of the descending pain control system.

PHYSICAL THERAPY

Physical therapy is often successfully used both for treating pain and improving function.[21] However, the physiological mechanisms underlying these beneficial effects have not been sufficiently assessed in experimental models and clinical studies. It is, for example, unclear which neuronal circuits are affected by physical therapy, or in which way transmitter/receptor systems (release, postsynaptic events) are involved.

For acute inflammation, cooling, inactivation and rest seem to be suitable. Since nociceptors are easily activated by mechanical stimuli such as movements and by warmth, these measures may preferably reduce the discharge rate of sensitized nociceptors. In the chronic phase of inflammation, warmth and mobilization seem to be more adequate. At this stage it is probably most important to restore function, as reduced function may contribute to pain. In particular it seems important to prevent atrophy of skeletal muscle and to keep affected joints mobile.

PSYCHOSOCIAL THERAPY

Demographic, psychological, social and economic factors are thought to play a role in the transition from acute to chronic pain. Consequently, pain therapy should also take into account these factors. The difficulty arises, however, in that the significance of single factors as predictors of chronic pain is still controversial. Some studies have found that sex, marital status, educational level and income are predictive for the development of chronic pain, whereas in other studies these factors failed to show predictive value.[22] There is good evidence that in some pain states the severity of acute pain is predictive for the development of chronic pain.[22, 23] Psychological factors, such as affective distress, anxiety and fear avoidance, current depression, lassitude, malaise, loneliness, personality disorders, abuse

---

PRACTICE POINTS

- Thoroughly document the characteristics of the pain suffered by the patient. Make inferences about the pathophysiological mechanism(s) involved.

- Think of the presence of peripheral *and* central sensitization. Removing peripheral sensitization might not completely solve the pain problem.

- Be aware that referred pain and secondary hyperalgesia may misguide you to the wrong origin of the problem.

- In the absence of damage in the painful tissue, suspect neuropathic pain.

- Investigate the putative role of psychosocial factors.

- Both peripheral and central sensitization involve multiple mediators. Attacking one of them may be insufficient for therapy.

- Inhibition of prostaglandin synthesis is still the standard therapy against peripheral and central sensitization. Both NSAIDs and selective Cox-2 inhibitors have their virtues and their drawbacks. In general, NSAIDs or selective Cox-2 inhibitors should be used first; opiates are reserved for strong pain.

- Opiates are still the strongest inhibitors of pain transmission. They must be used when Cox inhibitors are insufficiently effective. The prescription and therapeutic regimen of opiates require judgement by experts.

- Physical therapy is often beneficial, particularly for the recovery or maintenance of function in chronically affected tissues.

- Be aware that every therapeutic intervention (whether pharmacological, physical or surgical) may have (sometimes only) a placebo effect. This depends on the endogenous pain control system. Thus analgesia cannot solely be attributed to the molecular action of the drug, the physical phenomena of manipulation, or the surgery itself.

- NSAIDs, opiates and antidepressants may trigger or mimic the endogenous pain-control system. A possible effect of psychosocial therapy on this system must be kept in mind.

- Psychosocial factors may positively or negatively influence pain. The 'human' aspects of diagnosis and treatment must be considered as much as the 'biological' aspects.

of alcohol and other substances, maladaptive coping, passive cognition, perceived stress, stressful life events, disease conviction, perception of poor health, and perceived severity of illness or disability, have been identified as predictors in some studies, but often controversial results have been reported as well.[22] It seems necessary, nevertheless, to be aware of the potential influence of these factors in the development, maintenance and treatment of chronic pain.

SUMMARY

Inflammation of peripheral tissues or damage to peripheral nerves generally causes spontaneous pain, hyperalgesia, allodynia and referred pain. The generation and maintenance of these phenomena depend on peripheral sensitization (hyperexcitability of nociceptive fibres that supply the tissue) and central sensitization (hyperexcitability of neurons in the spinal cord and in supraspinal structures). Chronic pain not only results from prolonged sensitization of nociceptive neurons but also from the influence of social and psychological factors.

Drug treatment interferes with the activation and sensitization of the nociceptive system at several levels. NSAIDs and selective Cox-2 inhibitors reduce the synthesis of PGs, which contribute to peripheral and central sensitization. NSAIDs and selective Cox-2 inhibitors should be used in the first place to treat inflammatory pain. NSAIDs may cause gastrointestinal problems, and selective Cox-2 inhibitors putatively induce cardiovascular problems. Drugs against the ion channels, neurotransmitters, neuropeptides or cytokines that contribute to nociceptive sensitization are being developed. Opioids can be used in pain treatment when NSAIDs and selective Cox-2 inhibitors are insufficient. Opioids act mainly in the CNS where they inhibit the release of transmitters, hyperpolarize nociceptive neurons and increase descending inhibition. It is thought that side-effects such as tolerance and addiction are not a severe problem in proper use of opioids. Physical therapy may be useful for reducing pain and improving function. Finally, the use of psychosocial therapy should be considered, as chronic pain in particular is influenced by psychological and social factors. The placebo effect of therapeutic interventions should not be underestimated.

ACKNOWLEDGEMENT

Support of the Deutscher Akademischer Austauschdienst to H.V. is gratefully acknowledged.

RESEARCH AGENDA

- Further characterization of the mechanisms of action of mediators responsible for long-lasting peripheral sensitization. Development of compounds that effectively and safely block the synthesis or the action of, for example, tissue bradykinin, prostaglandins and cytokines, or block the activation of excitatory receptors for heat, hydrogen ions, PGs, etc.

- Further characterization of ion channels in nociceptive primary afferents. Development of compounds that effectively and safely block action potentials when these afferents have been modified by chronic disease.

- Further characterization of the mechanisms of action of mediators responsible for long-lasting central sensitization. Development of compounds that effectively and safely block, for example, spinal NMDA receptors, NK1 receptors, CGRP receptors, PG synthesis and PG receptors.

- Further characterization of the descending pain-control system. Development of centrally acting compounds and of psychosocial interventions that increase descending inhibition and decrease descending facilitation of nociception by this system.

- Characterization of the mechanisms of action (parenchymal, vascular, neural) of commonly used physical therapies. Development of means for the direct activation of such mechanisms.

- Development of standards for the selection and measurement of the effects obtained by physical therapy, so that such effects can be documented and the effectiveness of various methods can be compared.

- Characterization of the psychosocial factors that positively or negatively influence specific types of chronic pain. Development of strategies that respectively utilize and avoid such factors.

REFERENCES

1. Millan MJ. The induction of pain: an integrative review. *Prog Neurobiol* 1999; **57**: 1–164.
2. Talbot JD, Marrett S, Evans AC et al. Multiple representations of pain in human cerebral cortex. *Science* 1991; **251**: 1355–1358.
3. Treede R-D, Kenshalo DR, Gracely RH et al. The cortical representation of pain. *Pain* 1999; **79**: 105–111.
4. Vanegas H, Schaible H-G. Descending control of persistent pain: Inhibitory or facilitatory? *Brain Res Rev* 2004; **46**: 295–309.
5. Fields H. State-dependent opioid control of pain. *Nature Rev Neurosci* 2004; **5**: 565–575.
6. Schaible H-G. The neurophysiology of pain. In: Maddison PJ, Isenberg DA, Woo P et al. (eds), *Oxford Textbook of Rheumatology*, 2nd edn, vol. 1. Oxford Medical, Oxford, 1998, pp. 487–499.
7. Schaible H-G, Grubb BD. Afferent and spinal mechanisms of joint pain. *Pain* 1993; **55**: 5–54.
8. Woolf CJ. Evidence for a central component of post-injury pain hypersensitivity. *Nature (London)* 1983; **306**: 686–688.
9. McMahon SB, Lewin GR, Wall PD. Central hyperexcitability triggered by noxious inputs. *Curr Opinion Neurobiol* 1993; **3**: 601–610.
10. Vanegas H, Schaible H-G. Effects of antagonists to high-threshold calcium channels upon spinal mechanisms of pain, hyperalgesia and allodynia. *Pain* 2000; **85**: 9–18.
11. Schaible H-G. On the role of tachykinins and calcitonin gene-related peptide in the spinal mechanisms of nociception and in the induction and maintenance of inflammation-evoked hyperexcitability in spinal cord neurons (with special reference to nociception in joints). *Prog Brain Res* 1996; **113**: 423–441.
12. Vanegas H, Schaible H-G. Prostaglandins and cyclooxygenases in the spinal cord. *Prog Neurobiol* 2001; **64**: 327–363.
13. Svensson CI, Yaksh TL. The spinal phospholipase–prostanoid cascade in nociceptive processing. *Annu Rev Pharmacol Toxicol* 2002; **42**: 553–583.
14. Baba H, Kohno T, Moore KA et al. Direct activation of rat spinal dorsal horn neurons by prostaglandin E_2. *J Neurosci* 2001; **21**: 1750–1756.

15. Samad T, Moore KA, Sapirstein A et al. Interleukin-1β-mediated induction of COX-2 in the CNS contributes to inflammatory pain hypersensitivity. *Nature (London)* 2001; **410**: 471–475.

16. Lee K-M, Kang B-S, Lee H-L et al. Spinal NF-κB activation induces COX-2 upregulation and contributes to inflammatory pain hypersensitivity. *Eur J Neurosci* 2004; **19**: 3375–3381.

17. Ahmadi S, Lippross S, Neuhuber WL et al.. PGE₂ selectively blocks inhibitory glycinergic transmission onto rat superficial dorsal horn neurons. *Nature Neurosci* 2002; **5**: 34–40.

18. Kawasaki Y, Kohno T, Zhuang Z-Y et al.. Ionotropic and metabotropic receptors, protein kinase A, protein kinase C, and Src contribute to C-fiber-induced ERK activation and cAMP response element-binding protein phosphorylation in dorsal horn neurons, leading to central sensitization. *J Neurosci* 2004; **24**: 8310–8321.

19. Guo W, Wei F, Zou S-P et al. Group I metabotropic glutamate receptor NMDA receptor coupling and signaling cascade mediate spinal dorsal horn NMDA receptor 2B tyrosine phosphorylation associated with inflammatory hyperalgesia. *J Neurosci* 2004; **24**: 9161–9173.

20. Dubner R, Ruda MA. Activity-dependent neuronal plasticity following tissue injury and inflammation. *Trends Neurosci* 1992; **15**: 96–103.

21. Allan L, Zenz M. *Chronic Pain: A Review.* Excerpta Medica Medical Communications, Almere, 1999.

22. Turk DC. The role of demographic and psychosocial factors in transition from acute to chronic pain. *Prog Pain Res Manage* 1997; **8**: 185–213.

23. Kalso E. Prevention of chronicity. *Prog Pain Res Manage* 1997; **8**: 215–230.

24. Sawynok J. Topical and peripherally acting analgesics. *Pharmacol Rev* 2003; **55**: 1–20.

25. Campbell WB, Halushka PV. Lipid-derived autacoids. Eicosanoids and platelet-activating factor. In: Hardman JG, Limbird LE, Molinoff PB et al. (eds), *Goodman & Gilman's The Pharmacological Basis of Therapeutics.* McGraw-Hill, New York, 1996, pp. 601–616.

26. Vane JR, Bakhle YS, Botting RM. Cyclooxygenases 1 and 2. *Annu Rev Pharmacol Toxicol* 1998; **38**: 97–120.

27. Schaible H-G, Schmelz M, Tegeder I. Pathophysiology and treatment of pain in joint disease. *Adv Drug Deliv Rev* 2006; **58**: 323–342.

28. Eglen RM, Hunter JC, Dray A. Ions in the fire: recent ion-channel research and approaches to pain therapy. *Trends Pharmacol Sci* 1999; **20**: 337–341.

29. Caterina MJ, Schumacher MA, Tominaga M et al. The capsaicin receptor: a heat-activated ion channel in the pain pathway. *Nature (London)* 1997; **389**: 816–824.

30. Dray A, Perkins M. Bradykinin and inflammatory pain. *Trends Neurosci* 1993; **16**: 99–104.

31. Schaible H-G, Del Rosso A, Matucci-Cerinic M. Neurogenic aspects of inflammation. *Rheum Dis Clin North Am* 2005; **31**: 77–101.

32. Stein C, Yassouridis A. Peripheral morphine analgesia. *Pain* 1997; **71**: 119–121.

33. Bär K-J, Schurigt U, Scholze A et al. The expression and localization of somatostatin receptors in dorsal root ganglion neurons of normal and monoarthritic rats. *Neuroscience* 2004; **127**: 197–206.

34. Carlton SM, Du J, Zhou S et al. Tonic control of peripheral cutaneous nociceptors by somatostatin receptors. *J Neurosci* 2001; **21**: 4041–4049.

35. Carlton SM, Du J, Davidson E et al. Somatostatin receptors on peripheral primary afferent terminals: inhibition of sensitized nociceptors. *Pain* 2001; **90**: 233–244.

36. Helyes Z, Szabo A, Nemeth J et al. Antiinflammatory and analgesic effects of somatostatin released from capsaicin-sensitive sensory nerve terminals in a Freund's adjuvant-induced chronic arthritis model in the rat. *Arthritis Rheum* 2004; **50**: 1677–1685.

37. Warncke T, Stubhaug A, Jorum E. Ketamine, an NMDA receptor antagonist, suppresses spatial and temporal properties of burn-induced secondary hyperalgesia in man: a double-blind, cross-over comparison with morphine and placebo. *Pain* 1997; **72**: 99–106.

38. Dembo G, Park SB, Kharasch ED. Central nervous system concentrations of cyclooxygenase-2 inhibitors in humans. *Anesthesiology* 2005; **102**: 409–415.

39. Tegeder I, Niederberger E, Vetter G et al. Effects of selective COX-1 and -2 inhibition on formalin-evoked nociceptive behavior and prostaglandin E₂ release in the spinal cord. *J Biochem* 2001; **79**: 777–786.

40. Yaksh TL. Spinal systems and pain processing: development of novel analgesic drugs with mechanistically defined models. *Trends Neurosci* 1999; **20**: 329–337.

41. Tortorici V, Vanegas H. Antinociception induced by systemic or PAG-microinjected lysine-acetylsalicylate in rats. Effects on tail-flick related activity of medullary off- and on-cells. *Eur J Neurosci* 1995; **7**: 1857–1865.

42. Meng IA, Manning BH, Martin WJ et al. An analgesia circuit activated by cannabinoids. *Nature (London)* 1998; **395**: 381–383.

43. Egbunike IG, Chaffee BJ. Antidepressants in the management of chronic pain syndromes. *Pharmacotherapy* 1997; **10**: 262–270.

44. Benedetti F, Amanzio M. The neurobiology of placebo analgesia: from endogenous opioids to cholecystokinin. *Prog Neurobiol* 1997; **51**: 109–125.

Chapter 30

Recommendations for using opioids in chronic non-cancer pain

Eija Kalso, Laurie Allan, Paul L. I. Dellemijn,
Clara C. Faura, Wilfried K. Ilias, Troels S. Jensen,
Serge Perrot, Leon H. Plaghki and Michael Zenz

INTRODUCTION

Many doctors will be faced with patients who have chronic pain. Opioids such as morphine and fentanyl (which are full opioid agonists and classified as being on Step III of the World Health Organization analgesic ladder[1]) are now an established part of the care of patients with cancer and in palliative care settings, but they are still relatively new and unfamiliar in many areas for the treatment of chronic non-cancer pain. In most countries, the use of such opioids is controlled (e.g. a special prescription form is required and their storage and dispensing is regulated). Guidance is therefore needed about their use. This chapter aims to provide a framework for the development of national or local guidelines[2-5] but not to provide detailed advice about doses or formulations. It is designed to be a starting point for discussion and to be sufficiently flexible to gain practical acceptance in different regions. It aims to assist prescribers (whether in primary care or specialist settings) in the appropriate use of opioids in pain management.

One of the aims of the recommendations is to discuss the well-documented problems of undertreatment and avoidance of strong opioids, as well as to address possible problems of overuse or inappropriate use.[6-8]

The decision to initiate or terminate long-term opioid therapy should, ideally, involve a multidisciplinary pain clinic with experience in this field. However, in many cases this is not practical, since there are insufficient pain clinics to be able to evaluate every patient. In such circumstances, referral to a pain clinic would result in patients waiting unacceptably long periods for treatment. These recommendations, while emphasizing the central role of specialist teams, therefore recognize the fact that, in many cases, treatment decisions will have to be made by other doctors without the support of a specialist team. However, prescribing clinicians are encouraged to contact pain clinics, multidisciplinary teams or other colleagues if they are unsure about any aspects.

Patients with severe, continuous pain are not a homogenous group, and management will be more complex and problematic for some patients than others. Clinicians need to assess not only the likelihood of benefit from strong opioids, but also the potential for their misuse in each case. Other guidelines have recommended different approaches for patients considered at low or high risk of inappropriate use. However, we have not adopted this approach but, rather, recommend similar assessment, initiation and termination procedures for opioid therapy in both straightforward and problematic patients. Despite this common framework, treatment should be individualized for each patient and patients should be involved in treatment decisions.

Treatment of pain should be directed by the underlying cause. A clear-cut diagnosis of the cause of the pain seems to improve treatment outcome with opioids. A precise diagnosis of the cause of pain is the gold standard but this is often not attainable. Use of opioids without a clear diagnosis of the cause of pain is appropriate if the pain is severe and continuous, and is responsive to opioids.

Care should be individualized, and patients should be involved in treatment decisions. The consent process is useful for clarifying patient expectations and defining limitations of therapy. It can also be used to set out the consequences if compliance with medication is poor and to agree on the circumstances that will lead to treatment being stopped.

Division of pain into nociceptive and neuropathic may be outdated,[9] but is probably still helpful. Opioids are considered to be effective in nociceptive pain.[10-13] The efficacy of opioids in certain neuropathic pains has also been shown.[14–19] However, the benefit of opioids in terms of quality of life in long-term use is still a matter for debate. With the current state of knowledge, opioids should not be prescribed for chronic pain syndrome (idiopathic pain).

As pain is such a complex process, its control is multimodal. Chronic pain is likely to benefit from a combination of pharmacological and non-pharmacological therapies. Strong opioids should not be used as monotherapy, but in the context of a rehabilitation programme setting goals of improved physical and social function. The need for other pharmacological treatments (e.g. antidepressants) and non-pharmacological treatments (e.g. cognitive–behavioural therapy and physiotherapy) should be evaluated regularly. Careful assessment and optimization of other pain therapies will reduce the need for opioids.[20]

The patient's current pain level, quality of life and functional status should be assessed carefully at the start of treatment (baseline). Sustained-release strong opioids should be introduced in the context of a trial period of 3–4 months,[13, 21] during which time the dose is titrated. Long-acting, sustained-release opioids are usually the most practical preparations for dose titration. The maximum length of the trial period should be agreed by the physician and the patient. At the end of the trial period, the patient's pain level, the intensity of adverse effects, quality of life and functional status should be assessed again and compared to the baseline levels. In some cases, a pain diary is helpful to assess pain intensity and relief before and after treatment.

The use of an intravenous opioid infusion test can help to predict whether opioids will be beneficial. The negative predictive power of such tests is generally good, but a positive result may not predict long-term treatment success. If the test is performed in a double-blind fashion with saline, the placebo response can also be assessed. The assumption that a particular pain is unresponsive to opioids implies that the opioid dose has been individually titrated to the appropriate maximum level and that the opioid has reached the opioid receptor. Acute intravenous testing allows the opioid to be titrated to the level of dose-limiting adverse effects for each individual under safe and controlled circumstances. The potential analgesic effect of the particular opioid in a specific pain syndrome and for the individual patient can be assessed. However, intravenous testing is not able to determine the balance between analgesic effect and adverse effects in long-term opioid use. If the result of intravenous testing is positive (maximum pain relief with opioid minus placebo response is greater than 50%), the likelihood of long-term treatment being effective is about 50%. If the response to intravenous testing is negative, the odds for a positive treatment result are negligible.[15, 21] Intravenous opioid testing may save a bothersome opioid titration period of several weeks with initial gastrointestinal adverse effects for patients who are unlikely to benefit.

In most cases, however, opioid therapy is initiated without intravenous testing. A prolonged trial period with gradual dose increments of oral opioids and aggressive treatment of opioid-induced adverse effects has the advantage of achieving a balance between pain relief and adverse effects for the individual

patient. The balance between pain relief and adverse effects must be acceptable to the patient. Unless unwanted effects such as nausea, vomiting and constipation are treated immediately, many patients will stop opioid treatment in the early phase and not give it a fair trial. Most patients receiving strong opioids will require continuous prophylaxis against constipation, while tolerance to other adverse effects is likely to develop with continued treatment.[21]

The aim of treatment is to improve quality of life by relieving pain and improving functional status. Assessing a global measure such as quality of life ensures that both the beneficial and unwanted effects of treatment are taken into account. Relief of pain would be expected to be reflected in an improvement in quality of life, while the occurrence of adverse effects might decrease quality of life. However, clinical trials have shown that significant pain relief does not necessarily imply an improvement in physical function.[12] The optimum treatment will balance pain relief and adverse effects. The patient's views about the overall benefits of the treatment (in terms of analgesia, effects on functional status and quality of life, and any unwanted effects) should be determined and respected. A useful series of questions for pain assessment and a list of factors that may predict the outcome of opioid treatment are shown in Box 30.1. If the outcome of the trial treatment is unclear, a multidisciplinary pain clinic should be consulted.

Full assessment of psychosocial status and history is an important part of the assessment before treatment is initiated. It may be helpful to involve a psychologist or psychiatrist. If the patient has a history of psychiatric illness, a full psychiatric analysis should precede initiation of opioid therapy. Patients with a history of drug or alcohol abuse should be referred to a multidisciplinary pain clinic.

Alcohol or drug abuse is a relative (not an absolute) contraindication for opioid therapy. Such patients can develop pain that is suitable for treatment with opioids. It is important for pain to be treated promptly and controlled in such patients, otherwise it can reactivate the addictive behaviour. The complex nature of these cases is probably best handled by a multidisciplinary team, ideally including an addiction specialist. If a multidisciplinary team considers that a patient's compliance would be inadequate, the patient should not receive opioid therapy.

The efficacy of sustained-release opioids in the management of chronic pain has been demonstrated in randomized, controlled studies.[10–13, 21–24] Such preparations should be taken regularly (by the clock) rather than as needed.

Breakthrough pain may occur on movement in patients with spinal or vascular pain. The use of short-acting opioids (acting on the same receptor as the main therapy, i.e. pure μ agonists) should be considered carefully in such cases. As a rule, short-acting opioids should be avoided.

Opioid treatment is initiated at a low dose, and this dose is increased gradually if the patient reports unsatisfactory pain relief with acceptable or no adverse effects. The maximum dose is reached when the patient reports satisfactory pain relief or if unacceptable adverse effects persist despite symptomatic treatment. The optimum dose is essentially determined by the patient, who is the best judge of the balance between pain relief and adverse effects.

Thorough monitoring of treatment includes measuring not only pain relief and adverse effects, but also the patient's functional status and quality of life. Quality of life may be perceived as difficult to measure, but published rating scales or simple tools, such as visual–analogue scales, can overcome this. Absolute measures of quality of life or comparisons between patients are not the aim of such assessment. Rather, the aim is to use measures that compare the situation before and during opioid treatment for an individual patient.

Box 30.1. A useful series of questions for pain assessment and a list of factors that may predict the outcome of opioid treatment

Useful questions for assessing patients before opioid treatment

- Has a realistic attempt been made to diagnose the underlying cause of pain?
- Have other reasonable treatments been properly tested and exhausted?
- Does the patient have a history of mental illness, or substance or alcohol abuse?
- What is the patient's current functional status?
- What improvement in functional status is desired, and how will this be measured?
- Has the patient kept a pain diary?
- Does the patient understand and accept the goals of treatment?
- What is the patient's physical and psychosocial status?

Factors predicting outcome with opioid treatment

- Adverse (negative) predictors:
  - non-opioid-responsive pain type
  - evoked pain, paroxysmal pain or pain on weight bearing
  - history of drug or alcohol abuse
  - history of psychotic illness
  - patient without a clear idea or desire for functional improvement
- Positive predictors:
  - continuous pain with high pain intensity
  - clear-cut pain diagnosis
  - spontaneous pain
  - limited treatment period
  - positive outcome of intravenous opioid testing
  - younger age (fewer adverse effects)
  - patient accepts treatment goals
  - patient has kept a pain diary
  - patient makes attempts to maintain physical fitness
  - patient has good psychosocial status

Functional status, such as the ability to return to work, is an important goal of pain relief. However, functional goals must be individualized, and will depend on the patient. For example, return to work might be the most important outcome for a young woman with low-back pain, but the ability to sit comfortably might be an equally valid goal for an elderly man with hip pain.[25, 26] In some countries reimbursement is dependent on measurement of functional status.

Ideally, a single physician or members of one team should be responsible for the prescription of opioids and should monitor the outcome of treatment. Changes in treatment and/or dosage are best handled by this physician or team, who should also have information about the use of other drugs. Treatment by an individual physician ensures continuity of care and a good understanding of the patient's psychosocial background, but arrangements must be in place to ensure that patients are not left without pain control if access to specific physicians is not possible (e.g. during vacations or sickness).

For patients with a history of non-compliance or abusive behaviour, access should be restricted to one prescribing physician or team and one dispensing pharmacy. Such patients should not have the opportunity to 'shop around' different doctors for different drugs or to provide false information to obtain extra opioids.[27] The prescribing physician should monitor the patient's use of other drugs, such as recreational (illicit/lifestyle) drugs and alcohol, other analgesics and comedications. These should all be checked and recorded prior to starting opioid therapy.

In many areas, access to multidisciplinary teams or pain clinics is limited, and waiting lists for consultations may be long. This may mean that primary care physicians have to take responsibility for patient care and analgesic prescribing while they await referral. Box 30.2 suggests measures that should be taken with problem patients.

Patients have the right to be fully informed about the nature of their treatment and its possible benefits and harmful effects. Obtaining agreement from the patient about the conditions for stopping opioid therapy is as important as obtaining consent for the initiation of therapy. Agreeing a contract also shows that the patient is committed to the aims of treatment and understands that receiving opioid therapy entails certain responsibilities.

Box 30.2. Measures that should be taken with problem patients

Problem patients may require:

- Referral to a multidisciplinary team (including a psychologist and an addiction specialist)
- A contract/agreement
- A trial period of opioid therapy (e.g. 3 months):
  - with a predetermined, acceptable endpoint
  - with structured follow-up (e.g. efficacy, adverse effects, quality of life, drugs prescribed/consumed)
- One doctor, team and pharmacy

Topics that should be covered in a contract are shown in Box 30.3, and sample contracts and consent forms are available from other organisations.[4, 27–30]

Treatment may be stopped, or the dose reduced, if the patient experiences a significant improvement in the painful condition (e.g. improvement of the underlying disease), or a poor outcome of treatment (e.g. intolerable adverse effects). Treatment should be stopped in cases of poor compliance. Compliance problems might include uncontrolled dose increases or decreases, uncontrolled comedication or abandonment of non-pharmacological therapies.

SUMMARY

Guidelines should be based on available evidence, and this was the ambitious goal of this expert group. However, we soon realized that most of the key issues had to be discussed without evidence.[31] Several randomized, controlled clinical trials have been performed with opioids in some chronic pain conditions. However, the opioid responsiveness of many chronic pain conditions has not been assessed in controlled settings, and we know very little about the long-term (months to years) efficacy and adverse effects of opioids.

Our understanding of many basic factors, such as the mechanisms of pain, their relevance to the responsiveness to opioids and true differences between opioids, is still meagre. So is our understanding of pharmacogenetics and differences between individuals in pain perception and risk of addictive behaviour. Some specialists report successful treatment with methadone when other opioids have failed.[32] However, no clinical studies have been performed in this area. Another 'phenomenon' that is much discussed, but about which there is hardly

any evidence, is 'opioid rotation'.[33, 34] Another field for future research is the possibility of coadministering drugs that will increase the effectiveness of opioids or reduce their adverse effects, including the development of tolerance.

In these guidelines the patient is considered the 'key participant' in the management of his or her pain. The patient, together with the responsible physician, must take control of the pain. Pharmacists, pharmaceutical companies and society also have necessary and important contributions to make. The main object of guidelines such as these is to encourage the positive participation of all stakeholders in order to provide the maximum benefit to the patient.

DECLARATION OF INTERESTS

Eija Kalso, Laurie Allan, Leon Plaghki and Michael Zenz have participated in clinical studies on opioids sponsored by Janssen-Cilag and Purdue Pharma (Napp Laboratories). They have also lectured at meetings organised by these two pharmaceutical companies. Michael Zenz has also worked with Mundipharma, Braun and Astra. Paul Dellemijn has participated in clinical studies sponsored by Janssen-Cilag and has lectured at meetings organised by Janssen-Cilag and Pfizer. Troels S. Jensen has done consultancy for various medical companies including: GSK, Pfizer, Janssen-Cilag, Astra, Novartis, Pharmacia, and Schwartz. Clara C. Faura has lectured at a meeting organised by Janssen-Cilag. Wilfried Ilias has no financial interest in companies that market opioid analgesics.

Box 30.3. Topics that should be included in a patient contract*

- An explanation of the nature of the treatment and its possible beneficial and adverse effects
- Patients should inform the doctor/team if they take any other analgesic or medication for a psychiatric condition, or if they take alcohol or recreational (illicit/lifestyle) drugs
- Patients should not request prescriptions for analgesics from another doctor
- The medication should be taken only as prescribed, and never passed on to anybody else
- The medication should be kept in a safe place (out of the reach of children) and the police should be informed if it is stolen
- Patients need a written document from the doctor when travelling abroad and may be limited in the amount of opioid they can carry for their personal use (e.g. under the Schengen agreement).

*Adapted from guidelines issued by the National Academy for Medicines, Sweden.[4]

PRACTICE POINTS

- Sustained-release opioids administered at regular intervals are recommended for opioid maintenance analgesia in patients with chronic non-cancer pain.
- Test opioid treatment in each patient by dose titration during a trial period.
- Involve the patient by using an information and agreement form, setting out their rights and responsibilities, adapted to local and national medico-legal conditions.
- The primary goal of opioid maintenance therapy is to keep patients functional, with an improved quality of life.

RESEARCH AGENDA

- Large prospective follow-up studies with less restrictive inclusion criteria for opioid maintenance therapy are needed to match the reality of the clinic.
- Long-term observational studies are needed for assessing the safety of opioid maintenance therapy concerning hormonal and immune function, development of tolerance, increased pain sensitivity and addiction.

ACKNOWLEDGEMENTS

The meeting at which these recommendations were drawn up was funded by an educational grant from Janssen Pharmaceutica, who also provided funding for editorial assistance. We thank Elizabeth Wager (Sideview) for help in preparing the manuscript and Drs Jacques Meynardier and Sebastiano Mercadante who participated in the original meeting.

REFERENCES

1. World Health Organization. *Cancer Pain Relief.* WHO, Geneva, 1996.

2. American Academy of Pain Medicine. *The Use of Opioids for the Treatment of Chronic Pain,* 1996. Available at: http://www.painmed.org/productpub/statements/opioidstmt.html (accessed 27 August 2006).

3. Kalso E, Paakkari P, Stenberg I (eds). *Opioids in Chronic Noncancer Pain, Situation and Guidelines in Nordic Countries.* National Agency for Medicines, Finland, 1999.

4. National Agency for Medicines Sweden. Användning av opioider vid långvarig icke-cancerrelaterad smärta – rekommendationer. *Information Från Läkemedelsverket* 2002; **13**: 17–75.

5. Perrot S, Bannwarth B, Bertin P et al. Use of morphine in nonmalignant joint pain: the Limoges recommendations. The French Society for Rheumatology. *Rev Rhum Engl Ed* 1999; **66**: 571–576.

6. Large RG, Schug SA. Opioids for chronic pain of non-malignant origin – caring or crippling. *Health Care Anal* 1995; **3**: 5–11.

7. Melzack R. The tragedy of needless pain. *Sci Am* 1990; **262**: 19–25.

8. Zenz M, Willweber-Strumpf A. Opiodphobia and cancer pain in Europe. *Lancet* 1993; **341**: 1075–1076.

9. Woolf C, Bennett G, Doherty M. Towards a mechanism-based classification of pain? *Pain* 1998; **77**: 227–229.

10. Allan L, Hays H, Jensen N-H et al. Randomised crossover trial of transdermal fentanyl and sustained release oral morphine for treating chronic non-cancer pain. *BMJ* 2001; **322**: 1–7.

11. Caldwell JR, Hale ME, Boyd RE et al. Treatment of osteoarthritis pain with controlled release oxycodone or fixed combination oxycodone plus acetaminophen added to nonsteroidal antiinflammatory drugs: a double blind, randomized, multicenter, placebo controlled trial. *J Rheumatol* 1999; **26**: 862–869.

12. Moulin DE, Iezzi A, Amireh R et al. Randomised trial of oral morphine for chronic non-cancer pain. *Lancet* 1996; **347**: 143–147.

13. Roth SH, Fleischmann RM, Burch FX et al. Around-the-clock, controlled-release oxycodone therapy for osteoarthritis-related pain. *Arch Intern Med* 2000; **160**: 853–860.

14. Attal N, Guirimand F, Rasseur L et al. Effects of IV morphine in central pain. *Neurology* 2002; **58**: 554–563.

15. Dellemijn PLI, Vanneste JAL. Randomised double-blind active placebo-controlled crossover trial of intravenous fentanyl in neuropathic pain. *Lancet* 1997; **349**: 753–758.

16. Harke H, Gretenkort P, Ladleif HK et al. The response of neuropathic pain and pain in complex regional pain syndrome to carbamazepine and sustained-release morphine in patients pretreated with spinal cord stimulation: a double-blinded randomized study. *Anesth Analg* 2001; **92**: 488–495.

17. Huse E, Larbig W, Flor H et al. The effect of opioids on phantom limb pain and cortical reorganization. *Pain* 2001; **90**: 47–55.

18. Rowbotham MC, Reisner-Keller LA, Fields HL. Both intravenous lidocaine and morphine reduce the pain of postherpetic neuralgia. *Neurology* 1991; **41**: 1024–1028.

19. Watson CPN, Babul N. Efficacy of oxycodone in neuropathic pain. A randomised trial in postherpetic neuralgia. *Neurology* 1998; **50**: 1837–1841.

20. Maier C, Hildebrandt J, Klinger R et al. Morphine responsiveness, efficacy and tolerability in patients with chronic non-tumor associated pain – results of a double-blind placebo-controlled trial (MONTAS). *Pain* 2002; **97**: 223–233.

21. Dellemijn PLI, van Duijn H, Vanneste JAL. Prolonged treatment with transdermal fentanyl in neuropathic pain. *J Pain Symptom Manage* 1998; **16**: 220–229.

22. Caldwell JR, Rapoport RJ, Davis JC et al. Efficacy and safety of a once-daily morphine formulation in chronic, moderate-to-severe osteoarthritis pain: results from a randomized, placebo-controlled, double-blind trial and an open-label extension trial. *J Pain Symptom Manage* 2002; **23**: 278–291.

23. Milligan K, Lanteri-Minet M, Borchert K et al. Evaluation of long-term efficacy and safety of transdermal fentanyl in the treatment of chronic noncancer pain. *J Pain* 2001; **2**: 197–204.

24. Peat S, Sweet P, Miah Y et al. Assessment of analgesia in human chronic pain. Randomized double-blind crossover study of once daily Repro-Dose morphine versus MST Continus. *Eur J Clin Pharmacol* 1999; **55**: 577–581.

25. Follett KA. The fallacy of using a solitary outcome measure as the standard for satisfactory pain treatment outcome. *Pain Forum* 1999; **8**: 189–191.

26. Rowland M, Torgerson D. Understanding controlled trials: what outcomes should be measured? *BMJ* 1998; **317**: 1075–1080.

27. American Academy of Pain Medicine. *Long-term Controlled Substances Therapy for Chronic Pain. Sample Agreement,* 2001. Available at: http://www.painmed.org/productpub/statements/sample.html (accessed 27 August 2006).

28. American Academy of Pain Medicine. *Consent for Chronic Opioid Therapy,* 2002. Available at: http://www.painmed.org/productpub/statements/opioidconsent.html (accessed 27 August 2006).

29. Fishman SM, Bandman TB, Edwards A et al. The opioid contract in the management of chronic pain. *J Pain Symptom Manage* 1999; **18**: 27–37.

30. Gitlin MC. Contracts for opioid administration for the management of chronic pain: a reappraisal. *J Pain Symptom Manage* 1999; **18**: 6–8.

31. Jadad AD, Browman GP. The WHO analgesic ladder for cancer pain management. Stepping up the quality of its evaluation. *JAMA* 1995; **274**: 1870–1873.

32. Gardner-Nix JS. Oral methadone for managing chronic nonmalignant pain. *J Pain Symptom Manage* 1996; **11**: 321–328.

33. Do Quang-Cantagrel N, Wallace MS, Magnuson SK. Opioid substitution to improve the effectiveness of chronic noncancer pain control: a chart review. *Anesth Analg* 2000; **90**: 933–937.

34. Thomsen AB, Becker N, Eriksen J. Opioid rotation in chronic nonmalignant pain patients. *Acta Anaesthesiol Scand* 1999; **43**: 909–917.

Recommendations for using opioids in chronic non-cancer pain

Leon H. Plaghki

Although use of opioids for chronic non-cancer pain (CNCP) is growing in acceptance, the efficacy and safety of such therapy and the procedure for selecting patients are still matters of passionate debate. Based on recent published recommendations for using opioids in CNCP,[1–3] I briefly review the support in favour of and against such use, and stress some important factors in identifying appropriate candidates.

Enough evidence has been accumulated over the past two decades to chase away many old myths concerning opioid management for acute pain (e.g. postoperative pain) and cancer pain. However, regarding opioid maintenance analgesia for CNCP there is still a lack of evidence in many respects, and recommendations are based mainly on clinical practice. In a recent meta-analysis of 15 randomized, placebo-controlled studies addressing this problem[4] it became clear that:

- opioids can alleviate nociceptive and neuropathic pain in CNCP, but efficacy varies greatly among individuals
- no criteria have been identified for opioid sensitivity, implying that each patient needs to be tested individually
- important questions about addiction and tolerance remain unanswered because of the short follow-up periods
- the small number of patients and the highly restrictive inclusion criteria of published studies may impede the extrapolation of the findings to the reality in the clinic.

From these studies it is recommended that treatments should be tested in each individual and tailored to the individual's needs by dose titration during a trial period. There is large variation in responsiveness to opioids among patients. Minimal effective analgesic plasma concentrations for opioids vary among patients by factors of 5–10.[5] These differences in sensitivity can be patient related (age, gender, previous opioid exposure, emotional state, cognitive impairment, history of drug dependence/addiction, genetic factors), pain related (prior pain experience, pain intensity, presence of breakthrough pain, predominance of nociceptive versus neuropathic mechanism) or drug-related (e.g.

differences in pharmacokinetics, drugs with coupled N-methyl-D-aspartate (NMDA) blocking effect).

Sustained-release opioids administered at regular intervals are generally recommended. In recent systematic review articles, Chou et al.[6] and Furlan et al.[7] concluded that there was insufficient evidence to show that any long-acting opioid was better than another. The use of short-acting opioids should be avoided, or considered with great care for breakthrough pain in particular cases.

Adverse effects are common, and the most frequent are constipation, nausea, sedation, dizziness and itching. Because of the variability in responsiveness, a dose that can produce satisfactory pain relief with minimal side-effects in some patients might provide underdosing with failure of pain relief or overdosing with unbearable side-effects in other patients. Although it is frequently reported that most of these adverse effects have a tendency to resolve over time, other less well documented adverse effects[8, 9] may appear (e.g. amenorrhoea or impotence, primary hypoadrenalism, fatigue and amyotrophy). These effects must be monitored carefully and managed correctly. These adverse effects are among the reasons why in open-label, follow-up studies (up to 2 years) few patients continued to use opioids in the long term.

The safety of opioid maintenance therapy has not been properly addressed by any study.[2] As a consequence, long-term monitoring is mandatory for long-term effects on hormonal and immune function, development of tolerance, increased pain sensitivity and addiction. For all these reasons it is important to inform patients and their relatives of the benefits and potential risks of the treatment.

No criteria have been identified that allow the selection of CNCP patients for opioid treatment. The decision to start opioid treatment in CNCP is influenced by many factors that are patient related (e.g. mechanism of pain, severity of pain and disability, acceptance (or reluctance) for opioid therapy, trustworthiness and quality of psychosocial support) and physician related (e.g.

expertise with opioid maintenance analgesia, type of practice or accessibility to pain specialist, community regulatory rules), and most importantly the interaction between the two. It is generally accepted that the more chronic and complex the psychosocial history (e.g. litigation, conjugal conflict, history of addictive behaviour) the lesser the indication of opioid maintenance therapy in the process of rehabilitation. To involve the patient in his or her own treatment, it is highly recommended to use an agreement form, setting out the patient's rights and responsibilities.

Finally, it is important to stress that the primary goal of opioid treatment in CNCP is to keep patients functional, with improved quality of life, and not per se to obtain a reduction in pain intensity. The analgesic treatment is only one aspect of the overall process of rehabilitation.

REFERENCES

1. American Academy of Pain Medicine and American Pain Society. *The Use of Opioids for the Treatment of Chronic Pain*, 1997. Available at: http://www.painmed.org/productpub/statements/pdfs/opioids.pdf (accessed 27 August 2006).

2. Kalso E, Allan L, Dellemijn PLI et al. Recommendations for using opioids in chronic non-cancer pain. *Eur J Pain* 2003; **7**: 381–386.

3. The Pain Society. *Recommendations for the Appropriate Use of Opioids for Persistent Non-cancer Pain. A Consensus Statement of the Pain Society, the Royal College of Anaesthetists, the Royal College of General Practitioners and the Royal College of Psychiatrists*, 2004. Available at: http://www.britishpainsociety.org/opioids_doc_2004.pdf (accessed 27 August 2006).

4. Kalso E, Edwards JE, Moore RA et al. Opioids in chronic non-cancer pain: systematic review of efficacy and safety. *Pain* 2004; **112**: 372–380.

5. Camu F, Vanlersberghe C. Pharmacology of systemic analgesics. *Best Pract Res Clin Anaesthesiol* 2002; **16**: 475–488.

6. Chou R, Clark E, Helfand M. Comparative efficacy and safety of long-acting oral opioids for chronic non-cancer pain: a systematic review. *J Pain Symptom Manage* 2003; **26**: 1026–1048.

7. Furlan AD, Sandoval JA, Mailis-Gagnon A et al. Opioids for chronic noncancer pain: a meta-analysis of effectiveness and side effects. *Can Med Assoc J* 2006; **174**: 1589–1594.

8. Pechnick RN. Effects of opioids on the hypothalamo-pituitary-adrenal axis. *Annu Rev Pharmacol Toxicol* 1993; **33**: 353–382.

9. Rhodin A, Grondbladh L, Nilsson LH et al. Methadone treatment of chronic non-malignant pain and opioid dependence – a long-term follow up. *Eur J Pain* 2006; **10**: 271–278.

Index